Supportive care for the urology patient

Supportive care for the urology patient

Edited by

Richard W. Norman

Professor and Chairman
Department of Urology
Dalhousie University
Halifax
Nova Scotia, Canada

and

David C. Currow

Professor and Head
Palliative Care
Flinders University
Adelaide, Australia

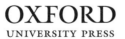
OXFORD
UNIVERSITY PRESS

OXFORD
UNIVERSITY PRESS

Great Clarendon Street, Oxford OX2 6DP

Oxford University Press is a department of the University of Oxford.
It furthers the University's objective of excellence in research, scholarship,
and education by publishing worldwide in

Oxford New York

Auckland Cape Town Dar es Salaam Hong Kong Karachi
Kuala Lumpur Madrid Melbourne Mexico City Nairobi
New Delhi Shanghai Taipei Toronto

With offices in

Argentina Austria Brazil Chile Czech Republic France Greece
Guatemala Hungary Italy Japan Poland Portugal Singapore
South Korea Switzerland Thailand Turkey Ukraine Vietnam

Oxford is a registered trade mark of Oxford University Press
in the UK and in certain other countries

Published in the United States
by Oxford University Press Inc., New York

British Library Cataloguing in Publication Data
Data available

Library of Congress Cataloging in Publication Data

Supportive care for the urology patient / edited by Richard W. Norman and David Currow.
(Supportive care series)
    Includes bibliographical references and index.
  1. Urinary organs–Diseases–Palliative treatment.
[DNLM: 1. Urologic Diseases–therapy.   2. Chronic Disease–therapy.
3. Palliative Care–methods.   4. Quality of Life.
WJ 166 S959 2005] I. Norman, Richard W.   II. Currow, David.   III. Series.
    RC900.5.S876 2005   616.6'06–dc22   2005006678

Typeset by Newgen Imaging Systems (P) Ltd., Chennai, India
Printed in Great Britain
on acid-free paper by
Biddles Ltd, King's Lynn

ISBN 0–19–852941–4 (Hbk: alk.paper)   978–0–19–852941–5

10 9 8 7 6 5 4 3 2 1

Preface to the Supportive Care Series

Supportive care is the multidisciplinary holistic care of patients with chronic and life-limiting illnesses and their families—from the time around diagnosis, through treatments aimed at cure or prolonging life, and into the phase currently acknowledged as palliative care. It involves recognising and caring for the side-effects of active therapies as well as patients' symptoms, co-morbidities, psychological, social and spiritual concerns. It also values the role of family carers and helps them in supporting the patient, as well as attending to their own special needs. Supportive care is a domain of health and social care that utilises a network of professionals and voluntary carers in a 'virtual team'. It is increasingly recognised by healthcare providers and governments as a modern response to complex disease management, but so far it can lay claim to little dedicated literature.

This is therefore one volume in a unique new series of textbooks on supportive care, published by Oxford University Press which has already established itself as a leading publisher for palliative care. Unlike 'traditional' palliative care, which grew from terminal care of cancer patients, supportive care is not restricted to dying patients and neither to cancer. Thus this series covers the support of patients with a variety of long-term conditions, who are currently largely managed by specialist and general teams in hospitals and by primary care teams in community settings. It will therefore provide a practical guide to supportive care of the patient at all stages of the illness, providing up-to-date knowledge of the scientific basis of palliation and also practical guidance on delivering high quality multidisciplinary care across healthcare sectors. The volumes, edited by acknowledged leaders in the specific field of each volume, will bring together research, healthcare management, economics and ethics through contributions from an international panel of experts of all disciplines. The underlying theme of all the books is the application of the latest evidence-based knowledge, in a humane way, for patients with advancing disease.

As Series Editors, we bring between us over four decades of research and clinical experience of acute medicine and palliative care. Our work has spanned St Christopher's Hospice and the Leicestershire Hospice in England—both of which have been inspirational leaders of traditional palliative care; the Academic Unit of Supportive Care at the University of Sheffield, England and the Harry Horvitz Center for Palliative Medicine in The Cleveland Clinic Foundation, USA. We have independently and jointly advocated the supportive care approach to cancer and other chronic disease management and are delighted to be collaborating on this series. We are both committed to delivering high quality of end-of-life care when it is necessary but we are constantly seeking to influence our colleagues in all relevant healthcare disciplines to adopt the principles of modern supportive care to benefit a wider range of patients at earlier stages of illness. We aim, through this series, to inform and inspire other doctors, nurses, allied health professionals, pharmacists, social and spiritual care providers and students, to improve the quality of living for all patients and families in their care.

2005

Sam Hjelmeland Ahmedzai
Professor of Palliative Medicine
Academic Unit of Supportive Care
The University of Sheffield
Royal Hallamshire Hospital
Sheffield, UK

Declan Walsh
Professor and Director
Harry Horvitz Center for Palliative Medicine
The Cleveland Clinic Foundation
Cleveland, Ohio, USA

The publishers would like to thank Kjersti Hjelmeland Brakstad for designing the covers for the Supportive Care Series.

Preface

Supportive care for the urology patient includes all aspects of optimizing quality of life and day-to-day functioning in patients suffering from significant urological symptoms. In the past, the emphasis has been on progressive malignancies, but, as we evaluated the variety of issues to consider, it is apparent that patients suffering from chronic non-malignant urological problems such as painful bladder syndrome or urinary incontinence would also benefit from a supportive care network. In many cases, medications or urological surgery offer real opportunities for improvement in comfort, physical activity, and social interaction even though cure is not possible. Realistic goals should always be set as the treatment strategy is being developed; discussion of the benefits, risks, and alternatives of each intervention should be a priority.

We believe that the importance of the patient's close interpersonal relationships, both emotional and physical, have been underestimated in the past. The relationship and family consequences of disturbances related to many of the conditions under consideration have a serious impact on patient morale and self-esteem. Obvious examples include the loss of interest in, or the ability to have, sex. In many cases, there are treatments which can help this component of patient care. It must also be recognized that while individuals other than the patient are often negatively affected by the underlying urological problem, these people can also be called upon to be part of the supportive care team.

As we edited chapters and topics, it became obvious that optimal supportive care would be best delivered by a specialized and motivated team that brings a cluster of different experiences and skills to the table. It is a surprise to see the large number of participants that may be required by one patient as he/she progresses through various stages of an illness. Since there are so many possible entry points into the world of supportive care for these patients, we wanted to be sure that all of these health care providers are aware of what the potential urological problems are, why each occurs, what can be done to help, and when they should seek wider team input.

Finally, this reference text would not have been possible without the enthusiastic support and participation by a variety of international contributors. This has allowed us to draw generously upon and meld international opinion and experience in our presentation of *Supportive care of the urology patient*.

Richard W. Norman
David C. Currow
2005

Contents

Contributors

Nora Albiger
Fellow, Division of Endocrinology,
University of Padova, Italy

Peter A M Anderson
Department of Urology, Dalhousie
University, Nova Scotia, Canada

Gregory G Bailly
Assistant Professor, Department of
Urology, Dalhousie University,
Nova Scotia, Canada

Rodney H Breau
Resident, Division of Urology, University
of Ottawa, Canada

Lorna Butler
Professor, School of Nursing and
Department of Urology, Dalhousie
University, Nova Scotia, Canada

Robert A Cummins
Professor of Psychology, Deakin
University, Victoria, Australia

David C Currow
Professor and Head, Palliative and
Supportive Services, Flinders University,
Adelaide, Australia

Darrel E Drachenberg
Urologic Oncologist, Assistant Professor
of Surgery and Director of Research,
University of Manitoba, Canada

M A Fischer
Assistant Clinical Professor, Division of
Urology, Department of Surgery and
Department of Obstetrics and
Gynaecology McMaster University,

Hamilton, Ontario, Canada; Andrology
Consultant, ISIS Regional Fertility Center,
Mississauga Ontario, Canada

John M Fitzpatrick
Professor of Surgery, University College
Dublin; Consultant Urologist, Mater
Misericordiae Hospital, Dublin, Ireland

Hugh Flood
Consultant Urologist, Midwestern
Regional Hospital, Limerick, Ireland

Jerzy B Gajewski
Department of Urology, Dalhousie
University, Nova Scotia, Canada

Ciaran F Healy
Senior House Officer, Department of
Surgery, Mater Misericordiae Hospital,
Dublin, Ireland

Nicholas J Hegarty
Specialist Registrar in Urology, Mater
Misericordiae Hospital, Dublin, Ireland

Florian Heid
Consultant Anaesthesiologist, Clinic of
Anaesthesiology, Johannes
Gutenberg-University Hospital, Mainz,
Germany

Carin V Hopps
Assistant Professor of Urology, Medical
College of Ohio, USA

Jürgen Jage
Professor of Anaesthesiology and Head
of Pain Service, Clinic of Anaesthesiology,
Johannes Gutenberg-University Hospital,
Mainz, Germany

Reena Karani
Assistant Professor; Director, Geriatrics
Consultation and Liaison Service, Mount
Sinai School of Medicine, New York, USA

Anna L D Lau
Assistant Professor, Department of
Rehabilitation Sciences, Hong Kong
Polytechnic University, Kowloon,
Hong Kong

Scott MacDiarmid
Department of Urology, Wake Forest
University, Winston-Salem, USA

Jane MacDonald
Registrar in Urology, Midwestern
Regional Hospital, Limerick, Ireland

Franco Mantero
Professor and Chairman,
Division of Endocrinology, University
of Padova, Italy

Villus Marshall
Surgical Specialty Unit, Royal Adelaide
Hospital, Australia

Catherine Martin
Renal Transplant Social Worker, Princess
Alexandra Hospital, Brisbane, Australia

Kamal Mattar
Urology Resident, University of
Manitoba, Canada

R Ashley McLellan
Department of Urology, Dalhousie
University, Nova Scotia, Canada

Diane E Meier
Professor of Geriatrics and Medicine,
Mount Sinai School of Medicine,
New York, USA

Alvaro Morales
Department of Urology, Queen's
University, Kingston, Canada

John P Mulhall
Associate Professor of Urology,
New York Weill Cornell University
Medical Center, USA

Aru Narayanasamy
Senior Health Lecturer, Queens
Medical Centre, University of
Nottingham, UK

David Nicol
Renal Transplant Unit, Princess
Alexandra Hospital, Brisbane, Australia

Lindsay E Nicolle
Professor of Internal Medicine and
Medical Microbiology, University of
Manitoba, Canada

Richard W Norman
Professor and Chairman, Department
of Urology, Dalhousie University,
Halifax, Nova Scotia, Canada

Allan B Patrick
Department of Urology, Dr Everett
Chalmers Regional Hospital, Fredericton,
Canada

Ernest Lawrence Rossi
Director of Ernest Lawrence Rossi
Foundation for Psychogenomic Research,
California, USA

Hans-Göran Tiselius
Professor of Urology, Huddinge
University Hospital; Division of
Urology, Karolinska Institutet,
Stockholm, Sweden

Paul Toren
Medical Student, Queen's University,
Kingston, Canada

Wendy Wobeser
Assistant Professor and Medical Director,
Clinical Immunology Clinic, Queen's
University and Kingston General
Hospital, Kingston, Canada

Zbigniew Wolski
Professor and Head, Department of
Urology, The Ludwig Rydygier Medical
College, Bydgoszcz, N. Copernicus
University, Poland

Chapter 1

Introduction to supportive care issues for the urology patient

Richard W. Norman

Recent technological advances in urology include the availability of a variety of new flexible endoscopic instruments, adoption of innovative operative approaches including laparoscopy, and the integration of robotics into patient care. There is a fear that these advanced interventions will supplant some of the art of medicine and forego the importance of the supportive care component of the health-care professional–patient relationship. While it is easy to appreciate the value of a successful curative operation, it is equally important that the patient and family understand the long-term consequences of a particular disease—benign or malignant—and that surgery and surgeons cannot correct all problems. It has become increasingly clear that successful management of most chronic urological conditions requires multidisciplinary input from a variety of different health-care professionals, all of whom bring special expertise and perspectives to the development of the optimal comprehensive treatment plan for a specific patient. In some cases, a few individuals may be involved; in others, it will be many (see Table 1.1). The goal is to be as inclusive as possible and to include all of those who may provide benefit to overall patient care. One must avoid the political debate over who owns emotional care of these patients.[1]

It is from within this context that the concept of supportive care for the urology patient arises as an add-on to the current understanding of the meaning of palliative care. The literature abounds with descriptions of the benefits of palliative care with the emphasis on active total care of patients whose disease is not responsive to curative treatment, and includes comprehensive, interdisciplinary care of patients and families facing a terminal illness, focusing primarily on comfort and support. Its goals are best described by the 2002 WHO definition of palliative care—an approach that improves the quality of life of patients and their families, facing the problems associated with life-threatening illness, through the prevention and relief of suffering by means of early identification and impeccable assessment and treatment of pain and other problems, physical, psychosocial and spiritual. Palliative care:

- provides relief from pain and other distressing symptoms;
- affirms life and regards dying as a normal process;

Table 1.1 Potential members of the urological supportive care team

Urologist
Medical oncologist
Radiation oncologist
Pharmacist
Palliative care—nurse and physician
Nursing—in-patient and out-patient
Enterostomal therapist
Social worker
Nutritionist
Homecare coordinator
Patient representative
Pastoral care worker
Volunteers
Others as required

- intends neither to hasten nor postpone death;
- integrates the psychological and spiritual aspects of patient care;
- offers a support system to help patients live as actively as possible until death;
- offers a support system to help the family cope during the patient's illness and in their own bereavement;
- uses a team approach to address the needs of patients and their families, including bereavement counselling, if indicated;
- will enhance quality of life, and may also positively influence the course of illness;
- is applicable early in the course of illness, in conjunction with other therapies that are intended to prolong life, such as chemotherapy or radiation therapy, and includes those investigations needed to better understand and manage distressing clinical complications.

Although palliative care is often defined in terms of its value for patients suffering from a specific cancer or its complications, this narrow meaning limits its applicability to a wide variety of other patient problems, which although not malignant in nature can also be the cause of impaired quality of life and interpersonal relationships. Supportive care builds upon these concepts by focusing on treatment given to prevent, control, or relieve complications and side-effects and to improve and maintain the patient's comfort, level of function, and quality of life; it is inclusive of those individuals suffering from chronic life-altering conditions which are benign or malignant.

A degree of semantic confusion surrounding the meaning of supportive care is compounded by the complex terminological morass encompassing a sweeping range of disciplinary, theoretical, and ideological distinctions and domains. While supportive care may refer to adjuvant therapies and psychosocial interventions, other terms like peer support, counselling and advocacy are often implicated as the non-technical or non-biomedical approaches. In fact, supportive care can refer to an array of activities, ranging anywhere from imparting a few encouraging words to running a structured therapeutic group discussion session, to conducting an individualized cognitive reframing intervention.[1] It is the common objective to bring in whatever support parameters may be required for an individual patient or family. Since there is a significant overlap and common goals for supportive and palliative care, a rigid definition to the exclusion of one over the other will benefit neither.

Both supportive and palliative care acknowledge that there is no cure for a specific medical condition. The decision to accept such care versus aggressive treatment (i.e. care versus cure) is often difficult for family members. Although it means accepting a poor prognosis or continued symptoms, it also means providing a very special kind of care to a loved one. This may range from a new goal of providing long-term day-to-day support and assistance with coping strategies or a peaceful, pain-free death in the presence of loved ones. The duration may be long-term over several years, or short-term, lasting days or weeks. Such help can be provided in the hospital, at home, or in a setting specializing in such care.

All of these points are especially important in urology where so many of the issues have traditionally had a very private personal nature to them. Fortunately times are changing, and it is now common to hear patients talking publicly about their concerns regarding such maladies as the embarrassment from urinary incontinence, the dyspareunia associated with interstitial cystitis, or the frustration caused by erectile dysfunction. Sometimes the condition is related to a primary urological problem or its treatment (e.g. urinary incontinence and erectile dysfunction after a radical prostatectomy) and, at others, it is secondary to another underlying problem or its treatment (e.g. bilateral ureteric obstruction from locally invasive cancer of the cervix). The increased awareness and openness surrounding these subjects are indications that they are important and deserve our attention.

The development of a functional supportive care programme will differ from institution to institution and may vary from an interested family physician consulting and coordinating health-care professionals as necessary to a complex well-organized and defined team with a framework to implement and maintain its different components. The latter includes processes to develop and monitor consistent standards of supportive care throughout the institution and identify and prioritize supportive care needs of patients, families, staff, hospital, and community. This implies acknowledgment of evidence-based guidelines recognizing the style and approach to care of each health-care discipline as well as standards, policies, and practices for assessment, care, and management of physical, emotional, psychosocial, spiritual, and financial distress through survivor-ship and coping or death and bereavement. In many, circumstances this will be no easy task. Our ageing population, and the associated health pitfalls that accompany it, demands that sufficient human and financial resources and initiatives be focused on these matters to assure success.

Supportive Care for the Urology Patient has been written to remove some of the mystique of urology for non-urological health-care professionals. It is expected that increased knowledge concerning chronic benign and malignant life-limiting urological conditions, and the various potential interventions surrounding them, will empower these key individuals to optimize their participation in the supportive care of these patients. At the same time, they should become aware of their own limitations and learn what urologists can and cannot offer—medically, surgically, and device-wise—so that discipline-specific assistance can be sought when needed. The best blend of the art and science of health care will yield the greatest positive impact on patient care and support.

Reference

1 Bultz BD, Thorne S, Fitch MI (2004). Who owns the emotional care of the cancer patient? *Oncol. Exchange* **3**: 32–5.

Chapter 2

Quality of life measurements

Robert A. Cummins and Anna L. D. Lau

Background

Quality of life measurement within the medical context takes a very different approach from that adopted by the social sciences. Within medicine the construct is referred to as health-related quality of life (HRQOL) which relies heavily on measuring symptoms of ill-health. Within the social sciences, quality of life is conceptualized as a global construct, positive in nature, encompassing, but not limited by, health. This chapter will explain and contrast these two views. It will become evident that these are serious logical and methodological issues concerning measurement of HRQOL, to the extent that the instruments may not be regarded as valid measures of quality of life as the term is generally understood. The global measures of subjective well-being, while valid and theoretically embedded, are also limited by their relative insensitivity to medical health. The reason for this insensitivity is proposed to be a homeostatic system that normally maintains subjective quality of life within a narrow positive range. The HRQOL scales are briefly reviewed and a new strategy is proposed that would allow the creation of a new family of scales to measure subjective quality of life within medical settings.

Introduction to quality of life measurement

The days when the single purpose of medicine was to preserve life are long gone. Increasingly, and appropriately, concern is being directed to the perceived quality of the preserved life. But the issue of how to conceptualize and measure such an abstract construct has yielded many views. Most importantly for this chapter, a schism has developed between the view developed within medicine and that within the social sciences.

Both forms of measurement rely on patient self-reports, but they are fundamentally different in terms of the type of information accessed. Within medicine, quality of life (QOL) is operationalized via the construct of HRQOL. This utilizes patient-reported symptoms. Consequently, an excellent level of HRQOL represents the absence of pathology as reported by the patient. Within the social sciences, on the other hand, QOL is operationalized by a construct called subjective QOL or subjective well-being (SWB). This utilizes patient-reported satisfaction with either their life as a whole or the compartments of their life (domains). Here, an excellent level of SWB represents a highly positive state of mind and satisfaction with life in general.

These two different views would be congruent if a lack of pathology was proxy for SWB, but it is not. No matter whether the pathology is subjective (e.g. perceived stress) or objective (e.g. degree of physical disability), pathology does not have a simple linear relationship to SWB.[1,2]

This chapter will examine some of the issues raised by measurement of HRQOL, after which the alternative conceptualization of SWB will be introduced, concentrating on the theory of SWB homeostasis. HRQOL scales relevant to sexual functioning and urinary incontinence will then be reviewed, followed by a suggestion that both forms of measurement could be usefully employed within a medical context.

Measuring quality of life

One of the crucial distinctions in measurement technology is that between objective and subjective variables. As has been stated, such different forms of measurement (e.g. physical health and satisfaction with health) do not form reliable linear relationships with one another.[1] Thus, they cannot be used to predict one another and cannot be validly combined into single scales of measurement. The reason for this separation is that SWB is actively managed by a homeostatic system, as will be explained later.

Not only are such variable combinations psychometrically invalid but they also confuse outcome with causation. This problem has been well articulated by Fayers et al.,[3] who distinguish between indicator and causal variables. Indicator variables (the perception of health quality) constitute the measured end-state. Causal variables are the patient symptoms that *cause* the end-state to change (e.g. urinary frequency, urgency and incontinence, etc.). Logically, then, it makes no sense to combine indicator and causal variables, yet this is precisely what HRQOL scales generally do. For example, the SF-36,[4] which is the most widely used generic HRQOL scale, combines limitations in ability to walk 100 m with a rating of current health, from excellent to poor.

It is unfortunate that this crucial distinction is not obvious from the normal analytical procedures that researchers apply to their data. This is especially so in a medical context where the symptoms are often severe enough to cause satisfaction to fall. In this situation both the indicator and the causal variable will correlate with one another and give the impression that their combination forms a coherent scale. If, however, the variable scores are derived from people in a non-pathological situation, their independence from one another will be evident.

There is a further problem in the use of medical symptoms to form scales of measurement. In their traditional context, symptoms are diagnostic of specific disorders. An increased production of leucocytes is diagnostic of infection not of diabetes. Moreover, the number of leucocytes is normally unrelated to the control of glucose metabolism, so it is inconceivable that someone would produce a scale of 'blood quality' that combined the average numbers of leucocytes and level of insulin into a single 'index'. Clearly, each measure has its own diagnostic utility, and this utility is obliterated by their combination. This logic also holds for the broadest picture of objective quality of life. Consider, for example, the person who is extremely wealthy, yet is in poor health and chronic pain, who has many excellent friends, yet lives in prison. The combination of such variables cannot be interpreted. Thus, each objective domain of life must be evaluated on its own, separate merits. There is no global construct of objective quality of life.

This principle of independence also holds at the level of functional systems. Consider urinary incontinence. There are several symptoms that may pertain to this condition such as wet and malodorous clothes, urinary urgency and frequency, requirement for use of protective pads, etc. A person who has incontinence may, or may not, have each of these symptoms, but once again, their diagnostic utility rests on their separate evaluation, not on some numerical average of their values.

Subjective well-being is quite different. Here the global construct can be captured through the single question 'How satisfied are you with your life as a whole?' Moreover, this global item can then be deconstructed into a minimal set of 'first level' domains which, together, comprise the global construct. For example, the seven domains of the Personal Wellbeing Index[5] are defined as satisfaction with standard of living, health, achievements in life, relationships, safety, connection to community, and future security. These domains form a robust single factor, which explains over half of the variance in 'life as a whole', and which therefore constitutes a useful measure of subjective QOL.

From this description, it is evident that medicine and the social sciences have taken very different paths in their conceptualization of quality of life. Since this chapter concerns measurement within urological settings, the HRQOL technology will now be examined in more detail.

Health-related quality of life

There are two kinds of HRQOL scales—generic and specific. The most widely used generic scale is the SF-36,[4] which is designed to measure HRQOL for diverse medical groups. One disadvantage of such scales is that their broad cover makes them insensitive to specific change. For example, an intervention may increase capacity to achieve a sturdy erection yet have little impact as judged through change in a generic HRQOL scale. Thus, condition-specific scales have been developed, which concentrate on symptoms relating to the body part or system in question.

The construction of all HRQOL instruments has been driven by the 1947 World Health Organization definition of health as a 'state of complete physical, emotional and social well-being'.[6] This global statement of philosophy then formed the basis of a 'consensus'[7] that HRQOL instruments 'should include physical, social and emotional functioning as well as perceptions of overall quality of life or general life satisfaction'.[8]

Defining HRQOL in this way has led to major problems of scale construction and the generation of data that are most uncertain in their interpretation. Perhaps not surprisingly, they have also been severely criticized (see, for example, the work of Leplege and Hunt[9] and Michalos[10]). Some of the contentious issues are as follows:

1 The 'consensus' statement adopted by test developers combines the global construct 'overall quality of life' with more specific concerns (e.g. physical functioning). This has caused the creation of scales that combine the scores from global items with the scores from items that represent some of their components. This makes no logical sense.

2 It has been pointed out[9] that 'Even if the WHO's definition of health as a hypothetical construct composed of physical, psychological, and social elements is to be accepted, this does not imply that quality of life is also composed of these dimensions . . . judgments about physical capacities and abilities have only relative objectivity. Thus, the observation that person A cannot walk as far as person B is merely a statement of fact, but if we extrapolate from this that person A has a poorer quality of life . . . this is a reinforcement of stereotypes that underlie discriminatory practices.' (p. 48). This concern also relates to the objective-subjective distinction mentioned earlier.

3 The term 'emotional functioning' is presumably intended to represent the affective component of subjective QOL. It is widely agreed that subjective quality of life comprises an interactive state of emotion and cognition. How, then, is such emotional functioning to be measured?
The answer should refer to the circumplex model of affect which, for well over a decade, has dominated the operationalization of affect (see, for example, Yik et al.[11]). This model depicts the affects on the circumference of a circle which is divided into quadrants by the axes of pleasant–unpleasant and activated–deactivated. Modified programs of factor analysis are used to position the specific affects with respect to one another in a highly predictable way, with the affective antonyms lying opposite one another. This model has been found sufficiently robust to seriously advance the understanding of affect, and especially its measurement, but, the HRQOL scales evidence no understanding of this important advance. Affects such as 'anxiety' or 'stress' are apparently selected at random to represent 'emotional functioning'. They are inadequate to perform this role.

4 The constructs of 'physical and social functioning' were presumably selected due to their connection to health and the important human need to feel connected to other people. Again, however, this choice disenfranchises other important areas which have just as much relevance for the human sense of well-being. These include such constructs as being productive, having self-esteem, feeling in control, and maintaining a sense of optimism.

A good perspective onto this disenfranchisement is provided by data from 11 surveys conducted in Canada.[10] These surveys included between them, 16 items of 'satisfaction' that were used to predict happiness. Various combinations of items were included in different surveys, but all included satisfaction with health. The top four predictors of happiness were found to be self-esteem (maximum $\beta = 0.38$), satisfaction with partner ($\beta = .30$), satisfaction with friendship ($\beta = 0.23$) and financial security ($\beta = 0.21$). Satisfaction with health was *never* the strongest predictor. Its maximum β was 0.18 and, in five out of 11 of the surveys its contribution was too low to enter the regression equation.

5 Finally, there is the issue of conceptual breadth. For example, a recent reviewer[12] states 'HRQOL narrows the QOL concept to aspects of life affected by a person's health condition and its treatment.' (p. 30). In confirmation of this view, another reviewer[13] describes generic HRQOL instruments as providing a 'summary health profile' while 'specialist instruments' focus on specific problems associated with a disease or area of functioning (p. 253). It is evident from such perspectives that the developed view of HRQOL is far more limited than the original intention of the 'consensus'[7] to include perceptions of overall quality of life.

In summary, HRQOL is a construct based on dubious premises. Let us now examine an alternative approach to quality of life measurement that has been derived through the social sciences.

Subjective well-being homeostasis

Early systematic research into the use of subjective indicators was heralded by two independent and major reports in the USA.[14,15] Both had used subjective indices of well-being with large population surveys, and both provided a detailed and insightful analysis of the resulting data. Numerous such surveys followed. In 1995, 16 estimates of population life satisfaction were assembled from surveys conducted in Western nations,[16] and it was reported that they averaged 75% of the scale maximum score (75%SM) with a standard deviation of just 2.5%SM. (The %SM is a standardized conversion of Likert-scale data projected on to a 0–100 scale.) In other words, the mean value from population surveys of subjective QOL, conducted in Western nations, can be predicted to lie within the narrow range of 70–80%SM. This result has been replicated on several occasions[17,18] and appears to be reliable.

In order to explain this narrow, positive range of values, a 'theory of subjective well-being (SWB) homeostasis' has been proposed.[17,19,20] This theory suggests that, in a manner analogous to the homeostatic maintenance of blood pressure or renal blood flow, subjective QOL is actively controlled and maintained by a set of psychological devices that function under the influence of personality (see Cummins and Nistico[19] for an extended description). The operation of these devices is most evident at the level of general, personal well-being. That is, homeostasis operates at a non-specific, abstract level, as exemplified by the classic question 'How satisfied are you with your life as a whole?' Because this question is so general, the response that people give reflects their core affect[21] which, it is proposed, is precisely the level at which the homeostatic system operates.

As one consequence of homeostasis, the level of satisfaction is remarkably stable. While unusually good or bad events will cause the SWB of individuals to change in the short term, over a period of time the homeostatic system will return this non-specific satisfaction with life to its previous level.[22,23,24] At the level of populations the degree of stability is extraordinary. This has been most clearly demonstrated by the application of the Australian Unity Wellbeing Index. Commencing in April 2001, quarterly surveys have been conducted with 2000 Australians, randomly chosen for each survey. Despite the occurrence of tumultuous international events during the intervening period, the population SWB, over the nine surveys conducted to the end of 2003, has varied from 73.2 to 75.9%SM, a range of just 2.7%SM.[5] Moreover, with the exception of the survey conducted immediately following 11 September, the population SWB has varied by less than 1% between adjacent surveys. Such stability is surely comparable to any measure of objective health status averaged across the population over a 3-year period.

It is also evident that the population SWB mean lies close to the three-quarters mark on the standardized 0–100 scale. This value represents the average 'set-point' for the average Australian. The normal range of individual values can be gauged from the within-survey standard deviation, which is about 12. Thus, using two standard deviations to describe the normative range around the mean of 75, it is apparent that the set-point of individuals may lie anywhere within the positive sector of the dissatisfied–satisfied scale (50 to 100%SM).

While this generalized sense of well-being is held positive with remarkable tenacity, it is not immutable. A sufficiently adverse environment can defeat the homeostatic system and, when this occurs, the level of subjective well-being falls below its homeo-static range. People who are suffering homeostatic defeat, experienced by such groups as carers of severely disabled family members living at home (54.5 ± 11.3%SM, Christensen et al.[25]) and people suffering chronic unemployment (50.4 ± 18.0%SM, Hepworth[26]), can experience marked upward shifts in subjective well-being if the circumstances of their lives improve allowing homeostasis to be restored. However, for people who are already maintaining a normally functioning homeostatic system, their levels of generalized subjective well-being will show little relationship to normal variations in their chronic circumstances of living. This is why the relationship between objective and subjective QOL is non-linear.

Abstract versus specific well-being

The homeostatic system, as described, has the role of creating a positive sense of well-being that is both non-specific and highly personalized. It is concerned only with the perceived well-being of the individual who is making this assessment and only in the most general sense. As one effect of this, people generally feel they are 'superior' to other people, or better than average.[23,27,28] They believe they are luckier, happier and more moral.[14] This is all part of the general 'positive bias' that is 'value added' by the brain to such thought processes and which leads, under the normal circumstances of living, to a generalized positive self-view.[29,30]

While the classic 'satisfaction with life as a whole' question is useful as an estimate of the homeostatic set-point, due to its high level of abstraction it cannot provide information about the components of life that also contribute, positively or negatively, to this sense of well-being. In order to acquire such information, questions need to be directed at satisfaction with life domains. There is converging agreement within the literature on the identification of the minimal set of domains that form the first-level deconstruction of personal well-being. One such approximation is offered by the Personal Wellbeing Index[5] which identifies seven domains, as has already been described. Theoretically, such a set should be sufficient to describe the entire 'life as a whole', and this case has been argued.[31] Moreover, the mean satisfaction score derived from the domains should approximate satisfaction expressed to 'life as a whole', and this too has been verified.[5] The domains' mean score and the life as a whole score are not, however, expected to be identical, due to the differing levels of abstraction in each.

While satisfaction with 'life as a whole' is proposed to approximate the homeostatic set-point, this is not so for the domains. Since questions at this level (e.g. How satisfied are you with your health?) are directed at broad but identifiable aspects of life, more specific information processing and affect linkage can be brought to bear on an evaluation of satisfaction. Consequently, the homeostatic influence on the satisfaction response will be diluted and the level of satisfaction will be allowed to vary either above or below the set-point. Because of this, when issues of ill-health arise, the domain of health will be more affected than the other domains due to the congruence of the information being processed. Moreover, due to its specificity, the domain of health will be more sensitive to such influence than will 'satisfaction with life as a whole' or the aggregate SWB derived from the combined domains.

This is all fairly intuitive. The more closely the elements of change match the reference to such items in the scale, the more sensitive will be the scale. Another determinant of sensitivity is the form of the response scale.

General measurement problems and solutions

Response scale sensitivity

The typical Likert scale offers five- or seven-choice points which, of itself, is hardly likely to exploit the discriminative capacity of most people in terms of their perceived well-being, but even this modest array of response choices is further reduced by the fact that subjective QOL data are normally confined to the positive side of bipolar scales, as has been described.[32,33] Consequently, because the majority of respondents are employing only half of the scale to register their judgement, Likert scales represent very blunt instruments by which to judge change in SWB.

A separate publication[34] has concluded that increasing the response options beyond seven points does not systematically detract from scale reliability, a conclusion shared by others.[35] So, since many people will have a discriminative capacity that exceeds the available response options, restricting people to such scales results in a loss of potentially discriminative data. However, there are some potential difficulties in generating expanded scales, and one of these involves the tradition of using category names.

Categorical naming

Likert[36] named all of his five scale categories, and the received wisdom is that categorical naming is a good idea. It is not. The use of such terms as 'good' does not ensure a standardized point of reference. For example, a 'good' house has very different meanings depending on a respondent's socioeconomic status, and high ambiguity in the allocation of values to scale categories has been documented for some time.[37] Additionally, there are other powerful reasons to avoid category naming.

The Likert scale makes the assumption that the psychometric distance between categories is equal. This aspect of scale construction is always dutifully portrayed as an equally spaced visual image, comprising marks on a horizontal line or a series of boxes. It may even be reinforced by a linear numbering system, for example from 1 to 7, with each successive integer corresponding to the next printed category, and then we add category names.

The clear implication is that these categorical names exhibit the same internal scaling as the printed scale and numbers suggest. This, however, is wrong, sometimes very wrong, and the data demonstrating this have been available for a considerable period of time.[38] A more recent review[34] has reported wide discrepancies in the values people give to the categorical names. We conclude that people have such varying interpretation of the numerical value accorded to category labels that their application in Likert scales detracts from the interval-nature of such scales.

In the area of HRQOL, Ware and Gandek[39] used the Thurstone method of equal-appearing intervals to calculate the following distances between category labels used in the SF-36[40] as follows: poor (1.0), fair (2.3), good (3.4), very good (4.3), and excellent (5.0). It can be seen that the distance between the lowest two categories (1.3) is about double that between the highest two categories (0.7). A separate investigation[41] found the separation of 'poor' and 'fair' to be 2.3, and that between 'good' and 'excellent' to be 1.1 units. It can be seen that the disparities between low and high adjacent category labels is in the same direction but of even greater magnitude. A more appropriate scale format is an 11-point, end-defined scale.

Justification for an 11-point, end-defined scale

The use of end-defined scales was pioneered by Jones and Thurstone in 1955.[37] They generated such a scale in relation to food preference, anchored by 'greatest like/dislike' (+4/−4), with a central category of 'neither like nor dislike' (0), and with the intermediate categories labelled only by their appropriate integer. So, do such scales produce data that are qualitatively different from conventionally labelled Likert scales?

The answer appears to be negative. Matell and Jacoby[42] used verbally anchored adjective statements related to civic beliefs, with the number of intervening points varying from two to 19. Apart from the fact that testing time increased with formats having more than 12 points, no differences were found on the proportion of scale utilized (more than three points) or in the proportion of 'uncertain' responses (more than five points). Similarly, the use of five-point[43] or six-point[44] scales has revealed no systematic differences between the data from end-defined and conventional Likert scales. From this it can be concluded that the end-defined format seems not to bias the data in any particular way. It is also interesting to note that an increasing number of recent authors (e.g. Hooker and Siegler[45] and Watkins *et al.*[46]) are using end-defined scales.

In summary, irrespective of whether the intention is to measure HRQOL or SWB, a critical feature of the response scale is to exploit discriminative capacity. This can best be achieved by the use of all 11-point, end-defined scale, which utilizes the 0 to 10 format that is a familiar form of rating within everyday life.

Questionnaires

The feature that all HRQOL scales share is that they are self-reports. They are completed by the patient independently of the physician, and are normally presented to the patient as a printed questionnaire.

General HRQOL scales

The most widely used generic scale is the SF-36.[4] HRQOL researchers generally have an extraordinarily high regard for this instrument as a 'gold standard', with many scale developers using the SF-36 for the purpose of validating their own 'QOL' instruments (e.g. Donovan *et al.*[47]). In fact there are many serious problems with both the construction and interpretation of this scale, as has been noted. However, this scale will not be further considered here. Instead, attention will be directed to the specific HRQOL scales concerned with either sexual functioning or urinary incontinence.

A general statement of evaluation

All of the scales that follow have received insufficient psychometric attention in relation to their validity, reliability, and sensitivity with different populations. Further, they all confuse the symptoms of incontinence or sexual dysfunction with quality of life, and make the incorrect assumption that the absence of pathology equates to quality of life. Since these problems are universal, no separate mention will be made in relation to specific scales. Other common issues concern the following, unless specified otherwise:

1 Unvalidated subscales: either the subscales have not been demonstrated to be independent from one another or an unsatisfactory factor analysis has been reported.

2 Mixed levels of measurement: all items forming subscales are not at the same level of specificity. For example 'worry about wetting myself' is a suitable item for a 'worry about incontinence' subscale. This, in turn, may be a useful subscale for a more general anxiety scale which, in turn, may form a subscale of depression. This logic is violated by the construction of subscales that combine 'I feel depressed' with 'I worry about wetting myself'.

Sexual function

Excellent reviews of sexual function scales are available.[48,49] The former located 24 scales of which 14 met the author's standards of reliability and validity. Just one of these has a title that clearly indicates its purpose to measure QOL:

◆ Quality of Life Measure specific to Men with Erection Difficulties (QOL-MED; Wagner *et al.*[50]). The 18 items for this scale were generated from interviews with men with erection difficulties. There are three subscales—emotional goals, values, and expectations.

Other scales that measure specific HRQOL in this area are as follows:

◆ Brief Male Sexual Function Inventory.[51] This 11-item scale has five subscales—sexual drive, erection, ejaculation, sexual problems, and overall satisfaction.

◆ Brief Sexual Function Index for Women.[52] Comprises 22 items that form seven subscales—sexual thoughts/desires, arousal, frequency of activity, receptivity/ initiation, pleasure/orgasm, sexual problems, and relationship satisfaction.

◆ Center for Martial and Sexual Health Questionnaire.[53] Comprises 18 items that form four subscales—erection, orgasm, desire, and satisfaction.

◆ Derogatis Sexual Function Inventory.[54] Comprises 245 items that measure a wide variety of sexual functions and dysfunctions. It also contains a global sexual satisfaction index.

◆ Female Sexual Function Index.[55] Comprises 19 items that form six subscales—desire, arousal, lubrication, orgasm, pain, and satisfaction.

◆ International Index of Erectile Function.[56] comprises 15 items forming five subscales—erectile function (six items), orgasmic function (two items), sexual desire (two items), intercourse satisfaction (three items), and overall satisfaction (two items). A brief five-item version has also been produced.[49]

The authors[56] report a factor analysis that confirms the five domains. However, three factors contain less than the minimum three items required to form an acceptable factor, so they cannot be regarded as reliable subscales. Moreover, the two items that form the 'overall satisfaction' domain are highly specific to the condition. They are—how satisfied have you been with your overall sex life/sexual relationship with your partner?

The five-item version concentrates on its function as a diagnostic instrument. The items were chosen for their ability to distinguish between men who have/have not got erectile dysfunction. This is a good example of a scale being less than its parts. The mean score is much less likely to be informative than an analysis of five separate questions pertaining to different aspects of the problem.

- Sexual Function and Quality of Sexual Life Questionnaire.[57] Despite the title, the authors are explicit that the aim of their scale is to measure 'sexual function and quality of life' (p. 315). This 42-item instrument comprises the four subscales of general health, sex life, sex and your health, and sexual relationships. These are referred to as 'sections' of the questionnaire. Yet these bear little coherent relationship to the 31 items that form the five discovered factors. These are labelled sexual function, general health, sexual effects of health problems, relationship intimacy, and erectile function. Only the 'general health' section and factor contain matching items. The other three sections contain items drawn from various factors and other items not included in the factor analysis. These inconsistencies are not explained.

  The content of the items is dominated by sexual problems and health problems. These appear in all four questionnaire sections. Interspersed within the sections are other items relating to other issues such as the quality of sex life, how attractive the respondent feels (women only), erection strength (male only), frequency of intercourse, and the level of sexual drive in their partner. Other items are effectively repeated in different sections (rating the quality of sex life).

- Sexual Functioning Questionnaire.[58] The authors indicate that their 13-item scale can be used to measure QOL. The items form four subscales—sexual frequency, erection quality, orgasm quality, and sexual satisfaction.

- Sexual Life Quality Questionnaire.[59] The 16 items form two factorially validated subscales of 'sexual QOL' (10 items) and treatment satisfaction for erectile dysfunction. The items are generated from the literature, qualitatively evaluated by men with erectile dysfunction, and subjected to routine psychometric analysis. Respondents to the sexual QOL subscale are asked to rate their experience of intercourse compared with how they felt prior to becoming impotent. This is probably an excellent method for enhancing instrument sensitivity. Their reduced adaptation level for the judgement of sexual performance and satisfaction, induced by the impotence, would mean they should be very sensitive to register improvement.

However, the recommended response scale does not capitalize on this, restricting the respondents to just four levels of improvement.

The sub-scale labelled 'quality of life' (p. 375) is a misnomer. However, it may be a valid measure of the construct 'subjective sexual QOL'.

Lower urinary tract symptoms

A recent review[8] identified and discussed 14 condition-specific QOL scales that concern urinary incontinence. However, many of these are little more than self-reports of symptoms or negative affect (e.g. bother or stress) associated with such symptoms. The others are as follows:

- American Urological Association Symptom Index[60] which is also called the International Prostate Symptom Score.[61] The original index comprises seven items, all of which are symptoms (e.g. frequency of urination). The authors make no claim for this as a measure of HRQOL. Okamura et al.,[61] however, have added a stand-alone 'QOL index' comprising the single item 'If you were to spend the rest of your life with your urinary condition just the way it is now, how would you feel about that' (delighted–terrible). The question is ambiguous. It confuses the rest of life with the urinary condition. Someone could have very positive feelings about their life yet be negative about their urinary condition.

- Benign Prostatic Hyperplasia Health-Related Quality of Life Survey (BPH-HRQOL; Epstein et al.[62,63]). This comprises 44 items forming six subscales. The authors[62] use the scale to assist with diagnosis.

- BPH Specific Quality of Life Scale.[64] These authors started with a 20-item scale comprising four subscales (physical, marital, social, global) designed by a 'group of experts'. This was administered to some 5500 patients and a principal component analysis was conducted. The authors provide no details of this analysis other than it detected two specific areas: sexuality (three items) and benign prostatic hyperplasia (BPH)-specific interferences with activities (four items). They also identified a 'third component represented by questions related to general QOL' (items not identified). From this they built a nine-item scale with three subscales: sexuality (three items), BPH-specific interferences (three items), and general QOL (three items—satisfaction with current life, energy–vitality, asthenia).

  A further factor analysis is required to test the integrity of the nine-item scale. Moreover, each of the subscales require further investigation to determine their optimal composition.

- European Organization for Research and Treatment of Cancer—Prostate Cancer Questionnaire (EORTC-PCQ).[65] This comprises the EORTC generic questionnaire with additional specific items. It has 30 items forming eight subscales—physical functioning, social role functioning, urological symptoms, fatigue, sexual function-ing, emotional functioning, social functioning, and pain.

♦ Incontinence Impact Questionnaire[66] is the modified form of a previous scale.[67] It contains 26 items forming three subscales—daily activities, social interaction, and self-perception. The aim of the first two subscales is to measure functional limitations associated with the condition. The self-perception subscale comprises four items—physical health, mental health, fear of odour, fear of embarrassment. This is a strange assortment of items.

A factor analysis of this scale was published in 1994.[68] The authors acknowledge the Incontinence Impact Questionnaire[66,67] as 'an earlier form of the measure' yet they include 30 items. They report four factors—physical activity (six items), travel (six items), social relationships (10 items), and emotional health (eight items). However, many of the items cross-load between factors at loadings up to 0.49. Moreover, the conceptual content of the factors does not make sense. 'Employment' is included in the travel factor, 'fear of embarrassment' is included in the social factor, while 'fear' and 'embarrassment' as separate items are included in the emotional health factor.

♦ Incontinence Quality of Life Instrument (I-QOL; Patrick et al.[69]). This scale comprises 22 items rated 'not at all' to 'extremely'. All items measured concern some aspect of the incontinence. Some address common behaviour (e.g. 'I have to watch what I drink'), some address negative affect attached to specific targets (e.g. 'I worry about wetting myself'), general temporal targets (e.g. 'I worry about my incontin-ence getting worse as I get older'), or the condition in general (e.g. 'Incontinence is always on my mind'), and some target non-specific negative affect (e.g. 'I feel depressed').

The instrument has three subscales—avoidance and limiting behaviour, psychosocial impacts, and social embarrassment. The types of items above are mixed through these subscales. So for example, psychosocial impacts contains both general items pertaining to the condition ('Incontinence is always on my mind'), general items of negative affect ('I feel depressed'), and items concerning specific targets ('I worry about having sex'). The problems of combining general and specific items has already been described.

Additional problems concern the placement of items. For example, the social embarrassment subscale contains the item 'I worry about my incontinence getting worse as I get older'.

The authors state that they 'identified three factors' but provide no details of item loadings. Thus, the adequacy of the proposed factorial structure cannot be evaluated. Their validation is against the SF-36 and the Psychosocial General Wellbeing Index.[70] No rationale is provided for choosing this latter scale. Their validation involves the total I-QOL score, not the subscales, and it correlates 0.15 to 0.48 with the SF-36 subscales and 0.18 to 0.48 with the Psychological General Wellbeing Index (PGWI) 'summary and subscale scores'. They conclude from this that the I-QOL shows 'good validity', which certainly overstates their case. The I-QOL shares 17.6% of the variance ($r = 0.42$) with the SF-36 subscale of psychological well-being.

Others authors[71] have used the I-QOL as a 'quality of life' measure. They report it is sensitive to patient-related incontinence severity. It correlated 0.73 with this score, and 0.55 with physician-rated severity of incontinence.

◆ International Incontinence Study—BPH Study Questionnaire.[47,72] This 31-item scale has three sections. Urinary symptoms are measured by 22 items, most of which also ask about the degree of 'bother' they cause. Sexual functioning is measured by four items, and 'condition-specific QOL' by six items. One publication[72] concerns only the symptoms part of the questionnaire. The other[47] reports an investigation into the six QOL items, all of which determine the degree of negative impact of urinary incontinence on feelings and behaviour. These six items do not relate to one another with sufficient strength to be considered a scale. Consequently, the authors refer to the two 'general' items, and their item 30 in particular, as being most useful 'to evaluate QOL' (p. 719). This asks 'Overall, how much do your urinary symptoms interfere with your life?' Other authors[73,74] have used such items as a QOL measure.

The other general item allows people to record positive emotion. 'If you had to spend the rest of your life with your urinary symptoms as they are now, how would you feel?' (perfectly happy–desperate). This is much closer to a true QOL index. If people have adapted to their symptoms they would probably respond to this in a similar manner to 'satisfaction with life as a whole'.

◆ King's Health Questionnaire[75] comprises 21 items combined in groups of one to five to form the King's Health Questionnaire—Quality of Life Index.[61] The index is validated against the SF-36. There is no possibility for the respondent to provide a positive view of their life. For example, in the 'domain' of personal relationships two items ask 'Does your bladder problem affect your relationship with your partner/sex life' scored from not at all (1) to a lot (4). The domain of 'social limitations' asks the same question in relation to 'family life'. It is most unlikely that a factor analysis would support such a distinction between domains. Other domains (e.g. incontinence severity) are a combination of objective (Do you wear pads to keep dry?) and subjective data (Do you worry in case you smell?).

Conclusions

It is evident that all of these instruments are based on condition-specific symptoms of the respective conditions. As such, they are based on items that otherwise are used to assist diagnosis and treatment, but here are combined to form an end-state called HRQOL. This end-state does not represent physical and mental health as positive experiences and nor does it represent SWB as conceived by the social sciences. Instead it represents a unique construct that has, as its optimal extent, a condition of health neutrality, where no symptoms of pathology are apparent to the patient.

Even ignoring the considerable psychometric difficulties that have been described, it is not clear why it is desirable to measure this particular end-state, which occupies some kind of middle ground between medical pathology and SWB. Our suggestion is that HRQOL measurement be abandoned, and that it be replaced with some combination of the following:

1 The conventional medical symptoms of pathology. These inform the medical diagnosis of a particular medical condition.

2 Subjective well-being. This informs about whether the medical symptoms are powerful enough to cause the normal positive state of well-being to be defeated. The seven-item Personal Wellbeing Index[5] could be used for this purpose.

3 Condition-specific satisfaction. We speculate that this new form of scale would inform about the extent to which the medical symptoms, perceived by the patient, were affecting the area of life involving the specific condition. The logic underpinning the development of such condition-specific instruments is as follows. It has been described how the seven domains of the Personal Wellbeing Index form the first-level deconstruction of satisfaction with 'life as a whole'. This process of scale derivation can be continued. Thus, the domain of 'health' can be deconstructed into satisfaction with fitness, bladder functioning, resistance to disease, etc. In turn, the domain of bladder function, now at a third level deconstruction, can be measured by a scale that might look like this: How satisfied are you with:

- the control you have over your bladder?
- your ability to finish urination without continued dribbling?
- your ability to postpone urination?
- the ease with which you commence urination?
- your sense of complete bladder emptying after urination?
- the strength of your urinary stream?

The above 'bladder functioning satisfaction scale' has the following advantages:

1 Its purpose is clear and it has high face validity.

2 The items will certainly scale together and exhibit good internal validity.

3 Its construction is theoretically driven. Multiple regression can be used to test whether each item contributes unique variance to the stem construct ('satisfaction with bladder functioning') and whether additional items should be added.

4 The scale is brief, due to the constraints of point 3 above.

The advantage of this set of three scales to medical practice would be as follows:

1 The physician can determine whether the symptoms are severe enough to affect general well-being (SWB). This, however, is a fairly insensitive indicator due to the functioning of SWB homeostasis. Certainly if it is found that SWB is below normal, then this is a very important signal of psychopathology (depression). However, it is possible for the patient to have normal SWB and yet to have below-normal condition-specific well-being.

2 The restoration of normative levels of condition-specific well-being could become the therapeutic goal, rather than the elimination of all symptoms of pathology.

3 A 'no treatment' decision could be made even in the presence of medical symptoms of pathology if the patient expressed normal levels of condition-specific well-being.

References

1 Cummins RA (2000). Objective and subjective quality of life: an interactive model. *Soc. Indic. Res.* **52**: 55–72.

2 Cummins RA, Eckersley R, Lo SK, Okerstrom E, Hunter B, Davern M (2004). *Australian Unity Wellbeing Index: Report 90 The Wellbeing of Australians—Owning a Pet.* Melbourne: Australian Centre on Quality of Life, School of Psychology, Deakin University (http://acqoldeakineduau/index_wellbeing/indexhtm).

3 Fayers PM, Groenvold M, Hand DJ, Bjordal K (1998). Clinical impact versus factor analysis for quality of life questionnaire construction. *J. Clin. Epidemiol.* **51**(3): 285–6.

4 McHorney CA, Ware JE, Raczek AE (1993). The MOS 36-item short-form health survey (SF-36): II Psychometric and clinical tests of validity in measuring physical and mental health constructs. *Med. Care* **31**: 247–63.

5 Cummins RA, Eckersley R, Pallant J, van Vugt J, Misajon R (2003). Developing a national index of subjective wellbeing: the Australian Unity Wellbeing Index. *Soc. Indic. Res.* **64**: 159–90.

6 World Health Organization (1947). *Definition of Health.* WHO, Geneva.

7 Berzon R, Hays RD, Shumaker SA (1993). Preface: international use, application and performance of health-related quality of life instruments. *Qual. Life Res.* **2**: 367–8.

8 Corcos J, Beaulieu S, Donovan J, Naughton M, Gotoh M, and Members of the Symptom Quality of Life Assessment Committee of the First International Consultation on Incontinence (2002). Quality of life assessment in men and women with urinary incontinence. *J. Urol.* **168**(3): 896–905.

9 Leplege A, Hunt S (1997). The problem of quality of life in medicine. *J. Am. Med. Assoc.* **278**(1): 47–50.

10 Michalos AC (2004). Social indicators research and health-related quality of life research. *Soc. Indic. Res.* **65**(1): 27–72.

11 Yik MSM, Russell JA, Barrett LF (1999). Structure of self-reported current affect: integration and beyond. *J. Pers. Soc. Psychol.* **77**: 600–19.

12 Kane RA (2003). Definition, measurement, and correlates of quality of life in nursing homes: toward a reasonable practice, research, and policy agenda. *Gerontologist* **43**(2): 28–36.

13 Nicholson P, Anderson P (2003). Quality of life, distress and self-esteem: a focus group study of people with chronic bronchitis. *Br. J. Health Psychol.* **8**(3): 251–70.

14 **Andrews FM, Withey SB** (1976). *Social Indicators of Well-being: Americans' Perceptions of Life Quality*. Plenum Press, New York.

15 **Campbell A, Converse PE, Rodgers WL** (1976). *The Quality of American Life: Perceptions, Evaluations, and Satisfactions*. Russell Sage Foundation, New York.

16 **Cummins RA** (1995). On the trail of the gold standard for subjective well-being. *Soc. Indic. Res.* **35**: 179–200.

17 **Cummins RA** (1998). The second approximation to an international standard of life. satisfaction *Soc. Indic. Res.* **43**: 307–34.

18 **Cummins RA** (2003). Normative life satisfaction: measurement issues and a homeostatic model. *Soc. Indic. Res.* **64**: 225–56.

19 **Cummins RA, Nistico H** (2002). Maintaining life satisfaction: the role of positive cognitive bias. *J. Happ. Stud.* **3**: 37–69.

20 **Cummins RA, Gullone E, Lau ALD** (2002). A model of subjective well being homeostasis: the role of personality. In: *The Universality of Subjective Wellbeing Indicators. A Multi-Disciplinary and Multi-National Perspective* (ed. E Gullone, RA Cummins), pp. 7–46. Kluwer, Dordrecht.

21 **Russell JA** (2003). Core affect and the psychological construction of emotion. *Psychol. Rev.* **110**(1): 145–72.

22 **Hanestad BR, Albrektsen G** (1992). The stability of quality of life experience in people with Type 1 diabetes over a period of a year. *J. Adv. Nurs.* **17**: 777–84.

23 **Headey B, Wearing A** (1989). Personality, life events, and subjective well-being: toward a dynamic equilibrium model. *J. Pers. Soc. Psychol.* **57**: 731–9.

24 **Suh E, Diener E** (1996). Events and subjective well-being: only recent events matter. *J. Pers. Soc. Psychol.* **70**: 1091–102.

25 **Christensen KA, Parris Stephens MA, Townsend AL** (1998). Mastery in women's multiple roles and well-being: adult daughters providing care to impaired patients. *Health Psychol.* **17**(2): 163–71.

26 **Hepworth SJ** (1980). Moderating factors of the psychological impact of unemployment. *J. Occup. Psychol.* **53**: 139–45.

27 **Headey B, Wearing A** (1988). The sense of relative superiority—central to well-being. *Soc. Indic. Res.* **20**: 497–516.

28 **Diener E, Suh EM, Lucas RE, Smith HL** (1999). Subjective well-being: three decades of progress. *Psychol. Bul.* **125**(2): 276–302.

29 **Taylor SE, Brown JD** (1988). Illusion and well-being: a social psychological perspective on mental health. *Psychol. Bull.* **103**: 193–210.

30 **Weinstein ND** (1989). Optimistic biases about personal risks. *Science* **246**: 1232–3.

31 **Cummins RA** (1996). The domains of life satisfaction: an attempt to order chaos. *Soc. Indic. Res.* **38**: 303–32.

32 **Watson GB** (1930). Happiness among adult students of education. *J. Educ. Psychol.* **21**: 79–109.

33 **Cummins RA** (1997). *Comprehensive Quality of Life Scale—Adult Manual*, 5th edn. School of Psychology, Deakin University, Melbourne.

34 **Cummins RA, Gullone E** (2000). Why we should not use 5-point Likert scales: the case for subjective quality of life measurement. *Proceedings of the Second International Conference on Quality of Life in Cities*, pp. 74–93. National University of Singapore, Singapore.

35 **Russell C, Bobko P** (1992). Moderated regression analysis and Likert scales: too coarse for comfort. *J. Appl. Psychol.* **77**: 336–42.

36 **Likert R** (1932). A technique for the measurement of attitudes. *Arch. Psychol.* **140**: 1–55.

37 Jones LV, Thurstone LL (1955). The psychophysics of semantics. *J. Appl. Psychol.* **39**: 31–6.

38 Cronbach LJ (1946). Response sets and test validity. *Educ. Psychol. Meas.* **6**: 475–94.

39 Ware JE, Gandek B (1994). The SF-36 Health Survey: development and use in mental health research and the IQOLA project. *Int. J. Ment. Health* **23**: 49–73.

40 Ware JE, Sherbourne CD (1992). The MOS 36-item short-form health survey (SF-36). *Med. Care* **30**: 473–81.

41 Spector PE (1976). Choosing response categories for summated rating scales. *J. Appl. Psychol.* **61**: 374–5.

42 Matell MS, Jacoby J (1971). Is there an optimal number of alternatives for Likert scale items? Study 1: Reliability and validity. *Educ. Psychol. Meas.* **31**: 657–74.

43 Wyatt RC, Meyers LS (1987). Psychometric properties of four 5-point Likert-type response scales. *Educ. Psychol. Meas.* **47**: 27–35.

44 Dixon PN, Bobo M, Stevick RA (1984). Response differences and preferences for all-category-defined and end-defined Likert formats. *Educ. Psychol. Meas.* **44**: 61–6.

45 Hooker K, Siegler IC (1993). Life goals, satisfaction, and self-rated health: preliminary findings. *Exp. Aging Res.* **19**: 97–110.

46 Watkins D, Adair J, Akande A, Cheng C, Fleming J, Ismail M, *et al.* (1998). Cultural dimensions, gender, and the nature of self-concept: a fourteen-country study. *Int. J. Psychol.* **33**: 17–31.

47 Donovan JL, Peters KTJ, Abrams P, Coast J, Matos-Ferreira A, Rentzhog L, *et al.* (1997). Using the ICSQoL to measure the impact of lower urinary tract symptoms on quality of life: evidence from the ICS-'BHP' study. *Br. J. Urol.* **80**: 712–21.

48 Daker-White G (2002). Reliable and valid self-report outcome measures in sexual (Dys)function: a systematic review. *Arch. Sex. Behav.* **31**(2): 197–209.

49 Rosen RC (2001). Measurement of male and female sexual dysfunction. *Curr. Psychiat. Rep.* **3**: 182–7.

50 Wagner TH, Patrick DL, McKenna SP, Froese PS (1996). Cross-cultural development of a quality of life measure for men with erection difficulties. *Qual. Life Res.* **5**: 443–9.

51 Laan E, Everaerd W (1998). Physiological measures of vaginal vasocongestion. *Int. J. Impot. Res.* **10**(Suppl. 2): S107–S110.

52 Taylor SE, Brown JD (1994). Positive illusions and well-being revisited: separating fact from fiction. *Psychol. Bull.* **116**: 21–7.

53 Corty EQ, Althof SE, Kurit DM (1996). The reliability and validity of a sexual function questionnaire. *J. Sex Marital Ther.* **22**: 27–34.

54 Derogatis LR, Melisaratos N (1979). The DSFI: a multidimensional measure of sexual functioning. *J. Sex Marital Ther.* **5**(3): 244–81.

55 Rosen RC, Capperlleri JC, Smith MD, Lipsky J, Pena BM (1999). Development and evaluation of an abridged, 5-item version of the international index of erectile function (IIEF-5) as a diagnostic tool for erectile dysfunction. *Int. J. Impot. Res.* **11**: 319–26.

56 Rosen RC, Riley A, Wagner G, Osterloh IH, Kirkpatrick J, Mishra A (1997). The international index of erectile function (IIEF): a multidimensional scale for assessment of erectile dysfunction. *Urology* **49**: 822–30.

57 Daker-White G, Crowley T (2003). Sexual function and quality of life in genitourinary medicine (GUM) outpatients and preliminary validation of a self-report questionnaire measure. *Qual. Life Res.* **12**: 315–25.

58 Glick HA, McCarron TJ, Althof SE, Corty EW, Willke RJ (1997). Construction of scales for the centre for marital and sexual health (CMASH) sexual functioning questionnaire. *J. Sex Marital Ther.* **23**(2): 103–16.

59 Woodward JMB, Hass SL, Woodward PJ (2002). Reliability and validity of the sexual life quality questionnaire (SLQQ). *Qual. Life Res.* **11**: 365–77.

60 Barry MJ, Fowler FJ, O'Leary MP, Bruskewitz RC, Hotgrewe HL, Mebust WK *et al.* (1992). The American Urological Association symptom index for benign prostatic hyperplasia. *J. Urol.* **148**: 1549–57.

61 Okamura K, Usami T, Nagahama K, Maruyama S, Mizuta E (2002). 'Quality of life' assessment of urination in elderly Japanese men and women with some medical problems using international prostate symptom score and King's health questionnaire. *Eur. Urol.* **41**: 411–19.

62 Epstein RE, Deverka PA, Chute DG, Lieber MM, Oesterling JE, Panser L *et al.* (1991). Urinary symptom and quality of life questions indicative of obstructive benign prostatic hyperplasia: results of a pilot study. *Urology* **38**: 20.

63 Epstein RE, Deverka PA, Chute CG, Panser L, Oesterling JE, Lieber MM *et al.* (1992). Validation of a new quality of life questionnaire for benign prostatic hyperplasia. *J. Clin. Epidemiol.* **45**: 143.

64 Lukacs B, McCarthy C, Grange JC (1993). Long-term quality of life in patients with benign prostatic hypertrophy: preliminary results of a cohort study of 7,093 patients treated with an alpha-1-adrenergic blocker, alfuzosin. *Eur. Urol.* **24**(1): 34–40.

65 da Silva FC, Fossa SD, Aaronson NK, Serbouti S, Denis L, Casselman J *et al.* and members of the EORTC Genitourinary Tract Cancer Cooperative Group (1996). The quality of life of patients with newly diagnosed M1 prostate cancer: experience with EORTC clinical trial 30853. *Eur. J. Cancer* **32**(1): 72–7.

66 Wyman JF, Harkins SW, Choi SC, Taylor JR, Fantl JA (1987). Psychosocial impact of urinary incontinence in women. *Obstet. Gynaecol.* **70**(3): 378–81.

67 Norton C (1982). The effects of urinary incontinence in women. *Int. Rehab. Med.* **4**: 9.

68 Shumaker SA, Wyman JF, Uebersax JS, McClish D, Fantl JA, for the Continence Program in Women (CPW) Research Group (1994). Health-related quality of life measures for women with urinary incontinence: the Incontinence Impact Questionnaire and the Urogenital Distress Inventory. *Qual. Life Res.* **3**: 291–306.

69 Patrick DL, Martin ML, Bushnell DM, Yalcin I, Wagner TH, Buesching DP (1999). Quality of life for women with urinary incontinence: further development of the incontinence quality of life instrument (I-QOL). *Urology* **53**: 71–6.

70 Wenger NK, Mattson ME, Furberg CD, Elinson J (1984). *Assessment of Quality of Life in Clinical Trials of Cardiovascular Therapies.* Le Jacg, New York.

71 Melville JL, Miller EA, Fialkow MF, Lentz GM, Miller JL, Fenner DE (2003). Relationship between patient report and physician assessment of urinary incontinence severity. *Am. J. Gynecol.* **189**: 76–80.

72 Donovan JL, Abrams P, Peters TJ, Kay HE, Reynard J, Chapples C *et al.* (1996). The ICS- 'BPH' study: the psychometric validity and reliability of the ICSmale questionnaire. *Br. J. Urol.* **77**: 554–62.

73 Bakke A, Malt UF (1993). Social functioning and general well-being in patients treated with clean intermittent catheterisation. *J. Psychosom. Res.* **37**(4): 371–80.

74 Brookes ST, Donovan JL, Peters TJ, Abrams P, Neal DE (2002). Sexual dysfunction in men after treatment for lower urinary tract symptoms: evidence from randomized controlled trial. *Br. Med. J.* **324**: 1059–61.

75 Kelleher CJ, Cardozo LD, Khullar V, Salvatore S (1997). A new questionnaire to assess the quality of life of urinary incontinent women. *Br. J. Obstet. Gynaecol.* **104**: 1374–9.

Chapter 3

Self-help strategies

Rodney H. Breau

Introduction

One of the most important, yet commonly overlooked, components of providing health care involves communication of information and provision of emotional support. Cancer patients expect to be informed, and report improved satisfaction and decreased anxiety when their physician is effective at providing information.[1–6] Clinicians strive to help patients understand and cope with disease; however, even refined communicators appreciate the minimal amount of information retained after a clinic appointment.[7–9] In a busy practice it is difficult to dedicate the time required to adequately educate and support each patient. For these reasons, patients and physicians often rely on supplemental resources as an adjunct to standard patient–clinician interaction.[3,10]

Some physicians are reluctant to accept self-help as an essential component of care. However, a large proportion of patients use these resources, and without proper guidance, are at risk of receiving erroneous advice and information. This chapter reviews self-help available to urology patients and provides specific suggestions pertaining to the development and dissemination of these resources. The attitude and awareness of the physician are discussed and a practical approach to incorporating self-help in clinical practice is presented.

Clinical case

Mr Smith, a 62-year-old man, and his wife arrive at your office visibly upset. He had a radical prostatectomy 3 years previously due to Gleason 8 prostate adenocarcinoma. Post-operatively he has experienced erectile dysfunction; however, his prostate-specific antigen (PSA) levels have been undetectable. His most recent serum PSA level was 0.08 mg/ml. The patient reports speaking with a prostate cancer support group member who was treated with brachytherapy and has not lost erectile function. Following this conversation Mr and Mrs Smith decided to search the internet. They now present with a stack of printed material. Among other issues, they want to know why he was not offered brachytherapy, why his free PSA has not been followed, and why he is not being treated with selenium, vitamin E and anti-androgen medication.

Defining self-help

'Self-help' is somewhat of a misnomer because the term implies that the patient independently seeks help with their disease. Although self-help is usually accessed voluntarily, we know that the majority of urology patients are referred to self-help by a third party.[11] The term self-help broadly refers to educational or emotional support gained from outside standard care offered by a physician.

Types of self-help currently available

A wide variety of self-help media is available to patients.[11–14] Traditionally, brochures, books, newsletters, videos, audio cassettes, telephone help lines, and support groups were used by urology patients. However, in recent years, interactive CD-ROMs and internet sites have been developed. Patient advocacy groups, professional associations, or pharmaceutical companies, provide the majority of resources. Availability and accessibility vary between diseases. Brochures are available for most urology patients and almost all types of self-help have been developed for those with prostate cancer and interstitial cystitis.[11] Self-help research has focused on support groups and internet sites; therefore, much of the discussion is devoted to these media.

Brochures

Brochures are the form of self-help most used by urology patients.[10,11] Patients prefer brochures because they are accessible, free, and require minimal effort to read. Since they can be developed and distributed at a low cost,[15–17] brochures are produced by many local and national urological associations. For these same reasons, pharmaceutical companies and special interest groups create information leaflets, commonly containing biased or inaccurate information. Not surprisingly, when brochures for prostate cancer patients were compared, it was found that the quality of content varied greatly.[18] Thankfully, tools that allow objective evaluation of information leaflets are currently in development and a group in Canada is structuring and modifying a prostate cancer booklet based on patient preference and feedback.[19,20] Information brochures on prostate and testicular cancer seem to improve knowledge and change screening behaviour.[21–26] However, minimal data for evaluating the efficacy of other urology brochures are available.

Physicians receive numerous brochures from different sources. A common error is to display all brochures in the office waiting room without proper review of their content. Some patients will take any brochure that may pertain to their disease or symptom. Clearly, this behaviour has the potential to provide patients with conflicting and confusing information. Health professionals must be selective when providing patients with brochures. A patient should only receive brochures from a health professional who is familiar with their illness. This affords an opportunity to discuss which aspects of the brochure are pertinent. Since brochures are so commonly used, they should contain a list of other forms of self-help that provide more detailed information and emotional support. The list of alternative self-help should contain specific details instructing patients on how to access the individual resources.

Books

Hundreds of books have been published for urology patients in the past two decades. Most are written by prominent physicians in various fields of urology. A significant number are written or co-authored by patients themselves. The books are widely available at bookstores and libraries. It is unrealistic to expect physicians to be familiar with all the available literature. It is, however, advantageous to be knowledgeable of at least one book for common urological conditions such as prostate cancer, urinary diversion, erectile dysfunction, and interstitial cystitis. Familiarization with the content of selected books will prepare the physician to respond to common concerns the book may elicit.

Books are commonly read by patients with prostate cancer and interstitial cystitis. In fact, if books specific to their illness were made available, over half of urology patients claim they would read them. Of those patients who read books about their disease, almost all reported them to be extremely useful.[11]

Newsletters and magazines

Several urology patient groups mail newsletters or magazines to communicate with their members. The patient is usually required to pay a membership fee to supplement publication and postal costs. Newsletters contain articles written by patients and health-care professionals giving advice on treatment and coping strategies. Updates on various advocacy and fund-raising initiatives are also included. A minority of urology patients receives newsletters; however, most patients would like to receive them if they were free.[11]

Patients report that newsletters are an effective means for communicating information.[11] However, since they are often supported by pharmaceutical companies or are unregulated, there is a risk of bias. Patients should be directed to newsletters that are regulated by a professional association. If a regulated newsletter does not exist, it is recommended a urologist receive the newsletter to screen for inaccurate content. Patients should be made aware that the information might be biased or not pertinent to their current situation.

Videos

Few urology patients have watched a disease-specific video, although many report they would like to if one were available.[10,11] Information seen on television has been shown to be better retained in the memory compared with information given in audio or printed form, especially by older adults.[27] However, when prostate cancer videos were evaluated it was found they were not effective at greatly increasing subjects' knowledge.[28,29] Interestingly, despite the lack of information retention, subjects felt more informed and better equipped to play an active role in treatment decision-making after seeing a video.

Telephone support lines

Telephone information and support lines have been used for various patient groups, including those with cancer.[30] It is likely that support lines would be helpful to patients with urological disease. Unfortunately, there is a considerable cost associated with maintaining this type of service. The cost of training help-line employees and associated litigation issues preclude their incorporation into the self-help armamentarium of most patients.

Support groups

A support group is a gathering of individuals who have similar issues affecting their quality of life. Patients suffering from cancer and other illnesses have established numerous support groups.[31,32] Most large towns and cities in North America have prostate cancer support groups affiliated to the Canadian Prostate Cancer Network, Man to Man (sponsored by the American Cancer Society), or Us Too (sponsored by the American Foundation for Urologic Disease). Hundreds of support groups are also available for patients with interstitial cystitis, usually sponsored by the Interstitial Cystitis Network. There are reports of independent support groups for patients with erectile dysfunction and testicular cancer, but these meetings are not available to most patients.[33,34] Despite the prevalence of support groups, it is important to remember that a proportion of patients do not have access to meetings because they live in remote areas or do not have suitable transport.

Group meetings are led by patients or professionals, and attempt to provide information, social support, and advice based on the collective experiences of peers.[31] There is considerable variation in the motives patient have for attending support group meetings. Prior to initiating a support group it is important to ask patients what they would like the meetings to provide. If the primary interest is information, meetings should be designed in a manner that facilitates dissemination of information. If, on the other hand, patients want to interact with other patients, the layout and agenda should be tailored to accommodate that objective. The vast majority of patients with prostate cancer cite information seeking as the principal reason for joining support groups, and this is reflected in meetings which are often lecture style with minimal opportunity for interaction between patients.[35,36] In contrast, interstitial cystitis groups seem to utilize the more traditional approach of round-table discussions for sharing ideas and experiences. While gender may influence the preferred support group format, inherent differences in disease probably also play a role. Disease characteristics such as social acceptance, chronicity, morbidity, and mortality may all influence the objectives of patients. Appropriately planned format and content will increase the likelihood of attaining patients' goals.

Support groups are used as platforms for patient advocacy. Individual groups often combine to form national and international patient associations. The associations actively pursue funding for research and lobby government for disease-specific legislation. Patient groups commonly initiate projects that serve to increase public awareness of their disease.[35,37–39] It is advantageous for physicians to recognize and collaborate with patient groups since they provide important services and have the common goal of improving patient well-being.

Seventy-seven to 90% of prostate cancer patients who attend support groups reported an improvement in knowledge of their disease and 86% reported an improvement in their ability to cope.[36,37,40] Furthermore, 89% of prostate cancer patients feel they are more involved in their treatment after attending support groups.[40] Unfortunately, there are no objective data available to determine if urology patients actually retain more information about their disease after attending support groups.

It is generally believed that support groups are useful;[31,40–46] however, only 13 to 29% of patients attend these meetings.[11,47] Lack of interest, inconvenience, embarrassment, and intimidation may contribute to the low rate of involvement in support groups.[11,48] Lack of awareness may also play a role in low attendance. Surveys have revealed that one-third of urologists do not advocate prostate cancer support groups,[8,46] and only half of prostate cancer patients are aware of the availability of self-help groups.[11,47] Nearly all interstitial cystitis patients and approximately 40% of erectile dysfunction and urinary diversion patients report they would join a support group if one were available.[11]

Those who join support groups seem to have a specific demographic profile.[49] The majority of patients who attend prostate cancer support groups are married, well educated, and within 5 years of diagnosis.[37,40,47,50,51] Black men have the highest incidence and mortality of prostate cancer;[52,53] however, far more White patients attend support groups than Black patients.[37,40,47] The demographics of other urology patients who attend support groups have not been adequately defined. It has been suggested that females are more likely to use support groups, since a higher percentage of breast cancer patients attend compared with prostate cancer patients.[31,47] It has also been postulated that low educational attainment and financial resources contribute to a lack of participation in cancer support groups.[49] However, a study of 120 urology patients failed to identify gender, educational level, and income as independent predictors of attendance at a urology support group.[11] It is important to ascertain why some people do not attend support groups. If possible, these issues should be addressed to allow equal access for all patients.

Internet websites

Internet websites began to proliferate exponentially in the mid 1990s. Currently, there are hundreds of thousands of websites containing information about virtually all urological ailments and diseases.[13,54–57] Medical websites are designed and operated by laypeople, patient groups, pharmaceutical companies, and medical institutions. Websites usually provide unrestricted access to the public and few regulations govern their content. As with support groups, much of the available literature on urology internet use pertains to prostate cancer.

As internet access has increased, many patients rely on websites for self-help. Surveys predict that over 50% of all patients and 27 to 35% of oncology patients use the internet for medical information.[58–60] Thirty-five to 43% of prostate cancer patients use the internet and a large percentage of those access websites for disease information.[10,61,62] Multivariate analyses have identified young age, high educational attainment, affluence, computer ownership, and computer literacy as positive predictors of internet self-help use.[10,11,61]

Computer access and literacy have been identified as limitations of internet self-help.[11,61,63] Indeed, a high percentage of young, affluent, and educated patients own home computers and use the internet for medical information. However, computer use is much lower in older patients, especially those from underprivileged socioeconomic areas. In some prostate cancer populations computer access has been estimated to be as low as 7 to 10%.[11,61] Presumably, as computers and the internet become more affordable, increased numbers of patients will use online resources.

As with all forms of self-help, the effectiveness of websites is improved by recognizing the needs of patients and developing resources to meet those needs. Prior to designing a self-help prostate cancer website, an Australian group surveyed their patients and identified services likely to be beneficial.[64] Fifty-nine per cent requested information on diagnosis and treatment, 49% requested a question post, 44% requested relevant news updates, and 22% requested a listing of available support groups. In follow-up, it was found the most accessed areas of the website were consistent with the patients' previously reported interests. In general, urology patients claim internet information is useful and some feel it influences their treatment decisions.[10,11]

Since the internet is not regulated, physicians and patients express concern about the accuracy of website content.[10,13,14,65–67] Several evaluation tools have been developed to assess the reliability of online medical information.[55,68–70] Many websites are of high quality,[66] but others are biased or inaccurate. A study of breast cancer websites concluded that only one of 20 was considered acceptable for accuracy of information.[71] Not surprisingly, patients are unable to differentiate between accurate and inaccurate information as the popularity of websites does not correlate with quality of content.[72–74]

The internet is an attractive medium for self-help since it is cost-effective, interactive, easy to update, accessible, and anonymous.[75] However, there is a considerable risk of receiving false information and it is important that patients are made aware of this risk. Few websites contain information references and, in fact, 40% of websites from academic institutions do not reference their content.[13] Some studies evaluating internet self-help have recommended quality websites;[55,56] however, for most diseases it is the responsibility of the individual health-care provider to screen self-help web pages and recommend those that are consistent with current standards of care. The endorsement of specific websites by urological associations would help discern what information should be trusted.[10]

Computer programs

Stand-alone and internet-integrated computer programs are currently being developed for patients with prostate cancer.[76–78] The programs are designed to provide individualized information based on the patient's disease characteristics. This has an advantage over internet resources since physicians can control the accuracy of information and only provide what is pertinent to the patient.[78] The drawback, when compared with internet sites, is the cost associated with developing and manufacturing CD-ROMs. Pilot studies report patients feel the computer programs are easy to use and helpful.[76,78] As access to computers and computer literacy continue to climb, this may be an effective means of providing information to patients.

Evaluating self-help

The ultimate goal of self-help research is to determine if utilization of these resources has an impact on patient outcome. Although some studies suggest that use of self-help resources improves quantitative outcome, such as survival,[41,42] this has not yet been proven. It is more likely that self-help enhances patient knowledge and aids in coping with illness, ideally resulting in improved patient satisfaction. However, to answer these questions we must control for confounding variables and reliably measure subjective outcomes, such as satisfaction. These challenges are difficult, if not impossible. Therefore, many of the data regarding self-help are cross-sectional or retrospective and lack the robustness to stand up to the statistical rigour expected of modern-day research. For the most part, snippets of information and a multitude of anecdotal reports are relied upon to guide self-help decision-making.

Identifying patients who will use self-help

The need for information and support varies between all patients.[11] In general, however, patients with chronic, poorly understood, or embarrassing illnesses tend to seek self-help. In addition, patients with disease or treatments that pose significant risk for morbidity or mortality tend to require support and information. In urology, self-help users most commonly have cancer, interstitial cystitis, erectile dysfunction, incontinence, or a urinary diversion.

Studies have attempted to identify patient characteristics which would allow us to predict those patients most and least likely to use self-help.[11,47,49,79–82] Not surprisingly, patients with higher education and income tend to use self-help more frequently than others. However, no study of urology patients has resulted in an absolute correlation between demographic characteristics and any component of self-help behaviour. We therefore should be cognizant of our inability to differentiate those who will and will not use self-help. As sociodemographic data are unreliable in identifying or predicting self-help use, it is impractical for clinicians to selectively refer self-help based on these characteristics.

Involvement of the family

Coping with disease is a shared experience between patients and their families.[83,84] In Chapter 6 the effect on the family and the importance of involving them in patient care is discussed. The patient's spouse is often the primary provider of emotional support, and in many cases is an active participant in provision of medical care.[85,86] Spouses want to participate in treatment decisions and patients value their partner's input.[86,87] When physicians involve family members, patients have displayed decreased anxiety and improved satisfaction.[88,89] The concept of partner contentment influencing patient well-being was highlighted in a study of post-prostatectomy cancer patients.[90] In that study, partner sexual satisfaction was more important than other sexual variables and urinary continence in predicting a patient's quality of life.

The burden on a patient's family is significant and often they need to be informed and supported.[91–93] Family members are relied upon to access information, and in some cases the spouse uses self-help more than the patient.[86,94] Directing family members to self-help resources is an important component of patient education. Although it has not been adequately studied, education may better equip one to care for a family member with disease. Moreover, self-help may be a valuable instrument to support those coping with the illness of a loved one.

Development of self-help

Self-help initiatives can be coordinated by anyone with a vested interest in patient care; however, the quality and effectiveness of the resource is dependent on contributions from several groups. Patients and their families should be surveyed to determine what information and support they require, nurses and psychologists should advise in areas of coping and emotional support, and urologists should be consulted to ensure the accuracy and relevance of the content. The involvement of urology professional associations is also beneficial since approval of worthy resources is a simple way of communicating to patients which materials are reliable.

Self-help projects may be funded by hospital institutions, professional associations, patient associations, or unrestricted grants from pharmaceutical companies. For common diseases, such as prostate cancer, private sector funding is readily available. In contrast, it can be difficult to attain sponsorship for illnesses with a low public profile, such as interstitial cystitis. Non-designated institutional funds should be reserved for projects designed to help patients with less-recognized disease.

For some illnesses, groups have developed similar types of self-help with comparable content. Redundant self-help projects are not an acceptable use of funds. Prior to producing self-help material, efforts should be made to ensure there are not pre-existing resources available from an alternative institution. Existing materials can often be used or modified to befit the intended patient population. Furthermore, it is important to identify which patient groups are in need of self-help since demand is not necessarily proportional to availability.[11]

Once need is identified, patients should be surveyed to determine the specific information and support they require and the form of self-help they prefer. The self-help resource should be designed to optimize the likelihood of meeting patient needs. A brochure should be the first mode of self-help established since it is most widely used and can direct patients to alternative forms of self-help. If an adequate brochure exists, other self-help media should be considered. Prior to embarking on a self-help project, funding that will support development, production, distribution, and modification must be secured.

All facets of health care are under fiscal restraint, and efforts should be taken to reduce unnecessary spending. Insufficient planning, failure to recognize available self-help material, poor utilization of professional expertise, inadequate solicitation of patient opinion, and improper allocation of funding all contribute to unsuccessful self-help projects. Figure 3.1 provides a stepwise approach to self-help development that incorporates the aforementioned recommendations.

Patient awareness and attitude of the physician

Friends, other patients, the media, and health-care workers appraise patients of self-help. Numerous family physicians and some urologists tend not to refer urology patients to self-help.[8,11,13] Physicians are often unaware of the existence of resources;[46,95,96] however, some physicians purposely do not recommend self-help because they feel that their patients do not require additional information or because they believe use of self-help use is harmful.[8,13,14,37,65,66,69,95–97] In general, doctors claim self-help is beneficial,[8,98] but many fear their patients will be misinformed or will encounter disgruntled patients, resulting in increased anxiety. Support groups and internet sources are believed to put the patient at highest risk since they are not routinely subject to the scrutiny of peer review or professional supervision. Patients commonly present with erroneous information, and physicians are concerned that other types of self-help will simply increase the risk of further confusing and upsetting their patients. A minority of urology patients access the self-help that is available, and the low levels of awareness reported by patients is concerning, especially as many would like to use such resources (Table 3.1). Physicians are responsible, at least in part, for lack of use and awareness.

The role of physicians in directing patients to self-help

As previously stated, urologists should be active participants in the development and distribution of self-help. However, non-urologists often independently or

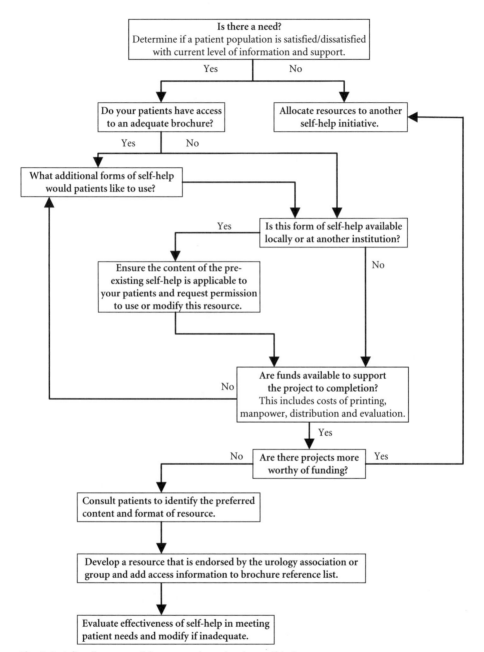

Fig. 3.1 A fiscally responsible approach to develop self-help resources.

Table 3.1 The proportion of patients who used, were aware of, or would definitely try self-help (modified from Breau et al.[11]).

Group/resource	n/N users (%)	Aware of resource (%)	Would try resource (%)
Prostate cancer			
Support group	6/22[†] (27)	63	34
Newsletter	5/30 (17)	20	60
Video	8/30 (27)	33	74
Book	7/30 (23)	33	60
Brochure	27/30 (90)	90	90
Internet	3/30 (10)	67	10
Interstitial cystitis			
Support group	6/21[†] (29)	53	89
Newsletter	3/30 (10)	20	90
Video	6/30 (20)	27	87
Book	9/30 (30)	37	97
Brochure	24/30 (80)	83	100
Internet	12/30 (40)	57	67
Erectile dysfunction			
Support group[‡]	—	—	37
Newsletter	1/30 (3)	7	66
Video	3/30 (10)	13	73
Book	1/30 (3)	7	53
Brochure	17/30 (58)	67	88
Internet	3/30 (10)	30	47
Urinary diversion			
Support group	3/23[†] (13)	37	40
Newsletter	3/30 (10)	20	73
Video	3/30 (10)	17	60
Book	1/30 (3)	3	66
Brochure	24/30 (80)	80	97
Internet	2/30 (7)	20	30

† Number who live within 1 hour of a support group location.

‡ Erectile dysfunction support groups were not available.

concurrently care for patients with urological disease and many patients seek the opinion and advice of physicians with whom they have long-standing, trusting relationships. Consistency of information is an important strategy to prevent patient confusion. The utilization of endorsed resources is a practical way to maintain consistency between physicians. To further improve self-help continuity, referral and consultation letters should include what types of self-help have been provided to the patient.

Integrating self-help in clinical practice

Many physicians are overworked and feel that they are unable to dedicate the time necessary to incorporate self-help advice into office visits. However, if physicians are aware of resources and have materials available, self-help will improve the effectiveness of clinic visits and reduce the amount of time required to communicate information.[99–101] After clinic visits, patients often express anxiety because they cannot recall or are confused by information they received. Supplying patients with basic literature and directing them to alternative sources of information is likely to reduce this anxiety and improve compliance with a treatment plan. Self-help material also provides answers to basic questions otherwise asked during follow-up appointments. The following recommendations should be adhered to when integrating self-help in clinical practice.

Self-help awareness

Health-care professionals who treat urological disease should be familiar with available resources. Philosophical variations in diagnosis and treatment will occur between geographical locations and patient populations. If possible, patients should be directed to resources that are endorsed by the applicable urological association. If these are not available, the local consultant urology group should provide specific self-help recommendations that coincide with current practice.

Provide self-help to all patients

Some patients do not want to know anything about their disease, others have an incessant need for information, but most fall somewhere between these extremes.[3,11,94,102,103] The majority of urology patients will read brochures, therefore they are the logical conduit for introducing self-help.[11] As previously described, an essential component of a brochure is a section referencing other forms of recommended self-help. These should be categorized by the medium used (internet sites, books, CD-ROMs, videos, support groups, etc.) and should include specific access instructions (web address, specific bookstores or libraries that carry the book titles, support group location and contact phone number, etc.). To avoid overwhelming patients, the list should not exceed three references for each type of medium. Short descriptions of each resource are helpful but not necessary.

Introduce self-help at initial consultation

The efficacy of self-help may depend on when the patient accesses it. It has been shown that prostate cancer patients who use self-help feel more involved in the treatment decision-making process.[10,28,40] It has also been suggested that patients involved in the decision-making process are more satisfied with outcomes, regardless of efficacy of treatment.[88–90] Providing self-help prior to treatment may indeed improve patient satisfaction, even though it may not improve objective results.

Ensure self-help is applicable to the patient

When self-help is introduced following treatment or establishment of a treatment plan, patients should be directed to specific resources that pertain to their clinical scenario. For example, providing a potential radical prostatectomy patient with information on prostate cancer screening is usually not helpful since the concerns of the patient relate to issues such as disease progression or treatment side-effects.

Self-help follow-up

During each follow-up appointment, the patient should be asked if they have sought information from sources other than their health-care providers. This is an opportunity to ensure that the patient is accessing reliable information or to remind patients of self-help that is available. Table 3.2 gives a list of mistakes commonly committed by physicians that lead to negative self-help experiences.

Clinical case discussion and conclusion

Use of self-help may be advantageous to the physician and patient. However, it is also important to recognize the potential harm caused by misinformation. We know that patients currently access medical information from external sources, and this

Table 3.2 Common errors in physician self-help behaviour

Displaying numerous brochures in the office waiting room
Not discussing self-help
Not including family in self-help discussion
Not offering self-help at the initial consultation
Not directing patients to specific resources
Not ensuring that the resources are accurate and pertinent
Not warning patients of the prevalence of inaccurate information
Relying too heavily on self-help to educate patients
Not asking if patients are using self-help resources
Assuming patients do not need information or emotional support

behaviour will probably increase in the future. Patients seek and demand information. Clinicians must decide if they wish to play an active or passive role in this aspect of care. Incorporating self-help into medical practice is not difficult, and if systematically approached it will improve patient knowledge and hopefully satisfaction.

The introductory clinical case described a patient who received reasonably successful treatment for prostate cancer. Despite the success of surgery, he and his wife sought information without guidance from a physician. They mistakenly associated prevention, screening, and non-applicable treatment options with his clinical situation. The couple also retrospectively considered primary treatments that would not have been reasonable options given his disease. It is plausible that this scenario could have been prevented if the patient and his wife were directed to self-help prior to treatment and if self-help follow-up had been regularly addressed.

It is imperative to be consistent and non-discriminatory in provision of self-help. Physicians cannot reliably recognize when patients are in need and it is difficult to predict who will, or will not, seek information and emotional support.[104] A misguided patient often receives inaccurate or non-applicable information that arouses feelings of fear and mistrust. Usually, the physician can assuage these fears and explain the rationale behind clinical decisions. However, doing so requires time and needlessly exposes patients to great amounts of anxiety. Referring patients to reliable self-help indirectly discourages use of harmful resources.

The objectives of this chapter were to give an overview of resources available to patients and reiterate the importance of involvement of the physician in directing patients to pertinent and applicable self-help. Knowledge is not necessarily associated with improved satisfaction. It is more likely that perception of knowledge is more important. It is rare that laypeople appreciate the intricacies of medicine that have taken the physician years of study and experience to understand. Invariably, self-help discussions address issues pertaining to patient autonomy. Self-help should be used as a tool to facilitate, not a replacement for, personal communication. Information that aids and fosters a patient's sense of control by emphasizing their role in the decision-making process could develop and enhance their feelings of empowerment. However, simply providing information and expecting patients to independently choose appropriate management should never be expected since this act undermines the value of physician training and erodes the foundation that is the basis of a trusting patient—doctor relationship.

References

1 Cassileth BR, Zupkis RV, Sutton-Smith K, March V (1980). Information and participation preferences among cancer patients. *Ann. Intern. Med.* **92**: 832–6.

2 Brody H (1985). Autonomy revisited: progress in medical ethics: discussion paper. *J. R. Soc. Med.* **78**: 380–7.

3 Sutherland HJ, Llewellyn-Thomas HA, Lockwood GA, Tritchler DL, Till JE (1989). Cancer patients: their desire for information and participation in treatment decisions. *J. R. Soc. Med.* **82**: 260–3.

4 Stiles WB, Putnam SM, Wolf MH, James SA (1979). Interaction exchange structure and patient satisfaction with medical interviews. *Med. Care* **17**: 667–81.

5 Smith CK, Polis E, Hadac RR (1981). Characteristics of the initial medical interview associated with patient satisfaction and understanding. *J. Fam. Prac.* **12**: 283–8.

6 Blanchard CG, Labreque BA, Ruckdeschel JC, Blanchard EB (1990). Physician behaviours, patient perceptions and patient characteristics as predictors of satisfaction of hospitalized cancer patients. *Cancer* **65**: 186–92.

7 Gray RE, Klotz LH, Iscoe NA, Fitch MI, Franssen E, Johnson BJ *et al.* (1997). Results of a survey of Canadian men with prostate cancer. *Can. J. Urol.* **4**: 359–65.

8 Crawford ED, Bennett CL, Stone NN, Knight SJ, DeAntoni E, Sharp L *et al.* (1997). Comparison of perspectives on prostate cancer: analyses of survey data. *Urology* **50**: 366–72.

9 Agre P, Kurtz RC, Krauss BJ (1994). A randomized trial using videotape to present consent information for colonoscopy. *Gastrointest. Endosc.* **40**: 271–6.

10 Pautler SE, Tan JK, Dugas GR, Pus N, Ferri M, Hardie WR *et al.* (2001). Use of the internet for self-education by patients with prostate cancer. *Urology* **57**: 230–3.

11 Breau RH, McGrath PJ, Norman RW (2003). Assessing self-help issues for patients with prostate cancer, interstitial cystitis, erectile dysfunction and urinary diversion. *BJU Int.* **92**: 736–40.

12 Sharp JW, Aviv L (1996). Patient resources for prostate cancer. *Cancer Pract.* **4**: 216–18.

13 Hellawell GO, Turner KJ, Le Monnier KJ, Brewster SF (2000). Urology and the Internet: an evaluation of internet use by urology patients and of information available on urological topics. *BJU Int.* **86**: 191–4.

14 Gomella LG (2000). The wild, wild Web: resources for counseling patients with prostate cancer in the information age. *Semin.Urol. Oncol.* **18**: 167–71.

15 Paul CL, Redman S, Sanson-Fisher RW (1998). Print material as a public health education tool. *Aust. N. Z. J. Public Health* **22**: 146–8.

16 Mottram DR, Reed C (1997). Comparative evaluation of patient information leaflets by pharmacists, doctors and the general public. *J. Clin. Pharm. Ther.* **22**: 127–34.

17 Funnell MM, Donnelly MB, Anderson RM, Johnson PD, Oh MS (1992). Perceived effectiveness, cost, and availability of patient education methods and materials. *Diabetes Educ.* **18**: 139–45.

18 Rees CE, Ford JE, Sheard CE (2003). Patient information leaflets for prostate cancer: which leaflets should healthcare professionals recommend? Patient Educ. Couns. 49: 263–72.

19 Rees CE, Ford JE, Sheard CE (2002). Evaluating the reliability of DISCERN: a tool for assessing the quality of written patient information on treatment choices. *Patient. Educ. Couns.* **47**: 273–5.

20 Feldman-Stewart D, Brundage MD, Van Manen L, Skarsgard D, Siemens R (2003). Evaluation of a question-and-answer booklet on early-stage prostate cancer. *Patient Educ. Couns.* **49**: 115–24.

21 Klein JF, Berry CC, Felice ME (1990). The development of a testicular self-examination instructional booklet for adolescents. *J. Adolescent Health Care* **11**: 235–9.

22 Wilt TJ, Paul J, Murdoch M, Nelson D, Nugent S, Rubins HB (2001). Educating men about prostate cancer screening. A randomized trial of a mailed pamphlet. *Eff. Clin. Pract.* **4**: 112–20.

23 Schapira MM, VanRuiswyk J (2000). The effect of an illustrated pamphlet decision-aid on the use of prostate cancer screening tests. *J. Fam. Pract.* **49**: 418–24.

24 Mahon SM (1995). Using brochures to educate the public about the early detection of prostate and colorectal cancer. *Oncol. Nurs. Forum* **22**: 1413–20.

25 Finney JW, Weist MD, Friman PC (1995). Evaluation of two health education strategies for testicular self-examination. *J. Appl. Behav. Anal.* **28**: 39–46.

26 Crawford SM, Littlejohn GM, Kamill PG (1991). Testicular self examination: evaluation of an educational leaflet. *Br. J. Gen. Pract.* **41**: 168–9.

27 Frieske DA, Park DC (1999). Memory for news in young and old adults. *Psychol. Aging* **14**: 90–8.

28 McGregor S (2003). Information on video format can help patients with localised prostate cancer to be partners in decision making. *Patient Educ. Couns.* **49**: 279–83.

29 Schapira MM, Meade C, Nattinger AB (1997). Enhanced decision-making: the use of a videotape decision-aid for patients with prostate cancer. *Patient Educ. Couns.* **30**: 119–27.

30 Carlsson ME, Strang PM, Lindblad L (1996). Telephone help line for cancer counseling and cancer information. *Cancer Pract.* **4**: 319–23.

31 Davison KP, Pennebaker JW, Dickerson SS (2000). Who talks? The social psychology of illness support groups. *Am. Psychol.* **55**: 205–17.

32 Cella DF, Yellen SB (1993). Cancer support groups: the state of the art. *Cancer Pract.* **1**: 56–61.

33 Clark A, Jones P, Newbold S *et al.* (2000). Practice development in cancer care: self-help for men with testicular cancer. *Nurs. Stand.* **14**: 41–6.

34 Meredith C (1985). ROMP: a self-help group for impotent men. *AUAA J.* **6**: 7–8.

35 Gray RE, Fitch M, Davis C, Phillips C (1997). Interviews with men with prostate cancer about their self-help group experience. *J. Palliative Care* **13**: 15–21.

36 Anderson PJ, Dowell CJ, Fairbrother G, Louey MA (1998). Prostate disease patients: planning services to meet their coping needs. *Urol. Nurs.* **18**: 195–7.

37 Coreil J, Behal R (1999). Man to Man prostate cancer support groups. *Cancer Pract.* **7**: 122–9.

38 Kaps EC (1994). The role of the support group, 'Us Too'. *Cancer* **74**: 2188–9.

39 Chin ALS, Fernsler JI (1998). Self-transcendence in older men attending a prostate cancer support group. *Cancer Nurs.* **21**: 358–63.

40 Gregoire I, Kalogeropoulos D, Corcos J (1997). The effectiveness of a professionally led support group for men with prostate cancer. *Urol. Nurs.* **17**: 58–66.

41 Fawzy FI, Fawzy NW, Hyun CS, Elashoff R, Guthrie D, Fahey JL *et al.* (1993). Malignant melanoma. Effects of an early structured psychiatric intervention, coping, and affective state on recurrence and survival 6 years later. *Arch. Gen. Psychiat.* **50**: 681–9.

42 Spiegel D, Bloom JR, Kraemer HC, Gottheil E (1989). Effect of psychosocial treatment on survival of patients with metastatic breast cancer. *Lancet* **2**: 888–91.

43 Calabrese DZ (1995). Prostate cancer groups: help, information, support. *Cancer Suppl.* **7**: 1897–9.

44 Kules AR, Axelrod A (1995). Utilizing effective group models for prostate cancer patients and their families. *Cancer Suppl.* **7**: 1892–6.

45 Sharp JW (1993). Expanding the definition of quality of life for prostate cancer. *Cancer* **71**: 1078–82.

46 Smith RL, Crane LA, Byers T, Nelson-Marten P (2002). An evaluation of the Man to Man self-help group in Colorado and Utah. *Cancer Pract.* **10**: 234–9.

47 Krizek C, Roberts C, Ragan R, Ferrara JJ, Lord B (1999). Gender and cancer support group participation. *Cancer Pract.* **7**: 86–92.

48 Weber BA, Roberts BL, McDougall GJ Jr (2000). Exploring the efficacy of support groups for men with prostrate cancer. *Geriatr. Nurs.* **21**: 250–3.

49 Bauman LJ, Gervey R, Siegel K (1992). Factors associated with cancer patients' participation in support groups. *J. Psychosoc. Oncol.* **10**: 1–20.

50 Steginga SK, Occhipinti S, Dunn J, Gardiner RA, Heathcote P, Yaxley J (2000). The supportive care needs of men with prostate cancer. *Psychooncology* **10**: 66–75.

51 Katz D, Koppie TM, Wu D, Meng MV, Grossfeld GD, Sadesky N *et al.* (2002). Sociodemographic characteristics and health related quality of life in men attending prostate cancer support groups. *J. Urol.* **168**: 2092–6.

52 Parker SL, Tong T, Bolden S, Wingo PA (1997). Cancer statistics, 1997. *CA Cancer J. Clin.* **47**: 5–27.

53 von Eschenbach A, Ho R, Murphy GP, Cunningham M, Lins N (1997). American Cancer Society guideline for the early detection of prostate cancer: update 1997. *CA Cancer J. Clin.* **47**: 261–4.

54 Mayor S (2003). Arsenal helps publicise testicular cancer website. *Br. Med. J.* **326**: 1282.

55 Lipp ER (2002). Web resources for patients with prostate cancer: a starting point. *Semin. Urol. Oncol.* **20**: 32–8.

56 London JW, Gomella LG (2000). Overview of the Internet and prostate cancer resources. *Semin. Urol. Oncol.* **18**: 245–53.

57 Sjogren D (1999). Urology sites on the Internet and search tips for Internet browsers. *AORN J.* **69**: 270–1.

58 Kalichman SC, Benotsch E, Weinhardt L (2001). Quality of health information on the Internet. *J. Am. Med. Assoc.* **286**: 2092–3.

59 Vordermark D, Kolbl O, Flentje M (2000). The Internet as a source of medical information. Investigation in a mixed cohort of radiotherapy patients. *Strahlenther. Onkol.* **176**: 532–5.

60 Chen X, Siu LL (2001). Impact of the media and the internet on oncology: survey of cancer patients and oncologists in Canada. *J. Clin. Oncol.* **19**: 4291–7.

61 Smith RP, Devine P, Jones H, DeNittis A, Whittington R, Metz JM (2003). Internet use by patients with prostate cancer undergoing radiotherapy. *Urology* **62**: 273–7.

62 Steginga SK, Occhipinti S, Gardiner RA, Yaxley J, Heathcote P (2002). Making decisions about treatment for localized prostate cancer. *BJU Int.* **89:** 255–60.

63 Duffy CC, McLernon NF, D'Orsogna LJ, Reagan S, Spry N, Joseph D *et al.* (2000). Internet use by radiation oncology patients: a pilot study. *Med. J. Aust.* **172:** 350–1.

64 Pinnock CB, Jones C (2003). Meeting the information needs of Australian men with prostate cancer by way of the internet. *Urology* **61:** 1198–203.

65 Larkin M (1999). Internet accelerates spread of bogus cancer cure. *Lancet* **353:** 331.

66 Biermann JS, Golladay GJ, Greenfield ML, Baker LH (1999). Evaluation of cancer information on the Internet. *Cancer* **86:** 381–90.

67 Markman M (2001). Cancer and the Internet: the good, the bad, and the very ugly. *Curr. Oncol. Rep.* **3:** 77–8.

68 Wilson P (2002). How to find the good and avoid the bad or ugly: a short guide to tools for rating quality of health information on the internet. *Br. Med. J.* **324:** 598–602.

69 Sacchetti P, Zvara P, Plante MK (1999). The Internet and patient education—resources and their reliability: focus on a select urologic topic. *Urology* **53:** 1117–20.

70 Gagliardi A, Jadad AR (2002). Examination of instruments used to rate quality of health information on the internet: chronicle of a voyage with an unclear destination. *Br. Med. J.* **324:** 569–73.

71 Berland GK, Elliott MN, Morales LS, Algazy JI, Kravitz RL, Broder MS *et al.* (2001). Health information on the Internet: accessibility, quality, and readability in English and Spanish. *J. Am. Med. Assoc.* **285:** 2612–21.

72 Markman M (1998). Cancer information and the Internet: benefits and risks. *Clev. Clin. J. Med.* **65:** 274–6.

73 Henson DE (1999). Cancer and the Internet. *Cancer* **86:** 373–4.

74 Meric F, Bernstam EV, Mirza NQ, Hunt KK, Ames FC, Ross MI *et al.* (2002). Breast cancer on the world wide web: cross sectional survey of quality of information and popularity of websites. *Br. Med. J.* **324:** 577–81.

75 Moul JW, Esther TA, Bauer JJ (2000). Implementation of a web-based prostate cancer decision site. *Semin. Urol. Oncol.* **18**: 241–4.

76 Jenkinson J, Wilson-Pauwels L, Jewett MA, Woolridge N (1998). Development of a hypermedia program designed to assist patients with localized prostate cancer in making treatment decisions. *J. Biocommun.* **25**: 2–11.

77 DePalma A (2000). Prostate Cancer Shared Decision: a CD-ROM educational and decision-assisting tool for men with prostate cancer. *Semin. Urol. Oncol.* **18**: 178–81.

78 Reis J, McGinty B, Jones S (2003). An e-learning caregiving program for prostate cancer patients and family members. *J. Med. Syst.* **27**: 1–12.

79 Volkers N (1999). In coping with cancer, gender matters. *J. Natl. Cancer Inst.* **91**: 1712–14.

80 Klemm P, Hurst M, Dearholt SL, Trone SR (1999). Gender differences on Internet cancer support groups. *Comp. Nurs.* **17**: 65–72.

81 Klemm P, Reppert K, Visich L (1998). A nontraditional cancer support group. The Internet. *Comp. Nurs.* **16**: 31–6.

82 Bui LL, Last L, Bradley H, Law CH, Maier BA, Smith AJ (2002). Interest and participation in support group programs among patients with colorectal cancer. *Cancer Nurs.* **25**: 150–7.

83 Butler L, Downe-Wamboldt B, Marsh S, Bell D, Jarvi K (2000). Behind the scenes: partners' perceptions of quality of life post radical prostatectomy. *Urol. Nurs.* **20**: 254–8.

84 Lewis FM (1990). Strengthening family supports. Cancer and the family. *Cancer* **65**: 752–9.

85 Breau RH, Norman RW (2003). The role of self-help groups in educating and supporting patients with prostate cancer and interstitial cystitis. *BJU Int.* **92**: 602–6.

86 Srirangam SJ, Pearson E, Grose C, Brown SCW, Collins GN, O'Reilly PH (2003). Partner's influence on patient preference for treatment in early prostate cancer. *BJU Int.* **92**: 365–9.

87 Davison BJ, Gleave ME, Goldenberg SL, Degner LF, Hoffart D, and Berkowitz J (2002). Assessing information and decision preferences of men with prostate cancer and their partners. *Cancer Nurs.* **25**: 42–9.

88 Phillips C, Gray RE, Fitch MI, Labrecque M, Fergus K, Klotz L (2000). Early postsurgery experience of prostate cancer patients and spouses. *Cancer Prac.* **8**: 165–71.

89 Dorey G (2001). Partners' perspective of erectile dysfunction: literature review. *Br. J. Nurs.* **10**: 187–95.

90 Perez MA, Skinner EC, Meyerowitz BE (2002). Sexuality and intimacy following radical prostatectomy: patient and partner perspectives. *Health Psychol.* **21**: 288–93.

91 Fergus KD, Gray RE, Fitch MI, Labrecque M, Phillips C (2002). Active consideration: conceptualizing patient-provided support for spouse caregivers in the context of prostate cancer. *Qual. Health Res.* **12**: 492–514.

92 Rees CE, Sheard CE, Echlin K (2003). The relationship between the information-seeking behaviours and information needs of partners of men with prostate cancer: a pilot study. *Patient Educ. Couns.* **49**: 257–61.

93 Rees CE, Bath PA (2000). Exploring the information flow: partners of women with breast cancer, patients, and healthcare professionals. *Oncol. Nurs. Forum* **27**: 1267–75.

94 Yakren S, Shi W, Thaler H *et al.* (2001). Use of the Internet and other information resources among adult cancer patients and their companions. *Proc. Am. Soc. Clin. Oncol.* **20**: 398a (abstract 1589).

95 Matthews BA, Baker F, Spillers RL (2002). Healthcare professionals' awareness of cancer support services. *Cancer Pract.* **10**: 36–44.

96 Gray RE, Carroll JC, Fitch M, Greenberg M, Chart P, Orr V (1999). Cancer self-help groups and family physicians. *Cancer Pract.* **7**: 10–15.

97 Fridinger F, Goodwin G, Chng CL (1992). Physician and consumer attitudes and behaviors regarding self-help health support groups as an adjunct to traditional medical care. *J. Health Soc. Policy* **3**: 19–36.

98 Carroll JC, Gray RE, Orr VJ, Chart P, Fitch M, Greenberg M (2000). Changing physicians' attitudes toward self-help groups: an educational intervention. *J. Cancer Educ.* **15**: 14–18.

99 Sandler DA, Mitchell JR, Fellows A, Garner ST (1989). Is an information booklet for patients leaving hospital helpful and useful? *Br. Med. J.* **298**: 870–4.

100 Webber D, Higgins L, Baker V (2001). Enhancing recall of information from a patient education booklet: a trial using cardiomyopathy patients. *Patient Educ. Couns.* **44**: 263–70.

101 McPherson CJ, Higginson IJ, Hearn J (2001). Effective methods of giving information in cancer: a systematic literature review of randomized controlled trials. *J. Pub. Health Med.* **23**: 227–34.

102 Davison BJ, Degner LF, Morgan TR (1995). Information and decision-making preferences of men with prostate cancer. *Oncol. Nurs. Forum* **22**: 1401–8.

103 Boberg EW, Gustafson DH, Hawkins RP, Offord KP, Koch C, Wen KY *et al.* (2003). Assessing the unmet information, support and care delivery needs of men with prostate cancer. *Patient Educ. Couns.* **49**: 233–42.

104 Sollner W, DeVries A, Steixner E, Lukas P, Sprinzl G, Rumpold G *et al.* (2001). How successful are oncologists in identifying patient distress, perceived social support, and need for psychosocial counselling? *Br J Cancer* **84**, 179–85.

Chapter 4

Role of the interdisciplinary team in urological supportive care

Reena Karani and Diane E. Meier

Introduction

Many urological diseases are complex and affect multiple dimensions of a patient's life. Therefore, no single discipline can be expected to meet the diverse medical and psychosocial needs of the patient and his or her family. Application of a comprehensive and integrated care plan that focuses on the whole patient and not just the disease state may improve satisfaction and outcomes. Such plans are best accomplished by communication and collaboration across the different health-care disciplines providing patient care. One important way to accomplish shared planning, decision-making, accountability, and responsibility for a patient and improve health-care delivery is through the use of team-based care.

Definition of teams

Over the years, many definitions of teams and teamwork have been offered. One simple definition offered by Beckhard is that a team 'is a group with specific tasks, the accomplishment of which requires the interdependent and collaborative efforts of its members'.[1] More broadly, however, a team may be described as a group of people with particular expertise and complementary skills that meet, share knowledge, create specific plans, and carry them out.

Background and outcomes of teams

Early interest in health-care teams began in the 1940s and early 1950s when the physicians Cherkasky and Silver advocated a team approach to delivering primary care services using a physician, a nurse, and a social worker. The team worked in caring for patients and families and emphasized the provision of health services and prevention.[2] In contrast to traditional physician-lead patient care plans, this model emphasized collaboration among all members of the team in determining goals and implementing plans to achieve them. The actual process of teamwork utilized by this model was, therefore, different from previous, more hierarchical models that involved physicians directing or delegating work to other health-care providers.

Subsequently, because of the escalating complexity and scope of patient problems as well as the emphasis on efficient and appropriate use of limited resources, health-care teams have become increasingly common. Some of the greatest strides in team care have occurred in the field of geriatric medicine.[3–5] Here, the intricacies and multiplicity of medical, social, and psychiatric problems faced by older adults have provided an ideal template for team-based model programmes of care. Beginning in the 1970s, the Department of Veterans Affairs and the Bureau of Health Professions in the United States of America funded several programmatic grants to promote interdisciplinary care and education in the field of geriatrics. Since then, many of these programmes have continued their commitment to teamwork and serve as training sites for new programmes wishing to develop and institutionalize such models of care. In addition to being widely used in geriatrics, teams have been developed in paediatrics, rheumatology,[6] palliative and hospice care, primary care health clinics, prostate assessment clinics,[7] and in-patient psychiatric units, among others.[8]

A driving force behind this increase in team-based care across settings and disciplines is the documented impact of the model on patient outcomes and system resources shown by various studies. A study of 1102 patient admissions to the medical wards of an acute-care teaching hospital in Cleveland, Ohio randomized 567 patients to receive interdisciplinary rounds (intervention group) and 535 to receive traditional rounds (control group).[9] The team included physicians, a nurse patient-care coordinator, a pharmacist, a nutritionist, and a social worker, and visited intervention patients daily. Results from this study showed that while no differences were observed in the rates of hospital death or discharge location, the intervention group had shorter mean lengths of hospital stay (5.46 versus 6.06 days, $p = 0.006$) and lower mean total charges (US\$6681 versus \$8090, $p = 0.002$). Further, a trial of 421 community dwelling stroke patients randomized to receive rehabilitation from a multidisciplinary stroke team versus routine care showed that the intervention group was significantly more satisfied with the emotional support they received and that their caregivers were more satisfied overall.[10] Similar beneficial effects of teams have been demonstrated with conditions such as diabetes, pain, chronic fatigue syndrome, and mental illness.[11–14]

Yet the mere formation of a health-care team does not guarantee that it will function well or improve clinical outcomes.[15] Effective team care involves some basic understanding of teamwork processes, a commitment to communication, and an interest in providing comprehensive care to patients. In the context of the urology patient, this chapter will review different types of teams, discuss the role of the team and its individual members, explore the phases of team development, review the principles of effective teamwork, and, finally, examine the variables that affect the quality and outcomes of teamwork.

Types of teams

Health-care teams may be classified into three types according to the disciplines represented and the degree of shared responsibility and leadership among team members.

Table 4.1 Different types of health-care team

	Description	Advantages	Disadvantages
A.1: Unidisciplinary team (e.g. paediatric urologists)	One discipline, agency, or department is represented. Individual identity is more important that integrated team identity. Leadership by rank or election	Team members 'speak the same language'. Security of one discipline. Final decision by one leader. Solutions have depth	Solutions lack breadth. No shared leadership
A.2: Interactive unidisciplinary team (e.g. urologists with different specialities such as paediatric, trauma, endo, or female urology)	One discipline, but different specialities, are represented. Issue- or expertise-based leadership	Team members 'speak the same language'. Solutions have depth	No shared leadership
B: Multidisciplinary team (e.g. urologist, social worker, nurse, stomal therapist etc.)	Multiple disciplines are represented. Members report to the group. Individual identity is more important that integrated team identity. Discipline specific care. Leadership by rank or election	Information from many perspectives. Independent decisions made simultaneously. Solutions have breadth	Team members 'speak different languages'. Solutions are not integrated. Solutions lack depth
C: Interdisciplinary teams (e.g. urologist, social worker, nurse, stomal therapist etc.)	Multiple disciplines are represented. Team develops goals for the patient and family. Members work interdependently. Leadership by issue and expertise	Integrated care plan is developed. Leadership is shared. Solutions have breath and depth	Discussions take time. Members must learn languages of multiple disciplines

Examples of unidisciplinary (UDTs), multidisciplinary (MDTs), and interdisciplinary (IDTs) teams may be found in various health-care settings (Table 4.1).

Unidisciplinary teams (UDTs)

Such teams generally comprise different personnel from the same discipline (e.g. paediatric urologists), although they may be further divided into interactive unidisciplinary groups. These interactive UDTs include people from one discipline who represent different speciality areas. An example is a group that includes urologists of varying specialities such as paediatric, endo, female and trauma urology.

Multidisciplinary teams (MDTs)

Multidisciplinary teams consist of people from different disciplines who develop treatment plans independently.[15] Generally in MDTs the highest-ranking team member (usually the physician) orders services and coordinates the care plan and there is little sharing of specific discipline goals among the members of different fields. In essence, the team members work in parallel with each other with the medical record often serving as the vehicle to share information.[16] Finally, the patient and family are often not considered a unit of service in this model, thus perpetuating an isolated disease-centered approach to care.[15]

Interdisciplinary teams (IDTs)

These teams comprise a group of people from different disciplines who assess and plan care in an interactive, interdependent, and collaborative manner.[15] The group establishes common goals and makes treatment plans in a coordinated, joint manner, but individual members maintain distinct professional responsibilities and have individual assignments.[17] Here, therefore, members share collective ownership of the care plan, and leadership varies depending on the issue at hand and on the expertise of various team members (also known as shifting leadership).[5] Since the patient and family are considered a unit, the treatment plan addresses the medical and psychosocial impact of the illness on the patient, his or her family, and their quality of life.

Since the IDT represents the most collaborative, coordinated, and complementary model of team care available, our further discussions will focus on this type of team.

Urology IDT members and their roles

The complexity of certain subgroups of urology patients, such as those with urological malignancies, neurological diseases affecting the genitourinary tract, or post kidney transplantation, necessitates the involvement of multiple disciplines in the IDT. A useful guiding principle in determining who participates in the IDT is to allow the problem to define the composition of the team and not vice versa.[15] Beginning with the urologist and adding when necessary primary care physicians, palliative care (symptom management and care coordination) experts, other physician specialists (radiation oncologists, infectious disease physicians, and pain management experts), nurses, dieticians, pharmacists, psychological support personnel, social workers and clergy, and physio, occupational, stomal, and sex therapists, such a team involves necessary personnel with varying areas of expertise to ensure comprehensive care of the patient. It is important to recognize that while some members comprise the core working-group of the team in all its efforts, others may be invited to participate on a case-specific basis.

Physicians

The role of physicians in the IDT includes sharing information and expertise about health, disease, potential complications, and prognosis as it relates to the patient being discussed. By communicating all the relevant medical history and health status information in a manner that is understandable to different disciplines, the physician creates the foundation of the care plan. Physicians of different specialities will then play varying roles during the interdisciplinary meetings.

Urologist

Since the primary problem requiring attention in these patients is urological, the role of the urologist on the IDT team is critical. In each discussion, he or she may present recent patient data along with recommended therapeutic choices. Because all medical aspects of the case must be fully understood by team members before a common care plan is developed, a urologist's skill in effective communication and achievement of consensus in consultation with the patient on the best mode of treatment becomes extremely important. In addition, this physician will often take the leadership role in treatment planning and symptom control for the patient.

Primary care provider (PCP)

The patient's PCP may have known the patient and his or her family for a period of time preceding the acute urological illness. Thus this provider's role on the IDT is to examine patient data and consider the benefits and burdens of therapeutic options in the light of other concurrent medical conditions, given their knowledge of the patient and his or her situation. In many instances, PCPs play a crucial role in clarifying the comprehensive goals of care for patients whom they have known over time and in continuing to provide a pivotal coordination role for health care.

Palliative care specialist

The palliative care specialist focuses on the amelioration of physical and psychological symptoms including alleviation of pain. In addition, she or he has expertise in the areas of advance care planning, comprehensive goals of care, and patient–family communication, and coordination of the care of complex patients with multiple co-morbidities across a wide range of care settings (such as home care, nursing home, hospital, and hospice). On the urology IDT, such specialists share information about the patient's symptom burden, details from family meetings, and critical recommendations for pain and symptom management. In addition, for patients desiring a solely palliative approach to a urological condition, these experts can take a leadership role in treatment and care planning that is concordant with the patient's directives.

Other physician specialists

Other physician specialists (radiation and medical oncologists and pain management experts) are valuable on a case-by-case basis in the supportive care of the urology patient. Radiation oncologists on an IDT can provide expertise on the use of radiation therapy as a palliative approach to advanced urological tumours and medical oncologists can recommend appropriate chemotherapy. Along with pain management and palliative care specialists, these physicians can develop a multicomponent treatment strategy to address a patient's pain and to coordinate decision-making.

Nurses

Among health-care providers, nurses have the most frequent and continuous bedside contact with patients whether in the hospital or the community. Therefore, their evaluation of a patient's status provides additional critical data for the IDT. Furthermore, since nurses act as advocates for patients, they often take a leadership role in patient education and support as well as in communication of IDT team plans to the patient and their family.

Dietitians

Dietitians play an important role in patient education following certain urological procedures. Dietitians can provide counselling regarding fibre, calcium, oxalate, protein, and salt intake to reduce the risk of recurrence in post-nephrolithiasis patients who have had calcium oxalate or uric acid stones. Patients with cachexia will require nutritional supplements and those with renal impairment will need dietary restrictions. In addition, these members of the IDT can evaluate a patient's nutritional status and determine more comprehensive dietary goals and regimens bearing the patient's urological condition and concurrent medical problems in mind.

Pharmacists

Urology patients are no different from other patients taking numerous medications. The role of a pharmacist on the IDT is to serve as an information resource for the patient as well as the team. By devising regimens that suit the medical and therapeutic needs of the patient, pharmacists play a leadership role in interdisciplinary care plan development. Finally, pharmacists have expertise in selecting pharmaceutical therapies that are easy to adhere to, tolerable, and safe.

Stomal therapists

A stomal therapist assesses, plans, and evaluates ostomy care in urology patients, most commonly after radical cystectomy and ileal diversion for bladder cancer. In addition to educating the patient on the care and management of a urostomy, such specialists play an important supportive role in helping patients adjust to the lifestyle changes that occur as a result of them.

Psychological support staff

Male and female sexual dysfunction, bladder incontinence, cancers, and other urological conditions have a significant psychological impact on patients. Therefore, a critical component of comprehensive urology care is the availability of psychological support services for patients as they adjust to major life transitions and stressors. Psychologists or psychiatrists can liase with members of the IDT to provide a detailed assessment of the patient and his or her family and thereafter to create a close follow-up plan.

Social workers

Social workers are trained to assess the impact of illness on patients and their families. Reaction to illness, the implications of ill health for a patient's life, and values and beliefs about health and medical care are only some of the areas evaluated by social workers. In addition, by communicating the strengths and difficulties faced by families as well as information about the physical and social resources available to a patient to the IDT, a comprehensive care plan can be created. Social workers frequently take a leadership role in coordinating finances and insurance benefits, obtaining out-of-hospital resources such as home health aides and durable medical equipment, and promoting insight into illness among patients and their families.

Pastoral care

While the religious, spiritual, and existential aspects of life often become more important to a person experiencing ill health, the health-care system rarely gives due attention to these needs. To address this need, the inclusion of clergy in the urology IDT is of significant importance. As staff trained to provide emotional support as well as counselling, interfaith clergy are invaluable resources to patients as well as members of the team. Issues of death and dying, goals of care, and patient strengths and needs are areas in which clergy can assume a leadership role in addressing. Finally, pastoral care workers can be one source of bereavement counselling and support to families after a patient's death.

Role of the team

Since the patient is the central focus of the IDT, the role of the team is to develop a management and follow-up plan that takes into consideration the patient's condition and symptoms, and the effect of these on the physical, psychological, and social well-being of the patient and his or her family. The priorities of treatment should be determined by the needs and wishes of the patient, and all members of the IDT should be involved in the diagnostic, therapeutic, and outcome evaluation phases of the case.

In order for the team to work together effectively, all professionals must balance their responsibilities, values, knowledge, skills, and even goals in patient care against their role as a team member in shared decision-making.[18] Achieving this balance is by no means simple, and teams often go through a series of developmental phases.

Phases of team formation

First labelled by Tuckman[19] and subsequently described by Drinka and Clark,[20] teams often move through four phases of development. The progression through these phases is not necessarily sequential, and a group often returns to a previous phase for a period of time and then moves out of it. Recognition of these phases is helpful in understanding the potential causes of team difficulties as well as in thinking about possible solutions to an issue confronting the team.

Forming

This is the creation phase of the group. Often, many members are uncertain about the purpose of the team, and therefore a few are active while many remain quiet and guarded. In this phase, conflict is not addressed in discussions. Interventions that are helpful during this period include icebreakers to share the formal and informal roles of members, as well as discussions on core membership and goals of the team. The organizational evolution of the team will change as members are added or removed to adapt to changes in the patient's problems.

Storming

Storming is characterized by conflicts over leadership and commitment and occurs during a period when team goals and member roles are being clarified. During this time of conflict, a functional leader often emerges and coalitions form among members. Some members may withdraw from the team at this point while others may feel anxious about continuing to participate. Eventually, there is a realization that everyone has the power of leadership and decision-making. Encouraging participation in developing constructive solutions to problems can help passive team members participate in discussions. In addition, informal leaders with skills to analyse problems and shape solutions may emerge and should be encouraged. By requiring respectful behaviour during all discussions, the team can ensure that professionalism is maintained.[18] Finally, by using conflicts as an opportunity for creative problem-solving, the team can encourage different members to assume leadership positions for various topics.

Norming

During this phase of team development, there is an attempt to establish common goals and overlaps become evident. Ground rules are established and strategies for sharing leadership are developed. Competition does occur among team members and some members begin to project blame and responsibility on others. Frustration about unachieved goals is expressed and conflicts are still present. Discussing goals and agreeing to them as a team is the first step in moving through the norming process of team development. By openly discussing role overlaps, the team can develop ground rules for duties and responsibilities of different members. Finally, using unachieved goals as an impetus, the group can develop strategies and solve problems for future cases. This joint effort may decrease competition among team members.

Performing

An emphasis on productivity and problem-solving characterizes this developmental stage. Self-initiated active participation becomes the norm, and because differences are appreciated members encourage and help each other. As a consequence, leadership moves between members depending on the issue. Team members have independent responsibilities and develop a commitment to the team. Conflicts are seen as part of the process of growth and used as an impetus for improvement. Reinforcing and praising informal leadership as well as scheduling time for feedback are important interventions during the performing phase of team development. Offering to provide mentorship is a way to include new members into the group.

Principles of effective teamwork

Once empowered by the institution and given the necessary resources, an IDT can begin the process leading to effective performance and team maintenance. Critical to this process are five areas that merit discussion.[21]

First is the establishment of open communication among members. This is vital, because in order to be an effective decision-making vehicle, the team must have a well-functioning intra-team and external information exchange mechanism.[22] While time, space, and opportunity for interaction are among the basic requirements for such communication, a well-designed record system, regularly scheduled meetings, and opportunities for the team to report to and communicate with institutional personnel are other important features that should be included. Finally, if each member of the team makes a concerted effort to avoid using buzzwords and discipline-specific jargon, misunderstandings that occur because of differences in approach and terminology may be reduced.

Clarification of the mission of the group and development of appropriate goals are the logical first steps in team development. While this step is both time- and energy-consuming, it is absolutely necessary in terms of future commitment and satisfaction of team members.[22] One recommended way to begin this process is to develop a broad mission statement that team members agree upon. Thereafter, clear, specific, and measurable goals and objectives along with a time line for achievement can be derived from this mission statement. This process by which team goals are defined and elaborated is an important part of team development and serves as a basis for establishing a plan of action and performance standards on a team.[22]

The next prerequisite for effective teamwork is a clear understanding by each team member of his or her role, responsibilities and function. Using the goals and objectives developed by the group, tasks and activities for each member can be negotiated. In order to de-emphasize issues of territoriality and ownership, wherever possible the differentiation of tasks (things to be done) should precede the negotiation of roles (who is to do them).[22] At the end of this process, it is important to confirm that each team member understands his or her roles as well as those of the other team members. Successful teams require energy and may have to interact with other teams.

In order for the team to function well and achieve its outcomes, team members must agree upon how decisions are made and understand how leadership is determined.

In IDTs, leadership shifts depending on the issues at hand and the skills of particular team members. By adopting a commitment to equal participation and responsibility from team members, this model becomes acceptable to team members over time. For clinical decision-making, the team member who best knows the issue and that aspect of the patient's care should have a major role in determining and carrying out the decision after consulting other members of the team.[22] This model is a departure from traditional norms that award decision-making power based on status or seniority. It has the potential weakness of not addressing the medico-legal issues of discipline-specific responsibilities that cannot be shared. There are also professional registration, licensing, and accountability issues which may override this concept.

The diversity of experiences and disciplines present in an IDT virtually ensure that conflict will arise. Data from the nursing and social work literature offer some well-documented sources of team conflict.[23] Differing personal and professional perspectives, role competition, variations in professional socialization processes, physician dominance of teams and decision-making,[24] role stereotyping or uncertainty, and differing interpretations of professional jargon[8] are common themes of conflict cited by team members. By accepting the inevitability of conflict, teams can focus on ways to confront and resolve differences. If the team is founded on the principles of open communication and mutual respect, conflicts can be seen as opportunities for creative problem-solving and innovation. Establishment of team rules and boundaries are critical. The presence of team members with conflict resolution and negotiation skills can make differences an opportunity for team success and satisfaction.[22]

Variables that influence successful teamwork

Three variables affect team development and performance: individual or personal, intra-team, and organizational.

Individual or personal variables

This refers to what an individual brings to a team and often such barriers become apparent when goals and roles have not been clarified before the team is formed.[15] Physicians may have a difficult time adjusting to the shared leadership approach of IDTs given their previous training and expectations. Individuals might not understand the necessity of collaboration and communication and continue to use the jargon exclusive to their field, for example. Further, team members may have been mandated to participate and therefore feel little commitment to the mission of the team. This, along with competing demands due to time pressures felt by individual members, can result in poor attendance or passive participation.

Intra-team variables

These barriers refer to the actual structure and processes of the team, and because of the sheer diversity of disciplines represented in IDTs it is not unreasonable to anticipate operating difficulties that emerge as a result. Ranging from unbalanced power dynamics as strong personalities claim control, to turf conflicts about how to handle particular situations, to differences in decisions, goals or responsibilities, intra-team barriers can often tear a team apart.

Organization variables

Since team care requires time, space, and personnel resources, it requires that the organizational culture be supportive of it. If the administration of the department and institution do not view IDT care as crucial and show a commitment to it, team members will be unable to have an impact on patient outcomes, implement quality improvement projects, or change practice standards at the institution.

Conclusion

In summary, teams allow health-care providers to develop comprehensive care plans that address the complex medical and psychosocial needs of patients. Moreover, such teams have been shown to improve both patient outcomes and utilization of system resources. For certain groups of complex urology patients facing serious illness, this model of collaborative care is appropriate. However, in order for the team to be effective, an understanding of team principles as well as a commitment to common goals and interprofessional communication is necessary. We hope that this practical review of teams in the context of urological care will encourage providers to apply these principles to the supportive care of their patients.

References

1 Beckhard R (1972). Organizational issues in the team delivery of comprehensive health care. *Milbank Mem. Fund Q.* **50**: 287–316.

2 United States Department of Health and Human Services (1995). *A National Agenda for Geriatric Education: White Papers*, pp. 12–80. United States Department of Health and Human Services, Rockville, MD.

3 Leipzig RM, Berkman CS, Ramirez-Coronado S (2001). Integrating housestaff into a geriatric interdisciplinary team. *Gerontol. Geriatr. Educ.* **21**: 63–72.

4 Robertson D (1992). The roles of health care teams in care of the elderly. *Fam. Med.* **24**:136–41.

5 Tsukuda RA (1990). Interdisciplinary collaboration: teamwork in geriatrics. In: *Geriatric Medicine*, 3rd edn (ed. CK Cassel, DE Riesenberg, LB Sorensen), pp. 668–75. Springer, New York.

6 van den Hout WB, Tijhuis GJ, Hazes JM, Breedveld FC, Vliet Vlieland TP (2003). Cost effectiveness and cost utility analysis of multidisciplinary care in patients with rheumatoid arthritis: a randomised comparison of clinical nurse specialist care, inpatient team care, and day patient team care. *Ann. Rheum. Dis.* **62**: 308–15.

7 Dasgupta P, Drudge-Coates L, Smith K, Booth CM (2002). The cost effectiveness of a nurse-led shared-care prostate assessment clinic. *Ann. R. Coll. Surg. Engl.* **84**: 328–30.

8 Barr O (1997). Interdisciplinary teamwork: consideration of the challenges. *Br. J. Nurs.* **6**: 1005–10.

9 Curley C, McEachern JE, Speroff T (1998). A firm trial of interdisciplinary rounds on the inpatient medical wards: an intervention designed using continuous quality improvement. *Med. Care* **36**(Suppl. 8): AS4–12.

10 **Lincoln NB, Walker MF, Dixon A, Knights P** (2004). Evaluation of a multiprofessional community stroke team: a randomized controlled trial. *Clin. Rehabil.* **18**: 40–7.

11 **The Diabetes Control and Complications Trial Research Group** (1993). The effect of intensive treatment of diabetes on the development and progression of long-term complications in insulin-dependent diabetes mellitus. *N. Engl. J. Med.* **329**: 977–86.

12 **Lynch RT, Agre J, Powers JM, Sherman J** (1996). Long-term follow-up of outpatient interdisciplinary pain management with a no-treatment comparison group. *Am. J. Phys. Med. Rehabil.* **75**: 213–22.

13 **Eaton KK** (1997). Cognitive behaviour therapy for the chronic fatigue syndrome. Use an interdisciplinary approach. *Br. Med. J.* **312**: 1097–8.

14 **Chandler D, Meisel J, Hu TW, McGowen M, Madison K** (1996). Client outcomes in a three-year controlled study of an integrated service agency model. *Psychiatr. Serv.* **47**: 1337–43.

15 (2001). Teams and teamwork. In: *Geriatric Interdisciplinary Team Training: The GITT Kit*, (ed. K Hyer, E Flaherty, S Fairchild, M Bottrell, M Mazey, T Fulmer), pp 12–23. The John A. Hartford Foundation, New York.

16 **Cooper BS, Fishman E** (2003). The interdisciplinary team in the management of chronic conditions: has its time come? In: *Partnerships for Solutions . . . Better Lives for People with Chronic Conditions*, pp. 2–19. Johns Hopkins University, Baltimore, MD.

17 **Young CA** (1998). Building a care and research team. *J. Neurol. Sci.* **160**(Suppl. 1): S137–S140.

18 **Van Norman G** (1998). *Interdisciplinary Team Issues.* Available at http://eduserv.hscer.washington.edu/bioethics/topics/team.html (accessed 24 January 2004).

19 **Tuckman BW** (1965). Developmental sequence in small groups. *Psychol. Bull.* **63**: 384–99.

20 **Drinka TJK, Clark PG** (2000). Developing and maintaining interdisciplinary health care teams. In: *Healthcare Teamwork: Interdisciplinary Practice and Teaching*, pp. 11–51. Greenwood Publishing Group, Westport, CT.

21 **Rubin IM, Beckhard R** (1972). Factors influencing the effectiveness of health teams. *Milbank Mem. Fund Q.* **50**: 317–35.

22 **Baldwin DC Jr, Tsukuda RA** (1984). Interdisciplinary teams. In: *Geriatric Medicine: Fundamentals of Geriatric Care*, 2nd edn (ed. CK Cassel, JR Walsh), pp. 421–35. Springer, New York.

23 **Leipzig RM, Hyer K, Ek K, Wallenstein S, Vezina ML, Fairchild S** *et al.* (2002). Attitudes toward working on interdisciplinary healthcare teams: a comparison by discipline. *J. Am. Geriatr. Soc.* **50**: 1141–8.

24 **Abramson JS, Mizrahi T** (1996). When social workers and physicians collaborate: positive and negative interdisciplinary experiences. *Soc. Work* **41**: 270–81.

Chapter 5

Psychological and spiritual support

Aru Narayanasamy

Introduction

This chapter considers psychological and spiritual support for chronically ill patients. In doing so, it develops an exposition on psychological and spiritual issues which are considered to be important for the well-being of individuals with chronic illness and those in the end stage of life. Specific strategies for maximizing psychological and spiritual support for patients going through the trajectory of chronic illness are identified and explained. This chapter also explores ethical issues surrounding psychological and spiritual support and the end of life. It is concluded that psychological and spiritual support, along with the ethical considerations dealt in this chapter are paramount in urology care.

Holism is a well-known notion used in health care to mean that there should be a balance of mind, body, and spirit for the maintenance of health in a person. This notion is based on the assumption that these parts are inseparable and function as an integral unit within the whole person with each dimension—mind, body, and spirit—affecting and being affected by others. Consequently, healing or illness at one level reverberate throughout the other levels. This perspective has implications for health care in that a good understanding of the knowledge, attitude, and skills required for the care of the total person, including the spirit, is needed.

The emerging literature on the subject of psychological and spiritual issues demonstrates an encouraging trend in that its significance is being addressed in a number of initiatives in health care. Advances in the efforts to meet patients' psychological and spiritual needs in palliative and terminal care are encouraging. However, attention to the spiritual and psychological support of patients requiring health-care intervention in urology is yet to be fully addressed in the theoretical and practice-based literature. According to Thomsen[1] medical education in the Western world has concentrated heavily on the more easily measurable aspects of the physical dimension in humanity and it has almost neglected to address the spiritual needs of patients. Learning about the spiritual needs of humanity has not been an active part of the medical curriculum, yet there is emerging evidence that patients have expressed needs which are typified as spiritual in nature.[2,3] This chapter is designed to address the many facets of spiritual and psychological support for patients.

Whether we are religious or not, we need to be in touch with our spirituality, the inner person in us. Sometimes our spirituality comes into focus when we face emotional stress, physical illness, or death.[4,5] However, in spite of the many advances and innovations in health care, there is still the concern that the provision of spiritual care for patients could be better. Emerging evidence suggests that there is scope to improve health-care practitioners' knowledge and skills related to professional education in spiritual care. Research studies consistently indicate that health carers are unable to give full attention to patients' spiritual needs because of poor role preparation in this area of care.[1,6–8]

Psychological and spiritual issues in chronic illness

According to the quality-of-life model, psychological and spiritual issues are important. These include life satisfaction, happiness, peace of mind, control, goal achievement, and a belief system.[9] However, in other models spirituality is subsumed within psychological well-being.[10,11] Patrick and Erickson[12] observed that religious beliefs influence well-being in some people and spiritual well-being may be sought by others as part of the treatment and care they receive. However, it is clear that considerable overlap exists between psychological and spiritual well-being. A separate coverage of each of these dimensions is provided in the following subsections.

Psychological issues

According to Schirm,[13] psychological well-being is paramount in the trajectory of chronic illness. Apart from affective aspects like happiness, satisfaction, goal achievement, or peace of mind,[14] the psychological dimensions include cognitive function.[12] Research findings suggest that the impact of cognitive dysfunction is more devastating for sufferers of chronic illness than functional losses or severe pain.[15] There appears to be a correlation between cognitive dysfunction and perceived quality of life. Consistent with other findings, Lawton et al.[15] found that in their quality of life research people usually expressed a desire to live a shorter time if that time is perceived to be of diminished quality.

Likewise, Ryan[16] demonstrated that psychological support designed to promote affective aspects of psychological well-being is considered to be important for enhancing quality of life for those who are housebound and receiving hospice care and their primary carers. In this study, primary carers appear to have attached more importance to nurses attempting to meet the psychological needs of these patients than they did for physical needs. Similarly, nurses themselves attached a lot of importance to psychological care in this study. Nurses typified psychological interventions as paramount by rating positively the following: offering assurance, listening, helping the client feel safe, and providing consistent nursing services.

The trajectory of chronic illness exerts an influence upon the quality of life for patients. Murdaugh[17] claims that those affected by HIV/AIDS attained a better quality of life when they had realistic expectations, modified job plans, or changed their goals to be concordant with their health status. Murdaugh concludes that in HIV/AIDS and other chronic illness there needs to be a balance between efforts and resources to ensure quality of life.

Further studies of chronic illness confirm the close interplay that exists between the affective aspects in the psychological domain and other quality-of-life domains. The cognitive–transactional model of stress and the psychoneuroimmunology paradigm establish that perceived stress, psychological functioning, quality of life, and somatic health are psychologically mediated by coping strategies and resources.[18–20] In a study of spirituality and psychological factors in persons living with HIV, Tuck *et al.*[18] assert that psychological well-being may lengthen life or enhance the quality of life of patients. It is therefore clear that spiritual and psychological support is central for the promotion of quality of life of patients. In another study, Engebretson *et al.*[21] found that clients participating in a cardiac rehabilitation programme showed marked improvement in physical function, a raised level of energy, and positive perceptions of their own health followed by declining anxiety, depression, and negative feelings. Studies of quality of life for survivors of cancer show that there is a close relationship between the psychological, spiritual, physical, and social domains.[13,22]

In summary, it is clear so far that there is sufficient evidence to suggest that psychological support is paramount for improving the quality of life of those who are chronically ill. In the next subsection spiritual issues are addressed.

Spiritual issues

Spirituality is a multidimensional word that defies a single definition. The word 'spiritual' is derived from the Latin *spiritualis*, of breathing of wind, and it embraces varieties of descriptions and definitions.[23,24] In the context of health, spirituality is viewed as an aspect of the holistic understanding of the person.[25–27] As seen earlier, the holistic notion holds the premise that an individual as a whole person is the integration of body, mind, and spirit, which are inseparable.

The holistic notion of spirituality

Stallwood[27] illustrates the holistic notion of spirituality in the conceptual model of the nature of a person. This model is a clear illustration of a person's wholeness. Stallwood explains that the individual, as an integrated whole, is composed of the body, mind (psychosocial), and spirit, and that these components are dynamically woven together, one part affecting and being affected by the other parts. Figure 5.1 depicts an adaptation of a model developed by Stallwood as an illustration of a person's wholeness. The outer circle represents the biological nature of an individual; the middle circle depicts the mind as having four elements—will, emotion, intellect, and moral sense; the innermost circle represents the spiritual nature. Alteration to any one of three components affects the other two components and, ultimately, the whole person.

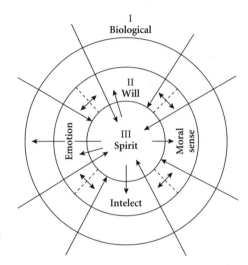

Fig. 5.1 Model of a person's wholeness.

There is a literature on health care which attempts to provide an emphasis on spirituality, from this holistic perspective. Such literature describes spirituality or spiritual life as:

+ the essence or life principle of person;[4,28]

+ a sacred journey;[29]

+ the experience of the radical truth of things[30] and ultimate values;[31]

+ giving meaning and purpose in life;[4,30,32,33]

+ relates to unconditional love;[4,7,34]

+ connectedness within oneself[35] and others;[33]

+ a life relationship or a sense of connection with mystery, a Higher Power, God, or Universe;[35,36]

+ as a belief that relates a person to the world;[37]

+ a quality that invokes a need to transcend the self in such a way that empowers, not devalues, the individual;[33]

+ inner dimension of being human attuned to the most valuable aspect of life that motivates and guides one's significant choices;[38]

+ being rooted in an awareness which is part of the biological make up of the human species.[39]

Research over the past 20 years suggests that spirituality is a human universal. Writing from a biological perspective, Hardy's[40] and Hay's[41] hypothesis is that religious awareness, or spirituality, is natural to the human species and has evolved because it has biological survival value. This hypothesis led to further studies on spiritual awareness in the United States, Britain, and Australia which consistently suggest that a significant number of the adult population believe they have been spiritually or religiously aware, at least from time to time.[39] According to Hay,[41]this spiritual awareness is normally described as:

- being aware of an emergent unfolding pattern of life, not imposed by themselves, that links them in a meaningful way with the rest of reality;
- being aware of the presence of God, typically in a way that helps them to relate creatively to the social context in which they find themselves;
- feeling a unifying presence in nature;
- feeling at one with or not different from the rest of reality.

All of these experiences can be described as forms of spirituality. That is, being aware of oneself in a holistic relationship with the rest of reality, which in a specifically religious experience in Western populations usually implies an awareness of God. Furthermore, according to Hay[41] research studies have consistently suggested that people who claimed to have undergone spiritual experience, compared with those who did not report such experience, appear to be:

- calmer and more stable,
- able to find more meaning in their lives,
- more concerned with issues of social justice,
- more tolerant of others,
- less materialistic,
- less conscious of status,
- less likely than others to be racially prejudiced.

These studies have further implications of specific importance for health care. Hay's[42] qualitative research reveals that people often experienced an intensity of spiritual awareness when they were undergoing stress related to emotion, physical illness or other forms of crisis. These experiences often remain a personal secret because of the fear that if others found out, they may become the subject of ridicule, be considered stupid or even mad.[43] According to Hay:[44] 'Quite often the initial breadth of a person's insight into God's presence dwindles and becomes constricted to little more than a source of private comfort in times of distress. This is to diminish spirituality.' [p. 134].

But even this privatized spirituality may be further constricted because the patient is unable to utilize its positive or healing aspects, through fearfulness, or the inability of health-care practitioners to integrate it into the patient's total care. It is highly likely that patients may trivialize or suppress their spiritual awareness if health-care practitioners appear to be unaware of these experiences or remain insensitive to patients' spiritual needs.

Definition of spirituality

In the light of the above understanding and for the purposes of this chapter, the following definition of spirituality is used: *spirituality is the essence of our being and it gives meaning and purpose to our existence.*

In summary, it is important to note that spirituality as a need comes into focus in illness when some sufferers face emotional stress, physical distress, or death; secondly, both religious and non-religious persons (atheists and agnostics) may express spiritual needs, in the sense of a need for meaning and purpose, identity, or a sense of harmonious interconnectedness; thirdly, spirituality as a concept is important in the caring context where health-care practitioners are frequently required to respond to their patients' spiritual needs.

Chronic illness

A body of knowledge related to chronic illness has emerged,[45,46] but the literature on spirituality and chronic illness is rather scarce. According to Lubkin and Larsen,[45] defining chronic illness is complex. Miller[46] refers to chronic illness as 'an altered health state that will not be cured by a surgical procedure or a short course of medical therapy'. The person with chronic illness may experience a range of impaired functioning involving the body, mind, and spirit and the perpetual illness-related demands on the self. Fieldman[47] considers chronic illness as a new/altered 'state of being' in that it is impossible for clients to view themselves and life as before. The illness permeates the person's whole being until it literally does not leave any part of life untouched. Chronic illness takes over the person's body, mind, and spirit, as well as relationships, roles, and lifestyle. Chronic illness is rarely completely cured or prevented.[45] Many chronically ill patients usually face some or all of the following: stigma, chronic pain, social isolation, altered mobility and fatigue, powerlessness, compliance or non-compliance, poor self-concept (body image and self-esteem), problems of sexuality, spiritual distress, and many other factors affecting their quality of life.

Researchers investigating spirituality and chronic illness have found spirituality to be a powerful resource for coping with health-related problems. Yates[48] found that religion acted as an important source of support for many patients. Baldree *et al.*[49] assessed the methods of coping used by 35 haemodialysis patients and found that hope, prayer, and trust in God were prominent coping mechanisms. In another study, Miller[46] found that arthritis patients reported a significantly higher level of religious well-being, defined as a sense of well-being in relation to God. Likewise, Johnson and Spilka[50] found that prayer and faith were extremely important resources for the majority of cancer patients who participated in their study.

In a study of spirituality and illness, Fernsler *et al.*[51] found that people with colorectal cancer in the sample who reported higher levels of spiritual well-being indicated significantly lower demands of illness (DOI) related to physical symptoms, monitoring symptoms, and treatment issues. In the light of their findings, these researchers suggest that a greater degree of spiritual well-being may help to mitigate the DOI as a consequence of colorectal cancer.

In a more recent focused study of spirituality and bone marrow transplantation, Cohen *et al.*[24] found that through personal stories, participants sought opportunities for reflections including adjustment to loss and resolutions. However, although the discourse on spirituality with regard to bone marrow transplantation is confined to one participant as a paradigm, it provides illuminating accounts. Spirituality and spiritual support from nurses appeared to have been instrumental to the adjustment and resolutions achieved by patients.

Having discussed the key features of spirituality and chronic illness in the light of emerging research findings, the psychological and spiritual needs of chronically ill patients are discussed in the next section.

Spiritual and psychological needs

The knowledge of spiritual and psychological needs is essential for spiritual care.[1,18,52] There is marked variation in the definitions of spiritual needs in the literature due to the influence of the belief systems and values of the various authors.[52,53] Spiritual needs are characterized by normal expressions of a person's inner being that motivates the search for meaning in all experiences and a dynamic relationship with others, self, and whatever the person values. Spiritual needs may be attained through faith, hope, love, trust, meaning and purpose, relationships, forgiveness, creativity, and experiences. These qualities are important for our holistic well-being in terms of meaningful existence. Some people achieve these via religious beliefs and practices.[33]

Terminal and chronic illness may leave a person in a state of imbalance or disharmony of mind, body, and spirit. Feelings of anger, sadness, guilt, and anxiety are often common following a period of disorganization and disruption. Despair and hopelessness may loom for the patient and his family. In their struggle with the impact of illness the patient and his or her family may feel separated from their usual support system. The patient's search for meaning in the disease may become apparent.

The patient's adaptation to his or her illness may mean new resolution, losses to be acknowledged, roles and expectations that have to be redefined. The illness not only has an impact upon the patient, but the patient's family has to share its effects. Although individuals' reactions to illness differ, many people struggle as a result of the disharmony of mind, body, and spirit. For some this means further spiritual growth or decline. The impact of an illness on a person compels them to turn in upon themself and reconsider their life. The illness becomes a spiritual encounter as well as a physical and emotional experience. Research into coping strategies suggests that in chronic illness many subjects indicated that they gained strength from their spiritual life.[46] The

Table 5.1 Spiritual and psychological needs

Spiritual needs	The need for meaning and purpose
	The need for love and harmonious relationship
	The need for forgiveness
	The need for a source of hope and strength
	The need for trust
	The need for expression of personal beliefs and values
	The need for spiritual practices, expression of concept of God or Deity, and creativity
Psychological needs	Fear/anxiety
	Anger management
	Time and attention
	Role change/adaptation
	Loss
	Positive self-concept (self-image and self-esteem)
	Relationships/conflict resolution
	Connection with family/significant others

source of strength included a renewed faith in God, prayer, a sense of peace resulting from prayer, and feeling God's love. Other strategies highlighted were meditation, receiving love and support from others, participating in church activities, and a life review.

For the purpose of this chapter an integrative approach is taken to address spiritual and psychological needs. However, the differences are illustrated in Table 5.1. The following may feature as spiritual needs in chronic illness:

1 The search for meaning and purpose:[52,54,55]

   • finding meaning and purpose;

   • finding meaning and purpose in illness and suffering;

   • searching and seeking motivation as to why and how to live.

2 Love and harmonious relationships:[52,56]

   • a universal need, especially love that is unconditional (no strings attached to it);

   • relationships with people, living harmoniously with people and their surroundings;

   • deriving inner peace and security from love and harmonious relationships.

3 Forgiveness:[52,57]

   • guilt is a universal human phenomenon that need to be ridden by forgiveness;

   • believers may seek forgiveness through their faith/religion; however, non-believers may not have such opportunities but still need to find the means to be forgiven.

4 Hope and strength:[1,52,58,59,60]

   • sources, religious or spiritual, that gives hope and strength to go on living and face the challenges of life.

5 Trust:[52]
  - emotional and physical security;
  - stable environment and living give security and peace.

6 Personal beliefs and values:[52,56]

  - life principles and values;
  - religious and cultural beliefs;
  - humanistic needs.

Spiritual needs at the end of life

There is evidence to support spirituality as a significant human experience during terminal illness.[55,61] In some instances a sense of spirituality acts as a resource in terminal illness. Spiritual well-being is related to low fear of death, low discomfort, decreased loneliness, emotional adjustment, and positive death perspectives among terminal cancer and other seriously ill patients.[46,56] The terminally ill patient facing death is likely to have the following spiritual needs: forgiveness/ reconciliation, prayer/religious services, spiritual assistance at death, and peace:

- Forgiveness/reconciliation: there may be the feeling of unaccomplished relationship in that the patient may not have been granted forgiveness. The patient may seek ways and means of achieving reconciliation and this may be reflected as wanting forgiveness and reconciliation with his or her God.

- Prayer/religious services: prayer, as indicated earlier, can be a source of comfort and strength. Religious services such as receiving sacraments and blessing of departures can all be very comforting to the patient and his or her family.

- Spiritual assistance at death: the presence of a significant person, including a doctor or nurse and/or religious advisor, at the bedside of a dying patient can be a very comforting spiritual assistance to the patient. This is an invaluable gift that can be given to a dying patient and his or her family.

- Peace: peace and tranquillity can be achieved through spirituality. All of the above needs contribute to spiritual well-being and this means attainment of peace and tranquillity.

In this section spiritual and psychological needs have been outlined. These include the need for meaning and purpose; the need for love and harmonious relationship; the need for forgiveness; the need for a source of hope and strength; the need for trust; the need for expression of personal beliefs and values; and the need for spiritual practice, expression of concept of God or Deity and creativity. These are by no means exclusive, but are commonly recognized as within the province of health care to incorporate spiritual and psychological support for patients at the end of their lives.

History taking/assessment for psychological and spiritual support

The following strategies may enhance spiritual and psychological support for patients.

History taking/assessment

According to Puchalski[62] a spiritual history taking offers practitioners the opportunity to understand their patients more holistically. Spiritual history as part of the assessment may provide insights into 'what gives meaning to a person's life'. Puchalski adds: 'The key element of the spiritual history is listening to what is important to the patient and being truly present to the patient. This is at the root of compassionate caregiving.' [p. 748].

Health-care assessment of psychological and spiritual needs includes obtaining detailed information about the patient's thoughts and feelings about the meaning and purpose of life, love, and relationship, trust, hope, and strength, forgiveness, expressions of beliefs, and values. However, assumptions or conclusions should not be drawn about spiritual needs on the basis of a patient's religious status as others who may not necessarily claim adherence to a faith may have spiritual needs. Furthermore, the health-care professional must remain sensitive to verbal and non-verbal cues from patients when carrying out an assessment. These cues might indicate a need to talk about spiritual problems.

Assessment of the patient's physical functioning may also provide valuable information for understanding their spiritual component. Such obvious considerations about a patient as his or her ability to see, hear, and move are important factors that may later determine the relevance of certain interventions. Also, psychosocial assessment data may serve a useful purpose in determining the patient's thought patterns, content of speech, affect (mood), cultural orientation, and social relationships. They may all provide the basis for identifying a need, or planning appropriate care, in conjunction with spiritual intervention.

The presence of religious literature, for example the Bible or Koran, gives an indication of a patient's concerns about spiritual matters. Objects like religious requisites such as pictures, badges, pins, or articles of clothing are symbolic of a patient's spiritual expressions. A patient may keep a religious statue or Deity to carry out his or her religious rituals. Schedules can be used to carry out spiritual assessment by observations:

- ◆ Observations of the ways in which the patient relates with 'significant others' (people close to the patient, friends, and others who matter to him or her) may provide clues to the spiritual needs. The quality of interpersonal relationships can be ascertained. Does the patient welcome visitors? Does their presence relax the patient or cause distress? Does the patient get visitors from the church or religious community?

- ◆ Observations of the above factors can lead to conclusions about patients' social support system. The social support system enables patients to give and receive love, and lack of such support may deprive patients of this need and leave them distressed.

The patient who has faith in God may feel estranged if he or she is cut off from their support network. Observations of a patient's environment and significant objects/symbols related to religious practice may give evidence of their spirituality.

The other area of assessment includes attention to three factors: sense of meaning and purpose, means of forgiveness, and source of love and relationship. Observations and routine conversations with patients can lead to valuable information about each of these factors. Observations may include:

- How does the patient deal with other patients?
- Does he or she ruminate over past behaviours or how has they been treated by other people?
- How does the patient respond to criticism?

If a patient responds with anger and hostility and blames others, these behaviours may suggest that they are unable to forgive themself with a consequent inability to tolerate anything that resembles criticism. The spiritual assessment must also look at the patient's ability to feel loved, valued, and respected by other people.

Giving psychological and spiritual support

Psychological and spiritual support should be given according to the indications of the individual, which may be unique and specific. The presence of active spiritual beliefs (in God or a 'higher being') and spiritual practices is a source of hope. These can enable patients to participate in specific practices and these may include praying, enlisting the prayers of others, listening to spiritual music and spiritual programmes on the radio or television, in religious activities, maintaining specific religious customs, and having visits from members and leaders of their spiritual community.

If, for example, the patient is part of a church or religious group, and their effect on the patient appears positive, the caring team can strengthen this contact. A patient who is accustomed to practices such as meditating, praying, or reading the Bible or other religious books should be given time and privacy. A visit by the patient's religious agent (pastor, rabbi, or others) can be arranged. For example, a nurse responded to a patient's spiritual needs by initiating religious care interventions:[63]

> The nursing team as a whole recognized towards the latter stage of patient's life that he became very aggressive and hostile. His relatives felt that this was due to lack of attention to his spiritual needs, and they admitted that the patient had been deeply religious until tragic events took over . . . It took time for the nursing team to sit with the family and patient to work out what was required, which led to eventual pastoral support. [p. 450]

However, not all patients may express their spiritual/religious needs explicitly. One nurse recounts how she addressed this need:[64]

> The patient has put his religion as atheist. A well-travelled person, spoke five different languages and was in the navy. Most people would have described him as 'know it all type of person'. In a

conversation he described a local Catholic priest fleetingly. Last few days of his life, he was frightened and someone remembered the priest, and I asked him, would he like me to contact the priest which he appreciated. The priest came and it turned out that the patient used to go to church a long time ago. I felt that the patient's need was to make peace with whatever he was frightened of. So, I tried to contact the priest, which took several phone calls and nearly all day to locate him. I eventually succeeded. The priest visited the patient several times and he [the patient] took communion and the last rite too. It appeared to me that he found some inner peace through this.

The practitioner can make it easier for the patient to talk about spiritual beliefs and concerns, especially about how these relate to his or her illness. The caring team may need to help the patient in their struggle and search for meaning and purpose in life. On the other hand, if the patient is trying to find a source of hope and strength, then it can be used in planning care.

The other aspects of support may include comfort, support, warmth, self-awareness, empathy, non-judgemental listening, and understanding. All these measures are the essence of a therapeutic relationship. An empathetic listener can do much to support a person who is spiritually distressed by being available when needed. For those patients suffering from loneliness, and expressing doubts, fears, and feelings of alienation, the presence of an empathetic person may have a healing effect.[65,66]

For some patients a powerful source of spiritual care and comfort can be prayer, scripture, and other religious reading.[1] All these may alleviate spiritual distress. Prayers as a source of help would help a patient develop a feeling of oneness with the universe or a better relationship with God, comfort the patient, and help relieve spiritual distress. A particular prayer could be selected according to the patient's own style of comfort and needs. Although health professionals may not all belong to the same faith as the patient, they could still support the patient in carrying out his spiritual beliefs.

Meditation, both religious and secular, can play an important role in the provision of psychological and spiritual support.[1,59] It enables patients to relax, clear the mind, and achieve a feeling of oneness with a Deity or the universe. Meditation also promotes acceptance of painful memories or decisions, and gathers energy and hope that may help the patient to face spiritual distress.

The use of music gives an inspirational and calming effect. A wide variety of religious, inspirational, and secular music may spiritually uplift a patient.

Giving psychological and spiritual support is a highly skilful activity. It requires education and experience specifically in spiritual and psychological support. Sufficient information is provided in this section to give readers a guide to spiritual and psychological support. It is imperative that the caring team observe the following during health-care interventions:

◆ do not impose personal beliefs (or lack of them) on patient or families;

◆ respond to a patient's expression of need with a correct understanding of their background;

♦ be sensitive to a patient's signal for spiritual and psychological support.

If a member of the caring team feels unable to respond to a particular situation of spiritual need, then he or she should enlist the services of an appropriate individual.

Health-care interventions should be based on an action which reflects caring for the individual. There is no cure without caring. Caring signifies to the person that he or she is significant, and is worth someone taking the trouble to be concerned about them. Caring requires actions of support and assistance in growing. It means a non-judgemental approach and showing sensitivity to a person's cultural values, physical preference, and social needs. It demands an attitude of helping, sharing, nurturing, and loving.

Hope-fostering strategy

Hope is something that we cannot easily give to another, but every effort can be made to support and encourage the hoping abilities of a patient. Health-care professionals such as doctors and nurses often are in an ideal position to foster or hinder hope. A caring relationship can be offered that permits, rather than stifles, the efforts of the patient to develop hope. The health-care professional can support the person who is testing his or her own beliefs or struggling with questions of fear and faith. Further encouragement can be given to patients to talk about their fears. Helping patients to relive their memories is another way of facilitating hoping. Memories of events when life's needs were met, when despair was overcome, and when failure was defeated, can all be used to encourage a patient to take a fresh view and face the future with confidence as part of spiritual recovery.

Herth[67] identifies hope-fostering strategies which could be used as part of spiritual care. She defines hope-fostering strategies as 'those sources that function to instil, support or restore hope by facilitating the hoping process in some way' [p. 1253]. Further strategies on fostering hope are shown in the box.

Hope-fostering strategies

Interpersonal connectedness

A meaningful and shared relationship with close ones and others including nurses is said to be a feature of interpersonal connectedness. For example, a harmonious and supporting relationship within the family offers the client hope and strength, which are fundamental parts of a person's spirituality. The willingness of nurses to share in a client's hope is a feature of this strategy.

Lightheartedness

Feelings of delight, joy, or playfulness are all features of lightheartedness and these may be communicated verbally or non-verbally. The nurse can enable clients to be

> **Hope-fostering strategies** *(continued)*
>
> lighthearted and this can be therapeutic in that it can provide a communication link between persons and a way of coping with deterioration in bodily function and confused emotions. It can be cathartic; in other words, it can provide a sense of release from the miseries of illness.
>
> ### Personal attributes
>
> The nurse can optimize clients' personal attributes of determination, courage, and serenity. Helping clients in their search for a sense of inner peace, harmony, and calm is one way of enabling the client to achieve serenity.
>
> ### Attainable aims
>
> Personal aims can be powerful means of achieving a sense of meaning and purpose and these often foster hope. The nurse who helps clients to search for meaning and purpose in life actually fosters hope. Helping clients and their families rework their aims and challenging their thoughts on to events or significant others are useful means of achieving a sense of hope.

Ethical issues

According to Beauchamp and Childress[68] four principles are involved in ethical decision-making. These include the following: respect for autonomy, beneficence, non-maleficence, and justice and fairness. Patients requiring psychological and spiritual support need ethical consideration in the light of these principles. According to Thomasma:[69] 'Speaking descriptively, autonomy can be viewed as a feature of individual identity and integrity'. Respect for patients' autonomy with regard to their spiritual beliefs and practices should be active on the agenda for medical intervention. However, some health-care practitioners coming from a strong religious tradition and conviction may find it difficult to provide spiritual support for patients who may not express adherence to any particular faith or religious beliefs. It is important that health-care practitioners do not attempt to proselytize patients to any particular faith or religious beliefs. Due care should be taken to ensure complete impartiality when approaching such patients. Such patients may be atheists or agnostics or humanists. However, as discussed earlier, my view is that we are all spiritual beings and have spiritual needs. Patients who claim to be humanists may have distinct needs based on the philosophy of humanism.

Humanists try to find meaning and purpose in life and attach great importance to scientific testing, reasoning, and discussion to arrive at facts.[70] They believe in the utilitarian ethical principle that the overall quality of life is important. They give consideration to the point that all people have natural potentials for understanding, caring, and cooperation, and an awareness of the consequences of their actions. These, they believe, motivate us to form relationships and govern behaviour towards others. Humanists believe that we should use these qualities to make life better for all of us.

Like Christians, Humanists tend to follow the 'golden rule', i.e. 'treat other people as you would like them to treat you'. Incidentally, this is shared by all the other world religions. The two fundamental moral principles of Humanists are happiness and tolerance.

Humanists share a common ground on moral problems, but give consideration to all possible consequences when discussing policies for action. Humanists hold beliefs in birth control and abortion, equal rights for everyone, voluntary euthanasia, and freedom of speech which are all dealt with in this way. Many people find humanism as an alternative to a 'theistic' or God-centred religion. In this respect, humanists play a part in multifaith groups and other groups that represent the views of non-religious people.

Furthermore, psychological and spiritual support should be based on sound principles and evidence about its beneficial effects. As suggested elsewhere, there is emerging evidence that spiritual and psychological support is beneficial to patients.[60,71,72] However, at the same time due care should be taken to avoid potential harm to patients as a consequence of ineffective spiritual and psychological support. Although in my view staff who are compassionate, caring, skilful communicators, committed, open, trustworthy, non-judgemental, and sensitive to patients' spiritual and psychological needs are best placed to provide support for patients, those staff requiring experience and training in spiritual and psychological support should be encouraged to seek courses or professional development. Readers wanting further information on strategies for such development for medical and health-care practitioners will find them in the works by Narayanasamy[52] and Thomsen.[1]

Confidentiality and veracity

The other challenging ethical areas for health-care practitioners are confidentiality and veracity.[73,74] Needless to say, respect for patients' confidentiality is paramount in a professional relationship. The guiding principle here is one that serves the best interests of the patient. However, where veracity has to be breached, it should be done in the best interests of the patient within the legal framework and the professional code of conduct. Informed consent should be sought in all matters involving disclosure of information about patients and medical interventions.

Ethics and the end-of-life issues

In this subsection the ethical issues surrounding death and dying are considered. However, clarity is required as to when life ends before exploring the ethical issues. Brainstem death is accepted as a defining measure of death in the industrialized world. In the UK, the process of confirming brainstem death has three phases:

1 Identifying the cause of the patient's coma and ensuring that it is not reversible, then ensuring that the coma is not due to any drug overdose or interaction, hypothermia, or metabolic disturbance.

2 Performing a standard range of physiological tests to ensure that all centres in the brain which control the body's vital functions are destroyed.

3 Ensuring that the patient cannot breathe when artificial supports are withdrawn.

According to Gert et al.[75] a patient in a persistent vegetative state (PVS) is usually 'regarded as living only in the most basic biological sense . . .'. Jennet[76] regards PVS as 'a merely physical life devoid of intellectual activity or social intercourse, incapable of growth and development but devoid of sensation and thought'.

Not so long ago in the UK, the case of Tony Bland stimulated much debate in the courts, including the decision in the House of Lord in England to stop life-sustaining treatment. The court ruled that this included artificial feeding and hydration, and allowed future treatment to be restricted to those measures which would allow him to die free from pain and with dignity. In Tony Bland's case the courts upheld that withdrawal of treatment could be in the person's best interest.

Euthanasia

Euthanasia remains a very emotive subject and continues to produce debates for and against. In many countries euthanasia is illegal. A doctor is not allowed to help patients to take their own life. In the UK euthanasia in which a doctor kills a patient directly is classed as murder and carries a mandatory life sentence. Suicide is self-administered euthanasia and it is legal in Britain. Under the 1961 Suicide Act it is an offence to help someone commit suicide with a penalty of up to 14 years imprisonment. In The Netherlands and the Northern Territories in Australia euthanasia is legal provided the doctors follow a set of clear guidelines and report the death to the coroner as euthanasia.[74] In fact The Netherlands was the first country to decriminalize euthanasia. However, Keown[77] suggests that cases such as that of Tony Bland and others raise serious ethical concerns in medicine. Keown highlights: 'This was, in sum, a hard case which made bad laws, largely by approving a consequentialist ethic radically inconsistent with the principle of the sanctity of life.'

In other words, Keown[77] suggests that just because the legal process allowed the ending of life in the case of Tony Bland it does not make it a good law as it goes against the principle of the sanctity of life. Those who oppose euthanasia and assisted death argue that these are unnecessary where there is sufficient provision for high-quality hospice and palliative care.

Assisted suicide

Like euthanasia, assisted suicide—that is, to assist a person to take their own life by providing the means or opportunity to end that life—remains both unlawful and unethical in the UK. The Voluntary Euthanasia Society believes that the time has now come for the medical profession to be open about this form of doctor assisted dying.[78] This is putting more pressure on some governments to legalize euthanasia. Dianne Pretty, a 43-year-old patient in the final stage of motor neurone disease raised public interest in the debate on euthanasia in the UK. She wanted her husband to assist her to commit suicide under the Human Rights Act but the House of Lords ruled unanimously in 2001 that Dianne Pretty did not have the right to commit suicide with the assistance of her husband.

The doctrine of double effect

An important ethical issue which must be taken into account when considering the ethics of the end of life, is the doctrine of double effect. This doctrine claims that a single act having two foreseen effects, one good and the other harmful (e.g. death), is not always morally prohibited if the harmful effect is not intended.[68,79] For example, if a person with terminal cancer is given a strong dosage of morphine for excessive pain and dies this is acceptable under the doctrine of double effect provided that death was unintended. According to Keown[79] the principle of double effect plays an important function in 'informing and guiding good palliative care and distinguishes it from euthanasia'. He implies that the principle remains an essential aspect of sensible medical ethics, good palliative practice, and sound criminal law. This means that the principle of double effect ensures that the ending of life is not the primary intention of medical practice.

Living wills

The issue of living wills or advanced directives of patients may pose ethical challenges for medical and health-care practitioners. According to Dimond[80] and Wilson,[81] living wills are valid in common law (that is judge-made, case law) in England, subject to the following conditions:

- The patient was mentally competent at the time the living will was made.
- The person made it clear that the living will should apply to all situations or circumstances that may arise at a later date.
- The person is now incapable of making any decisions because he/she is unconscious or otherwise unfit.
- The contents of the living will were witnessed.

As seen earlier, ethical issues surrounding the end of life and spiritual and psychological support may pose serious challenges to practitioners. The need to balance personal values with those of patients and their families in itself could be demanding on professionals but ethical decisions have to be made that bring the best possible consequences in terms of quality of life to patients who are facing the end of their life. Research is showing that both patients and professionals derive greater satisfaction when spiritual and psychological support is active on the caring agenda.[52]

Clinical evaluation

Evaluation is an activity that involves the process of making a judgement about outcomes of medical and health-care interventions. According to Rousseau[82] spiritual suffering is 'complex and nebulous and often difficult to assess'. Spiritual suffering increasingly may manifest as physical or psychological problems.[83,84]

The following questions may be helpful as part of an evaluation:

- Is the patient's belief system stronger?
- Do the patient's professed beliefs support and direct actions and words?
- Does the patient gain peace and strength from spiritual resources (such as prayer and minister's visits) to face the rigours of treatment, rehabilitation, or peaceful death?
- Does the patient seem more in control and have a clearer self-concept?
- Is the patient at ease in being alone? in having life plans changed?
- Is the patient's behaviour appropriate to the occasion?
- Has reconciliation of any differences take place between the patient and others?
- Are mutual respect and love obvious in the patient's relationships with others?
- Are there any signs of physical improvement?
- Is there an improved rapport with other patients?

Spiritual integrity is a key indicator of psychological and spiritual support. The person who has attained spiritual integrity demonstrates this experience through a reality-based tranquillity or peace, or through the development of meaningful, purposeful behaviour, displays a restored sense of integrity. O'Brien[85] comments that the measure of spiritual care should establish the degree to which 'spiritual pain' was relieved. Another view offered by Kim et al.[86] suggests that spiritual care may be measured by how disruption in the 'life principle' is restored. The contents of a patient's thoughts and feelings may also reflect spiritual growth through a greater understanding of life or an acceptance and creativity within a particular context.

Summary

In this chapter adequate discussion has been given of the importance of psychological and spiritual support for patients facing chronic illness. The ethical issues surrounding psychological and spiritual support and the end of life have been considered. It has been established that evidence suggests that psychological and spiritual issues need to be considered, and patients must be supported to attain a better quality of life whilst facing chronic illness or the end of their life. It is hoped that readers are guided in this chapter towards maximizing their role in psychological and spiritual support for their patients. Providing psychological and spiritual support for patients can be a rewarding experience for practitioners.

References

1 Thomsen R (1998). Spirituality in medical practice. *Arch. Dermatol.* **134**: 1443–6.
2 Koenig HG (2002). An 83-year old woman with chronic illness and strong religious health. *J. Am. Med. Assoc.* **288**: 487–93.

3 **Dossey L** (1993). *Healing Words: the Power of Prayer and the Practice of Medicine*. Harper, San Francisco, CA.

4 **Clark CC, Cross JR, Deane DM, Lowery LW** (1991). Spirituality: intergral to quality care. *Holistic Nurs. Pract.* **5**(3): 67–76.

5 **Murray RB, Zenter JB** (1989). *Nursing Concepts for Health Promotion*. Prentice Hall, London.

6 **Narayanasamy A** (1993). Nurses awareness and preparedness in meeting their patients' spiritual needs. *Nurse Educ. Today* **13**: 196–201.

7 **Ross L** (1997). *Nurses' Perceptions of Spiritual Care*. Avebury, Aldershot.

8 **Swinton J** (2001). *Spirituality and Mental Health Care*. Jessica Kingsley, London.

9 **Ferrans CE** (1996). Development of a conceptual model of quality of life. *Scholarly Inquiry for Nursing Practice* **10**(3): 293–304.

10 **Haberman MR, Bush N** (1998). Quality of life methodological and measurement issues. In: *Quality of Life: From Nursing and Client Perspectives* (ed. CR King, PS Hinds), pp. 117–39. Jones and Bartlett, Sudbury, MA.

11 **Padilla GV, Kagawa-Singer M** (1998) Quality of life and culture. In: *Quality of Life: From Nursing and Client Perspectives* (ed. CR King, PS Hinds), pp. 108–15. Jones and Bartlett, Sudbury, MA.

12 **Patrick DL, Erickson P** (1993). *Health Status and Health Policy: Quality of Life in Health Care Evaluation and Resource Allocation*. Oxford University Press, New York.

13 **Schirm V** (2002). Quality of life. In: *Chronic Illness*, 5th edn (ed. IM Lubkin, DP Larsen), pp. 181–201. Jones and Bartlett, Boston, MA.

14 **Ferrans CE** (1990). Developing of a quality of life index for clients with cancer. *Oncol. Nurs. Forum* **17**(3): 15–19.

15 **Lawton MP, Moss M, Hoffman C, Grant R, Ten Have T, Kleban MH** (1999). Health, valuation of life, and the wish to live. *Gerontologist* **39**: 406–16.

16 **Ryan PY** (1992). Perceptions of the most helpful nursing behaviours in a home-care hospice setting: caregivers and nurses *Am. J. Hospice Palliative Care* **9**(5): 22–31.

17 **Murdaugh C** (1998). Health-related quality of life in HIV disease: achieving a balance. *J. Assoc. Nurses AIDs Care* **9**(6): 59–71.

18 **Tuck I, McCain L, Elswick K** (2001). Spirituality and psychological factors in persons living with HIV. *J. Adv. Nurs.* **33**: 776–85.

19 **McCain NL, Smith JC** (1994) Stress and coping in the context of psychoneuroimunology: a holistic framework for nursing practice and research. *Arch. Psychiat. Nurs.* **VIII**: 221–7.

20 **Zeller JM, McCain NL, Swanson B** (1996). Psychoneuroimmunology: an emerging framework for nursing research. *J. Adv. Nurs.* **23**: 657–64.

21 **Engebretson TO, Clark MM, Niaura RS, Philips T, Albrecht A, Tilkemeier P** (1999). Quality of life and anxiety in a phase II cardiac rehabilitation programme. *Med. Sci. Sports Exercise* **31**: 216–23.

22 **Wyatt G, Kurtz ME, Liken M** (1993). Breast cancer survivors: an exploration of quality of life issues. *Cancer Nurs.* **16**: 440–8.

23 **Brown L** (ed.) (1993). *The New Shorter Oxford Dictionary*. Clarendon Press, Oxford.

24 **Cohen Z, Headley J, Sherwood GW** (2000). Spirituality and bone marrow transplantation: when faith is stronger than fear. *Int. J. Human Caring* Summer: 40–6.

25 **Carson VB** (1989). *Spiritual Dimensions of Nursing Practice*. W. B. Saunders, Philadelphia, PA.

26 **Shelly JA, Fish S** (1988). *Spiritual Care: The Nurses Role*. InterVarsity Press, Downers Grove, IL.

27 **Stallwood J** (1981). Spiritual dimensions of nursing practice. In: *Clinical Nursing* (ed. I Belland, J Passos), pp. 47–68. Macmillan, Basingstoke.

28 Colliton M (1981). The spiritual dimension of nursing. In: *Clinical Nursing* (ed. E Belland, JY Passos), pp. 901–1012. Macmillan, New York.

29 Mische P (1982). Toward a Global Spirituality. In: *The Whole Earth Papers*, No 16 (ed. P Mische), pp. 91–105. Global Education Association, East Grange, NJ.

30 Legere T (1984). A spirituality for today. *Stud. Formative Spirituality* 5: 375–85.

31 Cawley N (1997). Towards defining spirituality: an exploration of the concept of spirituality. *International Journal of Palliative Nursing* 3(1): 31–36.

32 Fitchett G (1995). Linda Krauss and the lap of God: a spiritual assessment case study. *Second Opinion* 20(4): 40–49.

33 Sherwood GW (2000). Spirituality and bone marrow transplantation: when faith is stronger than fear. *Int. J. Human Caring* Summer: 40–6.

34 Ellison CW (1983). Spiritual wellbeing: conceptualization and measurement. *J. Psychol. Theol.* 11: 330–40.

35 Reed P (1992). An emerging paradigm for the investigation of spirituality in nursing. *Res. Nurs. Health* 15: 349–57.

36 Granstrom SL (1985). Spiritual nursing care for oncology patients. *Top. Clin. Nurs.* 7(1): 39–45.

37 Soeken KL, Carson VJ (1987). Responding to the spiritual needs of the chronically ill. *Nurs. Clin. N. Am.* 22: 603–11.

38 Emblen JD (1992). Religion and spirituality defined according to current use in nursing literature. *J. Prof. Nurs.* 8(1): 41–7.

39 Narayanasamy A (1999). ASSET: a model for actioning spirituality and spiritual care education and training in nursing. *Nurse Educ. Today* 19: 274–85.

40 Hardy A (1979). *The Spiritual Nature of Man*. Clarendon Press, Oxford.

41 Hay D (1994). On the biology of God: what is the current status of Hardy's hypothesis? *Int. J. Psychol. Religion* 4(1): 1–23.

42 Hay D (1990). *Religious Experience Today*. London, Mowbray.

43 Hay D (1987). *Exploring Inner Space: Scientists and Religious Experience*. Mowbray, London.

44 Hay D (1996). Morals and religion. *The Tablet* 3: 132–3.

45 Lubkin M, Larson PD (2002). *Chronic Illness*, 5th edn. Jones and Bartlett, Boston, MA.

46 Miller JF (1983). *Coping with Chronic Illness*. F. A. Davies, Philadelphia, PA.

47 Fieldman DJ (1974). Chronic disabling illness. A holistic view. *J. Chronic Disab.* 22: 287–91.

48 Yates BC, Bensley LS, Lalonde B, Lewis FM, Woods NF (1981). The impact of marital status and quality of family functioning in maternal chronic illness. *Health Care Women Int.* 16: 437–49.

49 Baldree KS, Murphy SP, Powers MJ (1982). Stress identification and coping patterns in patients on hemodialysis. *Nurs. Res.* 31:107–10.

50 Johnson SC, Spilka B (1991). Coping with breast cancer: the roles of clergy and faith. *J. Religious Health* 30: 21–33.

51 Fernsler J, Kelman P, Miller MA (1999). Spiritual well-being and demands of illness in people with colorectal cancer. *Cancer Nurs.* 22: 134–40.

52 Narayanasamy A (2001). *Spiritual Care: a Practical Guide for Nurses and Health Care Practitioners*, 2nd edn. Quay Publishers, Dinton.

53 MacKinlay E (2001) *The Spiritual Dimensions of Ageing*. London: Jessica Kingsley.

54 Coyle J (2002). Spirituality and health: towards a framework for exploring the relationship between spirituality and health. *J. Adv. Nurs.* 37(6): 589–97.

55 Narayanasamy A (2002). Spiritual coping mechanisms in chronically ill patients. *Br. J. Nurs.* 11: 1461–70.

56 **O'Brien ME** (2003). *Spirituality in Nursing: Standing on Holy Ground.* Jones and Bartlett, Boston, MA.

57 **Macaskill A** (2002). *Heal the Hurt. How to Forgive and Move On.* Sheldon Press, London.

58 **Haase JE** (1987). Components of courage in chronically ill adolescents: a phenomenological study. *Adv. Nurs. Sci.* **9**(2): 9–64.

59 **Benson H, Stark M** (1996). *Timeless Healing: Power and Biology of Belief.* Simon and Schuster, London.

60 **Koenig HG** (2001). *Spirituality in Patient Care: Why, How, When and What?* Templeton Foundation Press, Radnor, PA.

61 **Narayanasamy A** (1995). Spiritual care of chronically ill patients. *J. Clin. Nurs.* **4**: 397–400.

62 **Puchalski CM** (1999). Taking a spiritual history: FICA. *Spirituality Med. Connect.* **3**: 1.

63 **Narayanasamy A, Owens J** (2001). A critical incident study of nurses' responses to the spiritual care of their patients. *J. Adv. Nurs.* **33**: 446–55.

64 **Narayanasamy A** (2004). Spiritual care of older people. Unpublished research report, University of Nottingham.

65 **Montgomery CL** (1991). The care-giving relationships: paradoxical and transcendent aspects. *J. Transpersonal Psychol.* **23**(2): 91–105.

66 **Montgomery CL** (1993). *Healing Through Communication; The Practice of Caring.* Sage, Newbury Park, CA.

67 **Herth K** (1990). Fostering hope in terminally ill people. *J. Adv. Nurs.* **15**: 1250–7.

68 **Beauchamp TL, Childress JF** (2001). *Principles and Biomedical Ethics,* 5th edn. Oxford University Press, New York.

69 **Thomasma DC** (1995). Beyond autonomy to the to the person coping with illness. *Camb. Q. Healthcare Ethics* **4**: 12–22.

70 **Narayanasamy A** (1998). Religious and spiritual needs of older people. In: *Promoting Positive Practice in Nursing Older People* (ed. A Pickering, J Thompson), pp. 128–51. Bailliere Tindall, London.

71 **Aldridge D** (2000). *Spirituality, Healing and Medicine.* Jessica Kingsley, London.

72 **Post S, Puchalski C** (2000). Physicians and patient spirituality: professional boundaries, competency, and ethics. *Ann. Intern. Med.* **132**: 578–83.

73 **Palmer M** (1999). *Moral Problems in Medicine.* Lutterworth, Cambridge.

74 **Mitchell KR, Kerridge IH, Lovat TJ** (1996). *Bioethics and Clinical Ethics.* Social Science Press, Wentworth Falls, NSW, Australia.

75 **Gert B, Culver CH, Clouser KD** (1997). *Bioethics: a Return to Fundamentals.* Oxford University Press, Oxford.

76 **Jennett B** (1993). The case for letting vegetative patients die. *Ethics Med.* **9**(3): 40–3.

77 **Keown J** (1993). Courting euthanasia? Tony Bland and the Law Lords. *Ethics Med.* **9**(3): 34–5.

78 **Langley T** (2002). The pro-choice view. http://news.bbc.co.uk/1/hi/health/background_briefings/euthanasia/1044776.STM

79 **Keown J** (1999). Double effect and palliative care: legal and ethical outline. *Ethics Med.* **15**(2): 53–4.

80 **Dimond B** (2002). Legal aspects of consent v23: Department of Health Guidelines. *Br. J. Nurs.* **11**: 331–4.

81 **Wilson L** (1999). *Living Wills,* Nursing Times Clinical Monographs Series no 7. Macmillan, London.

82 **Rousseau P** (2000). Spirituality and the dying patient. *J. Clin. Oncol.* **18**: 2000–2.

83 **Stolley JM, Koenig H** (1997). Religion/spirituality and health among elderly African Americans and Hispanics. *J. Psychosoc. Nurs. Ment. Health Serv.* **35**: 32–8.

84 Kuhn CC (1988). A spiritual inventory of the medical ill patients. *Psychiat. Med.* **6**: 87–100.

85 O'Brien ME (1982). Religious faith and adjustment to long-term hemodialysis. *J. Religion Health* **21**: 68–80.

86 Kim MJ, McFarland SK, McLane AM (1984). *Pocket Guide to Nursing Diagnosis.* Mosby, St Louis, MO.

Chapter 6

The patient and family

Lorna Butler

The inclusion of quality of life as an outcome measure in clinical research has become one of the major stimuli reshaping how health professionals incorporate the life-threatening nature and chronicity of various illnesses into the provision of care. Often referred to as supportive or rehabilitative care, the physical, social, emotional, informational, psychological, spiritual, and practical needs of individuals from diagnosis to palliation are now better understood, with interventions aimed at positively influencing adjustment. While there is a significant amount of literature on quality of life in chronic illness, in urology this research has been overwhelmingly situated within a treatment paradigm of prostate and testicular cancers, and more recently erectile dysfunction (ED). Health professionals have been cautioned about a narrow view of what constitutes a quality-of-life outcome when attention is focused on the disease.[1] The new knowledge generated from most of this research is related to heterosexual men and how their experiences influence their partner and the supportive role of family in providing physical and emotional care.

Thorne and Patterson[2] have suggested that both the patient and family perspectives are critical to understanding the real meaning of life when a chronic illness is experienced within a family context. While there are varying perspectives in the literature, one of the key factors identified as contributing to how individuals perceive their quality of life was managing the illness. This required that the patient and family members had access to information and were involved in decisions about care.[3]

Evidence-based care requires the translation of new knowledge to clinical practice. No longer can the response to illness be viewed as a disease-based assessment. The influence of psychosocial variables in shaping human responses and the capacity of individuals to respond to their circumstances are not necessarily related to the type or severity of the illness but include effective use of available resources, problem-solving abilities, and social support networks.[4] The economic burden of chronic illnesses on the health-care system requires innovation and creativity to effectively manage the high incidence of mortality and morbidity, given the aging population. The timing is ideal for health professionals to significantly alter the impending burden of illnesses such as prostate cancer and ED on the health-care system. This chapter will explore the state of the knowledge that supports health professionals in broadening their interpretation of care delivery to include psychosocial challenges, review the most recent findings on the patient–partner dyad as the focus of care, explore the influence of patient–provider communications in meeting the informational and decision-making needs of couples, and suggest possibilities of mobilizing existing resources to aid patient, partner, and family adjustment in the clinical practice setting.

Perceptions of quality of life as evidence building

Previously, quality-of-life measurement has been discussed within a urological context. For the purpose of this chapter the impact on intimate, interpersonal relationships will be the focus. There is comparatively little epidemiological data on sexual dysfunction as a health issue relative to the public interest generated by recent advances in pharmacological interventions for erectile dysfunction. The changing demographic profile of the population and the potential for patients to request varying treatment options demands that attention be given to resource allocation and a planned approach to service delivery that considers physical, social, and emotional determinants of health. Contrary to popular opinion, sexual dysfunction has been found to be more prevalent in women than men in United States.[5] Findings associate a poorer quality of life and strikingly more negative outcomes experienced by women then men. These results were from one of the two population-based assessments of sexual dysfunction reported since 1948.[6] The huge gap in new knowledge on the impact of sexual dysfunction limits our ability to make claims about risk assessment and supportive care for positive health outcomes.[5]

The experience of women

In the health literature breast and gynaecological cancers are the most frequently studied and published of all chronic illnesses. It is only within the last few years that attention has been given to how treatment can affect more than the physical aspect of losing a breast or an ovary to explore the invisible scars related to a woman's sense of herself as being feminine. To make a similar comparison within urology, interstitial cystitis (IC), commonly referred to as a woman's disease, has an impact on a woman's identity and quality of life. A sense of worthlessness, family responsibilities, relationships, and difficulty performing tasks and maintaining employment have all been described as problematic.[7] Women have indicated that the inability to diagnose IC has sometimes led to them being labelled as emotional or in poor mental health, compounding the distress already experienced. Similarly, women with breast cancer reported relationship quality, physical sexual functioning, psychological self, and feelings of self as female as key determinants for their well-being as women.[8] An unanticipated finding was the loss of sensation in the breast that was thought to contribute to a perception that reconstruction did not improve a woman's sense of sexual well-being.[8,9]

When the basis of an illness or associated morbidity is unknown the ability to predict, prevent, or manage the effects is compromised. The ambiguity created by an illness situation, determining why an event has occurred, gaining a sense of mastery through information, and maintaining a sense of self-esteem, present significant challenges to effective management.[10] How patients cope with the experiences of IC has received little attention in the literature. While there is a plethora of literature on adjusting to breast cancer, comparatively little exists to support patients who experience psychosocial distress and impaired functioning related to IC. Given the limitations of present treatment regimes for IC supportive care becomes a priority for care delivery.[10–13]

Women and their partners

To understand the meaning of life when a chronic illness is experienced, within the context of family relationships, attention should be given to exploring both the patient's and family members' perspectives.[2] Women with IC are reportedly well informed about how their illness is treated but are less well informed about the cause and why a cure does not seem to be achievable.[14] Women are frequently challenged by an inability to convince others, including health professionals, of the authenticity of their illness. Obtaining the necessary information for understanding and management is often left to the woman, who is also responsible for educating her partner and family. There is a decade of evidence in experiences of chronic illness about partner relationships, with communication frequently cited as problematic for women.[15] To what extent multiple treatment regimes compound these experiences is relatively unknown. What has been documented is the need to conceptualize the body as a social expression, an existential necessity, and a way of being in one's world rather than the traditional view of body image as the physical self.[16,17] Further, how an individual processes, retains, and compartmentalizes relevant information may be an attempt to recreate their life and their relationships given the uncertainty of their illness experience.[18] To support women who live with chronic urological problems involves ongoing adaptations and psychosocial adjustments specific to each woman's age, culture, and life circumstances.

The perspective of men as patients

Given the successful treatment of testicular cancer, long-term survivorship issues of quality of life and men's ability to adjust are relatively absent in the literature. While there is an absence of data from North American experiences, evidence suggests that sexual dysfunction and infertility remain as key morbidity concerns internationally.[19–23]

Prostate cancer affects more than the physical aspects of a man's life; self-esteem, self-image, masculinity, and sexuality are all affected.[24] Literature on quality of life with prostate cancer indicates that the physical side-effects of pain, incontinence, and sexual functioning are key determinants.[25–27] More recently, fatigue and issues related to quality of social life and psychological well-being have also been identified as important factors that influence the quality of life of men with prostate cancer.[28,29]

Sexual dysfunction has been identified as the primary complication of a radical prostatectomy, with ED occurring in up to 80% of men.[29–31] From the largest population-based study of 1291 patients, the ED rate 18 months after surgery was 59.9%.[30] If an erectile nerve-sparing radical prostatectomy is performed, the ED rate has been reported to be from 40–86% depending on the surgeon's expertise and whether one or both nerves were preserved.[32] There is a scarcity of studies that address the patient's perspective of the impact of ED on their view of themselves as a sexual being. For men, ED has been associated with a loss of manhood. When sexual functioning is altered, the feelings of loss of identity can be more devastating than the loss of ability to engage in intercourse.[30] Sexual function, potency, and physical appearance are intimately involved in the concept of self-esteem and may play as great a role as the physical disease in the impact of cancer.[31] It is during the follow-up and recovery period post-treatment when the impact of these side-effects is experienced, usually at home. Resources and information may not be readily available to men and their families outside the treatment clinics.

Urinary incontinence, a common problem induced by treatment interventions for prostate cancer, is given only cursory recognition in the literature, yet patients often view incontinence as significantly more disabling to their quality of life than impotence. The impact of urinary incontinence most often occurs when patients and their family members are at home following surgery. Patients and families are often left trying to manage the impact of this side-effect without adequate resources, information, or advice from health professionals. To better understand the impact of prostate cancer on the patient and his family members, and to develop the most appropriate interventions, health professionals in both hospital and community settings need to be aware of patients' and family members' potential discomfort in asking questions about sensitive topics such as incontinence and impotence.

The potential magnitude of concerns related to sexual health was revealed by a national survey of 965 Canadian men living with prostate cancer (120 with recurrent disease and 845 up to 5 years post-diagnosis). Fifty per cent experienced problems with sexual functioning and only 19% felt they had received adequate assistance from health professionals.[33] Unlike IC and testicular cancer, no references were found that explored sensation as a variable in the quality-of-life literature related to prostate cancer. Given that much of the literature on prostate cancer refers to screening, diagnosis, and treatment phases of the illness, timing may be a barrier in detecting these concerns. The impact of treatment on sexuality may take up to 6 months or a year to be experienced. During this time follow-up appointments vary and resources for support are scarce.[34] If sexual health is not being assessed then the knowledge needed to develop appropriate and relevant interventions for men with prostate cancer is lacking.

Men and their partners

Literature on the patient–partner dyad in urological diseases is rare. What has occurred is the consideration of sex roles for men with chronic illness and more recently the discussion of masculinity on men's health behaviours and adjustment to illness. While a diagnosis of testicular cancer may have psychological implications for sexual well-being, the extent to which a testicle is symbolically representative of one's sense of self as a man provides a more in-depth analysis of quality of life beyond body image.[20] Since the late 1980s there have been a number of studies that consistently report a group of men who are vulnerable to long-term changes in sexual health. The key recommendation has been for improved measures to support quality of life such as provision of information, counselling, and sexual rehabilitation. There has been relatively little suggested that would support health professionals in working with these men and their partners, particularly as intervention studies are needed.[35]

The first reported studies that considered the partners' perspectives in testicular cancer were in the late 1980s. Schrover and von Eschenbach[36] studied men treated by orchiectomy and retroperitoneal lymphadenectomy for non-seminomatous tumours. In addition to quality of erection, they included marital and sexual happiness as indicators of quality of life. Interestingly only the men's perspectives were sought, but these were considered proxies for their partners. Men reported low frequency of sexual activity, low sexual desire, erectile dysfunction, difficulty reaching orgasm, and reduced orgasmic intensity. These findings were not consistent with previous studies. The most significant contribution of this study was the reported change in sensation of orgasm. The men reported that infertility took its toll on relationships, particularly for young men who were married and had no children and those who were recently married. Approximately 25% felt the cancer hindered sexual satisfaction. A positive finding was that 47.4% of the men perceived that as a couple they now had a closer relationship with their partner.

Gritz et al.[37] were the first to include the perspective of the partner and considered the long-term (4 years post) effects of treatment for both seminomatous and non-seminomatous tumours. No differences were found by tumour type. The most striking finding was men's sense of being unattractive as a result of surgical scarring. Interestingly partners did not share this view but did comment on the physical impact chemotherapy had had on their husband's body. There were differences of opinion between the dyad as the men thought their wives would consider them less attractive. Men resoundingly underestimated their partner's positive response to physical appearance at least 50% of the time. The authors inferred that the women were being protective of men's feelings and did not want to expose their true feelings about the body changes. Such conclusions are speculative given that the women were also ambivalent about the need for reconstruction.

The findings of this study, while ground-breaking for its time, may have limited applicability given that most couples had long-term marriages (10 years or more) with children and thus issues of fertility may have been underrepresented. The couples agreed that frequency of intercourse was less, and that the men had a loss in sexual drive, although short term. Consistent with Schrover and von Eschenbach,[36] the couples reported an increase in intimacy which contributed to a more satisfactory relationship.

Having the partner as part of the illness experience supported adjustment. More recent findings continue to support both the men's and their partners' perceptions of decreased libido pre-treatment that intensifies during treatment and usually recovers within 3 months.[20] This highlights the treatment phase as a crucial time for ongoing informational support to men and their partners.

Over the last two decades the role of the partner has received attention as the treatment for ED has improved. Between 1982 and 2000, 26 references were found that mentioned partners or wives in the assessment and treatment of ED.[38] Global differences existed in the published papers. Men in Australia included partners, men in the UK attended treatment and counselling on their own, and men in the USA rarely discussed ED with their wives until the problem progressed and the wives initiated the treatment. Interestingly, the wives often blamed themselves for the distress and poor self-esteem of their husbands. The men thought that their wives viewed them as less of a man and were concerned with their own masculinity.

Most of the studies reviewed did not mention partner involvement with decision-making or type of treatment. While ED may in some settings be considered a family illness, it is imperative that men's choices are also respected and cultural variations acknowledged. Eighty-five per cent of patients were reportedly embarrassed and afraid to let their partners know about their treatment for ED.[39] These men did not want their partners to join in the treatment programme. For those women who did participate, 12% dropped out of the treatment programme indicating that in addition to being time-consuming they believed their husbands were acting differently towards them and their relationship. The change was thought to be related to men's attitudes of traditional, male sex roles.

The review provided very revealing information about the complexity of issues surrounding patient and partner participation in sexual health care. While men equated ED with masculinity, women did not equate their femininity with sex or sexual functioning. Although women did find ED to be annoying and at times disturbing, it was not viewed as a threat to their relationships with their husbands.[40] This is in contrast to more recent work where 40% of Australian men thought ED was detrimental to partners and 17% considered ending the relationship.[41] Maintaining relationships seemed to be associated with good communication and the strength of commitment to the relationship. Controversy arises for health professionals who believe that successful treatment for ED requires the active participation of couples such as use of devices or injections.

Both patients and partners prefer less invasive forms of treatment. Support is needed for the type of therapy chosen to assist couples in understanding changes that may occur, such as the lack of spontaneity and differences in sexual behaviours and sensations experienced. Recognition of the role of the partner and participation in the teaching may be integral to the successful treatment of ED. Since only one questionnaire was found that measured partner satisfaction, there is very little evidence to guide practice in relation to the roles and expectations of partners.[38]

Theoretical influences

In the early 1990s an NIH Consensus Conference on impotence examined the state of knowledge related to male sexual dysfunction.[42] The outcome has altered the way in which men's inability to achieve and maintain an erection has been conceptually applied for evidence-based practice and research. One of the most frequently referenced documents in this report replaces the disparaging word 'impotence' with 'erectile dysfunction', a term that more accurately reflects the difficulties associated with achieving an erect penis as one of many processes contributing to male sexual functioning. At the time the conference was held, little was known about the prevalence of erectile dysfunction in America, thus estimates were established based on data from the 1940s. The hallmark of this document was the breadth of inclusionary criteria that ranged from risk factors, clinical, psychological, and social impact of impotence, diagnostic information, efficacies and risks of behavioural, pharmacological, surgical, and other treatments, effective public and professional education, to future research. It was noted that available data overwhelmingly related to Caucasians, preventing any reference to race or ethnicity. In addition to various chronic illnesses and conditions contributing to ED, a major deficiency was poor sexual knowledge. This had a further impact on the distress experienced by couples in using different sexual techniques and in interpersonal relationships. The point that was highlighted was that the patient–partner dyad is essential to conducting a sexual history.[42]

The dominant perspective within the existing quality-of-life literature depicts sexual well-being as physical, and therefore an individual is either sexually functional or dysfunctional after an illness event. A critical analysis of the existing literature showed that empirical research supported the function/dysfunction measurement of sexuality. Missing from this literature is the views of patients in describing their lived experiences and how illness affects their lives as sexual beings. In our own research, men with prostate cancer have strongly objected to being considered dysfunctional sexual beings. This points out the gap between conceptualization and measurement tools. No existing instrument was found that reflected theoretical underpinnings emanating from the views of patients. To apply a dysfunction measurement would negate the substantive contributions that these men, as well as others, have made in challenging the views about ED as a measure of sexual well-being.[14,27]

While gender is clearly a distinguishing determinant in urological disease, ethnicity is not; thus outcomes tend to either be extrapolated from Caucasian findings or ignored. Most literature reflects the dominate culture of Western biomedicine upon which the health-care system in North America is structured. This ethnocentric perspective suggests that one set of values and beliefs will be used as the standard measure of health outcomes. Over the last 20 years numerous publications have recommended further study of variables that explain or predict the health behaviours and resultant health outcomes by ethnic origin.[43–48] The forum that much of the research continues to use remains in screening and diagnostic interventions. The impact of illness and its treatment continues to be evasive from a cultural perspective.

While significant advances are being made in the study of culture, translation of recommendations for culturally relevant interventions and educational materials that demonstrate cultural sensitivity in practice have yet to be designed. Knowledge about quality of life, and specifically sexual health, is in the early stages of development. Efforts to design and deliver culturally competent programmes that are accurate, appropriate, and acceptable to different cultures are critical.[49] It is through recognition of the mutual roles that members of cultural communities and health professionals share that health practice becomes culturally informed and culturally sensitive. Until this perspective is acknowledged, the ability to translate knowledge into culturally competent practice will remain research recommendations.[50]

Categories such as 'men' and 'women' are understood to be an ever-changing, complex, multiple, and contradictory collage of experiences that are politically and socially mediated.[51] Such a notion reflects the need for an alternative framework in which we can question established norms and break out of increasingly inadequate explanations that are incapable of grasping the complexities of people's lives and experiences and the cultures they create.[51] In response to the need for alternative analyses of people's lives, there has been an increasing awareness of the importance of gender as a fundamental and organizing factor of daily life.[52,53] Rarely do we understand the ways in which gender 'that complex of social meanings that is attached to biological sex, is enacted in our daily lives' (p. 3).[54]

The implications of such an understanding are significant for women and men, particularly for those who experience a challenge or change in their sexual identity as a consequence of illness. Such knowledge offers the hope of rendering visible how the experience of illness and related treatments affect women's and men's sense of themselves as gendered sexual beings. Given the reciprocal nature of masculinity and femininity, it is critical to explore sexual identity and meanings of sexual health for men and women as individuals and as partners in sexual relationships.[55] Women's experiences and practices can only be understood in relation to the experience and practices of men, and vice versa. Any hope for developing meaningful interventions consequently lies not just with men but with women as well.

Like all identity, sexual identity is culturally, socially, and politically mediated.[51,56] An understanding of the experience and meanings of masculinity and femininity for Black women and men is a necessary prerequisite to developing culturally sensitive interventions that will promote sexual health and well-being. Hearn and Morgan[57] suggest, however, that the experience of masculinity and femininity is not a uniform one and that there exist in society different forms and practices of masculinity and femininity. The dominant form of masculinity and femininity in Western society is based on the White, heterosexual, and middle-class.[56] Interventions aimed at meeting client needs in relation to sexual health and gender are consequently based on a limited understanding or standard that does not include Black, non-heterosexual, or poor populations.

Scientifically, it is important to advance our knowledge of the initial theoretical basis for determining sexual health. To measure the concept of sexual health and to test the emerging model in large samples, such as clinical trials, requires the development of instruments.

Patient–provider relationships

There is a pressing need for health professionals to focus on the experience of living with a body that has been threatened by disease, devastated by treatment, and forever changed. To consider only breast amputation and restoration ignores the lived experience of the woman whose body has the cancer. Yet curricula taught in both medical and health professional schools provide little opportunity to prepare clinicians for this aspect of care delivery.[58,59] The recent advances in pharmacological interventions for sexual dysfunction have just begun to raise an awareness of the extent of interest and demand for services in this area. In the absence of good epidemiological data, knowledge about the impact of sexual dysfunction on relationships and quality of life is scarce.[5] The changing social and cultural pressures relating to heterosexual behaviours have been given little consideration in clinical research examining the relationship of sexuality to a person's sexual health.[60]

Few health professionals are knowledgeable about the effects of cancer and its treatment on sexual health, and they may often be reluctant to talk about such issues. Most women will not initiate discussions concerning sexuality unless the opportunity is made available by the health professional with whom they interact.[61] It is critical to examine the likelihood of women with breast cancer experiencing barriers to the discussion of sexual health issues with their health professionals. To provide patient-centred care, health professionals must first learn what sexual health means to an individual, explore the changes that occur over time as treatment is completed, and identify strategies that will support an improved quality of life.

The effect of the experience of chronic illness, from diagnosis through treatment and palliation, on sexual health is just beginning to be researched. Evidence to date continues to reflect a more physical orientation of sexual dysfunction that is narrow in its perspective of a person's sexual identity. Patients and their partners are sending a message that while their sexual desire and performance is important, overall health as a sexual person is a much broader concept.[62] Health professionals particularly need to listen, as there was no definitive expectation that the health-care team views sexual health as significant to care delivery. Clinically, there is a need to incorporate sexual health in the nursing and medical care of urological patients. Ongoing education and mentors are needed to help in sexual health care—this includes assessing the degree of comfort and knowledge that health professionals bring to this type of discussion with patients and/or their partners.[63,64]

Patient and provider communications

The defining features that patients believe are representative of good communicators include an ability to explain what is happening and being willing to listen.[65] There is a wealth of communications research which ranges from identifying preference for information, involvement in treatment decision-making, use of decision aids, patient satisfaction, delivering bad news, to interventions involving communications training programmes. Clinical practice has experienced a major shift from the traditional paternalistic model of decision-making by the provider to shared decisions and information exchanges where patients are given the information and make an informed choice.[66] It is well known that delivering the message is only one component of communications. How patients interpret and translate that message in a way that is meaningful within the context of their own personal circumstances has an impact on what is understood.[67] It then becomes important to consider how providers' communication behaviours may influence quality of life. This is an important consideration, as measuring patient satisfaction is problematic in the clinical setting.[68]

Becoming skilled at communications requires more than knowledge gained from experience. Medical schools are now incorporating communications skills within their curricula. The impending burden of the baby boomers' accessing urological services is a strong incentive for implementing communications training. Increasing waiting lists for clinic appointments, queuing for surgical procedures, and access to speciality referrals such as radiation oncology departments are factors that affect patients' perception of supportive care within the health-care setting. Health professionals just entering the health-care setting need time to gain confidence in dealing with challenging situations.[69] Interventions to aid them to become skilled, effective communicators will strengthen their ability to at least acknowledge expectations and begin to build relationships with patients and families.

The diagnosis of life-altering and life-threatening illnesses is challenging for experienced as well as new health-care providers. Delivering bad news has been written about extensively in the communications literature. Oncologists have stated that the most challenging issues to communicate are related to disease progression. Treatment failure, palliative rather than curative options, and recurrence comprised the areas of greatest angst when initiating conversations.[70] Cancer patients value honesty in explaining the progress of their cancer and the available options.[71] Effective communication is grounded in delivering the bad news honestly and accurately. The skill of the clinician is their sensitivity in providing the message and assessing the patient's and partner's ability to hear the news.

Patients attending urology clinics will range in age. Those who are becoming independent with a new marriage, their own home, and a young family, are confronted with devastating changes that threaten their new-found independence. A lack of life experiences renders them vulnerable in weighing up options and readily identifying resources. Communications become grounded in relationship building and psychosocial care. The chronicity of many urological conditions and long-term approaches to symptom management, such as in IC, are compelling indicators for training in communication.

Providing patient and family care

It seems logical to assume that marital status would be a strong predictor of health, yet there has been little evidence to support any causal relationship. What appears to be an important indicator is the quality of relationships. Exacerbations, recurrences, and diminished treatment options do not occur in isolation from other life events. Much of what has been learned supports the need for careful assessment of relationships within the family context. Partners are at risk for both physical and psychological distress.[72] Women who have been in traditional, financially dependent roles and those who must assume caregiver functions tend to be more vulnerable.[73] To consider a patient's quality of life requires a broader understanding of family dynamics and support systems. Two strategies that have consistently been reported as essential for interventions are provision of information and support.[74] Partners need time to discuss their concerns without feeling guilty or insensitive to the one experiencing the illness. Family members worry about doing what is best and often have little knowledge of what that might mean. Extending care to the partner acknowledges the inclusion of their feelings and the impact that the illness experience has on their life.

Two major challenges for health professionals in urology are the impact of sexual health and incontinence on individuals and their partners. Scientifically, it is important to advance our knowledge of the theoretical basis for determining sexual well-being. Testing of emerging models is critical to building an evidence-based approach to understanding the experiences of patients as well as the impact on partners and family.

Quality of life is becoming an important outcome measure in treatment decisions. Health professionals are now able to readily translate research findings to treatment decisions in clinical practice. This acceptance of quality of life has provided an opportunity to introduce other psychosocial variables to clinical research. We are now finding out about the lived experience of incontinence. The next step is to move from descriptions of these effects to consider the impact of incontinence and associated distress on people's lives. To date most psychosocial concerns have been treated as secondary outcomes in clinical trials. To change policy, evidence is needed on the effect and the efficiency of supportive care interventions. Creating an evidence-based approach to supportive care in sexual health and/or incontinence would be a major contribution to clinical practice.

Messages embedded in the reports of numerous studies suggest that decreased desire and changes in sensation are perhaps more noteworthy than recognized. Very little is known about what a loss of desire means to an individual. Changes in sensation are just now being talked about by women receiving pelvic irradiation for gynaecological cancer, women with breast and nipple changes post-lumpectomy, and men with alteration in ejaculation. The relationships that health professionals create with patients and partners are themselves intimate, safe, and respectful of the couple. Listening to the messages is the first step. Supporting individual and couples to find meaning is the challenge.

References

1 Wellard S (1998). Constructions of chronic illness. *J. Int. Nurs. Stud.* **35**(1–2): 49–55.

2 Throne S, Patterson J (1998). Shifting images of chronic illness. *Image: J. Nurs. Scholarship* **30**(2): 173–7.

3 Gregory D, Way C, Hutchison T, Barrett B, Parfrey P. (1998). Patients' perceptions of their experiences with ESRD and hemodialysis treatment. *Qual. Health Res.*, **8**(6): 764–83.

4 Butler L, Love B, Reimer M, Browne G, Downe-Wamboldt B *et al*. (2002). Nurses begin a national plan for the integration of supportive care in health research, practice, and policy. *Can. J. Nurs. Res.* **33**(4): 155–69.

5 Laumann E, Paik A, Rosen R (1999). Sexual dysfunction in the United States: prevalence and predictors. *J. Am. Med. Assoc.*, **281**(6): 537–44.

6 Kinsey AC, Pomeroy WB, Martin CE (1948). *Sexual Behavior in the Human Female.* W. B. Saunders, Philadelphia, PA.

7 Bates P, Getz B, Gibbs E, Neu L, Pobursky J (2000). Clinical conversations: nurses who work with patients with interstitial cystitis. *Urol. Nurs.* **20**: 109–18.

8 Wilmoth M, Ross J (1997). Women's perceptions: breast cancer treatment and sexuality. *Cancer Prac.* **5**: 353–9.

9 Baron R (1997). Sensory alterations after breast cancer surgery. *Clin. J. Oncol. Nurs.* **2**(1): 17–23.

10 Draucker C (1991). Coping with a difficult-to-diagnose illness: the examples of interstitial cystitis. *Health Care Women Int.* **12**: 191–8.

11 Webster D, Brennan T (1998). Self-care effectiveness and health outcomes in women with interstitial cystitis: Implications for mental health clinicians. *Issues Mental Health Nurs* **19**: 495–519.

12 Webster D, Brennan T (1995). Use and effectiveness of psychological self-care strategies for interstitial cystitis. *Health Care Women Int.* **16**: 463–75.

13 Webster D, Brennan T (1995). Use and effectiveness of sexual self-care strategies for interstitial cystitis. *Urol. Nurs.* **15**: 14–22.

14 Butler L, Conner L, March S (2003). The meaning of quality of life and relationships for women living with interstitial cystitis. *J Sex Reprod Med* **3**(1): 9–14.

15 Cascarelli Schag A, Ganz P, Polinsky M, Fred C, Hirji K, Petersen L (1993). Characteristics of women at risk for psychosocial distress in the year after breast cancer. *J. Clin. Oncol.* **11**(4): 783–93.

16 Cohen M, Kahn D, Steeves R (1998). Beyond body image: the experience of breast cancer. *Oncol Nurs Forum* **25**(5): 835–41.

17 Young-McCaughan S (1996). Sexual functioning in women with breast cancer after treatment with adjuvant therapy. *Cancer Nurs.* **19**(4): 308–19.

18 Showers C, Abramson L, Hogan M (1998). The dynamic self: How the content and structure of the self-concept change with mood. *J. Person. Soc. Psych.* **75**: 478–93.

19 Arai Y, Kawakita M, Okada Y, Yoshida O (1997). Sexuality and fertility in long-term survivors of testicular cancer. *J. Clin. Oncol.* **15**(4): 1444–8.

20 Ozen H, Sahin A, Toklu C, Rastadoskouee M, Kilic C, Gogus A *et al.* (1998). Psychosocial adjustment after testicular cancer treatment. *J. Urol.* **159**(6): 1947–50.

21 van Basten J, Hoekstra H, van Driel M, Schraffordt Koops H, Droste J, Jonker-Pool G *et al.* (1997). Sexual dysfunction in nonseminoma testicular cancer patients is related to chemotherapy-induced angiopathy. *J. Clin. Oncol.* **15**(6): 2442–8.

22 Böhlen D, Burkhard F, Mills R, Sonntag R, and Studer U (2001). Fertility and sexual function following orchiectomy and 2 cycles of chemotherapy for stage I high risk nonseminomatous germ cell cancer. *J. Urol.* **165**: 441–4.

23 Peterson P, Shakkebæk N, Rørth M, Giwercman A (1999). Semen quality and reproductive hormones before and after orchiectomy in men with testicular cancer. *J. Urol.* **161**: 822–6.

24 Herr HW (1997). Quality of life in prostate cancer patients. *CA-Cancer J. Clin.* **47**: 207–17.

25 Kornblith AB, Herr HW, Ofman US, Schur HI, Holland JC (1994). Quality of life of patients with prostate cancer and their spouses: the value of a data base in clinical care. *Cancer* **73**(Suppl. 11): 2791–802.

26 Sharp JW (1993). Expanding the definition of quality of life for prostate cancer. *Cancer Suppl.* **71**(3): 1078–82.

27 Butler L, Downe-Wamboldt B, Marsh S, Bell D, Jarvi K (2001). Quality of life post radical prostatectomy: a male perspective. *Urol. Nurs.* **21**(4): 283–8.

28 Fossa SD, Aass N, Opjordsmoen S (1994). Assessment of quality of life in patients with prostate cancer. *Semin. Oncol.* **21**(5): 657–61.

29 Katz M, Rodin G, Devins G (1995). Self-esteem and cancer: theory and research. *Can. J. Psychiat.* **40**: 608–15.

30 Yabro C, Perry M (1985). The effect of cancer therapy on gonadal function. *Semin. Oncol. Nurs.* **1**(1): 3–8.

31 Stanford JL, Feng Z, Hamilton AS, Gilliland FD, Stephenson RA, Eley JW *et al.* (2000). Urinary and sexual function after radical prostatectomy for clinically localized prostate cancer: the prostate cancer outcomes study. *J. Am. Med. Assoc.* **283**: 354–60.

32 Steineck G, Helgesen F, Adolfsson J, Dickman P, Johansson J, Norlen B *et al.* (2002). Scandinavian prostate cancer group study number 4: quality of life after radical prostatectomy or watchful waiting. *N. Engl. J. Med.* **347**(11): 790–6.

33 Walsh P, Marschke P, Ricker D, Burnett A (2000). Patient-reported urinary continence and sexual function after anatomic radical prostatectomy. *Urology* **55**(1): 58–61.

34 Fitch M, Grey R, Franssen E, Johnson B (2000). Men's perspectives on the impact of prostate cancer: Implications for oncology nurses. *Oncol. Nurs. Forum* **27**(8): 1255–63.

35 Butler L, Downe-Wamboldt B, Marsh S, Bell D, Jarvi K (2000). Behind the scenes: partners' perceptions of quality of life post radical prostatectomy. *Urol. Nurs.* **20**(4): 254–8.

36 Schrover L, von Eschenbach A (1985). Sexual and marital relationships after treatment for nonseminomatous testicular cancer. *Urology* **25**(3): 251–5.

37 Gritz E, Wellisch D, Wang H, Siau J, Landsverk J, Cosgrove M (1989). Long term effects of testicular cancer on sexual functioning in married couples. *Cancer* **64**(7): 1560–7.

38 Dorey G (2001). Partners' perspective of erectile dysfunction: literature review. *Br. J. Nurs.* **10**(3): 187–95.

39 Lew-Starowicz Z (2000). Participation of patients' partners in the treatment of impotence. Proceedings of the 7th Biennial Asia-Pacific Meeting on Impotence 1999, Tokyo, Japan. *Int. J. Impot. Res.* **12**(2): S29.

40 Rust J, Golombok S, Collier J (1988). Marital problems and sexual dysfunction. *Br. J. Psychiat.* **152**: 629–31.

41 Lording DW, McMahon CG, Conaglen JV, Earle C, Gillman MP, Tulloch AGS (2000). Partners of affected men: attitudes to erectile dysfunction. Proceedings of the 7th Biennial Asia-Pacific Meeting on Impotence 1999, Tokyo, Japan. *Int. J. Impot. Res.* **12**(2): S16.

42 NIH Consensus Development Panel on Impotence (1993). NIH Consensus Conference. Impotence. *J. Am. Med. Assoc.* **270**: 83–90.

43 Denniston R (1981). Cancer knowledge, attitudes and practices among black Americans. *Prognost. Clin. Biol. Res.* **83**: 225–35.

44 Willis M, Davis M, Cairnes N, Janiszewski R (1989). Interagency collaboration: teaching breast self-examinatoin to black women. *Oncol. Nurs. Forum* **16**(2): 171–7.

45 Lovejoy N, Jenkins C, Wu T, Shankland S, Wilson C (1989). Developing a breast cancer screening program for Chinese-American women. *Oncol. Nurs. Forum* **16**(2): 181–7.

46 Price J, Colvin T, Smith D (1993). Prostate cancer: perceptions of African American males. *J. Natl. Med. Assoc.* **85**(12): 941–7.

47 Long E (1993). Breast cancer in African American women: review of the literature. *Cancer Nurs.* **16**(1): 1–24.

48 Myers R, Wolf T, Balshem A, Ross E, Chodak G (1994). Receptivity of African–American men to prostate cancer screening. *Urology* **43**(4): 480–7.

49 Collins M (1997). Increasing prostate cancer awareness in African American men. *Oncology Nurs. Forum* **24**(1): 91–5.

50 Kawage-Singer M (2000). Addressing issues for early detection and screening in ethnic populations. *Suppl. Oncol. Nurs. Forum* **27**(9): 55–61.

51 Lather P (1991). *Getting Smart*. Routledge, New York.

52 Messner M (1990). Men studying masculinity: some epistemological issues in sport sociology. *Sociol. Sports J.* **7**: 136–53.

53 Frank B (1993). The 'new men's studies' and feminism: promise or danger? In: *Men and Masculinities. A Critical Anthology* (ed. T. Haddad), pp. 333–43. Canadian Scholars' Press, Toronto.

54 Kimmel M, Messner M (1992). Introduction. In: *Men's Lives*, 2nd edn (ed. M. Kimmel, M. Messner), pp. 1–11. Maxwell Macmillan Canada, Toronto.

55 Pleck J (1992). Men's power with women, other men, and society. A men's movement analysis. In: *Men's Lives*, 2nd edn (ed. M. Kimmel, M. Messner), pp. 19–27. Maxwell Macmillan Canada, Toronto.

56 Connell RW (1996). New directions in gender theory, masculinity research, and gender politics. *Ethnoe* **61**(3/4): 157–76.

57 Hearn J, Morgan D (1990). Men, masculinities and social theory. In: *Men, Masculinities and Social Theory* (ed. J. Hearn, D. Morgan), pp. 1–18. Unwin Hyman, Boston, MA.

58 Waterhouse J (1993). Discussing sexual concerns with health care professionals. *J. Holistic Nurs.* **11**(2): 125–34.

59 McGarvey E, Peterson C, Pinkerton R, Keller A, Clayton A (2003). Medical students' perceptions of sexual health issues prior to a curriculum enhancement. *Int. J. Impot. Res.* **15**(suppl 5): s58–s66.

60 Few C (1997). The politics of sex research and constructions of female sexuality: what relevance to sexual health work with young women? *J. Adv. Nurs.* **25**: 615–25.

61 Nishimoto P (1995). Sex and sexuality in the cancer patient. *Nurse Practitioner Forum* **6**(4): 221–7.

62 Heymen E, Rosner T (1996). Prostate cancer: an intimate view from patients and wives. *Urol. Nurs.* **16**: 37–44.

63 Butler L, Banfield V (2001). Oncology nurses' view on the provision of sexual health in cancer care. *J. Reprod. Med.* **1**(1): 35–9.

64 Matocha LK, Waterhouse JK (1993). Current nursing practice related to sexuality. *Res. in Nurs. Health* **16**: 371–8.

65 Fellowes D, Moore, P (2003). Communication skills training for health care professionals working with cancer patients, their families and/or carers (Cochrane Review). *The Cochrane Library* **3**: 1–16.

66 Charles C, Gafni A, Whelan T (1999). Decision-making in the physicial-patient encounter: revisiting the shared treatment decision-making model. *Soc. Sci. Med.* **49**: 651–61.

67 Charles C, Redko C, Whelan T, Gafni A, Reyno L (1998). Doing nothing is no choice: lay constructions of treatment decision-making among women with early stage breast cancer. *Sociol. Health Illness* **20**: 71–95.

68 Arora NK (2003). Interacting with cancer patients: the significance of physicians' communication behavior. *Social Sci. Med.* **57**: 791–806.

69 Shilling V, Jenkins V, Fallowfield L (2003). Factors affecting patient and clinician satisfaction with the clinical consultation: can communication skills training for clinicians improve satisfaction? *Psychooncology* **12**: 599–611.

70 Baile WF, Lenzi R, Parker PA, Buckman R, Cohen L (2002). Oncologists' attitudes toward and practices in giving bad news: an exploratory study. *J. Clin. Oncol.* **20**(8): 2189–96.

71 Parker PA, Baile WF, de Moor C, Lenzi R, Kudelka AP, Cohen L (2001). Breaking bad news about cancer: patients' preferences for communication. *J. Clin. Oncol.* **19**(7): 2049–56.

72 Burman B, Margolin G (1992). Analysis of the association between marital relationships and health problems: an interactional perspective. *Psychol. Bull.* **112**(1): 39–63.

73 Morse S, Fife B (1998). Coping with a partner's cancer: adjustment at four stages of the illness trajectory. *Oncol. Nursing Forum* **25**(4): 751–60.

74 Northouse L, Peters-Golden M (1993). Cancer and the family: strategies to assist spouses. *Semin. Oncol. Nurs.* **9**(2): 74–82.

Chapter 7

The bioinformatics of integrative medicine in urology

Ernest Lawrence Rossi

The role of integrative approaches to supportive care in urology is as controversial today as at any time in the history of medicine. At present, however, we are witnessing the emergence of a new, unified scientific foundation that brings together the best of modern molecular medicine with the bioinformatics of integrative medicine. The basic idea is to explore how genes are expressed (genomics) in response to signals from the environment to generate the proteins (proteomics) and the physiological functions of the body and brain, which we ultimately experience as the dynamics of consciousness and culture. In this chapter, a bioinformatics approach is used to review the theory, research, and practice of integrative medicine in urology by the entire medical team as well as the patient, family, and general community.

A bioinformatics theory of integrative medicine

The supportive care of urology patients and their families involves their most intimate, personal, and subjective world of psychological experience. How does this mental world of psychological experience interact with the objective, material world of molecules, genes, cells, tissues, organs, drugs, surgery, and rehabilitation in urology? While it is believed that the molecular-genomic revolution initiated by Watson and Crick 50 years ago could serve as a scientific foundation for medicine, psychology, and culture, it has had almost no impact on the field of integrative medicine until recently.[1-4]

To understand how the molecular-genomic revolution could contribute to a new understanding of an integrative medicine of mind, body, and spirit we need to review a few basic concepts of bioinformatics. We recall that genes are molecules of DNA made up of long sequences of four nucleotides (adenine, cytosine, guanine, and thymine). The sequence of these nucleotides is a 'code' that determines the order in which amino acids will be strung together to build the structure of proteins, which determine the physiological functions of cells, tissues, and organs. When gene expression, i.e. gene transcription, is changed by physical trauma, toxins, or psychosocial stressors, for example, it means that the sequence of nucleotides is changed in mRNA during gene

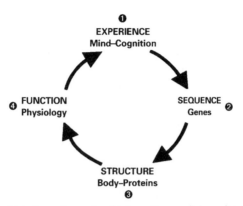

Fig. 7.1 The top-down bioinformatics cycle of integrative medicine wherein (1) psychological *experience* can modulate (2) gene *sequence*, (3) protein *structure*, and (4) physiological *function*. Modern molecular medicine, by contrast, focuses on the bottom-up direction of information transduction wherein genes, proteins, and physiological functions modulate psychological experience.

transcription so that the structure of proteins is changed leading to corresponding changes in physiological functions for good (e.g. a little stress can facilitate adaptation or healing) or for ill (e.g. too much trauma, toxins, or chronic stress results in dysfunction).

This linear relationship between sequence, structure, and function is the theoretical basis of the molecular-genomic revolution in biology that is now called 'bioinformatics'. To this textbook definition of bioinformatics I now add a fourth link so that human experience and consciousness can complete the bioinformatics cycle of information transduction between mind and body to bridge the so-called 'mind–body gap' as illustrated in Fig. 7.1.[1–6] It is of essence for integrative medicine to realize that the bioinformatics levels of sequence, structure, function, and experience are all expressions of information, which are related and capable of being translated into each other. This means that sequence, structure, function, and experience are different levels, forms, or classes of information that can be translated, transcribed, or transformed into each other (Fig. 7.1). From an information perspective this means that if you enter the bioinformatics cycle at any level with any of the diverse approaches of molecular or integrative medicine it is theoretically possible to modulate and possibly heal dysfunctions on any other level. This bioinformatics theory of integrative medicine takes the concept of information as the language of science very seriously.[7]

The top-down bioinformatics perspective of integrative medicine

Modern molecular medicine typically enters the bioinformatics cycle at the levels of sequence, structure, and physiological function with drugs, surgery, etc. This is called the 'bottom-up approach'. The molecular processes at the bottom are the foundation for the genomic, proteomic, physiological, and psychological experiences at the top. Many of the controversial approaches of integrative medicine, by contrast, typically enter the bioinformatics cycle on the top level of mind, consciousness, and human experiencing that is called the 'top-down approach'. It has been proposed that the simplest and most objective scientific way of understanding, measuring, and evaluating what is happening on all levels of the bioinformatics cycle is to use our currently evolving microarray technologies for measuring gene expression (genomics) and proteins (proteomics) associated with the mind–body–spirit approaches of integrative medicine. Patterns (or profiles) of gene expression and proteins can be used as a 'Rosetta stone' or measuring tool for evaluating all the seemingly different therapeutic approaches of modern molecular and integrative medicine. Because there are as yet no systematic programmes investigating this top-down bioinformatics theory of integrative medicine, however, we will proceed cautiously by outlining a series of hypotheses to guide current and future theory, research, and practice in urology. This bioinformatics theory of integrative medicine is supported with case histories that point to the type of research on the genomic and proteomic levels that will be required for the validation of the brief, practical, creative, and easy to learn integrative psychotherapeutic approaches presented in this chapter.

Hypothesis 1: a top-down bioinformatics theory is the essential foundation for understanding the complementary nature of integrative and modern molecular medicine

The top-down bioinformatics theory of integrative medicine complements the classical bottom-up approach of modern molecular medicine by exploring how psychological experiences can modulate gene expression, protein synthesis, and physiological functioning. Classical Mendelian genetics and its application to behavioural genetics and evolutionary psychology, for example, document the bottom-up approach of how genes modulate physiology and psychological experience. The new issue brought to light by the top-down bioinformatics cycle of Fig. 7.1 focuses on the reverse: How does psychological experience modulate gene expression, protein structure, and physiology? This surprising question is answered by Stahl in his text *Essential Psychopharmacology* :[8]

> But can behavior modify genes? Learning as well as experiences from the environment can give rise to changes in neural connections. In this way, human experiences, education, and even psychotherapy may change the expression of genes that alter the distribution and strength of specific synaptic connections. *Thus genes modify behavior and behavior modifies genes. Psychotherapy may even induce neurotropic factors to preserve critical cells and innervate new therapeutic targets to alter emotions and behaviors.* [p. 37, italics added]

Recent research extends Selye's concept of stress and the general adaptation syndrome on the physiological level to the proteomic and genomic levels.[9] Kaufer et al.[10] document how acute trauma and psychosocial stress facilitate changes in cholinergic gene expression on the genomic level. In related research, Meshorer et al.[11] describe how psychological stress modulates gene expression in humans experiencing post-traumatic stress disorder (PTSD) via stimulus-induced changes in alternative splicing of genes as follows:

> Traumatic stress is often followed by long-term pathological changes. In humans, extreme cases of such changes are clinically recognized a posttraumatic stress disorder (PTSD) . . . .*Stimulus-induced changes in alternative splicing [of genes] have recently emerged as a major mechanism of neuronal adaptation to stress, contributing to the versatility and complexity of the expression patterns of the human genome.*[p. 508, italics added]

This alternative splicing of genes induced by psychosocial stress is a clear example of how the top-down dynamics of psychological experience can modulate information encoded in the sequence of gene expression, which in turn modulates the structure of proteins, and the physiological functioning of the general adaptation syndrome in health and dysfunction in the bioinformatics cycle (Fig. 7.1). Rosbash and Takahashi[12] have noted that cancer can be a direct consequence of the stress-related disruption of circadian regulation via the period 2 (*PER 2*) gene. While there have been a number of studies relating a variety of integrated approaches to prostate cancer by stress reduction—such as the patient's cognitive coping style,[13] Zen meditation,[14] and mindfulness,[15] these outcome studies have not included the genomic and proteomic levels for a more complete bioinformatics analysis.[16]

Figure 7.2 is an illustration of what a more complete bioinformatics analysis stretched out over circadian time might look like. It illustrates the matching of bimodal circadian profiles of the bioinformatics cycle ranging from measures of the psychological experiences (therapeutic hypnosis), to the physiological functioning (body temperature), and the expression of behavioral state-related genes related to the being awake such as the period 1 gene (*PER1*, which is in the same family of genes implicated in cancer by Rosbash and Takahashi[12]) and sleep (*ARNTL*, formerly known as *BMAL1*). This matching of the bimodal bioinformatic circadian profiles of Fig. 7.2 is consistent with the hypothesis, but does not yet prove, that hypnosis can be used to modulate body temperature and gene expression for therapeutic purposes as is proposed by our top-down hypothesis of integrative medicine.[2–4] Systematic research is now required utilizing DNA microarray techniques to assess how the changing psychological states of waking, sleeping, dreaming, hypnosis and meditation, etc. can be efficacious in modulating the genomic and proteomic levels in integrative medicine. This bioinformatics approach provides new insights into the complex role of stem cells in the aetiology of cancer as well as healing and rehabilitation in the supportive care of urology patients.

The bioinformatics of stem cells in integrative medicine

Hypothesis 2: the bioinformatics of stem cells is a source of brain plasticity and rehabilitation as well as cellular pathology, such as cancer, at the genomic and proteomic levels accessible to the molecular dynamics of integrative medicine

New views of how stem cells, stress, gene expression, proteomics, brain plasticity, and healing as well as cancer are emerging in integrative medicine. Stress on all levels from

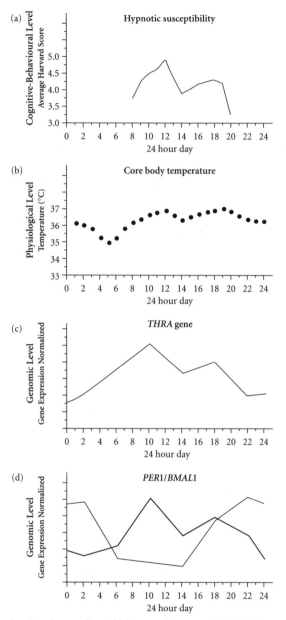

Fig. 7.2 Matching the circadian profiles of (a) hypnotic susceptibility, body temperature, and gene expression that illustrate the bioinformatic relationships between the cognitive-behavioural level, (b) the physiological level of core body temperature, and (c) the *THRA* gene associated with metabolism. Figure (d) shows how the circadian profile of the *PER1* gene, typical while awake, is similar to the *THRA* gene in (c) having a peak of expression about 90–120 min before the peak of hypnotic susceptibility and core body temperature around noon. By contrast, notice how the circadian profile of the *BMA11* (*ARNTL*) gene in (d), which is a marker for being asleep, is in *antiphase* (the opposite of) the awake profiles of *PER1* and *THRA* gene expression associated with peaks of core body temperature and hypnotic susceptibility. (From Rossi, 2004)

the psychosocial to the physical and traumatic leads to oxidation, injury, mutation, and malfunctioning on the genomic and proteomic levels. Some of the possible connections between the emerging bioinformatics of stem cells and integrative medicine can be summarized briefly.

New research on the cancer stem cell theory

Because normal stem cells in all tissues of the mature organism can replicate endlessly they have enough time to accumulate cancer-promoting mutations. While this theory of the origin of cancer via stem cells has been speculated upon about for 50 years, it was the more recent observation that testicular cancer cells had surface proteins like those of stem cells that led to much current research on the genomic theory of stem cells as potential 'bad seeds' for cancers of the prostate, breast, brain, blood, etc.[17,18] As noted above, however, research utilizing DNA microarrays is now required to assess whether integrative medicine could be efficacious in modulating the genomic and proteomic levels in cancer at the stem cell level.

Stem cells as Mother Nature's menders in rehabilitation

The presence of undifferentiated stem cells within injured tissues has been proposed as a general mechanism of recovery and rehabilitation from stress, trauma, and injury. Adult stem cells are self-replicating, multipotent cells that continue exist in adult tissues and that may be used as a source of 'spare parts' that can replace injured cells and tissues.[19] In this sense stem cells have been described as 'Mother Nature's menders' functioning as reserves within the brain and body.[20,21] It is hypothesized that the molecular messengers generated by psychosocial stress, injury, and disease can activate immediate early genes within stem cells so that they then signal the target genes required to synthesize the proteins that will transform (differentiate) the stem cells into mature well-functioning tissues. Healing via gene expression has been documented in self-renewing stem cells in the brain (including the cerebral cortex, hippocampus, and hypothalamus), muscle, skin, intestinal epithelium, bone marrow, blood, liver, heart, and the immune system.[22] Most of the integrative approaches to medicine purport to facilitate healing by reducing psychosocial stress, promoting relaxation and well-being; that such integrative approaches are efficacious at the genomic and proteomics levels of stem cell healing remains to be scientifically demonstrated.

Stem cells in neurogenesis and brain plasticity

Some of the most compelling evidence of a relationship between psychological experience and stems cells comes from the area of neurogenesis and brain plasticity.[23–25] Kandel, a Nobel laureate in medicine or physiology in 2000, discussed the implications of research on activity-dependent gene expression in the molecular genomics of memory, learning, and behaviour:[26]

> Insofar as psychotherapy or counseling is effective and produces long-term changes in behavior, it presumably does so through learning, by producing changes in gene expression that alter the

strength of synaptic connections and structural changes that alter the anatomical pattern of interconnections between nerve cells of the brain. As the resolution of brain imaging increases, it should eventually permit quantitative evaluation of the outcome of psychotherapy . . . .Stated simply, the regulation of gene expression by social factors makes all bodily functions, including all functions of the brain, susceptible to social influences. These social influences will be biologically incorporated in the altered expressions of specific genes in specific nerve cells of specific regions of the brain. *These socially influenced alterations are transmitted culturally. They are not incorporated in the sperm and egg and therefore are not transmitted genetically.* [p. 140, italics added]

Neuroscience research by Kandel and others[27–29] indicates that there are at least three classes of psychological experience that generate activity-dependent gene expression and brain plasticity via stem cell differentiation that have important implications for integrative medicine: novelty,[24,30,31] environmental enrichment,[28,32], and exercise.[29,33]

Activity-dependent gene expression facilitates the generation of functional neurons in the hippocampus of the brain, which encodes new memory, learning, and behaviour.[34,35] Most significantly for integrative medicine is how *brain plasticity* occurs in three neocortical association areas (prefrontal, inferior temporal, and posterior parietal cortex) that are involved in *behavioural plasticity* (that is, behavioural change) and associated transformations of *psychological experience*.[34,35] Gould et al.[34] conclude: 'These new neurons, which are continually added in adulthood, may play a role in the functions of association neocortex' (p. 548).

Stem cells in rehabilitation

It has been hypothesized that this process of activity-dependent gene expression and its consequent activity-dependent brain plasticity (synaptogenesis and neurogenesis) and stem cell healing is the molecular-genomic foundation of rehabilitative medicine and physical and occupational therapy as well as the many seemingly different approaches of integrative medicine.[2–4] Hood,[36] for example, has documented activity-dependent gene expression in mitochondria in skeletal, cardiac, and smooth muscle in response to physical exercise. We now need a systematic research programme to investigate the degree to which the many different approaches of integrative medicine, including touch,[37] can facilitate the novelty, environmental enrichment, and exercise which are required to evoke activity-dependent gene expression in stem cells of the body and brain to facilitate the bioinformatics cycle of healing.[4]

Of greatest interest for the practical applications of integrative medicine in urology is the 1.5 to 2 hour time frame within which new synapses develop in the brain. This relatively brief time frame means that urologists and all members of the medical team can expect that actual brain growth and the molecular dynamics of stem cell healing could be initiated at the synaptic level within a single therapeutic session. Once initiated, synaptogenesis in the brain and, presumably, stem cell healing in the body (e.g. the immune system) could, in the ideal case, continue for days, weeks, and months when the patient has been given an adequate way of facilitating their own healing. This leads us to our third major hypothesis of how an integrative approach in urology could be practiced with brief and relatively easy to learn creative psychotherapeutic approaches wherein patients learn how to solve their own problems privately in their own way.

Hypothesis 3: integrative medicine facilitates the construction and reconstruction of problematic memory, learning, behaviour, and symptoms during creative 'offline' replays of brain plasticity in the molecular dynamics of healing and physical rehabilitation

The integrative approaches to healing involve the repetition and creative replay of salient, stressful, and traumatic life experiences in what are typically called 'cultural traditions'. These cultural traditions may be of a spiritual, political, artistic, dramatic, humanistic, or so-called 'magical' and imaginative nature.[38–41] The value of creative replay in the reconstruction of human consciousness, memory, and problematic life experiences is currently recognized in the popular psychotherapeutic concept 'Every replay is a reframe'.[1] This concept finds neuroscience support by Shimizu et al.,[42] who demonstrate how the processes of repetition, recall, replay, and reconstruction are manifest in the transformations of consciousness, memory, and behaviour via the dynamics of brain plasticity. They conclude 'that *memory consolidation may require multiple rounds of site-specific synaptic modifications, possibly to reinforce plastic changes initiated during learning*, thereby making memory traces stronger and more stable.' (pp. 1172–3, italics added).

Cohen-Cory[43] provides more detail about the actual time parameters of such 'multiple rounds of site-specific synaptic modifications' or replay via activity-dependent synaptogenesis and brain plasticity:

> The anatomical refinement of synaptic circuits occurs at the level of individual axons and dendrites by a dynamic process . . . .As axons branch and re-model, synapses form and dismantle with synapse elimination occurring rapidly, in less than two hours . . . hippocampal neurons in which glutamate receptor function was altered demonstrated that synapse disassembly in the CNS occurs rapidly, within 1.5 hours after synapses are no longer functional. (p. 771)

It has been hypothesized that just as negative states of emotional arousal can evoke gene expression cascades leading to the synthesis of stress proteins and illness, so can the replay of positive psychological experiences initiate cascades of healing at the gene–protein level.[1–6,44] This implies that the replaying of positive creative human experiences of fascination, novelty, mystery, surprise, and insight experienced in the dramatic cultural rites of healing in many cultures could facilitate gene expression cascades leading to the synthesis of healing proteins.

This concept of positive, creative, therapeutic replay during 'offline' psychological states (rest, sleep, dreaming, daydreaming, meditation, prayer, etc.) as potentially important periods for integrative healing finds further support in the research of Lisman and Morris:[45]

> . . . newly acquired sensory information is funneled through the cortex to the hippocampus. Surprisingly, only the hippocampus actually learns at this time—it is said to be online. *Later*,

when the hippocampus is offline (probably during sleep), it replays stored information, transmitting it to the cortex. The cortex is considered to be a slow learner, capable of lasting memory storage only as a result of this repeated replaying of information by the hippocampus. In some views, the hippocampus is only a temporary memory store—once memory traces become stabilized in the cortex, memories can be accessed even if the hippocampus is removed. *There is now direct evidence that some form of hippocampal replay occurs . . . These results support the idea that the hippocampus is the fast online learner that 'teaches' the slower cortex offline.* [pp. 248–9, italics added]

Until recently such molecular-genomic mechanisms of brain plasticity during so-called 'offline' psychological states in rehabilitative healing and supportive care were not understood.[46] One of the most interesting lines of research has found that when experimental animals experience novelty, environmental enrichment and physical exercise, the *Egr1* gene (formerly *Zif268*) is expressed during their REM sleep.[47–49] *Zif-268* is an immediate-early and behavioural-state related gene that is associated with the generation of proteins and growth factors that facilitate brain plasticity. Ribeiro has most recently summarized his results as follows:[50]

The discovery of experience-dependent brain reactivation during both slow-wave (SW) and rapid eye-movement (REM) sleep led to the notion that the consolidation of recently acquired *memory traces requires neural replay during sleep . . . .*Based on our current and previous results, we propose that the 2 major periods of sleep play distinct and complementary roles in memory consolidation: pretranscriptional recall during SW sleep and transcriptional storage during REM sleep . . . .In conclusion, *sustained neuronal reverberation during SW sleep, immediately followed by plasticity-related gene expression during REM sleep, may be sufficient to explain the beneficial role of sleep* on the consolidation of new memories. [pp. 126–35, italics added]

Research reviewed above describing how novelty and enriched environments can initiate gene expression leading to the formation of brain plasticity is the basis of our hypothesis about positive, creative, therapeutic replay during offline periods as the essence of integrative healing illustrated in Fig. 7.3. This figure illustrates a continuum of integrative healing ranging from high to low states of circadian psychobiological arousal that is confirmed by many studies that suggest that different belief systems about cultural and so-called 'spiritual healing' of integrative medicine emphasize different parts of the same continuum[51,52] of the four-stage creative process, which we will now document with two case histories.

Case examples of the four-stage creative approach in urology

Case 1: amelioration of periurethral warts

A woman in her thirties experiencing a period of emotional transition and stress reports unusual sensations of burning and heat in her urethra and bladder. Medical examination indicates that she is having an outbreak of periurethral warts for the first time in her life. She claims she has had no new sexual partners for over 3 years and her current partner has been faithful.

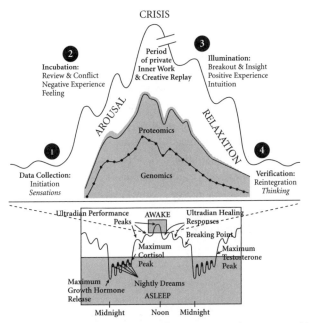

Fig. 7.3 The upper diagram outlines the classical four-stage creative process of integrative medicine as the utilization of one 90–120 minute basic rest–activity cycle (BRAC) that emerges from the genomics (redrawn from Levsky *et al.*, *Science* **297**: 836–40 (2002)) and proteomics levels (redrawn from Dill and Bromberg, *Molecular Driving Forces. Statistical Thermodynamics in Chemistry and Biology*. Garland Science, New York (2003)). The lower diagram summarizes the normal circadian (~24 hour) profile of alternating 90–120 minute ultradian (less than 20 hours) rhythms of waking and sleeping characteristic of Kleitman's 90–120 minute BRAC in a simplified manner. The ascending peaks of rapid eye movement (REM) sleep typical of nightly dreams every 90–120 minutes are illustrated with the more variable ultradian rhythms of activity, adaptation, and rest in the daytime. This lower figure illustrates how many hormonal messenger molecules of the endocrine system such, as growth hormone, the activating and stress hormone cortisol and the sexual hormone testosterone, as well as the urinary cycle (not shown) have typical 90–120 minute ultradian rhythms throughout the day (from Rossi[1]).

Stage 1: initiation by symptom scaling

The therapist initiates a therapeutic process by introducing her to symptom scaling: 'On a scale of one to ten where ten is the worst you have ever experienced that burning and heat and five is average, just how strong is your sense of burning and heat in your bladder and urethra right now?' She replies that the burning and heat is 'Seven right now', and crosses her legs with a facial grimace of distaste. The therapist asks her, 'Do you have the courage to really receive honestly just what you are feeling right now so you can fully experience what it leads to next?' This seemingly simple but novel question focuses her attention on her symptoms as bioinformatic signals that will eventually be transduced into healing and emotional insights as we shall soon see.

Stage 2: incubation and arousal

She responds with her impression that the symptom of genital warts is the source of the burning and heat she is feeling and it seems to be getting worst by the minute as she focuses on it with growing emotional fascination. The therapist supports this *novel* development by quietly murmuring an incomplete question, 'I wonder if you can allow that to continue until . . . ?' Her eyes close as she creatively replays, enriches, and exercises her psychological experience (facilitating brain plasticity?). Her body tenses and she leans forward slightly over the next 20 minutes or so as she hesitantly whispers the following bioinformatic transformations. '*Now the burning and heat are shifting around a little to my butt on the left cheek . . . now the burning and heat are moving through my body everywhere . . . its like a bad allergy . . . my head hurts . . . I feel like I should confess it all to my mother like I did as a kid . . . my right shoulder aches . . . Why is my right side trembling? . . . Why am I starting to cry? . . . Why do I still try to get approval from my mother even when she never gave it but only punished me instead? . . . I'm burning up with heat all over!*'

From a bioinformatics perspective the burning and heat she is experiencing indicates that she is going through a rather intense state of sympathetic system arousal as she experiences what has been traditionally called an 'emotional catharsis or crisis'. This is the state of 'arousal' illustrated as stage 2 of the creative cycle in Fig. 7.3. We speculate that the hormonal stress messenger molecules of the limbic—hypothalamic—pituitary—adrenal system are being released into the bloodstream where they travel to cells of the brain and body where they trigger receptors and initiate cascades of secondary messengers to signal the activation of immediate-early genes (IEGs). These IEGs turn on certain target genes to send their mRNA, blueprints for the cell's protein factories where stress and healing proteins are made.

Stage 3: illumination and insight

For a few tense minutes she continues with, '*Burning! Burning! I know . . . I know I have to leave* [her current boyfriend]. *I always knew it was only temporary, really, but now I really do have to leave . . . He punishes me too, even when he doesn't know it . . . my left knee is twitching uncontrollably . . . Can't you make it stop? . . . Oh, I'm tired of all this . . . I will leave . . . I'm getting sleepy . . . I feel warm . . . just warm now . . . I really have to leave*' [her boyfriend].

Her body sags back and she remains silent for about 3 or 4 minutes as her face gradually becomes calm, smooth, and relaxed. A profound bioinformatic transition is now taking place, which is indicated by the two line break just past the crisis peak in the upper diagram of Fig. 7.3. At this time no one really knows what is happening in this 'offline period of private creative inner work' at the moment of a cognitive-emotional breakthrough when she realizes that she must leave her boyfriend. The author originally proposed 'The neuropeptide hypothesis of consciousness and catharsis' to describe the dynamics of such creative moments.[53] From the psychobiological perspective, the arousal and relaxation phases of bioinformatic work are mediated by the release of messenger molecules such as ACTH and β-endorphin. The implication of more recent research suggests that immediate-early genes such as *FOS* and *JUN* are turned on in brain cells during emotional pain and arousal during the crisis of transition between stress and the release of relaxation hormones. This arousal may lead to the synthesis of new proteins that will facilitate brain plasticity by synthesizing new neural networks that will encode new psychological insight and healing in stage 3.

Stage 4: verification and reintegration

The therapist asks, '*What number describes what your level of comfort is now?*' Somewhat surprised she acknowledges that her symptoms are now at a level of 'one or two or maybe zero', that is, very close to complete comfort. From a bioinformatics perspective she has moved past her state of arousal and catharsis in stage two and emotional insight in stage three to a state of comfort, relaxation, and integrative healing in stage four that is so characteristic of what people typically feel when 'a job is well done'.

The therapist asks if she now knows what she has to do and she nods yes. She makes a few remarks about how she experiences a sense of relief in knowing that she now can make up her own mind with confidence about the important things in her life. She will leave her boyfriend and later she will tell others about it. A week later she reports that she has navigated the separation well, the warts have been treated, and the heat and burning sensations are gone. Microarray research on the genomic and proteomic levels is now required to document how this integrative medical approach modulated the bioinformatic state of her bladder and urethra so that her symptoms went into remission. A year later she remains symptom free and all available evidence indicates that her life was effectively 'turned around' in this single session.

Case 2: family dynamics and supportive care in urinary incontinence

For the past 3 years, while 'Gary' was playing during the day, he would have an 'accident' (urinary incontinence) and pass urine. He would then call his mother to come and take care of him. This could be very shaming for him at the school, day care, or even at home if he was playing with friends. Sometimes his mother could not get off work so the father would have to bring Gary some clean clothes. The family dynamics showed an overly strong coalition between Gary and his mother with Gary's father being distant and aloof from him. The father enjoyed Gary's brother more because, 'he's more into sports and cars like I am'. Such family dynamics indicated that more bonding was needed between Gary and his father.

Stage 1: initiating an 'offline' healing–rest–rejuvination

A few sessions were conducted with Gary and his father to help them relate together. In one session the father brought up the soiling issue. While we were discussing it Gary's eyes became moist, breathing deepened, and he began staring out the window. The therapist believed this withdrawal behaviour was at least in part related Gary's need to turn inward to cope with the shame he was experiencing. Since some of these withdrawal behaviours were similar to those that are naturally experienced when entering a natural 'offline' rest–rejuvenation period. However, the therapist reframed his obvious state of discomfort into an integrative healing response by saying, '*I notice you seem to be getting quieter in the last few minutes and you're not saying much while you're looking out the window. I wonder if that means you would really like to just rest a bit and be comfortable with your father. Just continue as you are Gary and see if it feels good to take a rest or maybe nap with your dad.*' Gary's eyes fluttered for a few minutes and then closed. The therapist signalled the father to put his arms around Gary as he snuggled close to his father.

Stage 2: healing incubation of father and son

The father then closed his eyes as the therapist stated, '*I wonder just how aware you both are doing just what you need to do to feel good together and solve your problem . . . take some time to enjoy it.*' After about 20 minutes they stirred, so the therapist said, '*Continue your good feelings together and know that good feelings can continue in the whole family when you enjoy being together. When something within you feels it has dealt with your problems as much as possible right now, will you find yourselves waking up refreshed and alert with a good stretch?*'

Stage 3: private period of creative integrative healing

After another few minutes they both opened their eyes and stretched. They commented how they had not really rested together like that since before Gary started school. Gary said, 'Even though it seemed kind of kooky I really feel good now'. A few minutes later Gary asked if he could use the bathroom, as he 'could now feel his bladder tingling'. He successfully passed urine under complete voluntary control and was obviously pleased with himself as he came out of the rest room and faced his father and the therapist with a broad smile.

Stage 4: continuing family and school 'offline healing'

Gary and his father were told to rest comfortably together this way whenever it 'felt right'. They agreed to this and Gary's school teacher was notified to let Gary lie down in the nurse's office during recess or lunch time when he asked. Gary later reported that such 'rest and napping' helped him feel what was 'going on' inside him when he needed to pass urine and he has not had an accidental voiding episode since. Recognizing the optimal therapeutic moment when Gary's shameful behaviour overlapped the typical withdrawal aspects of the normal 'offline' rest–rejuvenation phase of circadian behaviour was the key to facilitating the change that brought Gary and his father together in a comfortable bioinformatic state of healing.[54,55]

Summary

This chapter outlines a new bioinformatics model of integrative medicine that complements and is consistent with the molecular dynamics of modern medicine on the genomic, proteomic, physiological, and psychological levels. Much of integrative medicine remains controversial because the typical outcome research purporting to validate the top-down approaches of integrative medicine do not include the entire four-stage bioinformatics cycle of modern molecular medicine. We now need clinical–experimental research programmes that document the efficacy of integrative medicine with the currently emerging standards of validation via genomic and proteomic microarray technology.

References

1 **Rossi E** (2002). *The Psychobiology of Gene Expression: Neuroscience and Neurogenesis in Hypnosis and the Healing Arts*. W. W. Norton Professional Books, New York.

2 **Rossi E** (2004). Gene expression and brain plasticity in stroke rehabilitation: a personal memoir of mind-body healing dreams. *Am. J. Clin. Hypnosis* **46**(3): 215–27.

3 **Rossi E** (2004). A bioinformatics approach to the psychosocial genomics of therapeutic hypnosis. *Hypnos* **31**(1): 15–21.

4 **Rossi E** (2004). *A Discourse with Our Genes: The Neuroscience of Therapeutic Hypnosis and Psychotherapy*. Editris-S.A.S., Benevento, Italy.

5 **Rossi E** (2002). A conceptual review of the psychosocial genomics of expectancy and surprise: neuroscience perspectives about the deep psychobiology of therapeutic hypnosis. *Am. J. Clin. Hypnosis* **45**(2): 103–18.

6 **Rossi E** (2003). Gene expression, neurogenesis, and healing: psychosocial genomics of therapeutic hypnosis. *Am. J. Clin. Hypnosis* **45**(3): 197–216.

7 **Von Baeyer H** (2004). *Information: The New Language of Science*. Harvard University Press, Cambridge, MA.

8 **Stahl S** (2000). *Essential Psychopharmacology: Neuroscientific Basis and Practical Applications*. Cambridge University Press, New York.

9 **Selye H** (1974). *Stress Without Distress*. Signet, New York.

10 **Kaufer D, Friedman A, Seidman S, Soreq H** (1998). Acute stress facilitates long-lasting changes in cholinergic gene expression. *Nature* **393**: 373–7.

11 **Meshorer E, Erb C, Gazit R, Pavlovsky L, Kaufer D, Friedman A** *et al.* (2002). Alternative splicing and neuritic mRNA translocation under long-term neuronal hypersensitivity. *Science* **295**: 508–12.

12 **Rosbash M, Takahashi J** (2002). Circadian rhythms: the cancer connection. *Nature* **420**: 373–4.

13 **Petersson L, Nordin K, Glimelius B, Brekkan E, Sjödén P, Berglund G** (2002). Differential effects of cancer rehabilitation depending on diagnosis and patient's cognitive coping style. *Psychosom. Med.* **64**: 971–80.

14 **Yu T, Tsai HL, Hwang ML** (2003). Suppressing tumor progression of *in vitro* prostrate cancer cells by emitted psychosomatic power through Zen meditation. *Am. J. Chin. Med.* Summer: 3–25.

15 **Carlson L, Speca M, Patel K, Goodey E** (2003). Mindfulness-based stress reduction in relation to quality of life, mood, symptoms of stress, and immune parameters in breast and prostate cancer outpatients. *Psychosom. Med.* **65**: 571–81.

16 Graeber T, Eisenberg D (2001). Bioinformatics identification of potential autocrine signaling loops in cancers from gene expression profiles. *Nature Genet.* **29**: 295–300.

17 Al-Hajj M, Becker M, Wicha M, Weissman I, Clarke MF (2004). Therapeutic implications of cancer stem cells. *Curr. Opin. Genet. Dev.* **14**: 43–7.

18 Travis J (2004). The bad seed: rare stem cells appear to drive cancers. *Sci. News* **165**: 184–5.

19 McLaren A (2000). Cloning: pathways to a pluripotent future. *Science* **288**: 1775–80.

20 Pluchino S, Quattrini A, Brambilla E, Gritti A, Salani G, Dina G *et al.* (2003). Injection of adult neurospheres induces recovery in a chronic model of multiple sclerosis. *Nature* **422**: 688–94.

21 Vogel G (2000). Stem cells: new excitement, persistent questions. *Science* **290**: 1672–4.

22 Fuchs E, Segre J (2000). Stem cells: a new lease on life. *Cell* **100**: 143–55.

23 Sanai N, Tramontin AD, Quinones-Hinojosa A, Barbaro NM, Gupta N, Kunwar S *et al.* (2004). Unique astrocytes ribbon in adult human brain contains neural stem cells but lacks chain migration. *Science* **427**: 740–9.

24 Gage F (2000). Mammalian neural stem cells. *Science* **287**: 1433–8.

25 Kuwabara T, Hsieh J, Nakashima K, Taira K, Gage F (2004). A small modulatory dsRNA specifies the fate of adult neural stem cells. *Cell* **116**: 779–93.

26 Kandel E (1998). A new intellectual framework for psychiatry. *Am. J. Psychiat.* **155**: 457–69.

27 Lüscher C, Nicoll R, Malenka C, Muller D (2000). Synaptic plasticity and dynamic modulation of the postsynaptic membrane. *Nature Neurosci.* **3**: 545–67.

28 Kempermann G, Kuhn G, Gage F (1997). More hippocampal neurons in adult mice living in an enriched environment. *Nature* **386**: 493–5.

29 Van Praag H, Schinder A, Christie B, Toni N, Palmer T, Gage F (2002). Functional neurogenesis in the adult hippocampus. *Nature* **415**: 1030–4.

30 Eriksson P, Perfilieva E, Björk-Eriksson T, Alborn A-M, Nordborg C, Peterson D *et al.* (1998). Neurogenesis in the adult human hippocampus. *Nature Med.* **4**: 1313–17.

31 Kempermann G, Gage F (1999). New nerve cells for the adult brain. *Sci. Am.* **280**: 48–53.

32 Van Praag H, Kempermann G, Gage F (2000). Neural consequences of environmental enrichment. *Nature Rev.: Nature Neurosci.* **1**: 191–8.

33 Van Praag H, Kempermann G, Gage F (1999). Running increases cell proliferation and neurogenesis in the adult mouse dentate gyrus. *Nature Neurosci.* **2**: 266–70.

34 Gould E, Alison J, Reeves A, Michael S, Graziano S, Gross C (1999). Neurogenesis in the neocortex of adult primates. *Science* **286**: 548–52.

35 Gould E, Tanapat P, Reeves A, Shors T (1999b). Learning enhances adult neurogenesis in the hippocampal formation. *Nature Neurosci.* **2**(3): 260–5.

36 Hood D (2001). Plasticity in skeletal, cardiac, and smooth muscle. Invited review: Contractile activity-induced mitochondrial biogenesis in skeletal muscle. *J. Appl. Physiol.* **90**: 1137–57.

37 Schanberg S (1995). The genetic basis for touch effects. In: *Touch in Early Development* (ed. T. Field), pp. 67–79. Lawrence Erlbaum, New York.

38 Greenfield S (1994). A model explaining Brazilian spiritist surgeries and other unusual religious-based healing. *Subtle Energies* **5**: 109–41.

39 Greenfield S (2000). Religious altered states and cultural-biological transduction in healing. Paper presented at Congresso Brasilerio de Etnopsiciatria, Fortaleza CE, 28–30 September 2000. *Rev. Brasil. Etnopsiquiatr.*

40 Keeney B (1999–2000). *Profiles in Healing*, Vols 1–4. Ringing Rock Press, Philadelphia, PA.

41 Otto R (1923/1950). *The Idea of the Holy*. Oxford University Press, New York.

42 Shimizu E, Tang Y, Rampon C, Tsien J (2000). NMDA receptor-dependent synaptic reinforcement as a crucial process for memory consolidation. *Science* **290**: 1170–4.

43 Cohen-Cory S. (2002). The developing synapse: construction and modulation of synaptic structures and circuits. *Science* **298**: 770–6.

44 Rossi E (2003). The bioinformatics of psychosocial genomics in alternative and complementary medicine. *Forsch. Komplementärmed. Klass. Naturheilkd.* **10**: 143–50.

45 Lisman J, Morris G (2001). Why is the cortex a slow learner? *Nature* **411**: 248–9.

46 Strickgold R, Hobson J, Fosse R, Fosse M (2001). Sleep, learning, and dreams: off-line memory reprocessing. *Science* **294**: 1052–7.

47 Ribeiro S, Goyal V, Mello C, Pavlides C (1999). Brain gene expression during REM sleep depends on prior waking experience. *Learning and Memory* **6**: 500–8.

48 Ribeiro S, Mello C, Velho T, Gardner T, Jarvis E, Pavlides C (2002). Induction of hippocampal long-term potentiation during waking leads to increased extrahippocampal zif-268 expression during ensuing rapid-eye-movement sleep. *J. Neurosci.* **22**(24): 10914–23.

49 Ribeiro S (2003). Dream, memory and Freud's reconciliation with the brain. *Rev. Brasil. Psiquiatr.* **25**: 1–13.

50 Ribeiro S, Gervasoni D, Soares E, Zhou Y, Lin S, Pantoja J *et al.* (2004). Long-lasting novelty-induced neuronal reverberation during slow-wave sleep in multiple forebrain areas. *Public Library Sci. Biol. (PLoS)* **2**(1): 126–37.

51 d'Aquili E, Newberg A (1999). *The Mystical Mind: Probing the Biology of Religious Experience.* Fortress Press, Minneapolis, MN.

52 Glik D (1993). Beliefs, practices, and experiences of spiritual healing adherents in an American industrial city. In: *Yearbook of Cross-Cultural Medicine and Psychotherapy, 1992* (ed. W. Andritsky), pp. 199–223. Verlag für Wissenschaft und Bildung, Berlin.

53 Rossi E, Cheek D (1988). *Mind-Body Therapy: Methods of Ideodynamic Healing in Hypnosis.* Norton Professional Books, New York.

54 Rossi E, Nimmons D (1991). *The 20 Minute Break: Using the New Science of Ultradian Rhythms.* Zeig, Tucker and Theisen: Phoenix, AZ.

55 West A, Griffith E, Greenberg M (2002). Regulation of transcription factors by neuronal activity. *Nature Rev. Neurosci.* **3**: 921–31.

Chapter 8

The patient presenting with haematuria

Kamal Mattar and Darrel E. Drachenberg

Introduction

The patient presenting with haematuria may have no symptoms and may have been discovered on a routine urinalysis or may have obvious gross bleeding with clots and the difficulty voiding and fear that that entails. Although the latter may require aggressive acute management both may or may not portend serious underlying disease and need an organized investigative approach. This chapter will review in detail strategies for dealing with both situations.

Microhaematuria

The identification of microscopic haematuria may be the first sign of an underlying urological disease, yet the dilemma is that all healthy individuals excrete some erythrocytes in the urine. Thus, the ideal definition of significant microscopic haematuria should allow for the discrimination of essential haematuria which requires no further investigation and significant haematuria which requires further work-up to discern underlying pathology. The definition of microscopic varies from one to ten red blood cells per high-power field (RBCs/HPF). The Canadian and American Urological Associations recommend further investigation of patients who persistently have more than three RBCs/HPF in their urine. Most studies suggest a weak correlation between the degree of microscopic haematuria and the likelihood of detecting significant urological disease.[1,2] It is postulated that the presence of any degree of haematuria identifies patients at risk of serious urological disease. For instance, the risk of bladder tumours is two-fold higher in patients with microscopic haematuria than in those without.[3]

Epidemiology

Mass screening studies estimate the prevalence of microscopic haematuria to range from 0.18 to 16.1%.[1,3–5] The actual prevalence is influenced by a number of variables, which include the age and sex distribution of the population studied and the type and frequency of the screening test. Most studies report a higher prevalence of microhaematuria amongst male subjects, older patients, and referral-based populations.[6,7]

Aetiology

The source of the haematuria may be glomerular, upper urinary tract, or lower urinary tract in origin. The incidence of glomerular bleeding is difficult to ascertain, since not all patients screened for microhaematuria are evaluated for medical renal disease, and they are rarely subjected to renal biopsies. In a study of 165 patients (mean age 37.5 years) referred with isolated microscopic haematuria, renal biopsy abnormalities were found in 46.6% of patients.[8] The most common glomerular disorders were IgA nephropathy and mesangial proliferative glomerulonephritis (49/77 and 16/77, respectively). Therefore, glomerular disease is recognized as a common cause of persistent microscopic haematuria, particularly in patients aged less than 40. The diagnosis is important to establish because a significant number of patients progress to renal failure.

The presence of dysmorphic red blood cells or RBC casts and proteinuria on urine microscopy and analysis also helps confirm glomerular causes of haematuria. Another common medical cause of haematuria is papillary necrosis, a condition that should be considered in patients with diabetes mellitus, sickle cell disease, or patients known to be analgesic abusers.

Non-glomerular sources of haematuria, whether microscopic or gross, involving the kidney and upper urinary tract include malignant, infectious, and stone diseases. Lower urinary tract bleeding may arise from lesions in the bladder, prostate, or urethra. The causes of microhaematuria may be categorized into highly significant, moderately significant, or insignificant lesions, as shown in Table 8.1.[1,9] This categorization aids clinicians in prioritizing treatment of the underlying disease. Highly significant lesions are life-threatening or disabling to the patient, and usually require urgent intervention. Moderately significant lesions are not immediately life-threatening, but lead to significant morbidity if untreated. Insignificant lesions generally require treatment only if they are symptomatic. Urothelial cancer and renal cell carcinoma (RCC) are the most common life-threatening causes of haematuria (Figs 8.1 and 8.2). Renal cell carcinoma comprises a heterogeneous group of renal tumours with diverse histologies and differing underlying genetic mechanisms of tumourigenesis. Transitional cell carcinoma (TCC) accounts for more than 90% of urothelial tumours. The risk of TCC increases significantly beyond the age of 65, particularly when associated with specific risk factors that include cigarette smoking, exposure to chemicals used in the leather, dye, and rubber industries, abuse of phenacetin, and treatment with cyclophosphamide (Table 8.2).

Catheter-induced haematuria

Haematuria that occurs immediately following urethral catheterization is usually the result of urethral or bladder mucosal abrasion. It may also be related to the presence of local or systemic factors (e.g. urethral strictures, polyps, prostatic hypertrophy, or clotting abnormalities). Persistent gross haematuria induced by urethral catheterization is

Table 8.1 Lesions of the genitourinary tract associated with microscopic haematuria

Association	Lesion
Highly significant	Renal cell carcinoma
	Renal transitional cell carcinoma
	Ureteral transitional cell carcinoma
	Bladder cancer
	Prostate cancer
	Ureteral calculus
	Metastatic carcinoma
	Abdominal aortic aneurysm
Moderately significant	Renal calculus
	Bladder calculus
	Cystitis
	Pyelonephritis
	Symptomatic benign prostatic hyperplasia
	Vesicoureteral reflux
	Interstitial cystitis
	Bladder diverticulum
	Ureteropelvic junction obstruction
	Renal disease
	Prostatitis
	Urethritis
	Bladder papilloma
Insignificant	Renal cyst
	Asymptomatic benign prostatic hyperplasia
	Cystocele
	Overactive bladder
	Urethrotrigonitis
	Prostatic calculi
	Ureterocele
	Cystitis cystica/glandularis
	Bladder trabeculation
	Urethral polyp
	Renal cyst

uncommon. In studies of patients requiring catheterization, 44 to 67% developed transient catheter-induced haematuria.[10–12] The magnitude of the haematuria was very small, and only one patient developed gross haematuria. These data are helpful in differentiating haematuria caused by the catheter from that due to disease states. Thus, most clinicians will only evaluate gross haematuria if it persists beyond the initial stage, or after the catheter has been removed; microscopic haematuria is expected as long as the catheter is in place.

Some degree of gross haematuria is also a recognized risk following urinary drainage of a distended bladder by a catheter, occurring in 2 to 16% of patients.[13] The risk may increase the more rapidly the bladder is decompressed but is usually very mild and

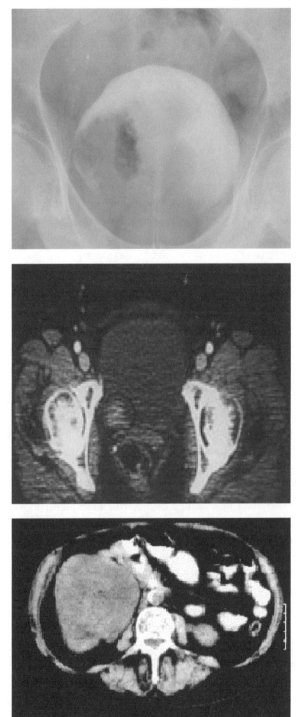

Fig. 8.1 Cystogram and appearance of a transitional cell carcinoma (TCC) in the bladder. Note the classic-appearing filling defect seen on the cystogram that is pathognomonic of TCC.

Fig. 8.2 Computed tomography (CT) appearance of renal cell carcinoma. Unequivocal enhancement of + 10 Hounsfield units aids in diagnosis. Note the invasion of the renal hilum with tumour that presented with gross haemauria in this patient.

Table 8.2 Risk factors for bladder cancer that should be elicited in a comprehensive history for patients presenting with haematuria

Smoking. Relative risk increase up to 50%

Occupational exposures: dyes—textiles, painters, hairdressers; associated with volatile chemical exposure

Chemical carcinogens: 2-naphthylamine, benzidine, 4-aminobiphenyl, nitrosamines

Analgesic abuse—phenacetin, NSAIDs?

Cyclophoshamide treatment—leukaemias, etc.

Pelvic irradiation

Genitourinary tuberculosis

Balkan nephropathy—upper tract transitional cell carcinoma

Schistosomiasis—*Schistosoma haematobium* (ova deposited in bladder wall and diffuse inflammatory reaction)

Chronic infection: indwelling Foley (5% of paraplegics develop bladder cancer)

Bladder calculi

Bladder diverticuli

Bladder exstrophy

Urinary diversion or augment with intestinal segments

Urachal origin

Endometriosis

Cystitis glanularis/pelvic lipomatosis

inconsequential; there is no need to partially empty the bladder and plug the catheter in a repetitive fashion; it should be allowed to drain freely.

Evaluation of microhaematuria

The evaluation of a patient with microhaematuria begins with a careful medical history and a focused physical examination. It is important to establish whether the micro-haematuria is asymptomatic or associated with irritative voiding symptoms suggesting a lower urinary tract cause or back or flank pain suggesting an upper tract one. Historical elements that should be elicited include a history of stones and risk factors for urological malignancy such as those mentioned for bladder cancer (Table 8.2), family history of urological malignancies, especially RCC given its genetic predisposition, and a determination of smoking history and the risk it imparts. A focused physical examination includes assessment of blood pressure, overall appearance looking for cachexia, assessment of peripheral lymphadenopathy, abdominal examination palpating for tenderness, masses and bladder distension, costovertebral angle for tenderness, as well as a digital rectal examination. A review of current medications with particular reference to the use of antiplatelet agents and systemic anticoagulants is important since anticoagulation therapy may aggravate any underlying cause of haematuria.[14] In a small series of patients evaluated for gross haematuria while receiving anticoagulation, tumours were found in 18% of the subjects.[15]

Urine dipstick testing is usually the test that picks up microscopic haematuria. The sensitivity of dipstick testing for blood in the urine is over 90%.[1,9,16] Practically, this may be too sensitive, since it detects as little as one to two RBCs/HPF. Positivity is the result of a peroxidase-like reaction that is catalysed by either free haemoglobin or myoglobin. The specificity of dipstick testing is lower because the presence of free myoglobin or haemoglobin in the urine without erythrocytes leads to false positive results. Consequently, a positive dipstick for blood should always be confirmed by microscopy of centrifuged urine for erythrocytes, leucocytes, casts, and bacteria. This can be done by centrifugation of 10 ml of urine specimen for 5 minutes at 2000 r.p.m. The supernatant is decanted, and the sediment is resuspended in the remaining urine by gently tapping the tube. A drop of the mixture is placed on a slide, a cover-slip is applied, and the specimen is examined under low- (10 $\times$) and high-power (40 $\times$) microscopy.

Most authorities suggest that if microhaematuria is absent on repeat testing, further evaluation is not indicated unless risk factors for urothelial cancer are present.[1,17,18] Transient microhaematuria may be due to urinary contamination with menstrual blood, dehydration resulting in increased erythrocyte concentration in the urine, sexual intercourse, vigorous exercise, or mild trauma. Alternatively, red-coloured urine may not indicate bleeding at all, since certain drugs (e.g. pyridium) and foods (e.g. beets and red berries) can discolour urine into shades of red.

Initial evaluation of the urine may also reveal concomitant proteinuria, which usually mandates a 24-hour urine collection to quantitate total protein excretion and creatinine clearance. The documentation of marked proteinuria, RBC casts, dysmorphic RBCs, or renal insufficiency warrants nephrological consultation. Urine culture is obtained to confirm or rule out urinary tract infection if pyuria or bacteriuria is present. Voided urine cytology has a 40 to 76% sensitivity in detecting bladder cancer.[1] It is especially important to evaluate urine cytology in low-risk patients with microhaematuria, since cystoscopy may not be indicated in this subgroup.[19–21] The specificity of urine cytology for transitional cell carcinoma (TCC) approaches 100%; therefore, positive cytology mandates further investigation until the location of the primary tumour is identified, whether upper or lower urinary tract.

Following the initial investigations, if a glomerular source of haematuria is considered unlikely, the upper urinary tract should be imaged. Excretory urography had traditionally been performed to examine the upper tracts for a source of bleeding (Fig. 8.3). Excretory urography provides clear visualization of the collecting system and ureters, thus it accurately reveals urothelial tumours of the upper urinary tract. However, TCC of the renal pelvis or ureter account for less than 10% of all upper urinary tract tumours in comparison with RCC, which accounts for the overwhelming majority of upper tract tumours.[9] Ultrasonography detects renal tumours better than excretory

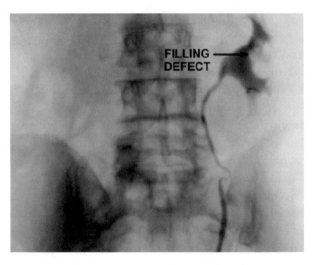

FILLING
DEFECT

Fig. 8.3 Contrast pyelography of upper tract transitional cell carcinoma demonstrating the pathognomonic finding of a renal pelvic filling defect.

urography. It can also accurately define hydronephrosis, which may be related to obstruction secondary to ureteric lesions, a finding that should prompt further investigations. Due to its equivalent efficacy and ease of performance, ultrasonography is currently recommended over excretory urography for upper urinary tract imaging in the investigation of most patients with microhaematuria.[1,17]

A positive finding at initial evaluation of the upper urinary tracts usually requires further imaging to better define the nature and extent of the disease. Computed tomography (CT) is a superior modality for imaging the kidneys, particularly for suspected tumours less than 3 cm in diameter (Fig. 8.2).[1,22,23] One study compared the efficacy of excretory urography, ultrasonography and CT in the detection of renal masses in patients with haematuria and found a relative insensitivity of excretory urography for detecting masses less than 3 cm (10 to 52% sensitivity) and of ultrasonography for masses less than 2 cm (26 to 60% sensitivity).[23]

Imaging of the upper urinary tract in patients with asymptomatic microhaematuria consists of excretory urography and/or renal ultrasound and is limited by a false negative rate of up to 16%.[6,22,24] Recent studies assert that helical CT accurately detects renal masses less than 3 cm, improves the characterization of such lesions, and categorizes various renal lesions into inflammatory, neoplastic, or cystic types. Thus, CT is superior to both urography and ultrasonography for the detection of renal parenchymal tumours. However, the role of CT in initial screening of asymptomatic microhaematuria is controversial due to its associated increased cost and morbidity, without substantially improved accuracy.[25] Most institutions reserve CT imaging for patients at high risk for malignant disease. CT also plays an important role in the evaluation of cases in which urographic or ultrasonographic results are equivocal, yet clinical suspicion of disease is high.

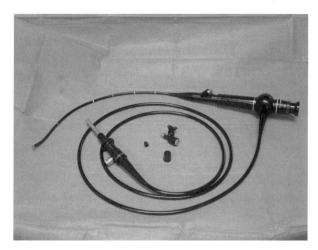

Fig. 8.4 Flexible cystoscopy is used to evaluate the urethra and bladder for pathological aetiology of haematuria.

Examination of the lower urinary tract is necessary if the source of haematuria remains undefined after investigating the upper tracts. Unfortunately, although voided urine cytology has a high sensitivity and specificity for the detection of a high-grade tumour somewhere in the urinary tract, its sensitivity for low-grade tumours is poor.[26] Unless a clearly defined lesion is detected in the upper tracts, cystoscopy must be carried out to confidently rule out malignant disease of the urethra and bladder. It is performed with a flexible cystoscope under local anaesthesia (Fig. 8.4). The American Urological Association guidelines for the evaluation of microscopic haematuria recommend cystoscopy for all persons who are older than 40 years of age.[17] In a study of 100 men under the age of 40 referred for evaluation of microscopic haematuria, no cases of urothelial cancer were identified by cystoscopy.[19] The literature provides even less support for cystoscopy in women under the age of 40 with asymptomatic microscopic haematuria, since women have a lower incidence of urothelial tumours.[20,21] Still, cystoscopic evaluation of the bladder is justified in all patients with microhaematuria and associated risk factors for bladder cancer, such as smoking, environmental exposure to carcinogens, or family history.

Despite evaluation of the upper and lower urinary tracts, the source of the haematuria will not be identified in the majority of patients. The positive predictive value (PPV) of asymptomatic microhaematuria for a serious and treatable urological lesion ranges from 0 to 2%.[21,27] An additional 18% of patients manifest a moderately significant urological lesion.[21] By contrast, more recent studies suggest that a full evaluation of microhaematuria—including repeat urinalysis, urine culture, urine cytology, intravenous urography, and/or ultrasonography and cystoscopy—will yield a cause for the haematuria in 32 to 100% of patients.[1,6,24] However, if the cause of microhaematuria is not identified after initial evaluation, further investigations are not indicated, unless new genitourinary symptoms develop or the degree of haematuria progresses.

Screening for microhaematuria

In the general population, testing for microhaematuria yields too low of a rate of significant urological disease to justify screening.[18,21] Thus, no major organization currently recommends screening for haematuria in asymptomatic adults.[28] Evidence from five population-based studies showed that haematuria screening in asymptomatic adults and subsequent evaluation yields serious and treatable urinary tract disease in less than 2% of patients.[4] Similarly, a large Japanese screening study of 823 adults with asymptomatic haematuria demonstrated that the PPV for urothelial carcinoma and RCC were 2.1% and 0.2%, respectively.[29] However, in the same study, male gender and age over 50 years increased the PPV for urothelial carcinoma to 6.2%. These results suggest that even though there is no role for screening for haematuria to detect RCC, it may be appropriate to detect urothelial carcinoma in men older than 50 years. Whether earlier detection of bladder cancer, as a result of screening, may result in better long-term outcomes remains unknown.

Gross haematuria

The presence of more than 100 RBCs/HPF signifies gross haematuria, because at this level blood is visually apparent in the urine. The discovery of frank blood in the urine is an alarming sign for patients and health-care professionals. Although the degree of haematuria may correlate with the likelihood of detecting an underlying disease, the presence of even a single episode of macroscopic haematuria warrants complete urological evaluation. Evaluation of the urinary tract should be promptly initiated in order to rule out serious urological disease, including malignancy. Macroscopic haematuria is caused by urological malignant disease in 17 to 27% of cases, mostly being TCC of the bladder.[30]

The approach to a patient with gross haematuria is similar to the evaluation of microhaematuria. On history, key characteristics of the haematuria may provide clues to the source of the bleeding. For instance, the timing of the haematuria during voiding—classified into initial, terminal, or total—may indicate the source of the bleeding. Initial haematuria is bleeding noted during the initial portion of the voided stream only, and it usually indicates urethral origin. Terminal haematuria occurs at the end of micturition during bladder neck contraction and it localizes the bleeding to the bladder neck or prostatic urethra. Haematuria that persists throughout the voided stream results from bleeding from the bladder or upper urinary tracts. If suprapubic pain or obstructive voiding symptoms are associated with the haematuria and clots, one should suspect clot retention. Renal colic in this scenario is usually the result of 'clot colic', i.e. sudden onset of ureteric obstruction secondary to a blood clot.

The presence of blood clots within the urine usually suggests a significant amount of bleeding and may warrant the insertion of a large 22–24F three-way (i.e. triple-lumen) catheter for manual irrigation of the bladder for clots with a Toomey syringe and then establishment of continuous bladder irrigation (CBI). The aim of CBI is to disrupt and evacuate blood clots from the bladder. With this conservative approach, gross haematuria resolves spontaneously in the majority of patients if all of the clots have been removed. Often this cannot be accomplished at the bedside and, if the bleeding persists or the catheter blocks repetitively from clots, the patient requires prompt endoscopic evaluation. Cystoscopy allows for irrigation and removal of all clots and potentially identifies the source of bleeding, whether it is from the urethra, bladder, or the upper urinary tract (i.e. if a jet of red urine is observed from a ureteric orifice). The latter is typically secondary to a renal cell carcinoma and is usually an indication for radical nephrectomy or renal artery embolization in patients who are not candidates for surgery. If the aetiology of the gross haematuria is still obscure after cystoscopy, imaging of the upper urinary tracts is indicated as discussed previously. If necessary, coagulation parameters should be corrected with vitamin K, plasma, platelets, and/or cryoprecipitate as indicated.

Following complete investigation of the urinary system, the aetiology of the haematuria remains obscure in many patients. Although appropriate follow-up of these patients is controversial, it is commonly accepted that no further investigations are needed.[30,31] Failure to find a cause after initial evaluation suggests a benign, self-limited process and patients should be reassured. In one study of 146 patients with unexplained macroscopic haematuria investigated up to 10 years following initial evaluation, only one patient had a missed tumour at follow-up and this was detected on further investigation for recurrent bleeding.[30] Although the chance of finding significant urological disease—after normal initial investigations—is unlikely, further investigation is warranted in patients who have recurrent bleeding or who develop new voiding symptoms. In addition, patients with risk factors for urological malignancies should undergo repeat cystoscopy and imaging, since progression of a missed lesion may be appreciated.

Intractable haematuria

Haemorrhagic cystitis is a disorder associated with diffuse bleeding from diseased bladder urothelium that manifests as intractable haematuria. The range of hemorrhage varies from mild to severe, where it can be life-threatening and its management remains a difficult clinical problem. Mild haemorrhage is associated with normal haemoglobin. Moderate haemorrhage is associated with a drop in haemoglobin and a transfusion requirement of less than six units of blood. Severe haemorrhage is defined by massive intractable bleeding requiring more than six units of blood. Haemorrhagic cystitis may be further categorized into acute or chronic. Acute bleeding from the bladder may arise from a severe infection, bladder carcinoma, or acute/chronic radiation cystitis. Chronic bleeding is a consequence of delayed radiation cystitis or cyclophosphamide-induced cystitis. The incidence of haemorrhagic cystitis following cyclophosphamide treatment is between 4 and 40%.[32]

Treatment of haemorrhagic cystitis

The initial management of any grade of haematuria begins with evacuation of all clots from the bladder and establishment of CBI as discussed previously. Intravesical therapy is considered when conservative therapy for intractable haematuria fails, and before surgical options are contemplated. The decision to use a particular treatment depends on the severity of the haematuria, the patient's health, anaesthetic requirement, and available therapies. Intravesical options for intractable haematuria include alum, formalin, or prostaglandin instillation, each of which has specific indications, modes of action, and complications.

Alum, either as potassium or ammonium aluminium sulphate, irrigation has been used successfully in the treatment of haemorrhagic cystitis[33,34] by acting as an astringent of protein precipitation at the bleeding cell surface. This leads to capillary vasoconstriction and decreased permeability. A typical application consists of closed irrigation with a 1 to 4% alum solution in sterile water at a rate of up to 1 l/h for 12 to 24 h.[35] High-flow irrigation through a large-bore triple-lumen catheter is maintained, since alum aggregates can precipitate and clog catheters. The main advantage of alum irrigation over other intravesical therapies is that it can be carried out at the bedside, without the need for anaesthesia. Aside from local bladder irritation, side-effects are minor and irrigation is well tolerated. Toxicity is low because alum has poor cellular permeability, so its action is limited to the cell surface and interstitial space. Nonetheless, acidosis, encephalopathy, and convulsions may be associated with toxic levels of serum aluminium (greater than 10 μmol/l); therefore, clinical monitoring and serum aluminium levels should be measured, particularly in patients with renal insufficiency.[35]

Due to serious complications, formalin instillations are reserved for patients who have failed more conservative measures.[36–38] Formalin is a fixative, and when it is instilled intravesically it acts by hydrolysing and precipitating cellular proteins of the bladder mucosa. It has an occluding effect on telangiectatic tissue and small capillaries. Prior to instillation, all patients must undergo cystography to exclude vesicoureteric reflux, since formalin can cause dramatic ureteric fibrosis and strictures. Formalin must be instilled under general or spinal anaesthesia because intravesical instillation is associated with significant bladder pain. Various protocols have been described for its instillation; however, the most important variable is the concentration of the formalin solution, which is closely related to the efficacy and complication rate of treatment. Concentrations ranging from 1 to 10% formalin solution have been described, although a 75% complication rate is associated with the 10% solution.[36] The complications are related to the fixative effect of formalin, and they include a small fibrotic bladder, urinary incontinence, vesicoureteric reflux, ureteric strictures, acute tubular necrosis, fistula formation, and bladder rupture.[35] In contrast, formalin concentrations of less than 4% are associated with a much lower complication rate.[38] Formalin may be either instilled up to bladder capacity or irrigated through and through for 15 minutes. Success rates for controlling massive haematuria are reported to be between 80 to 100%.[35]

Prostaglandins (PGs) have been used in the treatment of haemorrhagic cystitis secondary to cyclophosphamide therapy and after bone marrow transplantation.[35,39] Cyclophosphamide is an alkylating agent used in the treatment of malignancies and benign inflammatory conditions. The hepatic metabolite of cyclophosphamide is acrolein; it is excreted in the urine and causes haemorrhagic and ulcerative necrosis of the urothelium.[35] For prevention, 2-mercaptoethanesulphonic acid (MESNA), bladder irrigation, and hyperhydration with adequate diuresis are advocated.[40] MESNA is a thiol compound that reacts with acrolein, resulting in its detoxification.[41] Prophylactic intravesical instillation of PGs may also prevent haemorrhagic cystitis. It is postulated that PGs are cytoprotective by regulating a mucous barrier and stimulating platelet aggregation and vasoconstriction.[35] In patients with severe cyclophosphamide-induced haemorrhagic cystitis, intravesical PG therapy resolved the gross haematuria in one-half of the patients.[39] Although bladder spasms occurred in the majority of patients, there were no serious reactions and the treatment was well tolerated. Oral pentosan polysulphate can also be use to help replace the glycosaminogylcan layer of the bladder mucosa and stop the bleeding.

Embolization

Embolization of the bladder for the control of bladder haemorrhage was first reported in 1974.[42] Muscle fragments were used to occlude the internal iliac artery in a patient with severe bleeding from radiation cystitis. Since its initial description, the efficacy of therapeutic embolization in the control of severe haematuria has been reported to be greater than 90%.[35,43,44] The internal iliac artery is typically catheterized from the femoral artery and very selective control of bleeding points can be achieved by catheterizing the anterior branch of the internal iliac artery, or even the more distal superior and inferior vesical branches. Superselective embolization is believed to reduce the complications[45] which can include gluteal pain, distal embolization of the lower limb, or gangrene of the bladder.[35]

Hyperbaric oxygen

Hyperbaric oxygen reverses radiation-induced endarteritis by stimulating neovascularization of the bladder wall.[46–48] Cystoscopy after hyperbaric oxygen therapy shows resolution of haemorrhagic sites and telangiectasia.[49] Patients typically receive 100% oxygen in a hyperbaric chamber for 90 minutes daily for 20 to 40 treatments. Prospective studies evaluating the efficacy of hyperbaric oxygen therapy for severe haematuria suggest a resolution rate of up to 90%.[46–48] Major complications related to hyperbaric oxygen treatment are rare.

Surgical management

Very rarely, non-surgical measures fail to control intractable haemorrhagic cystitis, and surgical intervention may be indicated. Diverting the urine from the bladder mucosa may help. Complete supravesical urinary diversion via bilateral nephrostomy tubes or ileal conduit will promptly and consistently control life-threatening bladder haemorrhage.[50] However, the type of urinary diversion should be based on the general condition of the patient and the status of the primary disease. It is almost never necessary to remove the bladder.[50,51]

Conclusion

The presence of haematuria, either microscopic or gross, merits evaluation with a thorough history, physical examination, upper tract imaging, and lower tract endoscopy to rule out significant pathological entities that are potentially correctable. Haematuria that is intractable can be a significant challenge to health-care professionals and a variety of specialties may need to be involved including urologists, haematologists, radiologists, and medical/radiation oncologists. When a specific cause is identified its primary treatment should be expedited; when this is impossible or unsuccessful some of the strategies reviewed here should be tried. In many cases, prompt evaluation of patients with microscopic or gross haematuria may prevent progression to incurable malignant disease.

References

1 Grossfeld GD, Carroll PR (1998). Evaluation of asymptomatic microscopic hematuria. *Urol. Clin. N. Am.* **25**: 661–76.

2 Fracchia Ja, Motta J, Miller LS, Armenakas NA, Schumann GB, Greenberg RA (1995). Evaluation of asymptomatic microhematuria. *Urology* **46**: 484–9.

3 Hiatt RA, Ordonez JD (1994). Dipstick urinalysis screening, asymptomatic microhematuria, and subsequent urological cancers in a population-based sample. *Cancer Epidemiol. Biomarkers Prev.* **3**: 439–43.

4 Woolhandler S, Pels RJ, Bor DH, Himmelstein DU, Lawrence RS (1989). Dipstick urinalysis screening of asymptomatic adults for urinary tract disorders: I. Hematuria and proteinuria. *J. Am. Med. Assoc.* **262**: 1214–19.

5 Froom P, Ribak J, Benbassat J (1984). Significance of microhaematuria in young adults. *Br. Med. J. (Clin. Res. Ed.)* **288**: 20–2.

6 Messing EM, Young TB, Hunt VB, Wehbie JM, Rust P (1989). Urinary tract cancers found by homescreening with hematuria dipsticks in healthy men over 50 years of age. *Cancer* **64**: 2361–7.

7 Britton JP, Dowell AC, Whelan P, Harris CM (1992). A community study of bladder cancer screening by the detection of occult urinary bleeding. *J. Urol.* **148**: 788–90.

8 Topham PS, Harper SJ, Furness PN, Harris KP, Walls J, Feehally J (1994). Glomerular disease as a cause of isolated microscopic haematuria. *Q. J. Med.* **87**: 329–35.

9 Patrick CW (ed.) (2003). *Campbell's Urology*, 8th edn. Elsevier Science, New York.

10 Sklar DP, Diven B, Jones J (1986). Incidence and magnitude of catheter-induced hematuria. *Am. J. Emerg. Med.* **4**: 14–16.

11 Khoubehi B, Watkin NA, Mee AD, Ogden CW (2000). Morbidity and the impact on daily activities associated with catheter drainage after acute urinary retention. *BJU Int.* **85**: 1033–6.

12 Petursson SR, Weintraub M (1975). Incidence and range of microscopic hematuria in patients with indwelling urinary catheters. *Res. Commun. Chem. Pathol. Pharmacol.* **12**: 513–20.

13 Nyman MA, Schwenk NM, Silverstein MD (1997). Management of urinary retention: rapid versus gradual decompression and risk of complications. *Mayo Clin. Proc.* **72**: 951–6.

14 Van Savage JG, Fried FA (1995). Anticoagulant associated hematuria: a prospective study. *J. Urol.* **153**: 1594–6.

15 Avidor Y, Nadu A, Matzkin H (2000). Clinical significance of gross hematuria and its evaluation in patients receiving anticoagulant and aspirin treatment. *Urology* **55**: 22–4.

16 Ahn JH, Morey AF, McAninch JW (1998). Workup and management of traumatic hematuria. *Emerg. Med. Clin. N. Am.* **16**: 145–64.

17 Grossfeld GD, Litwin MS, Wolf JS Jr, Hricak H, Shuler CL, Agerter DC *et al.* (2001). Evaluation of asymptomatic microscopic hematuria in adults: the American Urological Association best practice policy—part II: patient evaluation, cytology, voided makers, imaging, cystoscopy, nephrology evaluation, and follow-up. *Urology* **57**: 604–10.

18 Tomson C, Porter T (2002). Asymptomatic microscopic or dipstick haematuria in adults: which investigations for which patients? A review of the evidence. *BJU Int.* **90**: 185–98.

19 Jones DJ, Langstaff RJ, Holt SD, Morgans BT (1988). The value of cystourethroscopy in the investigation of microscopic haematuria in adult males under 40 years: a prospective study of 100 patients. *Br. J. Urol.* **62**: 541–5.

20 Bard RH (1988). The significance of asymptomatic microhematuria in women and its economic implications: a ten-year study. *Arch. Intern. Med.* **148**: 2629–32.

21 Mohr DN, Offord KP, Owen RA, Melton LJ (1986). Asymptomatic microhematuria and urologic disease. A population-based study. *J. Am. Med. Assoc.* **256**: 224–9.

22 Lang EK, Macchia RJ, Thomas R, Ruiz-Deya G, Watson RA, Richter F *et al.* (2002). Computerized tomography tailored for the assessment of microscopic hematuria. *J. Urol.* **167**: 547–54.

23 Warshauer DM, Hammers L, Taylor C, Rosenfield AT (1988). Detection of renal masses: sensitivities and specificities of excretory urography/linear tomography, US, and CT. *Radiology* **169**: 363–5.

24 Murakami S, Igarashi T, Hara S, Shimazaki J (1990). Strategies for asymptomatic microscopic hematuria: a prospective study of 1,034 patients. *J. Urol.* **144**: 99–101.

25 O'Malley ME, Hahn PF, Yoder IC, Gazelle GS, McGovern FJ, Mueller PR (2003). Comparison of excretory phase, helical computed tomography with intravenous urography in patients with painless haematuria. *Clin. Radiol.* **58**: 294–300.

26 Wiener HG, Vooijs G P, van't Hof-Grootenboer B (1993). Accuracy of urinary cytology in the diagnosis of primary and recurrent bladder cancer. *Acta Cytol.* **37**: 163–9.

27 Howard RS, Golin AL (1991). Long-term followup of asymptomatic microhematuria. *J. Urol.* **145**: 335–6.

28 Grossfeld GD, Litwin MS, Wolf JS, Hricak H, Shuler CL, Agerter DC *et al.* (2001). Evaluation of asymptomatic microscopic hematuria in adults: the American Urological Association best practice policy—part I: definition, detection, prevalence, and etiology. *Urology* **57**: 599–603.

29 Sugimura K, Ikemoto SI, Kawashima H, Nishisaka N, Kishimoto T (2001). Microscopic hematuria as a screening marker for urinary tract malignancies. *Int. J. Urol.* **8**: 1–5.

30 Sells H, Cox R (2001). Undiagnosed macroscopic haematuria revisited: a follow-up of 146 patients. *Urol. Int.* **88**: 6–8.

31 Appleton GVN, Luthman GD, Charlton CAC (1986). A 5-year follow up of undiagnosed haematuria. *Br. J. Urol.* **58**: 6–8.

32 Levine L A, Richie JP (1989). Urological complication of cyclophosphamide. *J. Urol.* **141**: 1063–9.

33 Arrizabalaga M, Extramiana J, Parra JL, Ramos C, Diaz Gonzalez R, Leiva O (1987). Treatment of massive haematuria with alumnious salts. *Br. J. Urol.* **60**: 223–6.

34 Goel AK, Rao MS, Bhagwat AG, Vaidyanathan S, Goswami AK, Sen TK (2003). Intravesical irrigation with alum for the control of massive bladder hemorrhage. *J. Urol.* **133**: 956–7.

35 Choong SKS, Walkden M, Kirby R (2000). The management of intractable haematuria. *BJU Int.* **86**: 951–9.

36 Fair WR (1974). Formalin in the treatment of massive bladder hemorrhage. Techniques, results and complications. *Urology* **3**: 573–6.

37 Shah BC, Albert DJ (1973). Intravesical instillation of formalin for the management of intractable hematuria. *J. Urol.* **110**: 519–20.

38 Godec CJ, Gleich P (1983). Intractable hematuria and formalin. *J. Urol.* **130**: 688–91.

39 Levine LA, Jarrard DF (1993). Treatment of cyclophosphamide-induced hemorrhagic cystitis with intravesical carboprost tromethamine. *J. Urol.* **149**: 719–23.

40 Ballen KK, Becker P, Levebvre K, Emmons R, Lee K, Levy W *et al.* (1999). Safety and cost of hyperhydration for the prevention of hemorrhagic cystitis in bone marrow transplant recipients. *Oncology* **57**: 287–92.

41 Cohen MH, Dagher R, Griebel DJ, Ibrahim A, Martin A, Scher NS *et al.* (2002). U.S. Food and Drug Administration drug approval summaries: imatinib mesylate, mesna tablets, and zoledronic acid. *Oncologist* **7**: 393–400.

42 Hald T, Mygind T (1974). Control of life-threatening vesical hemorrhage by unilateral hypogastric artery muscle embolization. *J. Urol.* **112**: 60–3.

43 McIvor J, Williams G, Southcott RD (2003). Control of severe vesical haemorrhage by therapeutic embolisation. *Clin. Radiol.* **33**: 561–7.

44 Nabi G, Sheikh N, Greene D, Marsh R (2003). Therapeutic transcatheter arterial embolization in the management of intractable haemorrhage from pelvic urological malignancies: preliminary experience and long-term follow up. *BJU Int.* **92**: 245–7.

45 Olliff S, Thomas S, Karani J, Walters H (1990). Superselective embolization using a coaxial catheter technique. *Br. J. Radiol.* **63**: 197–201.

46 Bevers RF, Bakker DJ, Kurth KH (1995). Hyperbaric oxygen. *Lancet* **346**: 803–5.

47 Corman JM, McClure D, Pritchett R, Kozlowski P, Hampson NB (2003). Treatment of radiation induced hemorrhagic cystitis with hyperbaric oxygen. *J. Urol.* **169**: 2200–2.

48 Grim PS, Gottlieb LJ, Boddie A, Batson E (1990). Hyperbaric oxygen therapy. *J. Am. Med. Assoc.* **263**: 2216–20.

49 Rijkmans BG, Bakker DJ, Dabhoiwala NF, Kurth KH (1989). Successful treatment of radiation cystitis with hyperbaric oxygen. *Eur. Urol.* **16**: 354–6.

50 Berkson BM, Lome LG, Shapiro I (1973). Severe cystitis induced by cyclophosphamide: role of surgical management. *J. Am. Med. Assoc.* **225**: 605–6.

51 Okaneya T, Kontani K, Komiyama I, Takezaki T (1993). Severe cyclophosphamide-induced hemorrhagic cystitis successfully treated by total cystectomy with ileal neobladder substitution: a case report. *J. Urol.* **150**: 1909–10.

Chapter 9

The patient presenting with urinary retention

Nicholas J. Hegarty, Ciaran F. Healy, and
John M. Fitzpatrick

Introduction

During normal voiding the bladder empties completely. The inability to do so is
referred to as urinary retention. In acute urinary retention there is an inability to pass
any, or at most only small volumes of, urine. This is associated with severe lower
abdominal pain and represents one of the most common reasons for emergency urological hospital admission. It is the presence of pain that is used as the main feature in
distinguishing it from chronic urinary retention.[1] In chronic urinary retention the
ability to void is usually still present but a significant volume remains in the bladder at
the end of micturition. The symptom of overflow incontinence may be associated, and
generally there are pre-existing lower urinary tract symptoms (LUTS). There is often
very little discomfort other than a feeling of lower abdominal fullness. Unrelieved
chronic retention may progress to upper tract deterioration and renal failure.

Classification

Acute urinary retention is classified as spontaneous or precipitated. In spontaneous
urinary retention there is no definite predisposing cause. Generally there is a history of
lower urinary tract symptoms culminating in the retention episode, but this is not
invariably present. Precipitating causes are described below, but often occur with a
background of outflow obstructive symptoms.

Chronic urinary retention is subdivided into low-pressure chronic retention (LPCR)
or high-pressure chronic retention (HPCR) depending on urodynamic findings.[2] In
LPCR bladder pressures remain within the normal range both before and after filling.
It is usually secondary to bladder outlet obstruction, and high detrusor pressures can
be generated during voiding. Relief of obstruction is not urgent in that upper tracts are
not immediately under threat, with urinary tract infection (UTI) and acute retention
being the main risks. More conservative treatments, e.g. medical management, are
often initiated if symptoms are mild, followed by surgery if patients fail to improve or

as an initial treatment if symptoms are severe. A subset with LPCR will also have low detrusor pressure during voiding. This suggests bladder decompensation, which reduces the likelihood of successful voiding following surgery.[1] HPCR represents a more serious condition that, if untreated, results in upper tract dilatation with progressive renal impairment and hypertension.[3] Presentation may be masked by the silent nature of the urinary symptoms and the more pronounced nature of the renal impairment.[4] Once it is recognized and treated, however, the outcome for HPCR is generally good.[5]

Acute urinary retention

The aetiology of acute urinary retention (AUR) is often multifactorial. Bladder outflow obstruction (BOO) secondary to benign prostatic hyperplasia is the commonest cause. Urinary tract infection, constipation and faecal impaction, over-stretching of the bladder, excessive fluid intake, alcohol consumption, medications, sexual activity, debility, and bed rest can all contribute.[6] Areas of prostate infarction are frequently associated with urinary retention: Spiro and associates found evidence of infarction in 85% of prostates removed for AUR compared with 3% in prostates of men having surgery for symptoms alone.[7] Studies on TURP (transurethral resection of the prostate) specimens show an increased rate of infarction in AUR but not to the same degree as seen with open prostatectomy.[8] Retention can also occur as a result of impaired detrusor contractility. This may occur with bladder over-distension, anticholinergics, or as a result of a number of neurological disease processes.

Benign prostatic hyperplasia

Benign prostatic hyperplasia (BPH) is one of the commonest conditions associated with ageing in men, and is noted on autopsy in approximately 40% of men in their 50s and in up to 70% in their 60s.[9] BPH results in increasing pressure on the urethra and subsequent obstruction of the urinary flow. Patients often describe lower urinary tract symptoms (LUTS) as a result of difficulty in voiding (e.g. hesitancy, straining, weak stream, dribbling) and over-activity of the bladder (e.g. urgency, frequency, urge incontinence). LUTS suggestive of benign prostatic obstruction (BPO) are common in elderly men; in community-based surveys, approximately 25% of men describe LUTS (with a total International Prostate Symptom Score (IPSS) of >7).[10] There is a linear association with age, with the lowest incidence at age 45–49 and the highest incidence at the age of 75–79.[10] AUR is one of the most significant complications or long-term outcomes resulting from BPH. In the Olmstead County Study, the incidence of AUR per 1000 person-years increased from 2.6 for men in their 40 s to 9.3 for men in their 70s if they had mild symptoms, and from 3.0 to 34.7, respectively, if symptoms were more severe.[11] Along with age and symptom severity, the relative risk of AUR was greater in those with a flow rate less than 12 ml/s (3.9 times), and those with a prostate volume >30 ml (3 times). Factors that predispose to the occurrence of urinary retention in men with a diagnosis of BPH include age, prostate volume, serum prostate specific antigen (PSA) levels, and symptom severity.[12–14] The risk for recurrent AUR within 1 week of removal of a catheter is estimated as being 56 to 64%. This rises to between 76 and 83% in men with diagnosed BPH.[15–17] Most patients with BPH will opt for surgery as they do not wish to experience a further episode of AUR and even if they void successfully many will still require surgery for troublesome LUTS.

Drug-induced acute urinary retention

A number of medications predispose to the development of urinary retention. Principal amongst these are anticholinergics or drugs with anticholinergic side-effects such as antidepressants (especially tricyclic antidepressants, but other antidepressants may also decrease bladder contractility), antipsychotics, and antiparkinsonian drugs. Calcium channel blockers, opiates, and anaesthetic agents can also impair detrusor contractility.[18] Diuretics are thought to predispose to the development of retention by causing acute bladder over-distension.

Cannabis, opiates, and other recreational drugs as well as over-the-counter decongestants can precipitate an episode of retention. A number of cases have been reported in the literature describing urinary retention following the ingestion of ecstasy (3,4-methylenedioxymethamphetamine):[19,20] this acts by stimulating the release of monoamine neurotransmitters (serotonin, norepinephrine, and to a lesser extent dopamine). The resultant α-adrenergic stimulation causes sphincter contraction, while stimulation of β-adrenergic fibres reduces detrusor muscle contractility.

Postoperative acute urinary retention

Postoperative AUR is a well-recognized but poorly understood event. Its incidence is quoted as 4–25%, depending on the group studied. It occurs most frequently after lower urinary tract, perineal, anorectal, and gynaecological surgery. Contributing factors include sedation, general, spinal, and epidural anaesthesia, increased sympathetic stimulation, over-distension of the bladder by large quantities of fluid given intravenously, pain, and anxiety.[21] Studies suggest that α-adrenergic blockade can reduce the incidence of perioperative AUR in those at greatest risk,[22–24] but use in this regard is not as yet widely applied.

Infection

Urinary tract infection may predispose to urinary retention in a number of ways: cystitis reduces bladder contractility, prostatitis results in engorgement of the prostate and outflow obstruction, while the pain of urethritis may also impair voiding. The occurrence of UTI raises the possibility of incomplete emptying which will need to be assessed in deciding on treatment.

Table 9.1 Neurological diseases predisposing to urinary retention

Cerebrovascular accident
Brainstem infarct
Brain tumours (most commonly described lesions of the frontal cortex)
Acquired immunodeficiency syndrome
Acute disseminated encephalomyelitis
Reflex sympathetic dystrophy
Spinal cord injury
Spinal shock
Anogenital herpes simplex virus infection

Neuromuscular dysfunction

Urinary retention can occur in association with disease processes involving the central and peripheral nervous systems (a number of these are listed in Table 9.1). It may be the first manifestation of neurological disease, so a high index of suspicion should be maintained, particularly where the presentation appears atypical.

Chronic urinary retention

There is considerable overlap between the pathogenesis, clinical presentation, and treatment of acute and chronic urinary retention; however, a number of important differences do exist. Patients with chronic urinary retention (CUR) most commonly present with a bladder content of 1000 and 1500 ml, while bladder volumes up to 4 l have been described.[25] The patient can usually still pass urine, albeit with a large residual volume. The onset of CUR tends to be less dramatic and is often associated with only mild LUTS or it may even be asymptomatic in the early stages. The patient most commonly presents in one of three ways—incontinence, most notably at night (enuresis) from overflow in an insensitive bladder, renal failure due to back-pressure on the upper urinary tracts, or acute-on-chronic retention. In acute-on-chronic retention, the inability to pass urine is often considerably longer than in simple AUR and the amount of pain is less than expected for the size of the bladder. The distinction between straightforward AUR and acute-on-chronic retention is important not only from the point of view of diagnosis but also of the prognosis and subsequent management.[26]

Patient assessment

History

A full medical and surgical history is important in the evaluation of the patient with a focus on the urinary tract and allied areas of obstetrics and gynaecology in the female, lower gastrointestinal tract, and central and peripheral nervous systems. Specifically relating to the lower urinary tract is there any history of prior LUTS, and if so, their duration and severity. It is important to ask specifically about haematuria, any history of sexually transmitted disease or lower urinary tract infection or urethritis. A history of lower urinary tract instrumentation, trauma, or surgery should be recorded along with the results of these interventions in terms of lower urinary tract function.

The presence and severity of co-morbid medical illness is important to determine as it may contribute to the patient's condition and may also restrict the range of treatment options open to the patient. Similarly, a full list of prescribed and self-prescribed medications should be compiled. The level of family and social support available to the patient may also influence treatment options.

Physical examination

Normal bladder capacity in the adult is 400–600 ml. At approximately 500 ml the bladder reaches the upper border of the pubic symphysis. In the slim individual, however, the bladder may become palpable at 150 ml. The finding of bladder distension is usually apparent. In severe cases the distended bladder may be visible, particularly in slim individuals (see Fig. 9.1). The bladder is generally palpable as a mass arising out of the pelvis which is dull to percussion. Suprapubic tenderness is a feature of acute urinary retention. Though the diagnosis is usually apparent from the history and physical examination, difficulty can be encountered in examining obese patients and those with lower abdominal incisions from previous surgery. Palpably enlarged kidneys raise the possibility of obstructive uropathy. The findings on rectal examination are variable, with no direct correlation between the prostate size and the degree of obstruction. It remains important to rule out an advanced prostatic malignancy as the source of obstruction.

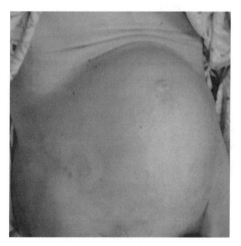

Fig. 9.1 Chronic urinary retention. Bladder distension extending to above the umbilicus. The patient presented with a markedly reduced urinary stream and overflow urinary incontinence.

Investigation

Basic investigations include measurement of serum urea, creatinine, and electrolytes. Ultrasound is a non-invasive means of confirming urinary retention and measuring residual urine volume, but where this is not readily available, urethral catheterization can be both diagnostic and therapeutic. Urine is collected for microscopy, culture, and sensitivity. Upper tract imaging is performed if obstructive uropathy is suspected. Urodynamics can be of use in determining whether retention is related to outflow obstruction or an atonic bladder.

Initial management of retention

The initial management of the patient with AUR is to relieve the considerable discomfort associated with this condition. This will often be regarded by the patient with more gratitude than any subsequent interventions. It is most simply done by the insertion of a urethral catheter. This involves cleansing the glans penis or vaginal introitus with disinfectant solution, the application of lubricating gel, usually combined with local anaesthetic and antiseptic and insertion of the catheter using a no-touch technique.

Due to the relatively short and straight course of the urethra, catheterization of the female is usually not difficult except in elderly women with an atrophic vaginal introitus. In this situation, it is imperative that the hips be well abducted and externally rotated, the labia be separated as much as is gently possible and the area be well-lighted. Even with optimal visualization, it still may be necessary to blindly pass the catheter along the middle of the anterior vaginal wall with a slight upward angulation in an attempt to identify the urethral meatus.

In the male increased sphincteric tone often impedes progression beyond the membranous urethra. Forceful attempts to advance a catheter beyond this may result in the formation of a false passage, rather, continuous gentle pressure should be maintained on the catheter until the patient relaxes the sphincter. This can sometimes be facilitated by asking the patient to bear down as if voiding. The size of catheter should be sufficient to allow drainage of the bladder but small enough to allow drainage of urethral secretions. Typically, a 16 or 18 Ch catheter is used, but a larger one, e.g. 20–22 Ch, will be required if there is coexisting haematuria. The choice of catheter material depends on whether long- or short-term catheterisation is anticipated. Other factors that influence the choice are price and risk of urethral stricture. The association of latex catheters and strictures has been suggested in historic series by the high rate of urethral stenosis in those catheterized with latex (43%) compared with 10% with PVC catheters.[27] In the early 1980s an epidemic of urethral strictures was seen in association with coronary artery bypass graft surgery. This was attributed in part to local urethral ischaemia,[28] but also to the use of latex rather than coated catheters.[29] Coated catheters result in a smoother surface and greatly reduce the contact between noxious agents in the catheter and the urethra. Currently Teflon- and silicone elastomer-coated catheters are the most widely used as they are considerably cheaper than pure silicone catheters. PVC catheters provide little in the way of tissue reaction, but are less comfortable than coated latex or silicone catheters and are therefore rarely used as indwelling catheters.

The choice of catheter design varies depending on the indication for catheterization. Indwelling catheters comprise two channels—a draining channel and a smaller balloon channel. Where irrigation is required a third channel is necessary, whereas single-channel catheters are used for self-intermittent catheterization, drainage prior to urodynamics, or measuring residual urine volume. A straight catheter is generally suitable for most catheterizations; however, when difficulty is encountered negotiating the angle of the bulbar urethra or where the prostatic urethra is deformed by intrusive prostatic enlargement or a transurethral resection (TUR) cavity a curved or coudé tip may be required.

The use of suprapubic catheterization is favoured by some in that, unlike urethral catheterization, it does not result in trauma to the urethra either on introduction or during the period of catheterization. This contributes to a lower incidence of urinary tract infection and stricture than an indwelling urethral catheter.[30] It can also be clamped to assess patient voiding while allowing residual urine volumes to be measured post-voiding. It does, however, require a higher degree of expertise to insert and risks damage to intra-abdominal viscera, particularly if there is a history of laparotomy. As it requires a full bladder, a definite diagnosis of urinary retention is needed before proceeding with trocar placement. However, most concerns arise for lack of familiarity with suprapubic catheters rather than technical difficulties associated with insertion.

The need for catheterization in chronic retention is not as urgent as with AUR. The complications of LPCR are principally those of urinary stagnation. Insertion of a catheter is associated with a high incidence of bacterial colonization and an increased risk of sepsis during subsequent manipulations. Thus in LPCR definitive surgery to the outflow obstruction is recommended as the first urethral intervention.[26] In HPCR back-pressure on ureters and kidneys may result in damage to the upper tracts. A period of catheterization prior to surgical intervention facilitates the potential reversal of obstructive renal impairment which may impart increased risks during surgery.

Post-obstructive diuresis may also occur following catheterization and relief of associated bilateral ureteric obstruction or obstruction of a single kidney. In these situations, it is important to be aware of this phenomenon and watch for it carefully by measuring the hourly urine output since the patient may quickly develop serious fluid and electrolyte abnormalities if the urine output remains >200 cm^3/h for several hours. Close monitoring of serum and urinary electrolytes with sufficient sodium and water replacement to maintain stability will usually allow the process to resolve spontaneously within 24–48 h. It is important that it is under control prior to any definitive treatment, since it will simplify fluid and electrolyte management in the post-operative period.

Chronic catheterization is frequently accompanied by haematuria, which may be heavy. The benefit of gradual decompression of the bladder referred to in older texts[31] is questionable as the source of bleeding following decompression is believed to be related to capillary changes occurring during ongoing obstruction rather than any phenomenon associated with catheterization.[32] Decompression of a chronically over-distended bladder may also allow regeneration of nerve and muscle pathways which will assist emptying following definitive treatment.

Outcomes in untreated urinary retention

In some patients with retention, micturition can restart following removal of the catheter, thus avoiding or at least deferring an operation. However, following trial without a catheter (TWOC), many are unable to void spontaneously and require recatheterization. Taube and Gajraj[33] looked at the success of TWOC in patients admitted with retention. This was successful in 17 of 60 patients (28.3%) the other 43 (71.7%) requiring recatheterization. Those patients most likely to benefit from a successful TWOC were those with a low residual volume of urine: 15 of 34 patients (44%) with residual volumes <900 ml were successful compared with 2 of 26 patients (8%) with a residual volume >900 ml. Other studies show a risk of recurrent retention of 56–64% within 1 week of TWOC.[15–17] When these patients are followed to 1 year, many of those who have initially voided successfully will have had a further episode of retention, or required surgery for severe LUTS.[17] In reviewing these data, Thorpe and Neal[34] suggested that TWOC be considered in those with a short, or no, previous history of LUTS and a residual urine volume <900 ml or where the precipitating cause was thought to be faecal impaction which has subsequently been treated or following discontinuation of drugs known to cause AUR. They suggest a 22–55% chance of successful voiding, though they acknowledge that there are no convincing data about the long-term outcome in these patients.[34] Based on these figures, many patients will opt for surgical treatment faced with a high probability of another episode of retention, or significant LUTS and the eventual need for surgery, whereas a significant proportion will still opt for more conservative means initially in the hope of avoiding the potential morbidity of surgery.[35]

Medical management

The availability of medical therapies that are effective without the complications and invasiveness of surgery has caused a considerable decline in the number of operations for LUTS in men and an increase in the prescription of medical therapy during the 1990s.[10] As mentioned, AUR is one of the main indications for transurethral resection of the prostate (TURP). However, TURP conducted as a result of AUR is associated with increased morbidity and perioperative mortality risk;[36] although these patients tend to be older and are less fit than those presenting for elective prostatectomy, this alone does not account for the increase in risk.

Alpha-blocking agents

The efficacy of α_1-adrenoreceptor antagonists in men with LUTS suggestive of BPH has traditionally been related to the blockade of the effect of norepinephrine on α_1-adrenoreceptors in the smooth muscle of the bladder neck, prostate, and prostatic capsule, with a subsequent reduction in the urethral resistance and the dynamic component of BPH. Caine and Perlberg[37] demonstrated that the increased prostatic urethral pressure in AUR could be reduced by adrenergic blockade and suggested this as an adjunct to bladder decompression in urinary retention and to increase the likelihood of spontaneous voiding after catheter removal. The effect of alfuzosin on the outcome of a TWOC following an episode of AUR was studied in a prospective double-blind study involving 81 patients with painful AUR related to benign prostatic obstruction.[38] Patients were randomly allocated to receive either alfuzosin SR, 5 mg twice a day (b.d.) ($n = 40$), or placebo ($n = 41$) for 48 h. Catheter removal occurred 24 h after the trial medication was started. A successful TWOC was noted in 55% of alfuzosin-treated patients compared with 29% in the placebo group. Kim et al.[39] studied the use of tamsulosin 0.4 mg given for at least 4 days prior to the removal of the catheter in 33 consecutive patients presenting with AUR. Eighty-eight per cent voided successfully, with 27% requiring TURP or clean intermittent self-catheterization (CISC) at 3-month follow-up. Shah et al.[40] treated 34 patients with alfuzosin SR 5 mg b.d. for a minimum of 36 hours prior to TWOC and continued for the duration of the study. At 2-year follow-up 68% of evaluable patients (19/28) had undergone TURP. It would appear from these data that alpha blockers assist in voiding in TWOC in the short to medium term; however, with longer follow-up the benefit is less pronounced. A potential secondary benefit proposed is that the higher rates of successful TWOC might allow surgery to be performed in more patients without indwelling catheters[41]—it would be hoped that this would reduce the risks associated with surgery; however, the value of this remains to be proved.

5α-reductase inhibitors

The 5α-reductase inhibitors finasteride and, more recently, dutasteride, which act by impeding the conversion of testosterone to dihydrotestosterone (which has considerably greater potency than testosterone in the prostate), have been shown to reduce prostate size in men with BPH. To achieve this, however, takes several weeks and take several months, thus their use as single agents in the setting of AUR is not appropriate. Potential side-effects of finasteride therapy include erectile dysfunction and loss of libido in less than 5% of men. They appear to have potential in combination with biodegradable stents[42] and their use with α-adrenergic blockade is being explored.

In summary, medical agents improve the rate of successful TWOC in patients presenting with AUR, but what proportion of patients they will prevent from needing surgery with long-term follow-up has yet to be determined.

Surgical management

Preparation of the patient for surgery

Many patients who present in retention have coexisting morbidities that need to be addressed in order to optimize their condition for planned or likely surgery. Opinions differ as to the timing of surgery—delaying of surgery does have the disadvantage of increasing likelihood of colonization of the urine from prolonged catheterization. Increased hospital stay is associated with expense and also increases the patient's risk of nosocomial infection, deep vein thrombosis, and other hospital-related illnesses. It does, however, allow for the complications of chronic retention and their relief to be addressed as well as any co-morbid illness to be addressed. It does also allow assessment of the likelihood of recovery of function following relief of obstruction and thus influence the decision to operate based on the likely benefits and inherent risks. Antiplatelet therapy or anticoagulants can be discontinued or modified to reduce the risk of significant bleeding post-operatively.

The correction of uraemia should facilitate the patient's overall capacity to undergo and recover from surgery, but in particular assist in haemostasis, while resolution of post-obstructive diuresis prior to surgery allows fluid and electrolyte balance to be controlled with greater ease.

The surgical options depend largely on the cause of retention, the fitness of the patient, and, to a lesser extent, the experience of the surgeon.[43] In bladder outflow obstruction the decision between open and transurethral surgery depends on the findings on cystoscopy, though the size of the prostate or any coexisting bladder pathologies can usually be determined on pre-operative examination and imaging.

Open surgery

Open prostatectomy is performed by either the transvesical or the retropubic route. Both involve enucleation of the area of prostatic enlargement (adenoma) either by opening the bladder or incising the prostate capsule, while leaving the surrounding rim of prostatic tissue and prostate capsule *in situ*. Haemostasis is achieved by controlling the prostatic vessels and a large-calibre catheter is left in the bladder until haematuria has resolved. Open prostatectomy differs from the more commonly encountered radical retropubic prostatectomy (for prostate malignancy) in that the entire prostate is not removed nor is the prostate capsule removed and thus a vesicourethral anastomosis is not required. Open surgery results in the most pronounced and most durable improvement in obstructive parameters: flow rates are seen to increase by 175%, symptomatic improvement is reported by 98% of patients, and the reported retreatment rate is only about 2%.[44] It does, however, require a more prolonged hospital stay and recuperation than other procedures and is associated with higher rates of bladder neck stricture, retrograde ejaculation, and erectile dysfunction than TURP.

Open prostatectomy is chosen in preference to TURP in very large prostates. It also allows for the removal of any coexistent large bladder calculi or bladder diverticulectomy if indicated and can be performed in those who are unsuitable to assume the lithotomy position, e.g. those with fixed hips secondary to osteoarthritis.

Transurethral resection of the prostate (TURP)

Transurethral resection of the prostate (TURP) is performed using a resectoscope which comprises a cystoscope with a diathermy loop attached at its under surface. This can be drawn toward the tip of the scope under vision to remove prostate chips. Cutting is accomplished using a low-power current while coagulation of bleeding vessels is achieved at higher power settings. The scope is positioned in the prostatic urethra and the prostate is cored out by sequential removal of chips of prostate from the luminal surface extending outward towards the capsule. This leaves a cavity within the prostate and thus relieves obstruction. The verumontanum represents the distal limit of surgery as resection distal to this risks injury to the external sphincter and urinary incontinence. Visibility is maintained during the procedure by irrigation with a non-conducting iso-osmotic fluid (usually glycine or sorbitol/mannitol). Excess absorption of irrigating fluid predisposes to dilutional hyponatraemia and the TURP syndrome (characterized initially by drowsiness and impaired mentation which may progress to seizures and coma). Avoidance of TURP syndrome requires a limit on resection time to between 40 and 60 minutes and thus TURP is not feasible in very large prostates. Symptom scores improve by an average of 82% following TURP, while maximum urinary flow rates increase by 125% compared with pre-operative values.[45]

Those with the greatest degree of bother pre-operatively are seen to derive most benefit from surgery.[45] This is consistent with the findings of Fowler et al.[46] who described significant symptomatic relief in 93% of men undergoing TURP with retention or severe symptoms pre-operatively, whereas 79% of those with moderate symptoms reported improvement. The results of surgery show a tremendous durability in the majority of patients, but re-operation is required in up to 10% within 8 years.[47] There is also a low (<1%) but definite mortality with TURP[48] and this is seen to further increase in patients who present for surgery in retention.[49] Other forms of morbidity, including bleeding requiring transfusion, urinary tract infection, urethral stricture, and incontinence (<1%), occur in 18%[48] of those undergoing TURP. Post-operative stay and peri-operative morbidity are also seen to increase in those presenting in retention.[49,50] Contributing to this is the tendency of patients in retention to be older and less fit than those presenting for elective prostatectomy, but poorer outcomes are seen in retention compared with age-matched controls.[49] TURP may also have an impact on sexual function in several ways. Estimates of new-onset erectile dysfunction vary greatly, but are thought to be of the order of 4–14%.[51] Retrograde ejaculation is reported by two-thirds and patients describe a reduction in sexual satisfaction. They do, however, describe increased sexual desire and overall satisfaction on the

International Index of Erectile Function following TURP,[52] which may relate to the improvement in urinary symptoms and will obviously improve in catheterized patients who can void post-TURP.

In summary, TURP provides significant and durable improvement in LUTS and indices of bladder emptying in the majority of patients. However, this is not without cost in terms of the requirement for hospital stay, general or regional anaesthesia, post-operative morbidity, and long-term effects on sexual function. It is for these reasons that there has been particular interest in the development of less invasive therapies, albeit in most incidences with reduced efficacy for the treatment of LUTS.

Less invasive surgical procedures

In the last 20–30 years a number of treatments have been proposed as less invasive means than TURP or open surgery for the relief of bladder outflow obstruction. The rationale for their development is to provide procedures that do not require hospital admission, that can be performed under local anaesthetic and/or sedation, and that have a lower side-effect profile than open surgery or TURP in terms of bleeding, retrograde ejaculation, or effects on erectile function and might also be possible in those unfit for surgery. Techniques that have been explored include a number of strategies that involve heating of the prostate with resultant destruction of prostate tissue and perhaps a reduction in the response to α-adrenergic stimulation in the bladder neck. Other techniques include transurethral vaporization of the prostate, transurethral incision of the prostate, laser ablation or resection techniques, and stenting of the prostatic urethra. There has been considerable enthusiasm from treating physicians and patients alike, especially in those with milder symptoms or with particular concerns about potency and fertility and those unfit for or unlikely to derive great benefit from surgery. This enthusiasm has on occasion overshadowed the primary aim of providing a treatment that has significant efficacy with durable results.[53] This is well illustrated in the experience with balloon dilation of the prostate. This involved the placing of a 35 mm balloon in the prostatic urethra, 1 cm proximal to the external sphincter. The catheter balloon was inflated to 4 atm of pressure and this maintained for 10 minutes. A urethral catheter was left *in situ* for 72 hours. Claims that this might replace TURP as a procedure that could be performed under local anaesthetic have not come to pass, and though symptomatic improvement was reported in the majority of patients,[54] this did not translate into objective improvement in flow parameters and few patients were shown to have a durable response.

Transurethral vaporization of the prostate

Transurethral vaporization of the prostate (TUVP) can be viewed as a modification of TURP, where a broader resection loop is used and higher energies are channelled through it to bring about charring and vaporization rather than resection of the prostate. It creates a similar resection cavity to TURP and both result in similar improvements in post-operative irritative symptoms, urinary infection, 1-year reoperation rate, and urethral stricture rate.[55] Haematuria and transfusion requirements are slightly less following TUVP as are catheter duration post-operatively and hospital stay, while operating time, post-operative urinary retention, erectile dysfunction, and urinary incontinence rates are slightly higher following TUVP.[55] There is less absorption of irrigation fluid than in TURP and a reduced bleeding tendency. It does not, however, provide satisfactory tissue for histological review and it takes longer to perform. It is effective in urinary retention, with 95% of patients in one report voiding satisfactorily post-operatively.[56]

Transurethral incision of the prostate

Transurethral incision of the prostate (TUIP) is another operative technique which has evolved to complement TURP and open prostatectomy. No tissue is resected, rather the prostate is incised using a single central or two lateral incisions[57,58] classically from below the ureteral orifices to the verumontanum at 5 and 7 o'clock, though techniques that spare the prostate–vesical junction have also been described. The incision is performed through the substance of the prostate down to the prostate capsule. The incision can be performed using a diathermy knife, resection loop, or laser and a urethral catheter is inserted for 24 hours after the procedure. Comparable results to TURP are obtainable in small prostates (estimated size of 20 g or less), with fewer complications in terms of post-operative bleeding, duration of catheterization and hospital stay, erectile dysfunction, and retrograde ejaculation.[59] Even lower rates of retrograde ejaculation are seen with preservation of the supramontanal 1 cm of prostatic urethra,[60] while laser incision means that TUIP can now be performed without the need for a catheter.[61]

Laser-based treatments

Laser-based techniques continue to evolve, and today offer a very real alternative to surgery.[62] Early contact techniques relied on vaporization of prostate tissue, while interstitial techniques resulted in ablation of tissue within the substance of the prostate. Both of these resulted in a high incidence of post-operative oedema of the prostatic urethra with associated irritative symptoms and often prolonged periods of post-operative urinary retention. Techniques that rely on prostate resection or enucleation do not suffer from these shortcomings. Laser resection involves performing multiple incisions in the prostate, dividing it into small pieces and removing them with a modified grasping forceps. Similar improvements in uroflow to TURP are seen, and resection in patients with retention is associated with return of voiding in over 90% of patients.[63] Unlike laser ablation, TUIP, and TUVP, laser resection provides tissue for histological assessment, though samples are inferior to those from TURP.[64]

Laser enucleation and morcellation is another technique, and is perhaps the endourological equivalent of open prostatectomy. It provides comparable outcomes to

TURP and can be performed in anticoagulated patients. Increases in prostate size increase the duration of the operation but is not in itself a limiting factor,[65] and this technique has been proposed as an alternative to open prostatectomy in very large prostates.[66] Laser enucleation takes 20–30% longer, but is associated with lower transfusion rates and shorter hospital stay than TURP.[67] A considerable drawback of laser treatments is the expense of purchasing dedicated equipment and laser probes. Some of this can be offset by applying its use to the treatment of stones and urothelial cancers and sharing equipment with other surgical disciplines.

Transurethral needle ablation

Transurethral needle ablation (TUNA) is generally performed under regional anaesthesia, though combined local and sedoanalgesia have been described.[68] The TUNA probe is a modified cystoscope that allows position in the urethra to be determined. There are two needles at the tip of the probe which are advanced at an angle (usually perpendicular) to the probe into the substance of the prostate to a depth determined either pre-operatively or intra-operatively on transrectal ultrasound. When in position, usually commencing just distal to the bladder neck, radiofrequency current is passed into the needles to cause a zone of surrounding tissue destruction. Needles are retracted and the scope positioned distally at the next treatment area. The number of treatments required depends on the size (principally the length) of the prostate and is generally between two and four. TUNA is believed to produce its effects both by tissue destruction and perhaps by reducing nerve receptors in the bladder neck.[69] Urinary retention occurs in 51% in the first 24 hours, so many recommend routine catheterization overnight following the procedure.[70] It results in a similar reduction in symptom score to TURP at 1-year review, but probably only provides half the increase in urinary flow rates seen with TURP.[71] Use has also been described in patients in retention with encouraging initial results;[72] however, despite this treatment being around for more than a decade, insufficient long-term data are available to recommend its use in retention.

Transurethral microwave therapy

Transurethral microwave therapy (TUMT) involves the delivery of microwave energy from a helical coil antenna located within a urethral delivery system. This is enclosed in a urethral catheter, the outer sleeve of which contains circulating water to allow surface cooling of the urethra to prevent urethral injury while allowing destruction of the underlying tissue. Positioning is monitored by ultrasound. Treatment is performed usually in a single 1-hour sitting in an out-patient setting under local anaesthesia. Rectal and urethral temperatures are monitored and limit the delivery of microwave energy. The efficacy is proportional to the amount of energy delivered and thus the temperature attained.

When used in patients presenting in acute retention, 63% were subsequently able to void;[73] however, effect on long-term outcome and the need for additional treatments or surgery is less clear.

Prostate stents

The application of stents to prevent restenosis after angioplasty in peripheral vascular disease has been practiced for several decades,[74] but has only more recently been applied to the lower urinary tract.[75,76] Stents are composed of a cylindrical wire mesh which is inserted in a collapsed state and then expanded within the prostatic fossa. Positioning is performed at cystoscopy and care is required with placement to avoid bridging the external sphincter which will result in incontinence or the stent protruding above the bladder neck into the bladder which will result in irritative symptoms.

Earlier studies describe the use of stents predominantly in those with urinary retention who were unfit for prostatectomy.[76] All men in this study were able to void successfully at a mean follow-up of 8 months, though one did describe severe irritative symptoms. The indication for stenting was subsequently extended to include high-risk surgical patients with severe LUTS.[77,78] In these groups mean peak flow rates improved by almost 50% and objective improvement was maintained with 2-year follow-up. Irritative symptoms were frequently reported following insertion, but these tended to improve within a few months. Side-effects described in those with stents included haematuria, UTI (epididimytis and prostatitis), and encrustation. With more extended follow-up, 13–40%[78,79] required removal of the stent. In most cases the stent can be removed cystoscopically, the principal indications for removal being detrusor instability, stent migration, and encrustation. However, others describe difficulties encountered in the removal of stents: it sometimes requires removal with a significant amount of the surrounding urethra or, where this is not possible, painstaking wire-by-wire removal,[80] indeed these procedures can sometimes be as demanding as the operation that stenting was meant to avoid. A number of modifications have been suggested, such as the use of more biocompatible materials, in particular nickel and titanium,[81] or the development of temporary stents.[82] Other causes of outflow obstruction for which stenting has been applied include recurrent urethral stricture[83] and detrusor–sphincter dyssynergia.[84] Their use in chronic retention is not associated with the same degree of success as acute retention, with 64% in one series either failing to void or requiring another treatment for incontinence.[82] Concerns about the long-term fate of stents, the frequent requirement for revision or removal, and the considerable expense of these devices has limited their application in BPH.

Long-term catheterization

The requirement for long-term catheterization should not be regarded as an endpoint, but rather as a challenge to maximize patient independence and minimize associated complications and discomfort. Unfortunately there are few well-designed studies to help guide the clinician in these goals. Fundamentals of catheter care include the use of sterile techniques during catheter insertion and maintenance of a closed drainage system. The use of biocompatible materials, e.g. pure silicone catheters, for prolonged catheterization is recommended. Attention to the position of the catheter bag is required (ensuring dependent drainage) and avoidance of traction on the catheter and trauma to the urethra. Cleansing of the meatus and surrounding area with unscented soap and water should be performed daily, while the patient should be encouraged to maintain sufficient fluid intake (e.g. >1.5 l/day). Many patients prefer the convenience and comfort of a supra-pubic rather than a urethral catheter for long-term drainage. Catheters should be changed at the appropriate interval, usually every 8–12 weeks but this may vary depending on the patient's tendency for catheter blockage. The need for on-going catheterization should also be reviewed at intervals in accordance with changes in the patient's status. Vigilance is needed to identify the development of and promptly treat complications of catheterization. Complications include bacteriuria, which is almost invariably present in prolonged catheterization. This does not in itself need treatment but can render the patient susceptible to urinary tract infection and bladder stone formation. Pyelonephritis, however, is a potentially life-threatening form of urinary tract infection and requires aggressive antibiotic treatment. Other complications associated with indwelling catheters include catheter encrustation and urethral erosion. An increased risk of squamous cell carcinoma is described in association with long-term catheterization.[85] This does not tend to occur until at least 10 years after the commencement of catheterization,[86] and as most patients with indwelling catheters have a limited life-expectancy this is usually not an issue. When it does occur, presentation tends to be with advanced disease and it carries a very poor prognosis.

Clean intermittent self-catheterization

Clean intermittent self-catheterization (CISC) has been described for the relief of urinary retention for centuries, but its use has only relatively recently achieved widespread clinical acceptance.[87,88] It involves the patient or his caregiver being instructed in the introduction of a small-calibre (typically 12 or 14 Ch) single-channel urethral catheter into the bladder. Usually it is performed four times per day, but may be required more frequently depending on the patient's urine output and bladder stability. Complications include the introduction of infection, urethral trauma, and stricture, though these are probably lower than with indwelling catheters. Other advantages over indwelling catheters include a greater degree of independence and the ability to assess the return of spontaneous voiding. It does require good hand–eye coordination, postural awareness, and motivation by the patient or caregiver and is not suitable for those with poor eyesight, poor dexterity, obesity, or restricted mobility. In general, however, it is extremely well tolerated even when it is required long term.[89] As with indwelling catheters, a number of case reports have described squamous cell carcinoma of the bladder in patients performing CISC[90] suggesting the need for periodic cystoscopic surveillance in those on CISC for more than 5 years. Though there are several other potential causes for haematuria in patients performing CISC, this should be investigated promptly and thoroughly if it does occur.

Urinary retention in women

Urinary retention in females is an uncommon clinical entity. In comparative studies its incidence is seen to be one-thirteenth that of male retention.[91] Neurological disease accounts for about a third of cases.[92] Other causes include bladder outflow obstruction secondary to bladder calculus, urethral stricture, diverticulum, caruncle, or extrinsic compression from a gynaecological tumour. Urinary retention is also encountered in pregnancy and the post-partum state. Other associated conditions include diabetes mellitus and cystitis. Urinary retention after hysterectomy has been reported, and is thought to be caused by deafferenatiation of the bladder wall and neck.[93] These patients respond well to sacral nerve stimulation. Initial management, as in the male, involves relief of retention. Outflow obstruction may be diagnosed on urethral calibration or cystoscopy. Other investigations include uroflow studies and renal and bladder scan. Disorders of bladder contractility may be demonstrated by cystometry, pressure-flow studies, and urethral pressure profilometry. CT and MRI of the sacral cord and lumbar puncture may be indicated in complex cases or where neurological disease is suspected. Frequently, however, no definite cause is found.[94] With further investigation including electromyography studies, a number of these will be found to have impaired relaxation and hypertrophy of the external sphincter.[95] These respond well to sacral nerve stimulation.[96] Definitive treatment of female retention is usually aimed at correcting the cause. Treatment of idiopathic urinary retention with CSIC is associated with a return to voiding in a significant proportion of women.[97]

Preventative strategies

A number of recent studies suggest that agents used in the medical management of BPH may also decrease the incidence of complications of this condition, notably a reduction in the incidence of urinary retention. Jardin and co-workers[98] reported that patients treated the α-adrenergic blocker alfuzosin had a 0.4% incidence of retention compared with 2.6% in the placebo group. The incidence of AUR was also lower in alfuzosin-treated patients compared with placebo in the pooled analysis of 11 studies: 0.3% versus 1.4% [38]. In a 4-year trial involving the 5α-reductase inhibitor finasteride in 3040 men AUR developed in 99 men (7%) in the placebo group and 42 men (3%) in the finasteride group.[12] In a second paper with 2-year follow-up, finasteride reduced the incidence of AUR by 61% in men with enlarged prostates (>40 ml) and by 47% in men with prostates sized <40 ml.[99] It also reported a decrease in the incidence of AUR by 63% in men with higher PSA levels (>1.4 ng/ml). The authors concluded that patients with larger prostates and higher PSA levels had an increased risk of AUR and were likely to derive the greatest benefit for the risk reduction observed with finasteride therapy. The more recently introduced 5α-reductase inhibitor dutasteride has also been associated with a significant reduction in the incidence of AUR and the need for prostate surgery.[100] With increased awareness as to the aetiology of this condition and a wider range of treatment options becoming available, identification and targeting of at-risk groups,[22] holds potential in preventing episodes of urinary retention.

Conclusion

Urinary retention represents an extremely common condition that has a great impact on patient well-being and also has huge social and financial implications. It may occur in isolation or, more frequently, in association with a variety of co-morbidities. Bladder decompression and prevention of upper tract deterioration are amongst the initial goals in the approach to this problem. Surgery remains the most effective means of relieving obstruction and preventing further episodes of retention in those fit for it. Several medical and less invasive surgical strategies show promise, increasing the number of patients who will have a successful trial without catheter. Long-term data are keenly awaited to see which of these treatments will result in durable patient benefit.

References

1 O'Reilly PH (1986). *Obstructive Uropathy*. Springer, New York.
2 Abrams PH, Dunn M, George N (1978). Urodynamic findings in chronic retention of urine and their relevance to results of surgery. *Br. Med. J.* **2**(6147): 1258–60.
3 George NJR, O'Reilly PH, Barnard RJ, Blacklock NJ (1983). High pressure chronic retention. *Br. Med. J.* **286**: 1780–3.
4 Jones DA, George NJ, O'Reilly PH, Barnard RJ (1987). Reversible hypertension associated with unrecognised high pressure chronic retention of urine. *Lancet* **1**(8541): 1052–4.
5 Jones DA, Gilpin SA, Holden D, Dixon JS, O'Reilly PH, George NJ (1991). Relationship between bladder morphology and long-term outcome of treatment in patients with high pressure chronic retention of urine. *Br. J. Urol.* **67**: 280–5.
6 Stimson JB, Fihn SD (1990). Benign prostatic hyperplasia and its treatment [review]. *J. Gen. Intern. Med.* **5**: 153–65.
7 Spiro LH, Labay G, Orkin LA (1974). Prostatic infarction: role in acute urinary retention. *Urology* **3**: 345–7.
8 Anjum I, Ahmed M, Azzopardi A, Mufti GR (1998). Prostatic infarction/infection in acute urinary retention secondary to benign prostatic hyperplasia. *J. Urol.* **160**: 792–3.
9 Berry SJ, Coffey DS, Walsh PC, Ewing LL (1984). The development of human benign prostatic hyperplasia with age. *J. Urol.* **132**: 474–9.
10 Fitzpatrick JM (2000). Facts and future lines of research in lower urinary tract symptoms in men and women: an overview of the role of a1-adrenoreceptor antagonists. *BJU Int.* **85**(Suppl. 2):1–5.
11 Jacobsen SJ, Jacobson DJ, Girman CJ, Roberts RO, Rhodes T, Guess HA *et al.* (1997). Natural history of prostatism: risk for acute urinary retention. *J. Urol.* **158**: 481–7.
12 McConnell JD, Bruskewitz R, Walsh P, Andriole G, Lieber M, Holtgrewe HL *et al.* (1998). The effect of finasteride on the risk of acute urinary retention and the need for surgical treatment in men with benign prostatic hyperplasia. Finasteride long-term efficacy and safety study group. *N. Engl. J. Med.* **338**: 557–63.

13 Kaplan S, Garvin D, Gilhooly P, Koppel M, Labasky R, Milsten R *et al.* (2000). Impact of baseline symptom severity on future risk of benign prostatic hyperplasia-related outcomes and long-term results to finasteride. The PLESS Study Group. *Urology* **56**: 610–16.

14 Meigs JB, Barry MJ, Giovannucci E, Rimm EB, Srampfer MJ, Kawachi I (1999). Incidence rates and risk factors for acute urinary retention: the health professionals follow-up study. *J. Urol.* **162**: 376–82.

15 Breum L, Klarskov P, Munck LK, Nielsen TH, Nordestgaard AG (1982). Significance of acute urinary retention due to infravesical obstruction. *Scand. J. Urol. Nephrol.* **16**: 21.

16 Klarskov P, Andersen JT, Asmussen CF, Brenoe J, Jensen SK, Jensen IL *et al.* (1987). Symptoms and signs predictive of the voiding pattern after acute urinary retention in men. *Scand. J. Urol. Nephrol.* **21**: 23–8.

17 Hastie KJ, Dickinson AJ, Ahmad R, Moisey CU (1990). Acute retention of urine: is trial without catheter justified? *J. R. Coll. Surg. Edinb.* **35**: 225–7.

18 Gray M (2000). Urinary retention. Management in the acute care setting. Part 2. *Am. J. Nurs.* **100**: 36–43.

19 Bryden AA, Rothwell PJN, O'Reilly PH (1995). Urinary retention with misuse of 'ecstasy'. *Br. Med. J.* **310**: 504.

20 Inman DS, Greene D (2003). 'The agony and the ecstasy': acute urinary retention after MDMA abuse. *BJU Int.* **91**: 123.

21 Tammela T (1995). Postoperative urinary retention—why the patient cannot void. *Scand. J. Urol. Nephrol.* **175**(Suppl. 1): 75–7.

22 Goldman G, Kahn PJ, Kashtan H, Stadler J, Wiznitzer T (1988). Prevention and treatment of urinary retention and infection after surgical treatment of the colon and rectum with alpha adrenergic blockers. *Surg. Gynecol. Obstet.* **166**: 447–501.

23 Cataldo PA, Senagore AJ (1991). Does alpha sympathetic blockade prevent urinary retention following anorectal surgery? *Dis. Colon Rectum* **34**: 1113–16.

24 Savona-Ventura C, Grech ES, Saliba I (1991). Pharmacological measures to prevent post-operative urinary retention; a prospective randomized study. *Eur. J. Obstet. Gynecol. Reprod. Biol.* **41**: 225–9.

25 Young TW, Mitchell JP (1968). Distension of the bladder leading to vascular compression and massive oedema. *Br. J. Urol.* **40**: 248–50.

26 Mitchell JP (1984). Management of chronic urinary retention. *Br. Med. J.* **289**: 515–16.

27 Keitzer WA, Abreu A, Navarro I, Banreuter E, Allen JS (1968). Urethral strictures: prevention with plastic indwelling catheters. *J. Urol.* **99**: 187–8.

28 Elihali MM, Hassouna M, Abdel-Hakim A, Teijeira J (1986). Urethral stricture following cardiovascular surgery: role of ureteral ischemia. *J. Urol.* **135**: 275–7.

29 Ruutu M, Alfthan O, Heikkinen L, Jarvinen A, Konttinen M, Lehtonen T *et al.* (1983). Unexpected urethral strictures after short-term catheterisation in open heart surgery. *Scand. J. Urol. Nephrol.* **18**: 9–12.

30 Horgan AF, Prasad B, Waldron DJ, O'Sullivan DC (1992). Acute urinary retention. Comparison of suprapubic and urethral catheterisation. *Br. J. Urol.* **70**: 149–51.

31 Blandy JP (1976). Benign enlargement of the prostate gland. In: *Urology* (ed. JP Blandy), pp. 889–90. Blackwell, Oxford.

32 Gould F, Cheng CY, Lapides J (1976). Comparison of rapid versus slow decompression of the distended urinary bladder. *Invest. Urol.* **14**: 156–8.

33 Taube M, Gajraj H (1989). Trial without catheter following acute retention of urine. *Br. J. Urol.* **63**: 180–2.

34 Thorpe A, Neal D (2003). Benign prostatic hyperplasia. *Lancet* **361**: 1359–67.

35 Kaplan S, Goluboff E, Olsson C, Deverka P, Chmiel J (1995). Effect of demographic factors, urinary peak flow rates, and Boyarsky symptom scores on patient treatment choice in benign prostatic hyperplasia. *Urology* **45**: 398–405.

36 Pickard R, Emberton M, Neal DE (1998). The management of men with acute urinary retention. *Br. J. Urol.* **81**: 712–20.

37 Caine M, Perlberg S (1977). Dynamics of acute retention in prostatic patients and role of adrenergic receptors. *Urology* **9**: 399–403.

38 McNeill SA, Hargreave TB, Geffriaud-Richouard C, Santoni J, Roehrborn CG (2001). Postvoid residual urine in patients with lower urinary tract symptoms suggested of benign prostatic hyperplasia: pooled analysis of eleven controlled studies with alfuzosin in general practice. *Urology* **57**: 459–64.

39 Kim HL, Kim JC, Benson DA, Bales GT, Gerber GS (2001). Results of treatment with tamsulosin in men with acute urinary retention. *Tech. Urol.* **7**: 256–60.

40 Shah T, Palit V, Biyani S, Elmasry Y, Puri R, Flannigan GM (2002). Randomised, placebo controlled, double blind study of alfuzosin SR in patients undergoing trial without catheter following acute urinary retention. *Eur. Urol.* **42**: 329–32.

41 McNeill SA (2001). Does acute urinary retention respond to alpha blockade therapy alone? *Eur. Urol.* **39**: 7–12.

42 Isotalo T, Talja M, Hellström P, Perttilä I, Välimaa T, Törmälä P *et al.* (2001). A double-blind randomized, placebo-controlled pilot study to investigate the effects of finasteride combined with a biodegradable self-reinforced poly L-lactide acid spiral stent in patients with urinary retention caused by bladder outlet obstruction from benign prostatic hyperplasia. *BJU Int.* **88**: 30–4.

43 Martin KW (1973). Prostatectomy: a discourse on the indications for and the choice of operation. *Ann. R. Coll. Surg. Engl.* **52**: 304–15.

44 McConnell JD, Barry MJ, Bruskewitz RC, Bueschan AJ, Denton SE, Holtgrewe HL *et al.* (1994). *Benign Prostatic Hyperplasia: Diagnosis and Treatment. Clinical Practice Guideline No. 8*, AHCPR publication no 94–0582. Agency for Health Care Policy and Research, Public Health Service, US Department of Health and Human Services, Rockville, MD.

45 Wasson JH, Reda DJ, Bruskewitz RC, Elinson J Keller AM, Henderson WG (1995). A comparison of transurethral surgery with watchful waiting for moderate symptoms of benign prostatic hyperplasia. The Veterans Affairs Cooperative Study Group on Transurethral Resection of the Prostate. *N. Engl. J. Med.* **332**: 75–9.

46 Fowler F, Wennberg J, Timothy R, Barry M, Mulley A, Hanley D (1988). Symptom status and quality of life following prostatectomy. *J. Am. Med. Assoc.* **259**: 3018–22.

47 Roos N, Wennberg J, Malenka D, Fisher E, McPherson K, Andersen T *et al.* (1989). Mortality and reoperation after transurethral resection of the prostate for benign prostatic hyperplasia. *N. Engl. J. Med.* **320**: 1120–4.

48 Mebust W, Holtgrave H, Cockett A (1989). Transurethral prostatectomy: immediate and postoperative complications. A cooperative study of 13 participating institutions evaluating 3855 patients. *J. Urol.* **141**: 243–7.

49 Thorpe AC, Cleary R, Coles J, Vernon S, Reynolds J, Neal DE (1994). Deaths and complications following prostatectomy in 1400 men in the northern region of England. Northern Regional Prostate Audit Group. *Br. J. Urol.* **74**: 559–65.

50 Styles RA, Ramsden PD, Neal DE (1991). The outcome of prostatectomy on chronic retention of urine. *J. Urol.* **146**: 1029–33.

51 Hegarty NJ, Fitzpatrick JM (2001). The non-surgical management of benign prostatic hyperplasia. In: *Comprehensive Urology* (ed. R Weiss, N George, P O'Reilly). Mosby International, London.

52 Gacci M, Bartioletti R, Figioli S, Sarti E, Eisner B, Boddi V *et al.* (2003). Urinary symptoms, quality of life and sexual function in patients with benign prostatic hypertrophy before and after prostatectomy: a prospective study. *BJU Int.* **91**: 196–200.

53 Fitzpatrick JM (1998). A critical evaluation of technological innovations in the treatment of symptomatic benign prostatic hyperplasia. *Br. J. Urol.* **81**(Suppl. 1): 56–63.

54 McLoughlin J, Keane P, Jager R, Gill K, Machann L, Williams G (1991). Dilation of the prostatic urethra with a 35 mm balloon. *Br. J. Urol.* **67**: 177–81.

55 Patel A, Fuchs GJ, Gutierrez-Aceves J, Andrade-Perez F (2000). Transurethral electrovaporization and vapour-resection of the prostate: an appraisal of possible electrosurgical alternatives to regular loop resection. *BJU Int.* **85**: 202–10.

56 Stewart SC, Benjamin D, Ruckle H, Lui P, Hadley R (1995). Electrovaporization of the prostate: New technique for treatment of symptomatic benign prostatic hyperplasia. *J. Endourol.* **9**: 413–16.

57 Orandi A (1985). Incision of the prostate (TUIP): 646 cases in 15 years—a chronological appraisal. *Br. J. Urol.* **57**: 703–7.

58 Orandi A (1987). Transurethral incision of the prostate compared with transurethral resection of the prostate in 132 matching cases. *J. Urol.* **138**: 810–15.

59 Edwards L, Powell C (1982). An objective comparison of transurethral resection and bladder neck incision in the treatment of prostatic hypertrophy. *J. Urol.* **128**: 325–7.

60 Ronzoni G, De Vecchis M (1998). Preservation of anterograde ejaculation after transurethral ejaculation of both prostate and bladder neck. *Br. J. Urol.* **81**: 830–3.

61 Cornford C, Biyani C, Powell C (1998). Transurethral incision of the prostate using the holmium:YAG laser: a catheterless procedure. *J. Urol.* **159**: 1229–31.

62 Fitzpatrick JM (2000). Will laser replace TURP for the treatment of benign prostatic hyperplasia? *Lancet* **356**: 357–8.

63 Kabalin JN (1997). Neodymium:YAG laser coagulation prostatectomy for patients in urinary retention. *J. Endourol.* **11**: 207–9.

64 Das A, Kennett KM, Sutton T, Fraundorfer MR, Gilling PJ (2000). Histological effects of holmium: YAG laser resection versus transurethral resection of the prostate. *J. Endourol.* **14**: 459–62.

65 Gilling PJ, Kennett K, Fraundorfer MR (2000). Holmium laser enucleation of the prostate for glands larger than 100 g: an endourologic alternative to open prostatectomy. *J. Endourol.* **14**: 529–31.

66 Moody JA, Lingeman JE (2001). Holmium laser enucleation for prostate adenoma greater than 100 gm: comparison to open prostatectomy. *J. Urol.* **165**: 459–62.

67 Tan AHH, Gilling PJ (2002). Holmium laser prostatectomy: current techniques. *Urology* **60**: 152–6.

68 Schulman CC, Zlotta AR, Rasor JS, Hourriez L, Noel JC, Edwards SD (1993). Transurethral needle ablation (TUNA): safety, feasibility, and tolerance of a new office procedure for treatment of benign prostatic hyperplasia. *Eur. Urol.* **24**: 415–23.

69 Zlotta AR, Raviv G, Peny MO, Noel JC, Haot J, Schulman CC (1997). Possible mechanisms of action of transurethral needle ablation of the prostate on benign prostatic hyperplasia symptoms: a neurohistochemical study. *J. Urol.* **157**: 894–9.

70 Ramon J, Lynch TH, Eardley I, Ekman P, Frick J, Jungwirth A *et al.* (1997). Transurethral needle ablation of the prostate for the treatment of benign prostatic hyperplasia: a collaborative multicentre study. *Br. J. Urol.* **80**: 128–35.

71 Bruskewitz R, Issa MM, Roehrborn CG, Naslund MJ, Perez-Marrero R, Shumaker BP *et al.* (1998). A prospective, randomised, 1-year clinical trial comparing transurethral needle ablation

(TUNA) to transurethral resection of the prostate for the treatment of symptomatic benign prostatic hyperplasia. *J. Urol.* **159**: 1588–94.

72 Millard RJ, Harewood LM, Tamaddon K (1996). A study of the efficacy and safety of transurethral needle ablation (TUNA) treatment for benign prostatic hyperplasia. *Neurourol. Urodyn.* **15**: 619–28.

73 Saranga R, Matzkin H, Braf Z (1990). Local microwave hyperthermia in the treatment of benign prostatic hypertrophy. *Br. J. Urol.* **65**: 349–53.

74 Dotter CT (1969). Transluminally-placed coilspring endarterial tube grafts: long-term patency in canine popliteal artery. *Invest. Radiol.* **4**: 329–33.

75 Fabian K (1980). Der intraprostatische 'Partielle Katheter' (Urologische Spirale). *Urologe A* **19**: 236–8.

76 Chapple C, Milroy EJG, Rickards D (1990). Permanently implanted urethral stent for prostatic obstruction in the unfit patient: preliminary report. *Br. J. Urol.* **66**: 58–65.

77 Milroy E, Chapple CR (1993). The UroLume stent in the management of benign prostatic hyperplasia. *J. Urol.* **150**: 1630–5.

78 Oesterling J, Kaplan S, Epstein H, Defalco A, Reddy P, Chancellor M (1994). The North American experience with the UroLume endoprosthesis as a treatment for benign prostatic hyperplasia: long term results. *Urology* **44**: 353–62.

79 Anjum M, Chari R, Shetty A, Keen M, Palmer J (1997). Long-term clinical results and quality of life after insertion of a self-expanding endourethral prosthesis. *Br. J. Urol.* **80**: 885–8.

80 Wilson TS, Lemack GE, Dmochowski RR (2002). UroLume stents: lessons learned. *J. Urol.* **167**: 2477–80.

81 Kaplan SA, Merrill DC, Mosely WG, Benson RC Jr, Chiou RK, Fuselier HA *et al.* (1993). The titanium intraprostatic stent: the United States experience. *J. Urol.* **150**: 1624–9.

82 Thomas PJ, Britton JP, Harrison NW (1993). The Prostakath stent: four years' experience. *Br. J. Urol.* **71**: 430–2.

83 Milroy E, Allen A (1996). Long-term results of UroLume urethral stent for recurrent urethral strictures. *J. Urol.* **155**: 904–8.

84 Shaw PJ, Milroy EJ, Timoney AG, el Din A, Mitchell N (1990). Permanent external striated sphincter stents in patients with spinal injuries. *Br. J. Urol.* **66**: 297–302.

85 Locke JR, Hill DE, Walzer Y (1985). Incidence of squamous cell carcinoma in patients with longterm catheter drainage. *J. Urol.* **133**: 1034–5.

86 Kaufman JM, Fam B, Jacobs SC, Gabilondo F, Yalla S, Kane JP *et al.* (1977). Bladder cancer and squamous metaplasia in spinal cord injury patients. *J. Urol.* **118**: 967–71.

87 Guttmann L, Frankel H (1966). The value of intermittent catheterisation in the early management of traumatic paraplegia and tetraplegia. *Paraplegia* **4**: 63–84.

88 Lapides J, Diokno AC, Silber SM, Lowe BS (1972). Clean, intermittent self-catheterization in the treatment of urinary tract disease. *J. Urol.* **107**: 458–61.

89 Diokno AC, Sonda LP, Hollander JB, Lapides J (1983). Fate of patients started on clean intermittent self-catheterization therapy 10 years ago. *J. Urol.* **129**: 1120–2.

90 Pattison S, Choong CM, Corbishley CM, Bailey MJ (2001). Squamous cell carcinoma of the bladder, intermittent self-catheterization and urinary tract infection-is there an association? *BJU Int.* **88**: 441.

91 Klarskov P, Andersen JT, Asmussen CF, Brennoe J, Jensen SK, Jensen IL *et al.* (1987). Acute urinary retention in women: a prospective study of 18 consecutive women. *Scand. J. Urol. Nephrol.* **21**: 29–31.

92 Deane AM, Worth PH (1985). Female chronic urinary retention. *Br. J. Urol.* **57**: 24–6.

93 Everaert K, De Muyunk M, Weyers S (2003). Urinary retention after hysterectomy for benign disease: extended diagnostic evaluation and treatment with sacral nerve stimulation. *BJU Int.* **91**: 497–9.

94 Fowler CJ (2003). Urinary retention in women. *BJU Int.* **91**: 463–4.

95 Fowler CJ, Christmas TJ, Chapple CR, Parkhouse HF, Kirby RS, Jacobs HS (1988). Abnormal electromyographic activity of the urethral sphincter, voiding dysfunction, and polycystic ovaries: a new syndrome? *Br. Med. J.* **297**: 1436–8.

96 Swinn MJ, Kitchen ND, Goodwin RJ, Fowler CJ (2000). Sacral neuromodulation for women with Fowler's syndrome. *Eur. Urol.* **38**: 439–43.

97 Murray K, Lewis P, Blannin J, Sjepard A (1984). Clean intermittent self-catheterisation in the management of adult lower urinary tract dysfunction. *Br. J. Urol.* **56**: 379–80.

98 Jardin A, Bensadoun H, Delauche-Cavallier MC, Attali P (1991). Alfuzosin for treatment of benign prostatic hyperplasia: The BPH-ALF Group. *Lancet* **337**: 1457–61.

99 Marberger MJ, Andersen JT, Nickel JC, Malice MP, Gabriel M, Pappas F *et al.* (2000). Prostate volume and serum prostate-specific antigen as predictors of acute urinary retention. Combination experience from three large multicentre placebo-controlled trials. *Eur. Urol.* **38**: 563–8.

100 Evans HC, Goa KL (2003). Dutasteride. *Drugs Aging* **20**: 905–16.

Chapter 10

The patient presenting with urinary incontinence

Hugh Flood and Jane MacDonald

Introduction

Urinary incontinence affects a broad spectrum of people and is not only detrimental to the patient's health and self-esteem but is a financial drain on the health budget. Supportive care and palliation become important when the patient is unfit or unsuitable for a curative procedure, e.g. the terminally ill or elderly, or the underlying condition is incurable, e.g. neuropathic patients. Urinary incontinence occurs when the lower urinary tract fails to store urine. The lower urinary tract is considered in two parts, the bladder and outlet (bladder neck and urethra), though both are functionally interdependent.

Broadly speaking, urinary incontinence is due to one or more of the following:

1 bladder overactivity (whether neuropathic or non-neuropathic),

2 stress incontinence due to sphincter weakness,

3 mixed incontinence due to a combination of (1) and (2),

4 abnormal fistulous connection between the urinary tract and adjacent organs (e.g. vagina or skin),

5 chronic retention with overflow incontinence.

Logical application of investigations, procedures, and devices begins with an understanding of the relevant anatomy, physiology, and pathophysiology of the lower urinary tract. (All relevant terms are used in accordance with the International Continence Society definitions.[1]).

Anatomy, physiology, pathophysiology and clinical presentation

The bladder

Anatomy

The urinary bladder has a capacity of approximately 500 ml in the adult. It lies directly behind the pubic bone in the pelvis. The base of the bladder is relatively immobile lying in the tough endopelvic fascia with ligaments connecting it to adjacent organs and the pelvic wall. The lateral walls of the bladder and urethra are clasped by the levator ani muscles of the pelvic floor and the dome is draped with peritoneum. This portion is relatively mobile and when distended rises up above the pubic bone and lies immediately behind the lower or suprapubic abdominal wall where it may be palpable when the bladder is distended.

The base of the bladder is commonly termed the trigone. The ureters enter at the trigone, conducting urine from the kidneys. The ureters pass obliquely through the detrusor muscle and this acts as a valve during contraction of the bladder preventing urine reflux into the upper tracts. The bladder neck is at the most dependant portion of the trigone and is contiguous with the urethra.

The bladder has two important layers. The outer layer is the detrusor which consists of smooth muscle fibres that are orientated in such a way that the bladder contracts as a whole and results in propulsion of the urine through the bladder neck and urethra. The detrusor has cholinergic receptors that when stimulated cause contraction. The inner mucosal layer is made of transitional cells that are unique in that the junctions between them are very tight rendering it relatively impermeable. The mucosa is loose and thrown into folds in the empty state but is stretched with filling.

Physiology

The bladder as a storage organ must act as a low-pressure reservoir. The pressure gradients between the upper tracts, the bladder, and the outlet are integral to urinary function and dysfunction. Urine (or any fluid) flows from high pressure to low pressure. Therefore the bladder must be able to store a reasonable volume of urine at pressures significantly lower than renal/ureteric peristaltic pressures of approximately 10 cmH$_2$O. Failure to do so results in functional ureteric obstruction, secondary reflux and bilateral hydroureteronephrosis. This may develop silently over time and cause end-stage renal failure.

On the other hand, the bladder must maintain pressures below the sphincteric closure pressure when it is acting as a reservoir or urinary incontinence will occur. To achieve this, the following are required:

1 Normal bladder wall compliance. Compliance and capacity form an integral relationship that is important to understand. As the bladder fills with urine, bladder pressure remains stable over a volume range of 0–500 ml. This is mainly due to the viscoelastic properties of its wall.[2] These properties are a function of muscular, neural, and connective tissue components. Normal compliance therefore approaches infinity (DV/DP) (Fig. 10.1).[3]

2 A stable detrusor muscle. The bladder contracts in response to activation of stretch receptors in the bladder wall whose afferent fibres run in the lateral spinothalamic tract of the spinal cord to the micturition centre in the pons. Influences from higher centers are mainly inhibitory. The pontine micturition centre works as a switch. It

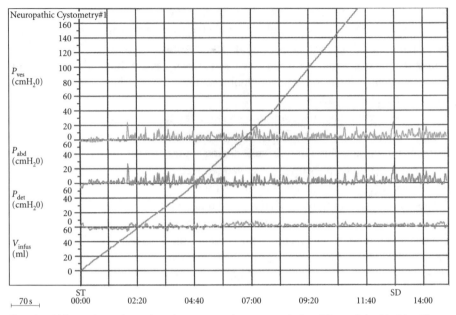

Fig. 10.1 This urodynamic tracing shows normal pressures during filling of the bladder. The line running obliquely shows increasing volume as the bladder is filled. The top trace shows the total pressure (abdominal plus intravesical). The middle trace shows intra-abdominal pressure. The bottom trace shows the abdominal pressure subtracted from the intravesical pressure representing true detrusor pressure (or subtracted pressure). The detrusor pressure remains consistently at 0 cmH$_2$O (calibrated) despite increasing volume as a result of normal compliance and stability of the detrusor muscle.

requires a certain level of afferent input and higher centre disinhibition to activate the micturition reflex. Thus the bladder contracts and empties to completion normally under voluntary control at a socially acceptable time and place. Involuntary contractions are abnormal and a common cause of urinary incontinence frequently associated with a sensation of urge.[4–6]

Pathophysiology

Poor-compliance, small-capacity bladder Particularly in patients with neuropathic bladder dysfunction or bladder fibrosis following radiotherapy, bladder compliance can be low resulting in a rapid rise in bladder pressure during filling. If sphincter pressure is normal or increased and the bladder continues to fill, intravesical pressure may exceed intraureteric/intrapelvic pressure causing functional obstruction of the upper urinary tract. Besides urodynamic assessment, this may be evidenced by bilateral hydronephrosis on ultrasound. The bladder pressure at which urethral leakage occurs is predictive of upper tract deterioration and a pressure greater than 40 cmH$_2$O is a critical threshold for renal injury.[7]

Small capacity and poor compliance usually coexist. These bladders have a low structural and/or functional volume resulting in frequency, urgency, and urge incontinence. Chronic inflammation of the bladder wall results in replacement of healthy collagen and muscle with inflexible fibrous tissue resulting in a small, poorly compliant bladder as seen in the following:

1 Permanent indwelling catheterization (urethral or suprapubic) is a potent cause of chronic inflammation and small contracted bladder. This explains some of the problems associated with permanent catheterization.

2 History of radiotherapy (often 15–20 years later) to any pelvic organ, e.g. prostate or cervix, increases the risk a small, contracted bladder.

3 Cystitis following cyclophosphamide can have a similar effect.

4 Chronic bladder denervation, particularly where intermittent catheterization has not been employed, may result in poor compliance and small capacity as in the patient with spinal cord injury, spina bifida, or multiple sclerosis.

Detrusor overactivity This term describes the bladder that contracts inappropriately, involuntarily, and often independently of volume (Fig. 10.2). There are two important subgroups:

1 The neurologically intact patient. In this group overactive bladder is characterized urodynamically by the finding of detrusor instability. Aetiology is predominantly idiopathic instability.

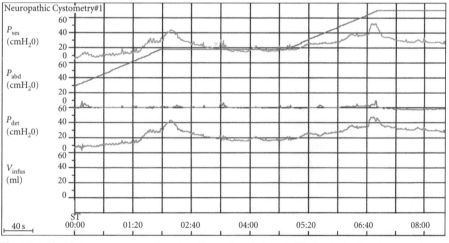

Fig. 10.2 The detrusor pressure rises steadily as the bladder is filled culminating in an end filling pressure of 30 cmH$_2$O. This reflects poor compliance of the detrusor muscle. The rise plateaus when filling is stopped in the middle section indicating that compliance is a function of volume. The intermittent peaks reflect unstable contractions (see also Fig. 10.3). These pressures reflect true detrusor pressure as they vary with total pressure while the rectal pressures remain consistently at 0 cmH$_2$O.

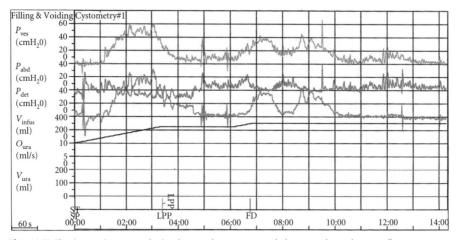

Fig. 10.3 The intermittent peaks in the total pressure and detrusor (or subtracted) pressure curves illustrate unstable contractions. Again they are independent of a stable rectal pressure. The compliance is normal (end filling pressure is 0 cmH₂O). Unlike compliance pressures, the pressures due to unstable contractions once initiated are independent of filling.

  2 The patient with a neurological deficit, e.g. congenital disorders affecting the sacral segments of the spinal cord (spina bifida), acquired disorders of the sacral spinal cord and peripheral nervous system (spinal cord injuries, multiple sclerosis), and disorders of the central nervous system (Parkinson's disease, cerebrovascular accident).

Detrusor underactivity Detrusor underactivity (Fig. 10.3) implies detrusor contractions of reduced strength or duration resulting in inefficient bladder emptying but not usually incontinence. However, when the detrusor is acontractile, overflow incontinence may result. There are two important subgroups:

  1 The neurologically intact patient, e.g. prostatic outlet obstruction or chronic detrusor failure.

  2 The neurologically abnormal patient. These are divided into congenital disorders, e.g. spina bifida, sacral agenesis, and acquired disorders, e.g. following abdominoperineal resection of the rectum or Wertheim's hysterectomy.

The outlet

The role of the outlet is to maintain continence at all ambient bladder pressures. Failure of the outlet to provide resistance results in stress urinary incontinence (e.g. leakage of urine during increased intraabdominal pressure such as laughing or coughing). Low outlet resistance can coexist with bladder overactivity leading to mixed incontinence.

The female outlet

Anatomy The female urethra is approximately 4 cm long, 1.5 cm of which is intrab-dominal. The bladder base and urethra are supported by the pelvic floor muscles and fasciae. The meatus is found just anterior to the vagina. The female sphincter is composed of smooth muscle throughout and specialized striated muscle enveloping the middle two-fourths of the urethra. The bladder neck is also known as the proximal sphincter. The distal sphincter comprises both smooth and specialized striated muscle components. Innervation of smooth muscle is both sympathetic and parasympathetic and the specialized striated muscle of the distal sphincter is innervated by pudendal somatic motorneurons arising in a special anterior horn nucleus (of Onuf) which is more resistant to some degenerative diseases of the anterior horn such as motor neuron disease.[8] It is worth noting that the urethral orifice can be inside the vagina on the anterior wall which can create problems with catheterization.

Physiology:

There are four main components to the continence mechanism:

1 Bladder neck or proximal (smooth muscle) sphincter.

2 Distal (mid-urethral) sphincter composed of smooth and specialized striated muscle.

3 Extrinsic muscles of the pelvic floor.

4 Non-muscular factors: turgidity (vascularity) of the submucosa, epithelial surface tension and urethral wall elasticity.

Components 1 and 2 are tonically active whereas 3 is phasically active either voluntarily or in a reflex fashion, e.g. with coughing. The smooth and striated muscle of the proximal and distal sphincters can be reflexly activated in response to bladder filling and other stimuli. Conversely, reflex relaxation occurs just prior to bladder contraction during voiding.

Pathophysiology Urethral compliance and coaption relies on vascularity and healthy collagen/elastin. Relative oestrogen deficiency in the post-menopausal woman is the most common cause of reduced coaption and elasticity. Examination often reveals thin vulval tissues that bleed easily on contact, i.e. atrophic vaginitis

Denervation of the sphincter, e.g. post-partum or following pelvic organ resection or urethral surgery, may result in stress urinary incontinence. Radiation may result in denervation and compromised tissue blood supply resulting in the so-called 'stovepipe urethra'. In this scenario there is failure of the urethra to coapt with leakage of urine at very low bladder pressures (also known as intrinsic sphincter deficiency). The result of this is leakage of urine with minimal exertion.[9] In these extreme cases, the urethral meatus orifice is constantly open, rigid, and pale.

One should remember that radiation is also a common cause of delayed (up to 20 years later) vesicovaginal fistulae and the clinical scenario of constant urinary leak may be difficult to distinguish from above by the casual examiner.

The male outlet

Anatomy The male urethra is approximately 20 cm long. It passes from the bladder neck and through the prostate and pelvic floor/perineum to the penis. As in the female there is a proximal smooth muscle continence mechanism at the bladder neck. Unlike the female there is a significant prostatic smooth muscle component. In men the distal mechanism lies distal to the verumontanum in the prostatic urethra and comprises smooth muscle and specialized striated muscle. This region varies in length between 0.8 and 2 cm. The sphincter is wrapped around the lower end of the prostate and here encompasses the urethra. The prostatic and sphincteric portion of the urethra is called the posterior urethra. From here the urethra passes into the bulb of the penis. The bulbar and penile portion is called the anterior urethra.

Physiology The bladder neck and the prostate provide a constant resistance during filling of the bladder. Both are important continence mechanisms but continence can be achieved with only one functioning sphincter, e.g. following transurethral prostatectomy when the bladder neck has been resected. The prostate and the length of the male sphincter urethra confer a more powerful continence mechanism than in the female urethra.

Pathophysiology Stress incontinence is clearly less common in the male and is either neuropathic or iatrogenic. If both bladder neck and sphincter function is lost, incontinence ensues. Radical prostatectomy for prostate cancer relies on careful reconstruction of the bladder neck and protection of the distal sphincter and its innervation to minimize the risk of stress incontinence, but stress incontinence occurs in all post-radical prostatectomy patients initially; it is persistently troublesome or severe in 10%.[10] In transurethral resection of the prostate for benign prostatic hyperplasia (BPH) the bladder neck is resected by definition. If the distal sphincter is inadvertently resected or was previously affected by disease (e.g. Parkinson's disease) incontinence may ensue. Malignant infiltration (e.g. from prostate cancer) of the sphincter also causes incontinence. History is the key to diagnosis. Neuropathic causes of sphincter injury include congenital abnormalities, e.g. spina bifida, and acquired disease, e.g. sacral spinal cord injury.

Urinary fistulae

A urinary fistula is an abnormal connection that develops between the bladder or urethra and the skin or an adjacent organ (e.g. vagina, rectum). It results in a constant leakage of urine from the affected organ or skin sinus and usually occurs in response to severe and chronic inflammation (e.g. radiation cystitis, diverticulitis of the sigmoid colon) or malignancy (e.g. cancer of the bladder, rectum, cervix). This is relatively rare but an important diagnosis not to miss. The clue is in the recognition of the at-risk groups and the constant (including nocturnal) and insensible nature of the leakage.

Investigation

Diagnosis begins with history and examination.

Basic investigations

Urinary retention

Urinary retention with overflow should be excluded in all patients. If the bladder is clearly palpable the patient should be catheterized. If not, then the post-void residual should be documented by ultrasound (ideally) or in and out catheter.

Examination of urine

Urinary infection can coexist with or exacerbate incontinence. A urine examination (including nitrites, leucocytes, and blood) is an inexpensive screening tool. If the dipstick test is negative then usually no further urinary testing is indicated. If the dipstick tests positive for nitrates and/or leucocytes, a specimen should be sent for microscopy and culture. This finding can also be indicative of a urinary tract stone.

Frequency/volume charts

Incontinence can be caused or exacerbated by excessive fluid intake, particularly of diuretic fluids like caffeine or alcohol. A frequency/volume chart allows assessment of frequency of micturition, day and nighttime urine production, average voided volume, functional bladder capacity, and whether polydipsia and polyuria are present. The patient is given a grid chart with a vertical time axis. He or she measures the volume at each void in a suitable graduated receptacle and (if required) the volume ingested to the nearest hour. For a 70 kg person 1500 ml per 24 hours is a reasonable 24-hour urinary output limit. When more than 33% of output occurs during the bedtime hours this constitutes nocturnal polyuria. Although somewhat cumbersome, this is an essential investigation and if necessary the information should be gathered by a caregiver.

Advanced investigations

Further investigations are invasive, expensive, and not indicated in all patients. The question that should be asked is: will this change my management? This is particularly important in the terminally ill when disruptive and uncomfortable investigations should only be imposed if they are likely to lead to clear patient benefit. A trial of anticholinergic therapy is reasonable in the patient with suspected bladder overactivity before any further investigations.

Plain abdominal film or bladder/renal ultrasound

Bladder stones can be a cause of irritation and cause incontinence. If the patient is at risk of forming bladder stones (e.g. a neuropathic bladder, chronic retention, or permanent indwelling catheter) then a plain film or pelvic ultrasound is indicated.

Urodynamic examination

Urodynamic testing is indicated when:

+ Anticholinergic therapy has failed (may have stress incontinence).
+ There is evidence of hydronephrosis or upper tract deterioration (may have poor bladder compliance).
+ Surgical reconstruction is being considered.
+ Surgical treatment has failed.
+ Diagnosis or follow-up of neuropathic bladder is needed.

An unstable contraction is identified by phasic contractions during bladder filling that continue even if filling is stopped (see Fig. 10.2) They are significant if the pressures are high enough to cause a sense of urgency, incontinence, and/or secondary vesicoureteric reflux. (The latter can be documented by using radiographic contrast as the filling medium with simultaneous fluoroscopy.)

Poor compliance is a steady increase in pressure in response to filling and is directly related to volume (see Fig. 10.3). Stress incontinence is identified by observing leakage from the urethra (directly or using fluoroscopy) during raised intra-abdominal pressures (coughing, straining). The pressures required to produce leakage are measured by recording abdominal and/or intravesical pressure using a fluid-filled or microtip catheter. The lower the abdominal pressure at which urinary leak occurs (abdominal leak point pressure) the more severe the incontinence.[11]

Studies of the upper tracts

The main reason to investigate upper tracts is to determine if high intravesical pressure responsible for the incontinence is also causing functional upper tract obstruction. If this is the case an ultrasound will show bilateral hydronephrosis. This combined with a rising creatinine indicates the aforementioned and makes a strong case for aggressive treatment if the prognosis warrants this. An example is the patient with spina bifida who has a poorly compliant bladder that only leaks at high intravesical pressure.

Cystoscopy

The role of cystoscopy in this setting is to rule out other pathology, e.g. stone, in the patient with an indwelling catheter or tumour in the patient with frank haematuria. This procedure can almost always be done with a flexible instrument that does not require anaesthesia.

Treatment

Chronic retention

Urinary retention with overflow must be ruled out or managed as described in Chapter 9.

Overactive bladder

Anticholinergic medication

The simplest treatment for detrusor overactivity is anticholinergic medication. The mechanism of action is cholinergic blockade. The drawbacks are limited efficacy and a side-effect profile that reduces patient compliance. The most common side-effect is a dry mouth due to blocking of the cholinergic receptors in the salivary glands. The aim of newer anticholinergic preparations is to improve the side- effect profile by increasing receptor specificity. Dry mouth can be counteracted using sweets, gum, or artificial saliva. Increasing fluid intake should be discouraged.

Fluid control

A frequency/volume chart will reveal excessive input/output. Generally, output should not exceed 1500 ml in 24 hours. If this is exceeded, input should be reduced accordingly. Avoidance of caffeine, alcohol, and diuretics is recommended. Treatable causes of polyuria should be addressed.

Desmopressin

Desmopressin is a synthetic form of antidiuretic hormone and is effective in reducing polyuria, particularly nocturnal polyuria and nocturnal enuresis. It should be restricted to patients younger than 65 years to avoid exacerbation of congestive heart failure and electrolyte disturbance.

Bladder augmentation

The gold standard surgical treatment for intractable overactivity is bladder augmentation. In essence, a segment of detubularized bowel is sewn into the bivalved bladder ('augmentation cystoplasty'). The bowel segment acts as a diverticulum, which increases capacity and compliance, absorbs contraction pressure, and may interrupt the spread of a detrusor contraction. There is no doubt that it is effective in resolving instability, particularly when the capacity is reduced. Subsequent loss of bladder contractility means the patient may need to catheterize themselves in order to empty. This is the case in most neuropathic and a significant percentage of non-neuropathic patients (men more than women). The decision to proceed with this surgery should not be taken lightly since the potential complications of a bowel/urine interface are considerable and include mucous excretion potentially causing outlet obstruction, stone formation, urinary infection, and a very small risk of malignancy. It is suitable for patients with reasonable performance status and life expectancy.[11]

An alternative operation is detrusor myectomy, where the muscular layer is stripped from the underlying mucosa which subsequently herniates acting as a diverticulum. It is effective in up to 75% of patients, particularly non-neuropathic ones, and avoids the complications of bowel in the urinary tract.[12]

Therapies under research

It is the aim of researchers to find a therapy more effective than anticholinergic medications and less traumatic than bladder augmentation. The following are some examples though none are in widespread clinical use as yet.

Intravesical instillation Intravesical instillation is a method that aims to increase the efficacy of agents in the bladder and avoid systemic effects. The earliest agents to be studies were anticholinergics (e.g. oxybutinin, atropine) and local anesthetics (e.g. bupivocaine, lidocaine (lignocaine)). Regardless of the variable efficacy in reducing sensation and increasing capacity, the limited duration of effect (less than 8 hours) precludes them from common clinical use.[13,14]

However, the efficacy of local anaesthetics in blocking afferent stimulation and thereby moderating efferent cholinergic activity has inspired a search for an agent that has a more enduring effect. Capsaicin and resiniferatoxin are two agents found to temporarily reduce the population of C-afferent fibres responsible for the afferent arm of the spinal micturition reflex, leading to increased bladder capacity and fewer incontinent episodes for up to 6 months. Resinoferotoxin has the significant advantage of being a non-irritant and therefore does not require a general or local anaesthetic for instillation. These agents have been shown to be particularly effective in patients with multiple sclerosis and spinal cord injury. The limitations are that this is only suitable for motivated patients of reasonable performance status who are able to self-catheterize and the efficacy is variable.[14]

Sacral neuromodulation Sacral neuromodulation acts on the efferent fibres of the spinal micturition reflex at the level of the sacral spinal cord (usually S3). The methods of sacral nerve modulation vary from surgical ablation to implantation of neurostimulator units.[15] The main limitations are the invasiveness of the procedures and the lack of specificity of the effect. That is, other pelvic organs also supplied by S3 and S4 can be adversely affected (e.g. reduced bowel motility, erectile function).

Cannabis extracts Initial trials researching the effects of cannabis extracts administered sublingually have shown promising results in terms of increasing the functional and anatomical capacity of the bladder mainly in neuropathic patients. These have stimulated larger trials which are currently awaiting publication.[16]

Botulinum toxin Botulinum toxin is a well-known neurotoxin that causes paralysis by blockade of the peripheral neuromuscular junction. Recent studies have investigated its therapeutic use in lower urinary tract dysfunction. A number of studies (albeit using small subject numbers) have shown that injection directly into the detrusor muscle of the overactive bladder leads to increased capacity and decreased number of incontinent episodes. It has been studied more extensively in neuropathic hyperreflexia than idiopathic instability, though more comprehensive investigations are in progress. Injection is a relatively simple transurethral procedure using local anaesthetic and the effect endures for up to 9 months. The patient must be prepared to self-catheterize after the procedure and there is a very small risk of serious systemic toxicity. It is not available for common clinical use at this stage.[17,18]

Treating causative and exacerbating factors

Indwelling catheters

The aetiologies underlying most high-pressure bladders are difficult or impossible to address (neurological disease, idiopathic instability). The exception to this is chronic inflammation secondary to an intravesical foreign body. The most common and the most potent of all foreign bodies is the permanent indwelling catheter which deserves special mention. The urethral catheter needs to be *in situ* for only a few days before the acute inflammatory reaction in the bladder wall is evident. The transitional mucosa develops bullous oedema around the contact point of the balloon and becomes friable. This acute inflammation may be troublesome since the trigone is usually involved. Early complications tend to persist as long as the catheter is in but are reversible on its removal. The most common are haematuria and bladder spasms causing intermittent intense suprapubic pain radiating to the penile tip and urine leakage around the catheter. (Note that penile tip pain is referred pain from the trigone and explains why a suprapubic catheter may cause penile tip pain.) The haematuria is rarely threatening and bladder spasm should be treated with anticholinergics rather than simple analgesia.

Late complications of long-term catheterization are common and are frequently more debilitating than the presenting incontinence. If life expectancy is less than 6 months then troublesome complications are unlikely and catheterization is reasonable to facilitate nursing care. If this is the case it is important that fluid intake is sufficient to avoid encrusting of the catheter and stone formation, and in contrast to the non-catheterized patient output volumes should exceed 2 l per day. Clearly the longer the life expectancy of a patient, the less acceptable permanent catheterization is.

Fibrosis in the bladder wall has irreversible effects on the viscoelestic properties of the bladder resulting in a small poorly compliant bladder. The consequences are constant leakage of urine around the catheter and the risk of upper tract deterioration. Increasing the catheter or balloon size or changing the catheter altogether has very little impact. Anticholinergics may improve things a little but as the underlying problem is structural, anything less than major surgery is weakly palliative.

As the bladder gets smaller, the inflamed wall and trigone has greater contact with the catheter balloon causing recurrent bladder spasm and chronic suprapubic/ penile tip pain.

When there is haematuria, recurrent or chronic, one must be careful to exclude other underlying pathologies when appropriate; however, chronic haematuria is common in long-term catheterization and seldom has a sudden impact on the haemoglobin level. It is distressing for the patient, however, particularly if the catheter becomes blocked with clots.

Colonization describes the adherence of an organism to a surface. Infection is when a pathogenic organism causes an inflammatory response in the biological host with clinical signs, e.g. haematuria and fever. Colonization of the urinary catheter is inevitable. It increases the risk of infection but it is not in itself an infection and should not be treated. In fact it is impossible to sterilize the catheter with antibiotics and the only treatment is to remove the catheter. Furthermore, shedding of red and white blood cells in the urine due to an inflamed bladder wall is similarly inevitable and does not necessarily denote an infection. Therefore, urinalyses and cultures are not helpful in diagnosing urinary infection in the presence of a catheter (or any foreign body). An infection should only be diagnosed and treated on the basis of clinical symptoms and signs.

It should be noted that suprapubic catheters have the same complications as urethral catheters with the exception of urethral erosion (see below). In fact, urine leakage around the suprapubic catheter can be more troublesome due to excoriation of the abdominal skin around the puncture site.

Urethral erosion is the endpoint in the natural history of chronic inflammation and ulceration of the urethra due to long-term urethral catheterization. It is clinically evident by full thickness erosion of the ventral wall of the urethra and penis or perineum (Fig. 10.4). It is relatively common at the penile meatus but can extend proximally to involve the entire penoscrotal urethra to a greater or lesser degree. Urethral erosion is clearly an indication for a suprapubic catheter. If the patient is at high risk, then it should be placed in the first instance (e.g. wheelchair-bound patients).

There are alternatives to indwelling urethral catheters and these include:

1 The condom drainage catheter. This device is a sheath that adheres onto the penis and is connected to the catheter tubing and bag. The sheath simply collects the urine, which then drains into the catheter tubing. It is important that the bladder

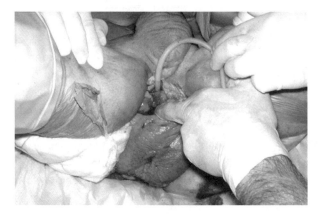

Fig. 10.4 This paraplegic man had a permanent urethral catheter for a number of years. The catheter has caused full thickness erosion of the bulbar urethra and perineal tissues. The erosion is evident between the scrotum above and the chronically inflamed tissues of the perineum below as shown by the surgeon's finger.

in this circumstance empties at low pressure and that the condom catheter is not being used to collect overflow urine from a bladder in retention. In some cases it is preferable to convert the obstructed lower urinary tract to an unobstructed and incontinent system that drains at low pressure into a condom catheter. The obvious example is the spinal cord injured patient with detrusor sphincter dysynergia. To avoid a permanent intravesical catheter, the sphincter function is obliterated. This is achieved by incising the sphincter muscle transurethrally ('sphincterotomy') or inserting a transsphincteric stent. The limitation of condom catheters is the tendency of the condom to fall off the penis, particularly if the penis is short and/or the patient is obese. A recent design modification addresses this by making the base of the sheath similar to a stoma bag, which adheres to the abdominal wall and scrotum around the base of the penis.

2 Clean intermittent self-catheterization (CISC). CICS is the ideal alternative to permanently attached or indwelling devices. Regardless of age and gender, as long as the patient has reasonable dexterity and vision, and can reach the perineum, the only things stopping them are the preconceived ideas of the patient and commonly the caregiver. The patient is taught to perform in/out urethral catheterization on themselves. This can usually be done in a single session with a continence advisor. The process is clean rather than sterile and the patient can use the same catheter many times, washing it in hot water between uses. Catheters are modified to facilitate ease of use, e.g. self-lubricating, angle tipped.

Permanent indwelling catheters are indicated to facilitate nursing care and patient comfort if the prognosis is limited. The lumen of the selected catheter should be large enough to minimize blockage but not so large as to be uncomfortable. A 16 to 18 gauge is usually suitable. The catheter ideally should be 100% silicone rather than latex coated with silicone. If the two are compared, the silicone catheter will have a larger lumen despite being the same outer calibre. This is because silicone can be more effectively machined and manipulated.

Bladder stones

Another common foreign body is the bladder stone, which develops if there is chronic stasis of urine or foreign body (such as an indwelling urethral catheter). If the patient is at risk of stones and develops exacerbation or a new onset of incontinence, a stone should be excluded. An annual plain film is reasonable in the at-risk groups. Surgical removal can usually be performed endoscopically.

Infection

Infective cystitis causes an acute and painful inflammation of the bladder wall. This creates a painful sensation of urgency at low urine volumes and to a certain degree instability. Therefore effective antibiotic treatment of a urinary infection can significantly palliate incontinence. Prophylactic treatment with long-term low-dose antibiotics may be indicated in the non-catheterized patient with recurrent bothersome urinary infections resistant to short courses of appropriate antibiotics. A prophylactic antibiotic should have a favourable side-effect profile and a low incidence of resistance, e.g. nitrofurantoin.

Cognitive impairment

A certain degree of cognition is required to cope with incontinence, particularly in accepting and using the anticontinence devices. Therefore minimizing confusion by treating reversible causes, facilitating a familiar environment, night-lights etc, reduces the burden of incontinence. A degree of cognition is required to void appropriately in time and space and therefore cognitive impairment can in itself be an aetiology of incontinence.

Stress urinary incontinence

Unlike the overactive bladder, stress urinary incontinence is usually amenable to curative surgery. The most common aetiology is loss of pelvic floor supports or intrinsic disease of the urethral wall. In these cases a pubovaginal sling operation is usually indicated but again requires a reasonable performance status. Another group is those with a structurally abnormal bladder neck and sphincter mechanism, whether it be congenital as in spina bifida or bladder extrophy or acquired as in men after radical prostatectomy. The surgical options are bladder neck reconstruction or insertion of an artificial urinary sphincter. Both of these are major undertakings and particularly in the former still leave the patient with a degree of incontinence that is unresolvable.

An alternative procedure to outlet surgery is injection of a bulking agent (transurethrally or transperineally) into the periurethral tissues. Biological materials (e.g. highly purified bovine collagen) superceded early synthetic materials which were associated with granuloma formation and distant migration. However, durability is a problem as biological materials tend to be reabsorbed with time. More recently synthetic agents have been refined and are usually composed of synthetic beads (e.g. silicone, zirconium oxide) of appropriate size to avoid migration suspended in a carrier gel. The material is injected submucosally under local anaesthetic and is appropriate for primary treatment in those not fit for general anaesthetic or as an adjunctive treatment if surgery results in partial response. The aim is for improvement rather than cure in many cases. The success rate is approximately 50–70% and multiple treatments are frequently required.[19] Pelvic floor exercises are reserved for mild cases of stress urinary incontinence due to urethral hypermobility.

Special groups

Children and adolescents

Children and adolescents with long-term incontinence often have other co-morbidities due to an underlying neurological disease. The very young are dependent on caregivers, usually a parent. Support and education of this person is integral part of the holistic care of the patient. As the child becomes an adolescent, the challenge is preparing them to take responsibility for their own care. Ideally, a balance is achieved between ensuring a high quality of self-management and maintaining the patient's enthusiasm and compliance during the social upheaval of adolescence. A multidisciplinary approach and community-based groups with an appropriate peer group are invaluable tools in the care of these patients.

The elderly

A common tendency is to underestimate the elderly person's ability to actively manage their own urinary tract and relegate them to permanent catheterization only to find that in a few months they are worse off. Regardless of age, an elderly person with reasonable cognition and dexterity can be taught to manage an external device with the correct instruction.

Spinal cord injuries

Prior to adequate management of the urinary tract in the spinally injured, renal failure was a common cause of premature death in this group. The primary goal is to maintain the bladder as a low-pressure reservoir without resorting to permanent catheterization. This can be a challenge, particularly if the patient is non-compliant or their dexterity precludes self-catheterization. Education of the patient and caregivers with ongoing motivational support and urinary tract review are the keystones to management.

The terminally ill

Clearly the aim is patient comfort and ease of nursing care. Investigation and management are balanced against the benefit to the patient, keeping in mind the prognosis.

Conclusion

The management of urinary incontinence in patients requiring palliative support can be easily reduced to three basic principles:

- Appropriate management of fluid intake and output.
- Avoidance if possible of indwelling urinary catheters.
- Selective use of invasive or minimally invasive procedures.

References

1 Abrams P, Cardozo L, Fall M, Griffiths D, Rosier P, Ulmsten U *et al.* (2002). The standardisation of terminology of the lower urinary tract function: report from the Standardization Subcommittee of the International Continence Society. *Neurol. Urodyn.* **21**: 167–78.
2 Van Mastright R, Coolsaet B, Van Duyl W (1978). Passive properties of the urinary bladder in the collection phase. *Med. Biol. Eng. Comput.* **16**: 471–82.
3 Klevmark B (1974). Motility of the urinary bladder in cats during filling at physiological rates: intravesical pressure patterns studied by a new method of cystommetry. *Acta Physiol. Scand.* **90**: 565.

4 Mundy AR, Thomas PJ (1994). Clinical physiology of the bladder, urethra and pelvic floor. In: *Urodynamics, Principles, Practice and Application* (ed. AR Mundy, TP Stephenson, AJ Wein), pp. 15–27. Churchill Livingstone, New York.

5 Wein A (1998). Pathophysiology and categorization of voiding dysfunction. In: *Campbells Urology*, 7th edn (ed. P Walsh, A Retik, A Wein), pp. 917–26. W. A. Saunders, Philadelphia, PA.

6 De Groat WC (1993). Anatomy and physiology of the lower urinary tract. *Urol. Clin. N. Am.* **20**(3): 383.

7 McGuire EJ, Woodside JR, Borden TA, Weiss RM (1981). Prognostic value of urodynamic testing in myelodysplastic patients. *J. Urol.* **126**: 205.

8 Schroder HDD (1981). Onufs nucleus X: a morphological study of a human spinal nucleus. *Anat. Embryol.* **162**: 443–5.

9 McGuire EJ, Fitzpatrick CC, Wan J, Bloom DA, Sanvordenker J, Ritchey ML (1993). Clinical assessment of urethral sphincter function. *J. Urol.* **150**: 1452–4.

10 Fowler FJ, Barry MJ, Lu-Yao G (1995). Effect of radical prostatectomy for prostate cancer on patient quality of life: result from a Medicare survey *Urology* **45**: 1007–15.

11 Greenwell TJ, Venn SN, Mundy AR (2001). Augmentation cystoplasty [review]. *BJU Int.* **88**(6): 511–25.

12 Leng W, Blalock HJ, Fredriksson W, English S, McGuire EJ (1999). Enterocystoplasty or detrusor myectomy? Comparison of indications and outcomes for bladder augmentation. *J. Urol.* **161**: 758–63.

13 Fowler C (2000). Intravesical treatment of overactive bladder. *Urology* **55**: 60–6.

14 Dasgupta P, Chandiramani V, Beckett A, Scaravilli F, Fowler C (2000). The effect of intravesical capsaicin on the suburothelial innervation in patients with detrusor hyper-reflexia. *BJU Int.* **85**: 238–45.

15 Janknegt R, Hassouna M, Seigal S, Schmidt RA, Gajewski JB, Rivas DA *et al.* (2001). Longterm effectiveness of sacral nerve stimulation for refractory urge incontinence. *Eur. Urol.* **39**: 101–6.

16 Wade D, Robbson P, House H, Makela P, Aram J (2003). A preliminary controlled study to determine whether whole-plant extracts can improve intractable neurogenic symptoms. *Clin. Rehab.* **17**: 21–9.

17 Harper M, Fowler CJ, DasGupta P (2004). Botulinum toxin and its applications in the lower urinary tract. *BJU Int.* **93**: 702–6.

18 Leippold T, Reitz A, Schurch S (2003). Botulinum toxin as a new therapy option for voiding disorders: current state of the art. *Eur. Urol.* **44**: 165–74.

19 Wilson T, Lemack G, Zimmern P (2003). Management if intrinsic sphincter deficiency in women [review]. *J. Urol.* **169**: 1662–9.

Chapter 11

The patient presenting with neurological disease affecting the urinary tract

Scott MacDiarmid

Neurogenic bladder dysfunction describes the abnormal changes in function of the bladder and urethra that result from lesions of their innervation, either within the central nervous system or the peripheral nerves of the lower urinary tract. Because of the complex innervation of the bladder, urethra, and pelvic floor, almost any neurological lesion may result in voiding dysfunction. Discrete neurological lesions at various levels within the nervous system usually affect the bladder and urethra in a relatively consistent fashion.

The goal of this chapter is to provide physicians with a functional working knowledge of neurogenic bladder dysfunction based on the location of the neurological lesion so they can better understand and anticipate the types of urinary problems their patients may suffer from as a result of neurological disease. The diagnosis, work-up, and management of patients with neurogenic bladder dysfunction are also presented. In addition, the concepts of high-pressure neurogenic bladder and autonomic dysreflexia are discussed since both entities can result in significant patient morbidity.

Neuroanatomy

Basic understanding of the neuroanatomy and neurophysiology of the bladder and urethra is germane to any discussion regarding neurogenic bladder dysfunction. Bladder filling and emptying is primarily a function of the peripheral autonomic nervous system, which in turn is controlled by the cerebral cortex.

Peripheral pathways

The autonomic and somatic nervous systems make up the peripheral innervation of the lower urinary tract.[1-4] The parasympathetic (cholinergic) efferent innervation originates in the intermediolateral region of the grey matter of the sacral spinal cord segments S2–S4 and exits as ventral nerve roots that ultimately become part of the pelvic nerve. The parasympathetic nerves primarily innervate the bladder body and dome and are responsible for voiding. Stimulation of the parasympathetics results in a coordinated bladder contraction and emptying.

In contrast, the sympathetic nervous system is responsible for bladder storage. The efferent sympathetic nerve fibres originate in the intermediolateral nuclei of the thoracolumbar spinal cord segments T11–T12 and L1–L2, which help form the superior hypogastric plexus and the right and left hypogastric nerves. The sympathetic (adrenergic) fibres primarily innervate the bladder base and proximal urethra. Sympathetic stimulation of α-adrenergic receptors located in the bladder neck and proximal urethra result in bladder neck closure facilitating bladder storage.

The external sphincter mechanism and pelvic floor musculature are innervated through the somatic nervous system by the pudendal nerve originating in the sacral spinal cord segments S2–S4. Somatic innervation of the external sphincter allows one to voluntarily stop the urinary stream.

Less is known regarding the sensory innervation of the lower urinary tract. Afferent pathways arise from bladder stretch receptors and from pain and temperature receptors in the bladder, urethra, and pelvic floor. The pelvic, pudendal, and hypogastric nerves transmit afferent messages to the spinal cord segments T10–L2 and S2–S4, where they ascend in the central nervous system.

Central pathways

The primary coordinating centre that controls vesicourethral function is located within the brainstem, specifically in the nucleus locus coeruleus of the pons.[5]

During bladder filling, stimulated stretch receptors send impulses up the spinothalamic tract of the spinal cord to the pontine micturition centre. From the pons, the messages descend in the spinal cord central canal and intermediolateral grey matter to the

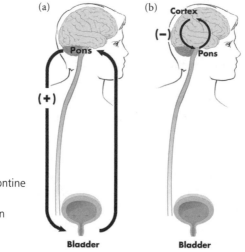

(a)
Pons
(+)

(b)
Cortex
(–)
Pons

Fig. 11.1 (a) The pontine micturition reflex. (b) Central inhibition of the pontine micturition reflex.

Bladder   Bladder

bladder, resulting in detrusor contraction (Fig. 11.1a). This is the primary reflex arc that coordinates bladder filling and emptying. The pontine centre synchronizes bladder contraction with relaxation of the urethral sphincter mechanism during voiding.

The cerebral cortex involved with bladder function is located primarily on the medial aspect of the frontal lobe and within the genu of the corpus callosum. Its primary effect on bladder function appears to be inhibitory (Fig. 11.1b). The frontal cortex inhibits the pontine voiding reflex facilitating bladder storage.[6]

Classification of neurogenic bladder dysfunction

Lesions resulting in neurogenic bladder dysfunction may be classified into supraspinal, suprasacral, and infrasacral, according to the level of the lesion with regard to the pontine micturition centre and conus, where a sacral voiding centre exists.[7–9] Supraspinal lesions include all lesions above the level of the brainstem and pons. Suprasacral lesions are all spinal cord lesions above the conus. Infrasacral lesions involve the conus or sacral roots and may be further subdivided into cauda equina lesions (within the spinal canal) and peripheral nerve lesions (outside the spinal canal). Neurological disease within each level tends to affect the bladder and urethra in a relatively consistent manner allowing the physician to better anticipate the patient's voiding dysfunction.

Supraspinal lesions

Patients with diseases of the cerebral cortex, including stroke, dementia, tumour, and Parkinson's disease commonly report bladder dysfunction. Regardless of the underlying pathology, diseases of the cerebral cortex adversely affect bladder function similarly. Central inhibition of the pontine micturition reflex is lost, resulting in uncontrolled reflex bladder contractions. Bladder instability secondary to neurological disease, once termed detrusor hyperreflexia,[10] is now called neurogenic detrusor overactivity (Fig. 11.2b).[11] An intact pons ensures normal coordination between the bladder and urethra, maintaining low and safe voiding pressures. Patients with supraspinal lesions do not develop high-pressure bladders which can threaten renal function and therefore do not need routine upper tract surveillance.

Patients with bladder instability secondary to supraspinal lesions most commonly report irritative voiding symptoms, including urinary frequency, nocturia, urgency, and urge incontinence. When sensory pathways are affected, they may not perceive bladder contractions as urgency but instead experience unconscious leakage. Many patients with supraspinal lesions also suffer from cognitive or functional impairment which may adversely affect their continence status.

Those with supraspinal lesions generally maintain voiding function and can volitionally empty their bladder efficiently. In those with impaired voiding, other causes should be considered including bladder outlet obstruction secondary to benign prostatic hyperplasia. Pre-existing bladder dysfunction is not uncommon in those who suffer

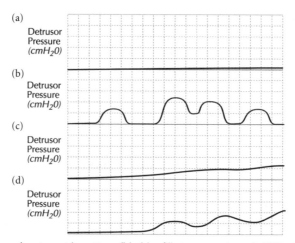

Fig. 11.2 (a) Normal cystometric pattern (bladder fills to approximately 500 ml without an associated rise in bladder pressure or involuntary bladder contraction). (b) Neurogenic detrusor overactivity (involuntary bladder contractions during bladder filling). (c) Loss of bladder compliance (gradual increase in bladder pressure associated with bladder filling). (d) Bladder instability in a 'stepping pattern' associated with loss of bladder compliance.

from neurological disease. Less commonly, supraspinal lesions can neurologically impair bladder contractility.

Spinal shock may occur in patients following an acute cerebral event such as stroke, surgery, or even severe concussion. Bladder contractility is temporarily impaired resulting in urinary retention. The duration of spinal shock is generally much shorter than that with spinal cord injuries, usually lasting for only a few days or weeks. During this period, urinary retention is best managed by either an indwelling or clean intermittent catheterization, depending on the patient's functional ability and support staff. A trial of voiding is generally delayed until the patient's mental and physical capacity improves.

Suprasacral lesions

Many patients with spinal cord lesions, including those with spinal cord injury, tumour, transverse myelitis, and multiple sclerosis, suffer from lower urinary tract symptoms secondary to neurogenic bladder dysfunction. The discussion of neurogenic bladder in patients with spinal cord lesions is usually directed to those with complete or near complete traumatic spinal cord injuries. Much of what is learned from these patients is transferable to those with other spinal cord conditions.

A period of spinal shock lasting a few weeks to months is common in patients following suprasacral spinal cord injuries. Loss of neurological activity below the level of the injury results in the inability of the bladder to generate a detrusor contraction, a condition referred to as detrusor areflexia, resulting in urinary retention. In the acute stage, patients are initially managed by indwelling catheterization or by intermittent catheterization performed by the nursing staff. When medically and neurologically stable, the patients are encouraged to perform self-catheterization.

Recovery from spinal shock is characterized by the gradual 'waking up' of the bladder and return of reflex activity. As is the case with supraspinal lesions, the bladder becomes hyperreflexic (Fig. 11.2b). The unstable bladder contractions are mediated through the sacral voiding centre, which is intact but separated from higher centres. Patients who are initially continent during the spinal shock phase often become incontinent as a result of the onset of reflex bladder activity. As the bladder recovers, its reflex contractions often become stronger, allowing for more efficient bladder emptying but possibly at the price of high bladder pressure. Baseline urodynamics is recommended 3 months following spinal cord injury in order to diagnose patients with high-pressure neurogenic bladder dysfunction.

High pressure neurogenic bladder dysfunction associated with supraspinal lesions

Patients with suprasacral lesions often lose the coordinating effect of the pontine micturition centre and develop detrusor sphincter dyssynergia (DSD). DSD is the involuntary contraction of the external sphincter during voiding and is pathognomonic for neurogenic bladder dysfunction (Fig. 11.3a,b).[10,12] The bladder contracts against a

(a)

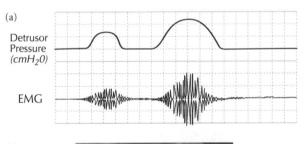

Detrusor
Pressure
(cmH$_2$0)

EMG

(b)

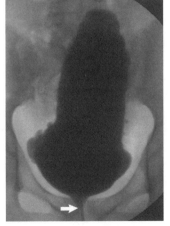

Fig. 11.3 (a) Detrusor sphincter dyssynergia (increase in electromyographic activity (EMG) during reflex bladder contractions). (b) Fluoroscopic evidence of detrusor sphincter dyssynergia (bladder is contracting against a closed external sphincter [see arrow]).

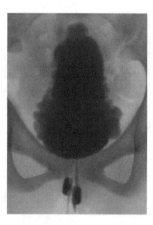

Fig. 11.4 A Christmas tree-shaped bladder secondary to high bladder pressure in a patient with neurogenic bladder dysfunction.

closed urethral sphincter resulting in high bladder pressures and inefficient bladder emptying. Patients with suprasacral lesions can also develop high bladder pressures secondary to poor bladder compliance (Fig. 11.2c).

High detrusor pressures secondary to DSD or poor bladder compliance may lead to both bladder and renal deterioration. It is generally accepted that sustained bladder pressures >40 cmH$_2$O are detrimental. The bladder wall thickens and loses its normal spherical shape, forming a 'Christmas tree-shaped' bladder with multiple diverticula (Fig. 11.4). Vesicourethral reflux, hydronephrosis, and renal insufficiency may develop as a result of elevated bladder pressures. The deterioration in bladder or renal function can occur silently over several years, or less commonly, acutely within months. Urodynamics are mandatory in order to measure bladder pressure and to identify patients who are at renal risk.

Infrasacral lesions

Infrasacral lesions involve the conus medullaris, the cauda equina, or the peripheral nerves that innervate the bladder and urethra (once termed lower motor neuron lesions).[13,14] Common causes include spinal cord injury, intervertebral disc disease, and lumbar spinal stenosis. The motor nuclei of the pelvic parasympathetics and pudendal nerves are situated within the conus medullaris, located approximately at the level of the T12 and L1 vertebral bodies. Thoracolumbar sympathetic nuclei in the conus medullaris also provide fibres that travel in the hypogastric nerves. Therefore, injury to the conus medullaris and cauda equina may affect bladder function variably, but the dysfunction primarily depends on the extent of injury to the parasympathetic innervation.

Infrasacral lesions most commonly result in a paralysed areflexic bladder. The normal reflex arc that exists between the bladder and conus medullaris is interrupted. The patient usually presents with obstructive voiding symptoms or urinary retention. Some patients, especially women, may empty by abdominal straining or suprapubic pressure. Others develop urinary incontinence due to overflow or stress incontinence secondary to a denervated and weakened urethral sphincter mechanism. The most characteristic finding on physical examination is sensory loss in the perineum and perianal area or on the lateral aspect of the foot.

Most patients with complete infrasacral lesions have large-capacity, low-pressure, poorly contractile bladders. For reasons not fully understood, a significant number of them lose bladder compliance and develop high-pressure systems. Urodynamics plays an important role in identifying this group of patients.

Although patients with complete infrasacral lesions develop detrusor areflexia and urinary retention, those with partial lesions are affected differently. Partial interruption of the sacral reflex arc often results in bladder instability. These patients typically preserve their voiding function but suffer from frequency and urge incontinence. Partial lesions are commonly seen in patients with lumbar disc disease.[14]

A number of distal cord reflexes exist that can help evaluate the intactness of the lower motor neuron reflex arc between the bladder, rectum, or perineum and the conus medullaris. These reflexes include the bulbospongiosus reflex (i.e. contraction of the anal sphincter stimulated by squeezing the glans penis), the anal wink (i.e. contraction of the anal sphincter stimulated by touching the inner aspect of the buttocks), and the presence or absence of rectal tone. The reflexes are absent in complete infrasacral lesions but present in partial lesions. In contrast, patients with suprasacral lesions have normal distal cord reflexes, although they may be temporarily absent for hours or days during spinal shock. It is noteworthy that the bulbospongiosus reflex is absent in a small percentage of normal men.

Diagnosis and work-up

A diagnosis of neurogenic bladder should be considered in patients who present with voiding dysfunction (Table 11.1). A high index of suspicion is often necessary in order to make the correct diagnosis. Voiding dysfunction is common among the millions of patients who suffer from neurological disease including those with stroke, diabetes,

Table 11.1 Patients suspected of neurogenic bladder dysfunction

Patients with neurological diagnosis or risk factors
Patients with neurological symptoms
Positive neurological examination
Clinical presentation 'out of the ordinary'
Detrusor sphincter dyssynergia
Characteristic cystometric patterns

Table 11.2 Symptoms suggestive of neurogenic bladder dysfunction

Loss/decreased sensation of:
perineum
genitalia
perianal
Poor sensation of the event of:
urination
defaecation
Urinary incontinence
Faecal incontinence
Erectile dysfunction
Sensory and motor deficits in lower extremities:
sciatica
numbness lateral aspect of foot

multiple sclerosis, lumbar disc disease, and Parkinson's disease. Approximately 1–10% of patients with multiple sclerosis present initially with voiding dysfunction and urinary incontinence.

The presence of neurological symptoms is suggestive of the diagnosis and should be ascertained during the initial evaluation (Table 11.2). The bowel, bladder, perineum, and lower extremities share common innervation from the sacral spinal cord which accounts for the associated neurological symptoms. Patients commonly report loss or decreased sensation in the perineum or genitalia. They may report urge or unconscious urinary or faecal incontinence as well as erectile dysfunction. Of course, many patients with neurogenic bladder also have positive motor or sensory findings of the lower extremities. The absence of neurological symptoms does not exclude the diagnosis of neurogenic bladder.

A focused neurological examination should be performed in all patients suspected of having neurogenic bladder dysfunction. The patient's general mental and ambulatory status, lower extremity neuromuscular function, and local neurological status should be assessed. Positive local findings include sensory loss involving the genitalia and perineum, reduced anal sphincteric tone, absent bulbospongiosus reflex, and inability to voluntarily contract the anal sphincter muscle. Palpation and inspection of the lower back and sacrum for dermatological stigmata of spinal bifida occulta or the presence of sacral agenesis are also important.

Clinical presentation 'out of the ordinary' may be the most important clue in making the diagnosis of neurogenic bladder. For example, a 40-year-old man who carries a urinal in his car because of urgency and fear of incontinence or a woman who reports incontinence since age 11 may have a neurogenic bladder.

Urodynamics are recommended in patients who are suspected to have neurogenic bladder dysfunction. Urodynamics (and video-urodynamics) characterize the bladder and urethral abnormality as well as measure bladder pressure.[15–18] The presence of detrusor sphincter dyssynergia is pathognomonic but is absent in many patients with neurogenic bladder dysfunction. In the absence of other causes, a number of cystometric patterns support the diagnosis. These include high-pressure instability, loss of bladder compliance, and sequential unstable contractions occurring in a 'stepping fashion' (Figs 11.2b–d). Many patients with neurogenic bladder demonstrate poor or absent bladder sensation during cystometery. The hyposensitive bladder is often associated with an abnormally high maximum cystometric capacity, poor bladder contractility, and high post-void residual urine volumes. Patients may not perceive bladder instability during bladder filling and demonstrate unconscious (also called reflex) incontinence. Video-urodynamics is preferable since fluoroscopy can identify the presence of bladder trabeculation, a Christmas tree-shaped bladder, vesicoureteral reflux, and detrusor sphincter dyssynergia. DSD is often more readily demonstrated radiographically than it is by an increase in electromyographic activity using patch electrodes due to their limited sensitivity in some patients.

With few exceptions, patients with suprasacral and infrasacral lesions are at risk of developing high-pressure bladders and should be evaluated with baseline and surveillance urodynamics as well as with renal imaging.[19] Most experts recommend a renal ultrasound in combination with a serum creatinine and plain radiograph of the abdomen and pelvis to screen patients for hydronephrosis and renal calculi. An intravenous pyelogram is useful but has the disadvantage of requiring a bowel prep which can adversely affect many patients with neurogenic bowel.[20] A computed tomography (CT) scan may be beneficial in selected patients.

In patients with spinal cord injuries, a baseline renal ultrasound is typically ordered at the time of the initial urodynamic evaluation 3 to 4 months following the injury. The urodynamics and ultrasound are generally repeated at 12 months. Long-term renal surveillance is recommended in nearly all patients.[21] Urodynamics are repeated annually or every alternate year, depending on the nature of the patient's bladder dysfunction, or until the urodynamic findings have stabilized. Other indications for urodynamics in patients with spinal cord injury include a change in voiding pattern, development of renal deterioration, recurrent urinary tract infections, or the new onset of autonomic dysreflexia.

Nuclear medicine scans can be very beneficial in the evaluation of patients with neurogenic bladder dysfunction. Renograms are sensitive in detecting renal scarring, obstructive hydronephrosis, and progressive renal deterioration. Neurogenic patients with non-obstructing hydronephrosis are most commonly followed by sequential ultrasounds in combination with a Lasix renogram.

Patients who have significantly recovered from a suprasacral or infrascral neurological lesion, and who are minimally symptomatic, should still be evaluated to rule out high bladder pressures and hydronephrosis, both of which can occur silently. Male patients with partial lesions notoriously report minimal voiding dysfunction in the face of high bladder pressures. Patients with supraspinal lesions are not at risk of developing high-pressure neurogenic bladders and do not require routine urodynamic and radiographic surveillance.

Neurosurgeons may request a neurourological and urodynamic assessment before spinal cord or brain surgery. This is especially important if the patient complains of symptoms suggestive of neurogenic bladder or if the risk of developing neurogenic dysfunction following surgery is high. The evaluation can provide an important baseline and play an important role in patient counselling pre-operatively.

Many newly diagnosed spinal cord injured patients are discharged from hospital or from rehabilitation units voiding spontaneously by reflex bladder contractions into an external appliance or condom catheter. Some of them are without urological follow-up. Unfortunately, some physicians mistakenly believe that patients are safely managed as long as they are proven to empty efficiently prior to discharge. This is true only if the patients reflex voids at low bladder pressures. Many spinal cord patients empty efficiently by generating high bladder pressures, which can result in renal deterioration. Safe bladder pressure can be only be determined by urodynamic evaluation.

Urologists are often asked to evaluate symptomatic patients for the presence of neurogenic bladder dysfunction. It is important to realize that in most cases the diagnosis is based on a number of non-specific factors and expert judgement rather than on pathognomonic signs or symptoms. The most important factor in making a diagnosis of neurogenic bladder is the presence of a temporal relationship between the neurological lesion and the patient's symptoms. For example, the development of urinary frequency and urge incontinence shortly following lumbar disc herniation or a stroke is highly suggestive of the diagnosis. Loss of sensation of bladder filling and decreased perineal or perianal sensation is similarly highly suggestive of a neurological process. Urodynamics plays a very important role but requires interpretive expertise to maximize its diagnostic potential. In patients without a neurological diagnosis, magnetic resonance imaging of the central nervous system and a neurological consultation is often necessary.

Specialized neurophysiological investigations, including nerve conduction studies, can be beneficial in diagnosing neurogenic bladder dysfunction in selected patients.[22] Nerve conduction studies are performed by the stimulation of a peripheral nerve and the monitoring of the time for a response to occur in its innervated muscle (motor latency). Latency studies test the integrity of nerve pathways, demonstrating prolonged latencies when there is injury to the nerve with associated demyelination. The most commonly tested latency in assessing neurogenic bladder dysfunction is the bulbospongiosus reflex. Although latency studies may be diagnostic in some patients, they require elaborate instrumentation and expert interpretation to be clinically beneficial; hence, their usage generally is limited to specialized neurophysiology centres.

Autonomic dysreflexia

Autonomic dysreflexia is the exaggerated sympathetic nervous system response which occurs in response to a noxious stimulus below the level of the injury in patients with

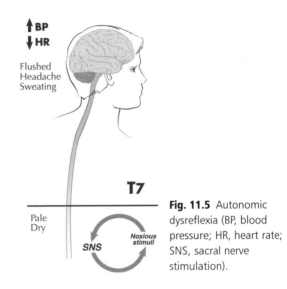

Fig. 11.5 Autonomic dysreflexia (BP, blood pressure; HR, heart rate; SNS, sacral nerve stimulation).

spinal cord injuries.[23] It occurs only in patients with lesions above T7, most commonly in patients with cervical spine injuries. The stimuli that most commonly trigger autonomic dysreflexia include an overdistended or high-pressure bladder, an overdistended rectum, and, in some cases, intercourse and labour.

A noxious stimulus stimulates a sympathetic reflex arc that causes vasoconstriction of the blood vessels below the level of the injury (Fig. 11.5). This results in paleness of the patient's skin below the injury and systemic hypertension. In response to the rapid rise in blood pressure, the patient's cardiovascular system attempts to compensate by reducing the heart rate and by causing peripheral vasodilatation above the level of the injury. For lower lesions, the vasodilatation response occurs within the splanchnic bed as well as in the head and neck and extremities, resulting in flushing above the level of the lesion and, in most cases, a less severe rise in blood pressure. In cervical spine injuries, most of the patient's blood vessels, including the splanchnic bed, are below the level of the injury and therefore are vasoconstricted. Very little compensatory reserve is available through vasodilatation. This results in a very rapid and severe rise in blood pressure which can be life-threatening.

Patients who suffer from autonomic dysreflexia typically complain of headache, as well as flushing and profuse sweating above the level of their injury. They often become pale below their lesion and bradycardic. Hypertension in a young spinal cord injured patient may be due to autonomic dysreflexia. Its primary treatment is the immediate removal of the noxious stimulus. Most commonly this entails changing a blocked catheter or stoppage of bladder filling during urodynamics or cystoscopy. For patients who do not respond quickly to these measures, administration of sublingual nifedipine or intravenous phentolamine is recommended. Prevention of autonomic dysreflexia by reducing the incidence of rectal and bladder overdistention and by controlling high bladder pressure plays an important role and can be accomplished by a comprehensive bowel and bladder management programme.

Treatment

Patients with neurogenic bladder are best managed by a well-designed bladder management programme tailored to the individual patient. The goals of therapy are to preserve renal function, to achieve adequate bladder emptying and urinary continence, and to minimize urological complications, including recurrent urinary tract infections and renal calculi (Table 11.3).[15,17] Consideration must also be given to optimizing patient independence.

Patients with suprasacral and infrasacral lesions are at increased risk of developing renal insufficiency from a number of factors including high detrusor pressure, vesicoureteral reflux, recurrent urinary tract infections and renal calculi.[24] Early diagnosis and careful long-term surveillance minimizes the likelihood in most patients.

In those who cannot void spontaneously, high bladder pressure is most often controlled by regular clean intermittent catheterization (CIC) in combination with anticholinergic medication.[25,26] Incontinence secondary to bladder instability is similarly controlled by self-catheterization and medical therapy. CIC effectively achieves bladder emptying and reduces the incidence of urinary tract infection by reducing bladder residual urine volumes.

Patients are generally instructed to catheterize during waking hours every 3–6 hours depending on the severity of their bladder dysfunction and treatment goals. Typically patients use a 14–18 French straight or coude tip catheter and utilize a 'clean' technique.[27] Many women prefer a short clear catheter since it can be easier to use and conceal. Urethral irritation resulting in discomfort, painful catheterization, or haematuria is not uncommon. A haematuria work-up including renal radiography and cystoscopy is recommended when non-traumatic sources of bleeding are suspected.

A number of factors must be considered when managing patients with clean intermittent self-catheterization. Many patients with cervical spine injuries, multiple sclerosis, or Parkinson's disease lack the necessary hand function needed to catheterize. Others are too obese or immobile to catheterize while sitting in a wheelchair and it is unrealistic to expect them to transfer to a bed or depend on others for assistance. Patients may also lack the cognitive ability or be unwilling to catheterize.

Table 11.3 Therapeutic goals in the management of neurogenic bladder

Preserve renal function
Achieve bladder emptying
Maximize urinary continence
Minimize urological complications (UTIs, calculi, autonomic dysreflexia)

When clean intermittent catheterization is not an option, patients are managed with an indwelling urethral or suprapubic catheter, or by urinary diversion with, for example, an ileal conduit. Long-term urethral catheterization should be avoided, especially in women, since it may cause urethral erosion or other urethral complications. Catheter-induced urethral erosion may occur within months and is a devastating complication. The placement of larger catheters in an attempt to prevent women from leaking around their catheter increases the erosion risk and should be avoided. Their incontinence is most commonly secondary to bladder instability and should be managed medically. A suprapubic catheter spares the urethra and is more desirable in sexually active patients. When properly managed, suprapubic catheterization has been shown to be a reasonable treatment alternative.[28] It is generally recommended to change long-term urethral or suprapubic catheters monthly and to perform weekly bladder irrigations in order to reduce the incidence of urinary tract infections and bladder calculi.

Anticholinergics are commonly used to control bladder pressure and treat incontinence secondary to neurogenic bladder instability. The most commonly prescribed medications include immediate (IR) and extended-release (ER) oxybutynin and tolterodine, and the oxybutynin transdermal delivery system, all of which have proven efficacy in patients with overactive bladder (Table 11.4).[29–33] Many neurogenic patients require higher dosages to control their symptoms and bladder pressure. O'Leary et al.[34,35] demonstrated that the majority of incontinent patients with multiple sclerosis and spinal cord injury chose a final dose of extended-release oxybutynin greater than 10 mg in order to maximize efficacy. Fortunately, higher dosages of anticholinergics are commonly well tolerated in this population of patients. The clinical efficacy of anticholinergics is generally measured by their effects on urinary incontinence. Dosages are increased or another anticholinergic is tried in an attempt to maximize continence. When anticholinergics are used to decrease bladder pressure urodynamics are often repeated while on medication in order to measure effectiveness.

Table 11.4 Anticholinergics commonly used for treatment of neurogenic bladder instability

Medication	Dosage
Oxybutynin ER	5–30 mg q.d.
Tolterodine IR/ER	2 mg b.i.d., 4 mg q.d.
Oxybutynin IR	2.5–5.0 mg b.i.d./t.i.d.
Hyocyamine	0.375 mg b.i.d.
Imipramine	10–75 mg b.i.d.
Oxybutynin transdermal	3.9 mg q.d.

IR, immediate release; ER, extended release; q.d., once a day; b.i.d., twice a day; t.i.d., three times a day.

A number of patients continue to be incontinent or have high bladder pressure in spite of frequent CIC and high-dose anticholinergic therapy. They can be effectively managed by bladder augmentation where the bladder is surgically enlarged using a detubularized segment of small or large intestine.[36] More recently, patients with refractory high-pressure bladders have been successfully treated with botulinum toxin type A cystoscopically injected into the bladder wall. Schurch et al.[37] demonstrated excellent short-term efficacy and impressive urodynamic effects in spinal cord injured patients injected with 300 units.

Male patients with urinary retention secondary to detrusor sphincter dyssynergia (DSD) but who cannot perform CIC have a number of options to facilitate bladder emptying. During a sphincterotomy,[38] the external sphincter muscle is surgically incised along its length, relieving the obstruction. A short metallic stent, called a Urolume stent, may be placed cystoscopically across the external sphincter and is highly effective in treating DSD.[39] Botulinum toxin can also be injected into the sphincter, resulting in a chemical sphincterotomy.[40] Following successful management of DSD, patients then reflex void into an external appliance or condom catheter. Such procedures require careful patient selection and may render patients totally incontinent during all activities, including showering and intercourse, and should be used judiciously.

The same goals of therapy apply to the management of neurogenic patients with suprasacral or infrasacral lesions who are able to void spontaneously and empty efficiently. Anticholinergics may be necessary to control high bladder pressure and can be highly effective in managing incontinence due to bladder instability. Some patients with poorly contractile bladders empty by abdominal straining or by credé manoeuvres. Female patients who strain to urinate may predispose themselves to the future development of stress incontinence. α-adrenergic antagonists may reduce urethral resistance and facilitate bladder emptying but are effective only in a minority of cases.

Patients with urinary frequency and urge (or unconscious) incontinence secondary to a supraspinal lesion are best managed by a combination of behavioural therapy and medication. Commonly, patients are instructed to void according to a schedule, for instance, every 90 minutes to 2 hours, in order to empty their bladder before their involuntary reflex bladder activity results in incontinence. Anticholinergic medications suppress involuntary bladder contractions, and, in many patients, are highly effective. Physiotherapy and rehabilitation play an important role by improving functional status, which in turn can benefit continence. Severely debilitated patients who are refractory to therapy may be best managed by long-term indwelling catheterization.

Conclusion

Patients with neurological disease commonly suffer from neurogenic bladder. The type of bladder and urethral dysfunction is dictated primarily by the location of the lesion within the central or peripheral nervous system, not by the disease itself. Urodynamics plays an important role in characterizing the type of vesicourethral dysfunction and is necessary in order to diagnose high bladder pressure. Preserving renal function, achieving continence, minimizing urological complications, and optimizing quality of life are among the goals in managing patients with neurogenic bladder. Fortunately, the majority of patients can be safely and effectively managed by a properly designed bladder management programme tailored to the individual.

References

1 **Cardenas DD** (1992). Neurogenic bladder evaluation and management. *Phys. Med. Rehabil. Clin. N. Am.* **3**: 751–63.

2 **Bradley WE, Timm GW, Scott FB** (1974). Innervation of the detrusor muscle and urethra. *Urol. Clin. N. Am.* **1**: 3–27.

3 **Fletcher TF, Bradley WE** (1978). Neuroanatomy of the bladder—urethra. *J. Urol.* **119**: 153–60.

4 **Wein AJ, Barrett DM** (1988). Peripheral innervation of the lower urinary tract. In: *Voiding Function and Dysfunction—A Logical and Practical Approach* (ed. DK Marshall), pp. 45–52. Yearbook Medical Publishers, Chicago, IL.

5 **Carlsson CA** (1978). The supraspinal control of the urinary bladder. *Acta Pharmacol. Toxicol.* **43A** (Suppl. II): 8–12.

6 **Wein AJ, Barrett DM** (1988). Central nervous system influences on the lower urinary tract. In: *Voiding Function and Dysfunction—A Logical and Practical Approach* (ed. DK Marshall), pp. 77–103. Yearbook Medical Publishers, Chicago, IL.

7 **Bradley WE, Chou S, Jarkland C** (1967). Classifying neurologic dysfunction of the urinary bladder. In: *The Neurogenic Bladder* (ed. S Boyarski), pp. 139–46. Williams and Wilkins, Baltimore, MD.

8 **Krane RJ, Siroky MB** (1979). Classification of neuro-urologic bladder disorders. In: *Clinical Neuro-urology*, 2nd edn (ed. RJ Krane, MB Siroky), pp. 143–58. Little, Brown, Boston, MA.

9 **Wein AJ** (1981). Classification of neurogenic voiding dysfunction. *J. Urol.* **125**: 605–9.

10 **Abrams P, Blaivas JG, Stanton SL, Andersen JT** (1998). Standardization of terminology of lower urinary tract function. *Neurourol. Urodyn.* **7**: 403–27.

11 **Abrams P, Cardozo L, Fall M, Griffiths D, Rosier P, Ulmsten U** *et al.* (2002).The standardisation of terminology of lower urinary tract function: report from the Standardisation Sub-committee of the International Continence Society. *Neurourol. Urodyn.* **21**: 167–78.

12 **McGuire EJ, Brady S** (1979). Detrusor-sphincter dyssynergia. *J. Urol.* **121**: 774–7.

13 **Blaivas J, Chancellor M** (1996). Cauda equina, infections, and other spinal diseases. In: *Atlas of Urodynamics* (ed. J Blaivas, M Chancellor), pp. 192–201. Williams and Wilkins, Baltimore, MD.

14 **Appell RA** (1993). Voiding dysfunction and lumbar disc disorders. In: *Problems in Urology: Neurourology and its Role in Urologic Disease: Part II* (ed. DF Paulson), pp. 35–40. Lippincott, Philadelphia, PA.

15 **MacDiarmid SA** (1999). The ABCs of neurogenic bladder for the neurosurgeon. *Contemp. Neurosurg.* **21**: 1–8.

16 **Galloway NTM** (1989). Management of neurogenic bladder in spinal cord injury. In: *Problems in Urology—Neurourology* (ed. DF Paulson), pp. 40–3. Lippincott, Philadelphia, PA.

17 **Benevento BT, Sipski ML** (2002). Neurogenic bladder, neurogenic bowel, and sexual dysfunction in people with spinal cord injury. *Phys. Ther.* **82**: 601–12.

18 **Chancellor MB, Kiilholma P** (1992). Urodynamic evaluation of patients following spinal cord injury. *Semin. Urol.* **10**: 83–94.

19 Linsenmeyer TA, Culkin D (1999). APS recommendations for the urological evaluation of patients with spinal cord injury. *J. Spinal Cord Med.* **22**: 139–42.

20 Hoffman WW, Grayhack JT (1960). The limitations of the intravenous pyelogram as a test of renal function. *Surg. Gynecol. Obstet.* **110**: 503.

21 Kuhlemeier KV, Lloyd LK, Stover SL (1985). Long-term follow-up of renal function after spinal cord injury. *J. Urol.* **134**: 510–13.

22 Snooks SJ, Swash M (1994). Neurophysiological techniques for assessment of pelvic floor and striated sphincter muscles and their innervation. In: *Urodynamics—Principles, Practice and Application* (ed. AR Mundy, T Stephenson, AJ Wein), pp. 183–94. Churchill Livingstone, New York.

23 Karlsson AK (1999). Autonomic dysreflexia. *Spinal Cord* **47**: 383–91.

24 McGuire EJ, Woodside JR, Borden TA, Weiss, RM (1981). Prognostic value of urodynamic testing in myelodysplastic patients. *J. Urol.* **126**: 205–9.

25 Wein A, Raezer D, Benson G (1976). Management of neurogenic bladder dysfunction in the adult. *Urology* **8**: 432–43.

26 Herschorn S (1989). The management of neurogenic bladder dysfunction. In: *Problems in Urology—Neurourology* (ed. DF Paulson), pp. 23–39. Lippincott, Philadelphia, PA.

27 Wyndaele JJ (2002). Intermittent catheterization: which is the optimal technique? *Spinal Cord* **40**: 432–37.

28 MacDiarmid SA, Arnold EP, Anthony A, Palmer NB (1995). Management of spinal cord injured patients by indwelling suprapubic catheterization. *J. Urol.* **154**: 492–4.

29 Appell RA (1997). Clinical efficacy and safety of Tolterodine in the treatment of overactive bladder: a pooled analysis. *Urology* **50**: 90–6.

30 Appell RA, Sand P, Dmochowski R, Anderson R, Zinner N, Lama D *et al.* (2001). Prospective randomized controlled trial of extended-release oxybutynin chloride and tolterodine tartate in the treatment of overactive bladder: results of the OJBECT Study. *Mayo Clin. Proc.* **76**: 358–63.

31 VanKerrebroeck P, Kreder K, Jonas U, Zinner N, Wein A (2001). Tolterodine once-daily: superior efficacy and tolerability in the treatment of the overactive bladder. *Urology* **57**: 414–21.

32 Diokno AC, Appell RA, Sand PK, Dmochowski RR, Gburek BM, Klimberg IW *et al.* (2003). Prospective, randomized, double-blind study of the efficacy and tolerability of the extended-release formulation of oxybutynin and tolterodine for overactive bladder. Results of the OPERA Trial. *Mayo Clin. Proc.* **78**: 687–95.

33 Dmochowski RR, Davila GW, Zinner NR, Gittelman MC, Saltzstein DR, Lyttle S *et al.* (2002). Efficacy and safety of transdermal oxybutynin in patients with urge and mixed urinary incontinence. *J. Urol.* **168**: 580–6.

34 O'Leary M, Erickson JR, Smith CP, Cannon TW, Fraser M, Boyd M *et al.* (2002). Changes in voiding patterns in multiple sclerosis patients with controlled release oxybutynin. *Int. J. MS Care* **4**: 116–19.

35 O'Leary M, Erickson JR, Smith CP, McDermott C, Horton J, Chancellor MB (2003). The effect of controlled release oxybutynin on neuorgenic bladder function in spinal cord injured patients. *J. Spinal Cord Med.* **26**: 159–62.

36 Webster GD (1998). Cystoplasty management of the intractably hostile neurogenic bladder. In: *Problems in Urology—Neurourology* (ed. DF Paulson), pp. 102–21. Lippincott, Philadelphia, PA.

37 Schurch B, Stohrer M, Kramer G (2000). Botulinum-A toxin for treating detrusor hyperreflexia in spinal cord injured patients: a new alternative to anticholinergic drugs? Preliminary results. *J. Urol.* **164**: 692–7.

38 Reynard JM, Vass J, Sullivan ME, Mamas M (2003). Spincterotomy and the treatment of detrusor-sphincter dyssynergia: current status, future prospects. *Spinal Cord* **41**: 1–11.

39 Chancellor M, Gajewski J, Ackman C, Appell RA, Bennett J, Binard J *et al.* (1999). Long-term follow-up of the North American multicenter UroLume trial for the treatment of external detrusor-sphincter dyssynergia. *J. Urol.* **161**: 1545–50.

40 Schurch B, Hauri D, Rodic B, Curt A, Meyer M, Rossier AB (1996). Botulinum-A toxin as treatment of detrusor-sphincter dyssynergia: prospective study in 24 spinal cord injury patients. *J. Urol.* **155**: 1023–9.

Chapter 12

The patient presenting with sexual dysfunction

Carin V. Hopps and John P. Mulhall

Introduction

Sexual dysfunction is a medical problem affecting a vast number of both men and women. In 1992, an NIH Consensus Development Panel on Impotence was held to assess evidence-based data in an effort to clarify issues of epidemiology, risk factors, diagnosis, treatment, and education relative to sexual dysfunction.[1] The term *impotence* was replaced by *erectile dysfunction* (ED), defined as the consistent inability to obtain and/or maintain an erection sufficient for satisfactory sexual relations. The panel also recognized ED as an important public health problem that deserved attention, both in terms of research support and in terms of willingness of physicians to address sexual matters, as sexual dysfunction is associated with significant mental stress affecting an individual's interpersonal relationships. Over a decade has passed since the meeting of the Consensus Panel, which published its insightful findings 5 years prior to the introduction of sildenafil citrate (Viagra™, Pfizer, NY, USA), and a tremendous amount of insight has been gained into the epidemiology, aetiology, evaluation, and treatment of ED. The widespread attention that this disorder has received is perhaps best reflected in the volume of sildenafil citrate used since its introduction to the market in 1998. This first oral phosphodiesterase (PDE) inhibitor to become commercially available for treatment of ED has been prescribed for more than 20 million men worldwide by over half a million physicians and has annualized sales in excess of $1.7 billion.[2]

Prevalence

Many studies have determined the prevalence of ED in the general population, and while the prevalence amongst studies varies, they are consistent in concluding that ED is a disease process that is widespread and that it increases as men age.[3–5] The Massachusetts Male Aging Study (MMAS) was an early sentinel study that determined the prevalence of ED in 1709 healthy non-institutionalized men within the general population.[6] This was a community based, random sample, observational survey of men aged 40 to 70 years that demonstrated a combined prevalence of minimal, moderate, and complete impotence of 52%, while the prevalence of complete impotence tripled from 5 to 15% between the ages of 40 and 70 years. According to the MMAS, an estimated 40% of respondents experienced ED at age 40, whereas 67% reported difficulty by age 75. A longitudinal study performed over a 9-year period on a cohort of men enrolled in the MMAS found that the incidence rate of new-onset ED was approximately 26 cases per 1000 men per year.[7] As in the initial MMAS study, ED was strongly related to age and was elevated among subgroups of men with diabetes, heart disease, hypertension, and a lower level of education. Extrapolation of data from multiple studies suggests that ED affects in excess of 100 million men worldwide.

It has been recognized that sexual dysfunction is common in women as well, affecting 25 to 63% of women.[8,9] Analysis of data from the National Health and Social Life Survey of 1749 women and 1410 men has shown that sexual dysfunction is more prevalent for women (43%) than for men (31%) and is associated with various demographic characteristics such as age and level of education.[10] Importantly, this study demonstrated that sexual dysfunction correlates with negative experiences in sexual relationships and overall well-being, emphasizing the significance of this health concern to the general public.

Despite the prevalence of ED, only 10% of men with sexual dysfunction present to a physician for evaluation and treatment.[1] While 85% of adults would like to discuss sexual function with their physician, 71% believe the physician lacks time or interest to address this issue, 68% of adults are concerned that they will embarrass their physician and 76% think that no treatment is available for them.[11] Moreover, the failure of physicians to inquire about sexual function is a source of dissatisfaction for many patients. Eighty-five per cent of patients believe that physicians should initiate discussion regarding ED, and 74% of patients feel less than satisfied by their physician's attempt to discuss sexual matters.[12] Physicians may hesitate to initiate discussion of sexual function because of embarrassment, discomfort with terminology, lack of training, or underestimating the importance of diagnosing sexual dysfunction. However, the diagnosis of ED may then lead to recognition of serious health problems with which it is associated such as diabetes and hypercholesterolaemia. Perelman stresses the need for physicians who care for patients with sexual dysfunction to consider the psychological and behavioural aspects of the patient's diagnosis and management in addition to the organic causes and risk factors, emphasizing that the integration of sex therapy and other psychological techniques with pharmacotherapy in the office practice will improve effectiveness in treatment of ED.[13]

Risk factors

Erectile dysfunction is classified as psychogenic, organic, or a mix of psychogenic and organic. While ED has a primary organic cause in 80% of men, most cases have a mixed organic/psychogenic aetiology.[14] Psychogenic ED may be caused by factors such as performance anxiety, a strained relationship, lack of sexual arousability, and overt psychiatric disorders such as depression and schizophrenia. Both depression and the treatment for depression are risk factors for sexual dysfunction. Antidepressants such as tricyclics, monoamine oxidase inhibitors, selective serotonin reuptake inhibitors (SSRIs), and lithium significantly impair sexual function including not only potency but also libido and ejaculation. The most commonly prescribed antidepressants are the SSRIs. A large non-randomized study of psychiatric patients taking different SSRIs determined that the incidence of new-onset sexual dysfunction was 20% overall; the most common sexual side-effects were delayed orgasm, anorgasmia, and hypoactive sexual desire.[15] Patients with depression may not take the initiative to discuss issues of sexuality with a physician, and thus the impetus for discussion remains with the physician in many cases.

Multiple lifestyle factors, medical conditions, medications, physical disabilities, and psychosocial issues have been identified as risk factors for sexual dysfunction. Age >40 years, smoking, excessive alcohol consumption, excess weight or obesity, and substance abuse are all lifestyle issues associated with the development of sexual dysfunction.[16,17] The most unavoidable risk factor, increasing age, correlates with a progressive decline in sexual function. As men age, the time between onset of sexual stimulation and erection increases, erections are less rigid, ejaculation is less forceful, ejaculatory volume decreases, and the refractory period between erections lengthens.[18] A large review of the literature on smoking and its relationship to ED showed that a strong correlation exists between smoking, coronary artery disease, atherosclerosis, and ED.[19] The mechanism of injury for smokers may be impairment of endothelium-dependent smooth muscle relaxation as well as contribution of risk to atherosclerotic and vascular disease. In addition, the likelihood of moderate or complete ED in men who smoke may be increased by two-fold, though the prevalence of ED was no different in former smokers when compared with non-smokers, suggesting that injury incurred from smoking may be reversible with smoking cessation.

Among the most common medical conditions associated with sexual dysfunction are diabetes, dyslipidaemias, hypertension, coronary artery disease, peripheral vascular disease, and pelvic irradiation. Vascular disease promotes penile arterial insufficiency and potentially veno-occlusive dysfunction resulting in ED. Hypertension causes arteriosclerotic lesion formation within the pelvic vasculature, and certain antihypertensive drugs affect compliance of the erectile tissue resulting in a functional venous leak (described below).[20] Of patients with a history of recent myocardial infarction (MI), 64% reported ED in the pre-MI period.[21] Eighty per cent of men with the four main arterial risk factors (i.e. diabetes, smoking, hyperlipidaemia, and hypertension) have organic impairment of erection.[22] Diabetes mellitus results in vasculopathy and autonomic neuropathy, both of which contribute to the development of ED in this population. Twelve per cent of men with newly diagnosed diabetes have ED,[23] while up to 35–75% of men with diabetes ultimately develop ED,[24] and nearly all men with autonomic diabetic neuropathy suffer from ED.[25]

Lower urinary tract symptoms (LUTS) associated with benign prostatic hyperplasia (BPH) such as urinary frequency, urgency, nocturia, incomplete emptying, intermittency, weak stream, and straining have been identified as age-independent risk factors for development of ED.[26] It is hypothesized that a common pathophysiological mechanism such as increased pelvic α-adrenergic tone in association with bladder outlet obstruction may cause the occurrence of both LUTS and ED such that the two disease processes coincide as men age. Animal models of partial bladder outlet obstruction have demonstrated increased cavernosal smooth muscle tone and impaired capacity for relaxation, supporting the role of increased pelvic sympathetic tone in the pathogenesis of concomitant BPH and ED.[27]

Neurological disorders are frequently the cause of sexual dysfunction. These include Alzheimer's disease, Parkinson's disease, epilepsy, multiple sclerosis, stroke, traumatic brain injury, and spinal cord injury. These medical issues may result in diminished libido, altered genital sensation or corruption of the neurological tract that is necessary for sexual function. Distressing psychosocial and interpersonal issues associated with these health problems may also impart a psychogenic component to sexual dysfunction.

Other medical conditions commonly associated with sexual dysfunction are sickle cell anaemia, rheumatoid arthritis, cancer, cancer treatments, menopause, hypogonadism, hypothyroidism, Peyronie's disease, hysterectomy, pregnancy and post-partum recovery, trauma or surgery to the pelvis (such as radical prostatectomy) or spine, vascular surgery, and chronic renal insufficiency. While androgen deficiency in men decreases nocturnal erections and libido, erection in response to visual sexual stimulation is preserved in men with hypogonadism, demonstrating that androgen is not essential for erection.[28] Diminished erectile function, libido, and fertility are observed in men with chronic renal insufficiency; hypogonadism, vascular insufficiency, use of multiple medications, peripheral neuropathy, and stress may be causative.

Multiple medications are known to cause severe sexual dysfunction. From a medical standpoint, this is a significant concern as high side-effect profiles correspond with poor drug compliance. The most common medications known to cause ED are antihypertensive and antidepressant medications. Diuretics, especially thiazides frequently used for the initial management of hypertension, mediate their effect through alterations in cellular ion channels which ultimately affects smooth muscle relaxation in the corpora cavernosae. β-blockers decrease β_2 vasodilation, potentiating unopposed α_1-induced vasoconstriction within the corpora cavernosa, inhibiting erection. α-blockers are rarely associated with ED, though they have been linked to priapism and ejaculatory dysfunction. H_2-receptor blockers resemble anti-androgens and are associated with hyperprolactinaemia, possibly causing diminished libido and erectile function through this mechanism.[29] Large amounts of alcohol can cause sedation, decreased libido, and sexual dysfunction, while chronic alcoholism can cause hypogonadism and neuropathy, potentially affecting genital innervation.[30] Additional drugs associated with sexual dysfunction include anti-androgens, anticonvulsants, cytotoxics, ketokonazole, lipid-lowering agents, neuroleptics, phenothiazenes, progestin-dominant birth control pills, and sedatives.[31]

Evaluation

Because ED may be the presenting sign for medical co-morbidities such as diabetes, neurological disease, vascular disease, dyslipidaemia, hypertension, and coronary artery disease, a thorough evaluation, including multidimensional history, physical examination, and laboratory tests when indicated, is warranted.

History taking

A detailed psychosocial, medical, and sexual history is the necessary first step in evaluation for sexual dysfunction. To initiate discussion and concomitantly assess the presence and severity of ED, patients may be administered the Sexual Health Inventory for Men (SHIM) questionnaire. The SHIM is an abbreviated version of the International Index of Erectile Function (IIEF) questionnaire, a validated tool that assesses in detail erectile function, intercourse satisfaction, orgasmic function, sexual desire, and overall satisfaction. With a careful history, signs of psychogenic ED may be revealed. These may include abrupt onset of ED at a young age or ED that is specific to one partner only or a distinct situation. The presence of normal nocturnal and masturbatory erections suggests psychogenic ED, as does an individual's susceptibility to stress, anxiety, depression, or psychosis.[32]

The sexual history begins with inquiry regarding the onset of sexual dysfunction, status of function before onset, the status since, level of libido, and whether any degree of curvature is present indicative of Peyronie's disease. The degree of penile tumescence that can be achieved is assessed on a scale. We prefer a numerical scale from 0 to 10, where 0 represents the flaccid state and 10 represents maximal tumescence (5–6 necessary for penetration). The patient is asked about the presence and quality of nocturnal erections and masturbatory erections in addition to those achieved with intercourse and if the duration is sufficient for completion of intercourse. The medical and surgical history is obtained with questions aimed at risk factors for sexual dysfunction described above, such as a history of cardiovascular disease, perineal or back trauma, or surgery in addition to medication or drug use.

Physical examination

While a general examination of the patient is performed, attention is focused on factors that may contribute to sexual dysfunction. The patient's body habitus is assessed for secondary male sex characteristics such as normal body hair distribution and lack of gynaecomastia. Femoral and lower extremity pulses are examined and a focal neurological examination performed. The testicles are assessed for normal size and consistency.

Normal testicular volume measures 15 to 25 cm^3 and the consistency should be firm.[33] Small, soft testes are associated with either primary testicular failure (intrinsic defect in spermatogenesis) or secondary testicular failure, caused by endocrine abnormalities or extrinsic factors such as the use of exogenous androgens or exposure to heat and gonadotoxins. The penis is evaluated for penile plaques located within the tunica albuginea of the corpora cavernosa suggestive of Peyronie's disease. In addition to measuring stretched penile length (normal mean is 12.4 cm),[34] the quality of stretch is assessed to predict extent of smooth muscle fibrosis within the corpora. Finally, a digital rectal examination is performed for evaluation of the prostate.

Laboratory studies

Laboratory tests may be used to elucidate risk factors that contribute to sexual dysfunction. Low serum testosterone levels are associated with hypogonadism and diminished libido. Serum testosterone peaks in the morning, and therefore blood should be drawn before 10 a.m. To evaluate for systemic disease, a complete blood count, urinalysis, serum creatinine, glucose, and lipid profile may be obtained. In diabetics, a haemoglobin A1c test can determine effectiveness of recent glucose management, indicating the extent to which glucose control must be modified for optimization. A prostate-specific antigen (PSA) level is also drawn in men who meet the age criteria for prostate cancer screening.

Nocturnal penile tumescence and rigidity testing

Evaluation and determination of the aetiology of sexual dysfunction can be difficult and no single test can provide this information. Nocturnal penile tumescence and rigidity (NPTR) monitoring, however, can help to differentiate psychogenic from organic ED in an objective, non-invasive manner. Men with normal erectile function experience three to five erections while sleeping, 80% of these erections occurring during REM sleep.[35,36] Men with psychogenic ED are likely to have physiological erections during sleep in the absence of organic factors. The RigiScan (Timm Medical Technologies, Eden Prairie, MN) can be transported home by the patient and used for up to three monitoring sessions, each up to 10 hours in duration. The device consists of two loops, one of which is placed at the base and one at the distal aspect of the penis, and a battery-powered logging device that is strapped to the patient's thigh. It records penile circumference every 15 s and rigidity every 3 minutes. When circumference increases by more than 10 mm, rigidity monitoring increases to every 30 s. In this manner, tumescence, rigidity, and duration of each event are recorded; this information is downloaded and printed in graphic form for interpretation. Men without risk factors associated with sexual dysfunction or in whom psychogenic ED is suspected may benefit from NPTR evaluation such that the appropriate treatment modality is selected.

Colour duplex Doppler ultrasonography

Colour duplex Doppler ultrasonography (CDDU) is an excellent modality for visualization of cavernosal vessels and measurement of blood flow. It is used to assess arterial insufficiency, cavernous venous occlusive disease, high- and low-flow priapism, and extent of Peyronie's disease prior to a planned operative procedure. It is *imperative* that this diagnostic modality be used following intracavernosal injection to induce a bedroom quality erection. Peak systolic (PSV) and end diastolic (EDV) velocities of the cavernosal arteries are determined. PSV < 25 cm/s suggests the presence of arterial disease, while EDV > 3–5 cm/s suggests venous leak (failure of the veno-occlusive mechanism) especially when associated with normal PSV. During normal erection (described in greater detail below), the smooth muscle within the corpora cavernosa dilates, arterial flow increases, and venous flow through the tunical albuginea of the corpora cavernosa is obstructed, allowing the corpora to fill with blood at high pressure resulting in erection. Venous occlusion may be impaired by processes such as Peyronie's disease, congenital venous anomalies, or traumatic injury.

The extent of venous leak may be further investigated with dynamic infusion cavernosometry and cavernosography, an invasive technique requiring placement of two large-bore needles in the corpora cavernosa, one for saline infusion and one for pressure monitoring. Following administration of an intracavernosal medication to induce maximal smooth muscle relaxation (such as Trimix), the maintenance flow rate, or saline flow rate necessary to maintain an intracavernosal pressure of 150 mmHg, is determined. A maintenance flow rate less than 3 ml/min is considered normal and greater than this is indicative of venous leak. Cavernosography is performed with infusion of contrast with radiographic imaging for visualization of the site of venous leak. This study is reserved for patients who are candidates for venous ligation or crural ligation surgery.

Penile arteriography provides excellent anatomical assessment of the penile vasculature, but is associated with complications and difficulty in performing the procedure due to interindividual anatomical variation and correlation with erectile function. Selective internal pudendal arteriography is therefore reserved for those individuals who have had traumatic perineal injuries and are candidates for penile revascularization procedures.

Treatment of erectile dysfunction

Although ED is highly prevalent in society and significantly affects quality of life, treatment options are multiple and diverse, such that nearly all men are able to achieve an erection of sufficient rigidity for intercourse following appropriate evaluation and treatment. Treatment options are categorized into three lines of therapy.[37] First-line therapy entails the reversal of modifiable risk factors, psychological support, and use of oral therapies. Second-line therapy consists of the vacuum device, transurethral therapy and intracavernosal injection, while third line therapy is surgical intervention including placement of a penile prosthesis and penile revascularization surgery.

First-line therapy

Reversal of modifiable risk factors

Studies done to assess efficacy of oral treatment for ED are typically conducted in groups of men without identifiable risk factors for ED. Very few studies have examined treatment outcome in men for whom modifiable risk factors have been reversed. Guay and colleagues assessed the efficacy and safety of sildenafil citrate in a population of men with organic risk factors in whom these factors were managed by medication and/or lifestyle modification prior to treatment with sildenafil.[38] ED was reversed in approximately 15% of cases when medical management of heart disease or hypertension was altered such that erectolytic medications or risk factors such as smoking were modified. Furthermore, this study demonstrated an overall successful intercourse rate (with risk factor modification and sildenafil use) of 82%, a rate that is greater than that observed when sildenafil is used without risk modification. This study highlights the importance of not only treating previously identified risk factors, but also screening for potential risk factors to optimize response to treatment.

Phosphodiesterase type 5 inhibitors

Erectile response begins with release of nitric oxide (NO) from non-adrenergic non-cholinergic (NANC) nerve terminals and from endothelial cells in response to sexual stimulation. NO activates the cytoplasmic enzyme guanylate cyclase to convert guanosine triphosphate (GTP) to cyclic guanosine monophosphate (cGMP), a second messenger that mediates smooth muscle relaxation, which allows blood to fill the corpora cavernosae and effect penile erection. cGMP is degraded by type 5 phosphodiesterase (PDE5), limiting the capacity for continued smooth muscle relaxation. Inhibition of PDE5 prevents the degradation of cGMP, thereby promoting erection. The first oral PDE5 inhibitor to enter the market was Viagra™, introduced in 1998, and subsequently, vardenafil (Levitra™, Bayer AG, Leverkusen, Germany and GlaxoSmithKline plc, Middlesex, UK) and tadalafil (Cialis™, Lilly ICOS LLC, Indianapolis, IN and Bothell, WA, USA) have become available as well.

Double-blind, placebo-controlled studies of sildenafil use in men with ED of organic, psychogenic, or mixed aetiology have demonstrated successful intercourse rates of 65–69% for all attempts at intercourse compared with 20–22% of those receiving placebo.[39,40] Men with lesser severity of ED exhibit the best response to sildenafil, whereas men with no spontaneous erectile function are less likely to respond to the drug.[41] In phase III clinical trials, both vardenafil and tadalafil significantly increased the percentage of successful intercourse attempts in a dose-dependent manner (up to 65% and 75%, respectively) when compared with placebo (32% for both).[42,43] Both have been shown to significantly enhance erectile function across a wide range of ED severities and medical co-morbidities.[44,45] Overall, the responder rate and magnitude of response with vardenafil and tadalafil are similar to those of sildenafil. The adverse event profile for the three PDE5 inhibitors is similar. Adverse events include headache, dyspepsia, facial flushing, nasal congestion, and visual disturbances. Tadalafil is associated with a low incidence of back pain and myalgia, the exact mechanism of which is unclear. As with all PDE5 inhibitors, side-effects appear to improve with continued use of the medication.[42,43]

PDE5 inhibitors have established themselves as an integral component of oral ED management. In the absence of head to head trials, the relative role of each of these agents is as of yet undefined. When compared to sildenafil, vardenafil is distinguished by its biochemical potency and tadalafil by its prolonged half-life (17.5 hours). However, the clinical correlates of these factors can only be defined with use in the general ED population.

Apomorphine

Apomorphine SL (Uprima™, TAP Pharmaceuticals, Lake Forest, IL, USA) is a sublingually administered dopamine receptor agonist that has been approved in Europe. It is a centrally acting, non-opioid dopaminergic agonist, acting predominantly on the hypothalamic medial pre-optic area and the paraventricular nucleus. Stimulation of dopamine receptors in these regions is associated with oxytocinergic discharge into the spinal cord, which eventuates in penile vascular and corporal smooth muscle relaxation. Placebo-controlled parallel arm investigation of apomophine SL has demonstrated statistically significant differences in the percentage of attempts resulting in successful intercourse between placebo (33%) and increasing doses of apomorphine (45–51%).[46] Recent data suggests that apomorphine SL is most effective in men with short-term ED who have some preservation of erectile function.[47] Sublingual administration of this agent has two benefits: rapid absorption (70% of responders obtain an erection firm enough for intercourse within 20 minutes) and circumvention of hepatic metabolism thereby avoiding drug or food interaction.

The most common side-effects observed with apomorphine SL are nausea, headache and dizziness; these symptoms tend to subside with continued use of the medication.[46,48] Within the dose range approved in Europe (2–3 mg), vasovagal syncope (non-cardiogenic) occurs rarely (<0.2%) and is usually associated with a prodrome of nausea, sweating, and dizziness.[46,48] The exact role of this agent in the management of sexual dysfunction must further be refined.

Second-line therapy

Transurethral

The first pharmacological approach to the management of ED was introduced in the early 1980s as penile injection therapy. Over a decade later in 1995 regulatory agency approval of prostaglandin E_1 (alprostadil) *intracavernosal* therapy (Caverject™, Pharmacia, Kalamazoo, MI, USA) was obtained. A formulation of *transurethral* alprostadil (Medicated Urethral System for Erection or MUSE™, Vivus, Menlo Park, CA, USA) received approval in 1997. Alprostadil is a synthetic form of naturally occurring prostaglandin E_1 (PGE-1). It effects erection through interaction with membrane-bound receptors that activate adenylate cyclase, thereby increasing intracellular levels of cAMP, resulting in cavernosal smooth muscle relaxation and cavernosal artery dilation.[49] MUSE is the only intraurethral treatment modality that is approved for treatment of ED at this time. Transurethral application circumvents administration of the medication with a needle into the corpora cavernosa and relies upon urethral absorption of a semisolid pellet of alprostadil applied with a 3.2 cm applicator that is inserted through the urethral meatus. MUSE was administered to 1511 men with chronic ED from various organic causes in a double-blind placebo controlled trial.[50] In this study, men who responded to MUSE in the office setting were randomized to either drug or placebo for 3 months at home. Sixty-five per cent of men in the MUSE arm reported erections that were sufficient for intercourse compared with 19% of those in the placebo arm. Notably, only men who responded to MUSE in the office setting were included in the controlled portion of the trial; overall, however, a response rate of 44% was observed. The most common side-effect was mild penile pain (11%) and rare hypotension.

Intracorporal injection therapy

Penile injection therapy was the first form of pharmacological treatment for ED and remains the most consistently effective form of treatment. In addition to Caverject™, a second preparation of alprostadil, Edex™ (Schwarz-Pharma, Monheim, Germany), became available in 1998. Off-label combinations of vasoactive medications are also used effectively for intracavernosal injection therapy. Trimix contains PGE-1, papaverine, and phentolamine, whereas Bimix contains papaverine and phentolamine. Papaverine is an alkaloid derived from *Papaver somniferum* (opium), though it is not closely related to the other opium alkaloids in its structure or pharmacological actions. Papaverine is a non-specific phosphodiesterase inhibitor that increases levels of cAMP and cGMP leading to an efflux of calcium from the cell and subsequent smooth muscle relaxation within the corpora cavernosa resulting in erection. It is also used as a vasodilator, especially for cerebral vasodilation. Phentolamine mesylate is a non-selective α-adrenergic antagonist used in the treatment of hypertension and hypertensive emergencies, phaeochromocytoma, vasospasm of Raynaud's disease and frostbite, clonidine withdrawal syndrome, and peripheral vascular disease in addition to ED. Use of papaverine and phentolamine in combination is recommended to increase effectiveness while reducing side-effects associated with higher-dosage single-agent use.[51]

Patients who do not respond to oral therapy have been shown to respond very well to intracavernosal injection. A study of men with ED who did not respond to Viagra and underwent treatment with intracavernosal alprostadil (Edex™) showed that 90% reported significant improvement in the percentage of intercourse attempts in which penetration was successful and 85% in the percentage of attempts that erection could be maintained for completion of intercourse.[52] Thus, intracavernosal alprostadil was found to be efficacious and safe in men who failed initial therapy with sildenafil. Similarly, a crossover, randomized, open label multicentre study comparing the efficacy, safety, and patient preference of MUSE with intracavernosal alprostadil (Edex™) showed that Edex™ more often resulted in an erection sufficient for sexual intercourse (83% versus 53%), more patients using Edex achieved at least one erection sufficient for intercourse (92% versus 62%) and more patients were able to attain at least 75% of erections sufficient for intercourse with Edex use (75% versus 37%).[53] This study also demonstrated that patient and partner satisfaction were greater with intracavernosal alprostadil, and more patients preferred this form of therapy, proving that it is an excellent choice for treatment if oral therapy fails or for those patients in whom oral therapy is contraindicated.

Vacuum constriction device

For men with ED who are not candidates for treatment, are unwilling to attempt treatment, or have failed treatment with oral, intraurethral, or intracavernosal pharmacological agents and either choose not to proceed with penile prosthesis placement or are poor surgical candidates, the vacuum constriction device (VCD) is an additional option for treatment. The VCD consists of a suction cylinder and pump that induce erection by generating negative pressure to distend and fill the corporal sinusoids. A constriction band is placed at the base of the penis to maintain the erection by preventing venous return when the pump is removed. The erection induced is different from a physiological erection as the portion of the penis proximal to the constriction band is flaccid, potentially producing a pivot effect. The constriction ring should not be kept in place for longer than 30 minutes to avoid ischaemia to the corpora cavernosae. The penis may feel cooler than body temperature, the skin may appear cyanotic, and the ejaculate may be trapped by the ring. Additional complications of use include penile petechiae, ecchymosis, initial penile pain, discomfort from the ring, ejaculatory difficulty, discoloration of the glans, and penile numbness.[54,55] A benefit of the VCD includes constriction of the corpus spongiosum and consequent engorgement of the glans improving glanular insufficiency.

Patient selection is integral when assessing effectiveness of the device. Patients who have psychogenic impotence generally do not have success with use of the VCD. A questionnaire-based retrospective study of men with ED using the VCD reported that at a median of 29 month follow-up, 70% of the group used the VCD on a regular basis and patient and partner satisfaction were 84% and 89%, respectively.[56] While this outcome appears promising, only 57% of patients initially enrolled in the study responded with a follow-up questionnaire, and the possibility that those who were lost to follow-up were predominantly non-responders cannot be excluded. Another retrospective study found that 20% of patients rejected the device outright initially, 31% rejected the device after 16 weeks, and a long-term dropout rate of approximately 7% was observed (over a mean of 10.5 months), while 42% of patients used the device long term (median 27.6 months).[57] For patients who are partial responders to other types of treatment, such as oral therapy and intraurethral alprostadil, use of the VCD in combination with these agents may allow conversion to a response adequate for intercourse. For men with severe vascular disease, fibrosis of erectile tissue secondary to priapism, failed placement of penile prosthesis, and those with a penile prosthesis in place with suboptimal tumescence, the VCD may play an important role as well.

Third-line therapy

Patients who do not respond to first-line oral therapy or to the second-line treatment options detailed above are candidates for penile prosthesis placement. Rigorous patient selection and pre-operative education are imperative to optimize chances for a good outcome with prosthesis placement. The patient must be familiar with the mechanics of the device and must have adequate manual dexterity to operate an inflatable device. Infection and malfunction of the device are the main risks associated with the procedure. Patients are cautioned that a mild reduction in penile length may be observed post-operatively, the glans usually remains flaccid and it may take 6 to 12 months until the patient is satisfied with the quality of erection. Both malleable and inflatable devices are available. While malleable devices are easier for the surgeon to implant and for the patient to use (requires limited manual dexterity), they result in a persistently rigid penis that does not approximate normal rigidity or flaccidity. A malleable prosthesis is difficult to conceal and is susceptible to erosion. For these reasons inflatable devices, either two-piece or three-piece, are preferred. Two-piece devices consist of two cylinders, each of which is placed into a corporal body, and a pump (containing a limited reservoir) that is positioned in the scrotum, and the three-piece device has in addition a large-volume fluid reservoir that is placed in the space of Retzius. Of these, the three-piece prosthesis most approximates natural erection when fluid is pumped from the reservoir through the pump into the cylinders for intercourse and thereafter the fluid is drained from the cylinders back into the reservoir to achieve flaccidity. Patients who are not good candidates for placement of a three-piece device are predominantly those who have had previous surgical procedures such as radical cysto-prostatectomy and radical prostatectomy, as the space of Retzius is scarred and autoinflation of the prosthesis (from high pressure on the reservoir) is a risk if adequate space for the reservoir cannot be developed.[58] In addition, placement of the reservoir is difficult in men who have had renal transplant surgery, bilateral inguinal herniorrhaphies, and pelvic radiation; in this population a two-piece device is appropriate.

For various inflatable devices, infection rates of 1.8 to 6% and mechanical failure rates of 2.5 to 4.2% are reported.[59–62] Overall, both patient and partner satisfaction rates are high. Levine reported that 96.4% of men who underwent penile prosthesis surgery had erections suitable for coitus while overall patient and partner satisfaction was 96.4% and 91.2%, respectively and 92.9% of patients and 90.1% of partners would recommend the device to others.[62] This study also demonstrated that patients had a high level of confidence in the device: 91% were satisfied and 83% were very satisfied with the device overall. Another study used validated instruments (the IIEF and EDITS questionnaires) to assess the chronology of efficacy and satisfaction profiles in men undergoing penile prosthetic surgery, and found that satisfaction increased in the year following implant surgery with significant improvements observed in the second half of the first year.[63] Placement of a penile prosthesis has been shown to alleviate concern about the ability to achieve and maintain an erection suitable for intercourse, increase the frequency of sexual intercourse, and improve satisfaction in sexual relations, demonstrating significant improvement in the psychosexual well-being of patients implanted with multicomponent penile devices.[64]

Female sexual dysfunction

Analysis of data from the National Health and Social Life Survey showed that 43% of women suffer from sexual dysfunction, which represents a largely uninvestigated yet significant public health problem with a major impact on quality of life and interpersonal relationships.[10] In this survey that included 1749 women between the ages of 18 and 59 years, 32% lacked interest in sex, 26% were unable to achieve orgasm, 16% experienced pain during sex, 23% found sex not pleasurable, 12% were anxious about performance, and 21% reported trouble with lubrication. Low sexual desire, arousal disorder, and sexual pain were found to be strongly associated with low feelings of physical and emotional satisfaction and diminished happiness. Women with sexual dysfunction most commonly presented with multidimensional complaints, early in the fifth decade of life with depression as a co-morbid factor.

The female sexual response, initially described by Masters and Johnson in 1966, was modified by Kaplan in 1974 to include the coordination and integration of sexual desire, arousal, orgasm, and satisfaction.[65,66] In 1998, the first Consensus Development Panel on Female Sexual Dysfunction was convened by the Sexual Function Health Council of the American Foundation for Urologic Disease to develop a consensus-based definition and classification system for female sexual dysfunction that would include psychogenic and organically based disorders.[9] The new classification scheme includes disorders of sexual desire, sexual arousal, orgasm, and sexual pain; the definition of each based on the consensus panel report is shown in Box 12.1.

Box 12.1 **Classification system of female sexual dysfunction[9]**

Sexual desire disorders

- Hypoactive sexual desire disorder: the persistent or recurrent deficiency (or absence) of sexual fantasies/thoughts and/or desire for or receptivity to sexual activity, which causes personal distress.
- Sexual aversion disorder: the persistent or recurrent phobic aversion to and avoidance of sexual contact with a sexual partner, which causes personal distress.

Sexual arousal disorder

- The persistent or recurrent inability to attain or maintain sufficient sexual excitement, causing personal distress, which may be expressed as a lack of subjective excitement, or genital (lubrication/swelling) or other somatic responses.

Orgasmic disorder

- The persistent or recurrent difficulty, delay in, or absence of attaining orgasm following sufficient sexual stimulation and arousal, which causes personal distress.

Sexual pain disorders

- Dyspareunia: the recurrent or persistent genital pain associated with sexual intercourse.
- Vaginismus: the recurrent or persistent involuntary spasm of the musculature of the outer third of the vagina that interferes with vaginal penetration, which causes personal distress.
- Non-coital sexual pain disorder: recurrent or persistent genital pain induced by non-coital sexual stimulation.

Aetiology

Just as multiple risk factors predispose men to development of ED, medical problems in women may contribute to sexual dysfunction. Vascular disease associated with coronary artery disease, previous myocardial infarction, hypertension, and diabetes may contribute to impaired arousal, as clitoral and vaginal blood flow may be compromised.[67] Neurological disorders affecting pudendal sensory and motor nerves or the autonomic nervous system, such as spinal cord injury, multiple sclerosis, stroke, or peripheral neuropathy secondary to diabetes may result in dysfunction. Endocrinopathies in addition to diabetes such as hyperprolactinaemia, thyroid or adrenal disorders, oestrogen or androgen deficiency may be causative as well.

Androgens are important mediators of female sexuality, and a decline in serum androgen levels is observed in women as they age, contributing to diminished sexual desire, arousal, and orgasm.[8] Oestrogen deficiency contributes to decreased vaginal lubrication and gradual genital atrophy, both of which contribute to sexual dysfunction. Gynaecologialc aetiologies include a history of hysterectomy and oophorectomy, sexually transmitted diseases, and age relative to menopause. Medications such as anti-depressants and birth control pills, autoimmune disorders, arthritis, renal insufficiency, bladder or bowel disease, and breast cancer are additional causative factors for female sexual dysfunction.[67] Psychogenic sexual dysfunction may be caused by intrapersonal conflicts, such as those associated with religious, social, or cultural restrictions, issues of abandonment, trust, control, or safety. Interpersonal conflicts may also play a role as can a history of sexual inexperience or sexual abuse. Finally, significant life-stressors such as family illness, death, financial, or employment problems may compromise sexual function.[67]

Evaluation

A thorough history and physical examination are integral components of evaluation for sexual dysfunction in women. The topic of sexuality can be approached initially with questions about the patient's menstrual cycle and can be pursued with directed questions regarding change in sexual activity and satisfaction associated with intercourse. The Female Sexual Function Index is a validated questionnaire that assesses six domains of sexual function and may be used to distinctly define areas in which the patient has concerns. A general physical examination is performed with focus on pelvic examination. Laboratory tests, such as serum electrolytes, complete blood count, thyroid function, prolactin, free and total testosterone, follicle-stimulating hormone, luteinizing hormone, sex hormone binding globulin, and estradiol levels, are assessed as indicated. Vaginal photoplethysmography may be performed to measure vascular engorgement within the vaginal wall, though an absolute standard of measurement has not been determined.[9] Measures of genital blood flow (using colour duplex Doppler ultrasonography), vaginal lubrication, vaginal compliance and elasticity, and genital sensation are all currently under investigation to achieve validated and standardized assessment modalities.[8]

Treatment

A great deal of investigation is ongoing in the relatively new field of female sexual dysfunction. While a detailed review of the literature on treatment of female sexual dysfunction is exhaustive, those treatment modalities most commonly utilized are discussed for a general overview.

Hormone replacement therapy

Both oestrogen and testosterone appear to be important components of the female sexual response cycle. Oestrogen deficiency leads to diminished vaginal lubrication and eventual thinning of the vaginal wall mucosa and atrophy of the smooth muscle layer. Systemic oestrogen replacement is associated with improved clitoral sensitivity, increased libido, and decreased dyspareunia, while topical therapy with a vaginal estradiol ring (Estring™, Pharmacia Upjohn, Kalamazoo, MI) or vaginal estradiol tablets (Vagifem™, Novo Nordisk A/S, Bagsvaerd, Denmark) may relieve pain and dryness.[8]

Low testosterone levels in women are associated with a decline in sexual arousal, genital sensation, libido, and orgasm.[8] Total testosterone less than 20 pg/dl and free testosterone less than 0.9 pg/dl are considered low in women. Patients who have premature ovarian failure, or iatrogenic, natural, or surgical menopause are candidates for androgen replacement. Hormone replacement therapy with oestrogen plus androgens has been found to provide greater improvement in psychological (e.g. lack of concentration, depression, and fatigue) and sexual (e.g. decreased libido and inability to have an orgasm) symptoms than does oestrogen alone in naturally and surgically menopausal women.[68] Both hormones may be administered as esterified oestrogens/methyltestosterone tablets (Estratest or Estratest-H.S., Solvay Pharmaceuticals, Brussels, Belgium). Transdermal testosterone preparations (gel and patch) are currently under investigation for appropriate dosage in women and preliminarily have resulted in enhanced sexual function and well-being in well-defined populations, presenting a promising new approach for providing physiologically based androgen therapy.[69] Potential side-effects of androgen replacement include weight gain, clitoral enlargement, facial hair, hypercholesterolaemia, and liver damage.

Phosphodiesterase type 5 inhibitor

The mechanism of increased blood flow to the vagina and clitoris and smooth muscle relaxation with subsequent engorgement of the clitoris appears to be mediated by NO and guanylate cyclase production of cGMP, an effect that is limited by breakdown of cGMP by PDE5.[70] A randomized, double-blind placebo-controlled study on the safety and efficacy of sildenafil citrate treatment of Female Sexual Arousal Disorder (FSAD) in 202 post-menopausal women with normalized serum estradiol and free testosterone concentrations demonstrated that use of sildenafil was safe and resulted in significant improvements in sexual arousal, orgasm, intercourse, and overall satisfaction with sexual life in post-menopausal women with FSAD who did not have concurrent hypoactive sexual desire disorder.[71]

Eros vacuum therapy device

The EROS-CTD™ (Clitoral Therapy Device, Urometrics, Anoka, MN) is a small, hand-held, battery-powered device with a small suction cup that is applied to the clitoris and applies gentle suction, thereby increasing genital blood flow. The device has been shown to significantly improve clitoral sensation, lubrication, the ability to achieve orgasm, and sexual satisfaction.[72] The increase in vaginal lubrication is hypothesized to occur secondary to clitoral engorgement induced by the vacuum and subsequent activation of an autonomic reflex that triggers arterial vasodilation with an increase in transudate and lubrication.

Treatment of orgasmic disorder must be tailored to individual aetiology. For example, patients taking SSRIs may develop orgasmic dysfunction as a side-effect of the medication, and in this case the medication should be stopped or adjusted. Appropriately selected patients may benefit from hormone replacement therapy, while others with complex causes of orgasmic dysfunction such as emotional trauma or sexual abuse may require referral to a sex therapist for thorough evaluation and treatment.

For appropriate treatment of dyspareunia, the aetiology must first be determined, possibly requiring the performance of laparoscopy for correct diagnosis.[67] Improvement in pain may be observed with use of a lubricant for intercourse. Women with genital atrophy may benefit from local hormone replacement with Estring™ or Vagifem™. Vaginismus can be treated with progressive muscle relaxation and vaginal dilatation with success rates as high as 90%.[73] Patients that do not respond to this type of treatment may require referral to a sex therapist.

Conclusions

The patient presenting with sexual dysfunction requires, and benefits from, thoughtful consideration. Discussion of sexual dysfunction can be difficult for both the patient and for the physician, though discussion of this medical problem is extremely important. Sexual dysfunction is the source of significant personal and interpersonal distress and has considerable impact on an individual's well-being. The multiple risk factors for sexual dysfunction can be identified when the patient presents allowing timely diagnosis and treatment of concomitant medical conditions such as coronary artery disease and diabetes ultimately averting further morbidity. Overall, treatment options for the patient with sexual dysfunction are diverse and successful. Although a great deal of progress has been made in discovering physiological mechanisms involved in both male and female sexual function, continued research efforts are necessary not only to understand the disease process on a molecular level, but also to optimize treatment modalities that will maximally enhance patient quality of life.

References

1 NIH Consensus Conference (1993). NIH Consensus Development Panel on Impotence. *J. Am. Med. Assoc.* **270**: 83–90.

2 Pfizer Inc., NY, USA. Data on file.

3 Braun M, Wassmer G, Klotz T, Reifenrath B, Mathers M, Engelmann U (2000). Epidemiology of erectile dysfunction: results of the 'Cologne Male Survey'. *Int. J. Impot. Res.* **12**(6): 305–11.

4 Kubin M, Wagner G, Fugl-Meyer AR (2003). Epidemiology of erectile dysfunction. *Int. J. Impot. Res.* **15**(1): 63–71.

5 Nicolosi A, Moreira ED Jr, Shirai M, Bin Mohd Tambi MI, Glasser DB (2003). Epidemiology of erectile dysfunction in four countries: cross-national study of the prevalence and correlates of erectile dysfunction. *Urology* **61**(1): 201–6.

6 Feldman HA, Goldstein I, Hatzichristou DG, Krane RJ, McKinlay JB (1994). Impotence and its medical and psychosocial correlates: results of the Massachusetts Male Aging Study. *J. Urol.* **151**(1): 54–61.

7 Johannes CB, Araujo AB, Feldman HA, Derby CA, Kleinman KP, McKinlay JB (2000). Incidence of erectile dysfunction in men 40 to 69 years old: longitudinal results from the Massachusetts male aging study. *J. Urol.* **163**(2): 460–3.

8 Berman JR, Goldstein I (2001). Female sexual dysfunction. *Urol. Clin. North Am.* **28**(2): 405–16.

9 Basson R, Berman J, Burnett A, Derogatis L, Ferguson D, Fourcroy J *et al.* (2000). Report of the international consensus development conference on female sexual dysfunction: definitions and classifications. *J. Urol.* **163**(3): 888–93.

10 Laumann EO, Paik A, Rosen RC (1999). Sexual dysfunction in the United States: prevalence and predictors. *J. Am. Med. Assoc.* **281**(6): 537–44.

11 Marwick C (1999). Survey says patients expect little physician help on sex. *J. Am. Med. Assoc.* **281**(23): 2173–4.

12 Metz ME, Seifert MH Jr (1990). Men's expectations of physicians in sexual health concerns. *J. Sex Marital Ther.* **16**(2): 79–88.

13 Perelman MA (2003). Sex coaching for physicians: combination treatment for patient and partner. *Int. J. Impot. Res.* **15**(Suppl. 5): S67–S74.

14 Lue TF (2000). Erectile dysfunction. *N. Engl. J. Med.* **342**(24): 1802–13.

15 Keller Ashton A, Hamer R, Rosen RC (1997). Serotonin reuptake inhibitor-induced sexual dysfunction and its treatment: a large-scale retrospective study of 596 psychiatric outpatients. *J. Sex Marital Ther.* **23**(3): 165–75.

16 Bacon CG, Mittleman MA, Kawachi I, Giovannucci E, Glasser DB, Rimm EB (2003). Sexual function in men older than 50 years of age: results from the health professionals follow-up study. *Ann. Intern. Med.* **139**(3): 161–8.

17 Greiner KA, Weigel JW (1996). Erectile dysfunction. *Am. Fam. Physician* **54**(5): 1675–82.

18 Masters WH, Johnson VE (1977). Sex after sixty-five. *Reflections* **12**: 31–43.

19 McVary KT, Carrier S, Wessells H (2001). Smoking and erectile dysfunction: evidence based analysis. *J. Urol.* **166**(5): 1624–32.

20 Muller SC, el-Damanhoury H, Ruth J, Lue TF (1991). Hypertension and impotence. *Eur. Urol.* **19**(1): 29–34.

21 Wabrek AJ, Burchell RC (1980). Male sexual dysfunction associated with coronary heart disease. *Arch. Sex Behav.* **9**(1): 69–75.

22 Virag R, Bouilly P, Frydman D (1985). Is impotence an arterial disorder? A study of arterial risk factors in 440 impotent men. *Lancet* **1**(8422): 181–4.

23 Whitehead ED, Klyde BJ (1990). Diabetes-related impotence in the elderly. *Clin. Geriatr. Med.* **6**(4): 771–95.

24 Ellenberg M (1971). Impotence in diabetes: the neurologic factor. *Ann. Intern. Med.* **75**(2): 213–19.

25 Zonszein J (1995). Diagnosis and management of endocrine disorders of erectile dysfunction. *Urol. Clin. North Am.* **22**(4): 789–802.

26 Blanker MH, Bohnen AM, Groeneveld FP, Bernsen RM, Prins A, Thomas S *et al.* (2001). Correlates for erectile and ejaculatory dysfunction in older Dutch men: a community-based study. *J. Am. Geriatr. Soc.* **49**(4): 436–42.

27 Chang S, Hypolite JA, Zderic SA, Wein AJ, Chacko S, DiSanto ME (2002). Enhanced force generation by corpus cavernosum smooth muscle in rabbits with partial bladder outlet obstruction. *J. Urol.* **167**(6): 2636–44.

28 Bancroft J, Wu FC (1983). Changes in erectile responsiveness during androgen replacement therapy. *Arch. Sex Behav.* **12**(1): 59–66.

29 Wolfe MM (1979). Impotence on cimetidine treatment. *N. Engl. J. Med.* **300**(2): 94.

30 Miller NS, Gold MS (1988). The human sexual response and alcohol and drugs. *J. Subst. Abuse Treat.* **5**(3): 171–7.

31 Benet AE, Melman A (1995). The epidemiology of erectile dysfunction. *Urol. Clin. North Am.* **22**(4): 699–709.

32 Sadovsky R, Dunn M, Grobe BM (1999). Erectile dysfunction: the primary care practitioner's view. *Am. J. Manag. Care* **5**(3): 333–41; quiz 342–3.

33 Prader A (1966). Testicular size: assessment and clinical importance. *Triangle* **7**: 240.

34 Wessells H, Lue TF, McAninch JW (1996). Penile length in the flaccid and erect states: guidelines for penile augmentation. *J. Urol.* **156**(3): 995–7.

35 Fisher C, Gross J, Zuch J (1953). Cycle of penile erections synchronous with dreaming (REM) sleep. *Arch. Gen. Psychiat.* **12**: 29.

36 Karacan I, Goodenough DR, Shapiro A (1966). Erection cycle during sleep in relation to dream anxiety. *Arch. Gen. Psychiat.* **15**: 183.

37 Padma-Nathan H (2000). Diagnostic and treatment strategies for erectile dysfunction: the 'Process of Care' model. *Int. J. Impot. Res.* **12**(Suppl. 4): S119–S121.

38 Guay AT, Perez JB, Jacobson J, Newton RA (2001). Efficacy and safety of sildenafil citrate for treatment of erectile dysfunction in a population with associated organic risk factors. *J. Androl.* **22**(5): 793–7.

39 Goldstein I, Lue TF, Padma-Nathan H, Rosen RC, Steers WD, Wicker PA (1998). Oral sildenafil in the treatment of erectile dysfunction. Sildenafil Study Group. *N. Engl. J. Med.* **338**(20): 1397–404.

40 Padma-Nathan H, Steers WD, Wicker PA (1998). Efficacy and safety of oral sildenafil in the treatment of erectile dysfunction: a double-blind, placebo-controlled study of 329 patients. Sildenafil Study Group. *Int. J. Clin. Pract.* **52**(6): 375–9.

41 Marks LS, Duda C, Dorey FJ, Macairan ML, Santos PB (1999). Treatment of erectile dysfunction with sildenafil. *Urology* **53**(1): 19–24.

42 Hellstrom WJ, Gittelman M, Karlin G, Segerson T, Thibonnier M, Taylor T *et al.* (2002). Vardenafil for treatment of men with erectile dysfunction: efficacy and safety in a randomized, double-blind, placebo-controlled trial. *J. Androl.* **23**(6): 763–71.

43 Brock GB, McMahon CG, Chen KK, Costigan T, Shen W, Watkins V *et al.* (2002). Efficacy and safety of tadalafil for the treatment of erectile dysfunction: results of integrated analyses. *J. Urol.* **168**(4, Pt 1): 1332–6.

44 Goldstein I, Young JM, Fischer J, Bangerter K, Segerson T, Taylor T (2003). Vardenafil, a new phosphodiesterase type 5 inhibitor, in the treatment of erectile dysfunction in men with diabetes: a multicenter double-blind placebo-controlled fixed-dose study. *Diabetes Care* **26**(3): 777–83.

45 Saenz de Tejada I, Anglin G, Knight JR, Emmick JT (2002). Effects of tadalafil on erectile dysfunction in men with diabetes. *Diabetes Care* **25**(12): 2159–64.

46 Dula E, Keating W, Siami PF, Edmonds A, O'Neil J, Buttler S (2000). Efficacy and safety of fixed-dose and dose-optimization regimens of sublingual apomorphine versus placebo in men with erectile dysfunction. The Apomorphine Study Group. *Urology* **56**(1): 130–5.

47 Schulman C, Sleep D (2002). Duration of erectile dysfunction prior to treatment influences the response to apomorphine SL. *Annual Meeting of the American Urological Association, Orlando, FL, May 29, 2002.* Abstract LB39 http://aua.agora.com//abstractviewer/av_view.asp.

48 Mulhall JP (2002). Sublingual apomorphine for the treatment of erectile dysfunction. *Expert Opin. Investig. Drugs* **11**(2): 295–302.

49 Palmer LS, Valcic M, Melman A, Giraldi A, Wagner G, Christ GJ (1994). Characterization of cyclic AMP accumulation in cultured human corpus cavernosum smooth muscle cells. *J. Urol.* **152**(4): 1308–14.

50 Padma-Nathan H, Hellstrom WJ, Kaiser FE, Labasky RF, Lue TF, Nolten WE *et al.* (1997). Treatment of men with erectile dysfunction with transurethral alprostadil. Medicated Urethral System for Erection (MUSE) Study Group. *N. Engl. J. Med.* **336**(1): 1–7.

51 Stief CG, Wetterauer U (1988). Erectile responses to intracavernous papaverine and phentolamine: comparison of single and combined delivery. *J. Urol.* **140**(6): 1415–16.

52 Shabsigh R, Padma-Nathan H, Gittleman M, McMurray J, Kaufman J, Goldstein I (2000). Intracavernous alprostadil alfadex (EDEX/VIRIDAL) is effective and safe in patients with erectile dysfunction after failing sildenafil (Viagra). *Urology* **55**(4): 477–80.

53 Shabsigh R, Padma-Nathan H, Gittleman M, McMurray J, Kaufman J, Goldstein I (2000). Intracavernous alprostadil alfadex is more efficacious, better tolerated, and preferred over intraurethral alprostadil plus optional actis: a comparative, randomized, crossover, multicenter study. *Urology* **55**(1): 109–13.

54 Nadig PW, Ware JC, Blumoff R (1986). Noninvasive device to produce and maintain an erection-like state. *Urology* **27**(2): 126–31.

55 Witherington R (1985). The Osbon Erecaid system in the management of erectile impotence. *J. Urol.* **133A**: 306.

56 Cookson MS, Nadig PW (1993). Long-term results with vacuum constriction device. *J. Urol.* **149**(2): 290–4.

57 Derouet H, Caspari D, Rohde V, Rommel G, Ziegler M (1999). Treatment of erectile dysfunction with external vacuum devices. *Andrologia* **31**(Suppl. 1): 89–94.

58 Ghaly SW, Mulhall JP (2002). Penile prostheses: device types, selection, and reliability. In: *Atlas of the Urologic Clinics of North America* (ed. JJ Mulcahy), pp. 153–162. W. B. Saunders, Philadelphia, PA.

59 Goldstein I, Newman L, Baum N, Brooks M, Chaikin L, Goldberg K *et al.* (1997). Safety and efficacy outcome of mentor alpha-1 inflatable penile prosthesis implantation for impotence treatment. *J. Urol.* **157**(3): 833–9.

60 Govier FE, Gibbons RP, Correa RJ, Pritchett TR, Kramer-Levien D (1998). Mechanical reliability, surgical complications, and patient and partner satisfaction of the modern three-piece inflatable penile prosthesis. *Urology* **52**(2): 282–6.

61 Montorsi F, Rigatti P, Carmignani G, Corbu C, Campo B, Ordesi G *et al.* (2000). AMS three-piece inflatable implants for erectile dysfunction: a long-term multi-institutional study in 200 consecutive patients. *Eur. Urol.* **37**(1): 50–5.

62 Levine LA, Estrada CR, Morgentaler A (2001). Mechanical reliability and safety of, and patient satisfaction with the Ambicor inflatable penile prosthesis: results of a 2 center study. *J. Urol.* **166**(3): 932–7.

63 Mulhall JP, Ahmed A, Branch J, Parker M (2003). Serial assessment of efficacy and satisfaction profiles following penile prosthesis surgery. *J. Urol.* **169**(4): 1429–33.

64 Tefilli MV, Dubocq F, Rajpurkar A, Gheiler EL, Tiguert R, Barton C *et al.* (1998). Assessment of psychosexual adjustment after insertion of inflatable penile prosthesis. *Urology* **52**(6): 1106–12.

65 Masters WH, Johnson VE (1966). *Human Sexual Response*. Little Brown, Boston, MA.

66 Kaplan HS (1974). *The New Sex Therapy*. Brunner/Mazel, New York.

67 **Phillips NA** (2000). Female sexual dysfunction: evaluation and treatment. *Am. Fam. Physician* **62**(1): 127–36, 141–2.

68 **Sarrel PM** (1999). Psychosexual effects of menopause: role of androgens. *Am. J. Obstet. Gynecol.* **180**(3, Pt 2): S319–S324.

69 **Mazer NA, Shifren JL** (2003). Transdermal testosterone for women: a new physiological approach for androgen therapy. *Obstet. Gynecol. Surv.* **58**(7): 489–500.

70 **Berman JR, Berman LA, Lin H, Flaherty E, Lahey N, Goldstein I et al.** (2001). Effect of sildenafil on subjective and physiologic parameters of the female sexual response in women with sexual arousal disorder. *J. Sex Marital Ther.* **27**(5): 411–20.

71 **Berman JR, Berman LA, Toler SM, Gill J, Haughie S** (2003). Safety and efficacy of sildenafil citrate for the treatment of female sexual arousal disorder: a double-blind, placebo controlled study. *J. Urol.* **170**(6, Pt 1): 2333–8.

72 **Billups KL, Berman L, Berman J, Metz ME, Glennon ME, Goldstein I** (2001). A new non-pharmacological vacuum therapy for female sexual dysfunction. *J. Sex Marital Ther.* **27**(5): 435–41.

73 **Rosen RC, Leiblum SR** (1995). Treatment of sexual disorders in the 1990s: an integrated approach. *J. Consult. Clin. Psychol.* **63**(6): 877–90.

Chapter 13

The patient presenting with androgen deficiency

Alvaro Morales

Introduction

The care of the hypogonadal male patient presents two very different scenarios: on the one hand we have the obvious (albeit not always so obvious) congenital abnormalities such as occur with Kleinfelter's syndrome or the iatrogenically castrated man suffering from advanced prostate cancer. On the other, we have the progressive, slow decline in androgen production associated with ageing. This chapter will deal exclusively with the latter. In the former, the need for treatment is either clearly evident or indisputably contraindicated. The issues related to hypogonadism of ageing are not so obvious and there remains a great deal of controversy on its significance, the specificity of its clinical manifestations, the accuracy of its biochemical diagnosis, and the safety of its treatment. Some of these concerns are justified; many, however, are based on obsolete information or erroneous extrapolation of the effects of hormone replacement in women.

This chapter provides current and updated information on the care of the ageing hypogonadal man from diagnosis to treatment options and monitoring. In most cases these aspects of care are straightforward. The informed clinician has the responsibility to either refer appropriately or to manage effectively and safely the patient with late-onset hypogonadism (LOH), also known as androgen decline in the ageing male (ADAM). At the risk of appearing redundant, it is, however, important to emphasize that only symptomatic late-onset hypogonadism (SLOH) needs to be treated. The man without sequelae from low levels of serum testosterone requires follow-up but not necessarily androgen replacement or supplementation.

Diagnosis

Clinical

The clinical diagnosis of LOH is easily missed for various reasons. Prominent among them is lack of awareness by the physician but also because the manifestations (Table 13.1) are not all present, are frequently subtle, and progress so slowly over the years that the patient himself may not be aware of their occurrence. Most commonly,

Table 13.1 Clinical manifestations of symptomatic late-onset hypogonadism

Decreased in sexual interest and performance
Tiredness
Depression
Irritability
Anaemia
Osteoporosis
Sarcopenia

however, they are attributed to the unavoidable process of ageing, about which there are only limited options. Although this is true, ageing associated with hypogonadism can be treated effectively so as to ameliorate some of the infirmities of growing old.

The importance of a proper history and physical examination holds true here. A number of questionnaires currently available are useful as screening tools but continue to be employed, unfortunately, not only as diagnostic but also as treatment outcome instruments. This practice is to be discouraged.

It is important to emphasize that many of the manifestations described in Table 13.1 can be difficult or impossible to distinguish from other conditions such as depression or hypothyroidism. Although the presence of one or more signs or symptoms is important, the clue for accurate diagnosis relies on the physician's ability to interpret the significance of the clinical manifestations and biochemical findings indicating one or more possible hormonal abnormalities. This point needs to be emphasized: the asymptomatic patient with LOH does not necessarily require treatment. By the same token, a man with evident manifestations of the syndrome and ambiguous biochemistry may be a candidate for therapy.

Biochemical

Much confusion reigns in this area. The basic evaluation includes a serum testosterone (T) determination. For consistency and accuracy (due to the pulsatile and circadian pattern of T production), the sample should be taken in the morning, between 7 and 11 a.m. Although little dispute exists about this, the controversy begins with the issue of which assay best reflects the individual degree of androgenicity in a cost-effective manner. Current views are summarized as follows:

1 Total T. This test is available in most clinical biochemistry laboratories. It is automated, consistent, easy to perform, and inexpensive. In the vast majority of situations, it is satisfactory for the initial evaluation. The physician, however, must be aware that because of increases in sex hormone-binding globulin (SHBG) associated with some conditions, including healthy ageing, the results may be misleading,

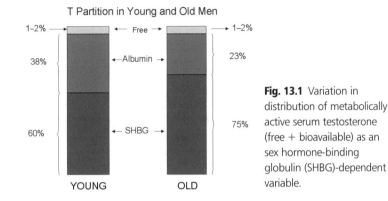

Fig. 13.1 Variation in distribution of metabolically active serum testosterone (free + bioavailable) as an sex hormone-binding globulin (SHBG)-dependent variable.

i.e. a total T in the presence of elevated SHBG may be within the normal range but a significant proportion of T will not be available at the tissue level (Fig. 13.1).

2 Free T. This test measures the fraction of T that is unbound to albumin and globulin and is the most accurate index of a man's androgenicity. This is an accurate statement as long as the performing laboratory conducts the assays by the methods of equilibrium dialysis or ultracentrifugation. This methodology is cumbersome, demands expertise, and is costly. It is rarely done. Unfortunately, most laboratories carry out a 'free T' test by radioimmunoassay that is automated, cheaper, and notoriously inaccurate. The physician ordering a 'free T' should be aware of the method used and interpret the results accordingly.

3 Calculated free T. In order to circumvent the vagaries and expense of free T determination, Vermeulen et al.[1] devised a method for measuring free T based on a complicated formula using the results of the serum levels of total T and SHBG. The reader does not need to bother with the intricacies of the formula which is easily accessible on the web (www.issam.ch). By entering the results of the two assays (total T and SHBG) and the results of the calculated free T (cFT) can be calculated. Several studies have shown this method to be as accurate (as a measure of metabolically active T in peripheral blood) as either free T or bioavailable T.

4 Bioavailable T. Here the amount of T circulating free together with that loosely bound to albumin is measured. When done by experienced individuals (unfortunate it is not an automated methodology) it represents a reliable assessment of a man's levels of biologically active T in serum (an important point since at present there are no reliable methodologies to assess availability of any form of testosterone at tissue level).

5 Free androgen index. This is the quotient of total T over SHBG. It is simple but unreliable and is not recommended.

6 Repeated measurements. If the biochemistry does not initially support the clinical impression, the testing should be repeated. Morley et al.[2] unambiguously showed

that there are large intra-individual variations in the levels of serum T over time. The clinic should lead the biochemistry and not, as frequently happens, the other way around.

When biochemical hypogonadism is documented, it is wise to consider assessment of the hypothalamics–pituitary–gonadal (H–P–G) axis. This will establish the type of hypogonadism: primary (testicular), secondary (pituitary), or tertiary (hypothalamic). The results are helpful in deciding therapeutic strategy.

Treatment

Testosterone

Treatment of hypogonadism should not be initiated in the absence of reliable clinical and biochemical diagnostic evidence; in other words, a fairly firm diagnosis of the condition. The combination of signs and symptoms, the serum levels of hormones, and the knowledge and experience of the physician are the relevant factors determining the need for androgen replacement therapy (ART). Low levels of testosterone by themselves are not sufficient reason to initiate treatment, i.e. there must be a defined need to improve one or more aspects of the patient's quality of life. Equally important is the value of the T serum values, since they show marked intra-individual variation over time and are not necessarily a reliable reflection of events at tissue level. The astute physician may need to consider ART in the presence of borderline T levels.

Treatment may need to be tailored to the manifestations present in each individual case. The approach will be different in a man with the sequelae of osteoporosis compared with a man whose main complaint is sexual dysfunction. In the former, a long-term plan is needed while for the latter a relatively short period of treatment may be sufficient to establish therapeutic significance. Regardless of the primary manifestation, treatment is generally for life and the patient should be informed of such commitment from the outset.

The production of testosterone by the testicles is pulsatile in nature and, except in the elderly, follows a circadian and, perhaps, a seasonal rhythm. Although the availability of new forms of testosterone delivery represent an important improvement in the pharmacokinetics and pharmacodynamics of therapeutic androgen substitution, none of them can replicate the patterns of androgen production by the testis. This situation may have a bearing on some of the adverse effects of testosterone supplementation. Such side-effects may be due to the appearance of non-physiologically high/low levels of T, over reduction of T into 5α-dihydrotestosterone (DHT) or the aromatization of T into oestrogen. A combination of these factors or their relative ratios may also play a role. Furthermore, the route of administration matters, e.g. transdermal administration of T is associated with high DHT levels. This is also the case with oral testosterone undecanoate which circumvents a first pass through the liver through its absorption from the gut along with the fats via the thoracic duct, thus avoiding the liver toxicity observed with other oral T preparations. Probably a fair amount of T still arrives via the portal vein in the liver and causes a significant decline in the production of SHBG.[3] While documentation is much clearer for oestrogens, it seems likely that androgens also exert different metabolic effects depending on their route of administration.

Commercial preparations

With the notable exception of the 17-α alkylated preparations, currently available preparations are generally (with some peculiar variations) safe and effective. The choice depends, primarily, on issues of perceived safety, efficacy, cost, convenience, and patient's and physician's choice (Table 13.2). Each preparation offers advantages and drawbacks:

1 Injectable testosterone preparations have the longest history of use and are the least expensive. They are, however, inconvenient, i.e. there is the need for injection at regular, frequent intervals, they commonly produce a 'roller-coaster' effect, and they are more prone to induce polycythaemia.

2 Oral testosterone undecanoate is safe and effective although it may require doses above those recommended by the manufacturer. It needs to be taken with food to avoid the first passage through the liver and is not available in the United States. Oral alkylated preparations exhibit the potential for liver toxicity and have been banned from many countries, although they are still available in the United States.

3 Testosterone patches are safe and effective when applied in the evening. Some men find them unacceptable because they produce skin irritation in about 30% of users and are visible.

4 Testosterone gels are available in a variety of formulations. They circumvent the problem of skin irritation but precautions need to be taken to avoid passage to a second party through skin contact.

5 Buccal applications are the newest preparations in the North American market. Satisfactory levels of serum testosterone are achieved but experience with this form of delivery is still very limited.

Table 13.2 Available testosterone preparations

	Generic name	Trade name	Dose
Injectable	Testosterone cypionate	Depo-testosterone cypionate	200–400 mg every 2–4 weeks
	Testosterone enanthate	Delatestryl	200–400 mg every 2–4 weeks
Oral	Testosterone undecanoate	Andriol	120–240 mg daily
Transdermal	Testosterone patch	Androderm	2.5–5 mg daily
	Testosterone gel	Testim	50–100 mg daily
	Testosterone gel	Androgel	5–10 g daily

It needs to be emphasized that exogenous administration of androgens directly affects the negative feedback mechanisms of the hypothalamics–pituitary–gonadal axis. Chronic testosterone supplementation will eventually shut off endogenous androgen production by the gonads. Therefore, even in cases of partial androgen production—as seen with the ageing process—full therapeutic substitution is usually required.

The selection of a T preparation depends on several factors. All commercial preparations, apart from the methylated ones, are safe. The choice, therefore, is made on the basis of efficacy, patient tolerance and convenience, physician's familiarity, and, depending the specific regional situation, cost (Table 13.3.).

Other androgens

The use of other androgens in the treatment of hypogonadism is in its infancy. The two most frequently used are dehydroepiandrosterone (DHEA) and dehydrotestosterone (DHT). The former has been the subject of a great deal of speculation and is currently available as an over-the-counter 'nutritional supplement' in the United States. Their current status in the armamentarium is summarized below.

DHEA

A great deal of enthusiasm was generated following a randomized, placebo-controlled, crossover trial of a small group of men and women with low levels of DHEA who received nightly oral administration of either 50 mg DHEA or a placebo for a period of 3 months.[4] In the subjects receiving DHEA the serum levels of this hormone as well as testosterone reached levels expected in the young adult range. Clinically there was an increase in the sense of well-being reported by most (>60%) subjects after 12 weeks of DHEA administration whereas fewer than 10% reported any change after placebo. However, no changes were evident in the domain of sexual interest. Another placebo-controlled study of 39 men receiving 100 mg DHEA daily for 3 months resulted in no effect on well-being and sexual function.[5] Artl et al.[6] in a controlled trial did not find significant differences in those receiving 50 mg DHEA for 4 months in well-being or sexual function as compared with those taking placebo. It should be noted, however, that none of these patients had sexual dysfunction, a somewhat unusual situation considering that they were all over 50 years old. The largest controlled study available is the one conducted by Beaulieu et al.[7] (on 140 men and 140 women) in which they did not detect a difference in sexual function between the DHEA and placebo groups among the men. This contrasted with the effect of the hormone in the female counterparts.

It is important to emphasize here that exogenous DHEA is readily and extensively metabolized into other sex steroids. This process interferes with the ability to accurately define the efficacy of DHEA *per se* as opposed to the effect of its converted metabolites. Clinically this is not a major concern but it contributes to the confusion that exists regarding the true value of DHEA in improving sexual function. In addition, its biological effects may be exerted locally in tissues by DHEA or its metabolites, under the mechanisms appropriately designated as intracrinology by Labrie *et al.*[8]

Dihydrotestosterone (DHT)

Available studies in hypogonadal men show that DHT maintains sex characteristics, increases muscle mass, and improves sexual function without significant increases in prostate size.[9] In fact, in elderly men, DHT administration resulted in a 15% decrease in prostate size.[10] This effect has been ascribed to the lack of aromatization of DHT to estradiol, therewith reducing the hypothesized synergism between androgens and oestrogens on the prostate. In a more recent study of 3 months' duration, percutaneous DHT administration to ageing men[11] caused no effect on circulating estradiol levels or prostate disease markers such as serum prostatic specific antigen (PSA), prostate symptom scores, or prostate volume. In another recent trial[12] DHT was administered also by the transdermal route for 6 months to a group of ageing men. A reduction of plasma estradiol was noted, but again effects on the prostate were not observed. There were no were detrimental effects on lipid profiles. Erectile function was improved in the active compound group as measured by the International Index of Erectile Function (IIEF). On the basis of the above findings, DHT cannot be dismissed as a potentially useful androgen for the ageing male, but a number of the same issues raised above, in regards to testosterone, have to be addressed in future studies. For instance, DHT could be used as a single agent instead of testosterone in hypogonadal men with erectile dysfunction (ED) or in combination with other drugs, as discussed above.

DHT gel is available at a dose of 125–250 mg/day which yields plasma DHT levels comparable to physiological T levels; more recently it has been shown that in healthy elderly males, a lower dose of 32–64 mg/day yields comparable levels.

Selective androgen-receptor modulators (SARMS)

There has been increasing interest and experience with the use of selective oestrogen receptor modulators (SERMS) in women. Concerns heightened by the report of the Women's Health Initiative (WHI)[13] on the detrimental effects from the use of hormone replacement therapy in post-menopausal women has intensified the search for alternatives to traditional oestrogen/progesterone combinations. Whether or not the findings of the WHI will withstand the passage of time, further experience, and additional statistical review remain to be seen. The therapeutic potential of SERMs in women may set the stage for the development of selective androgen receptor modulators (SARMs). The availability of these molecules with their diversity of ligands provides the opportunity to explore their clinical usefulness.[14]

A great deal of interest exists on the use of androgens that will spare the most prominent adverse effects of testosterone supplementation. At present, the number of agents for clinical use is extremely limited. DHT (see above) not being aromatizable, and as such partially sparing effects on the prostate, can be considered an earlier SARM.

A more evolved, but still rudimentary, SARM undergoing clinical trials, is 7α-methyl-19-nortestosterone (MENT).[15] Its potency is higher that that of T by a factor of 10 and it does not undergo 5α reduction which may or may not be an advantage for its effects on the prostate. However, it retains its capacity to be aromatized to estradiol and has antigonadotrophic properties and anabolic effects on muscles. It maintains sexual function in hypogonadotrophic men. Its effects on the prostate are less pronounced.[16]

Hyperprolactinaemia

Although not a steroid hormone, prolactin has to be included among the hormones to be considered in the assessment and care of men with hypogonadism. Prolactin is a relatively frequent cause of hypoactive sexual desire and its overproduction is commonly associated with hypogonadism which may or may not resolve after adequate treatment of the hyperprolactinaemic state. If low levels of testosterone and clinical manifestations of hypogonadism persist after successful treatment of a prolactinoma, testosterone supplementation is indicated, together with continuation of medical treatment, i.e. dopaminergic agonists, of the pituitary adenoma.

Patient follow-up

This represents the most important aspect in the care of the hypogonadal man under treatment because androgen administration can cause potentially significant and occasionally serious adverse effects. The issues of highest concern refer to prostatic, cardiovascular, and haematological safety. Less frequently, the appearance of fluid retention, exacerbation of sleep disorders, gynaecomastia, or, rarely, adverse mood swings may require reassessment of the instituted treatment.

Prostatic safety

Safety issues demand special consideration regarding androgens and the prostate gland. Although the pathogenesis of benign prostatic hyperplasia (BPH) is still poorly understood, there is evidence that androgens and, more specifically, dihydrotestosterone are necessary for benign prostatic growth. The risks of androgen therapy, listed later on in this chapter, are widely accepted. The most prominent concern about androgen use relates to prostatic safety and several publications have addressed this topic recently. It is well established that hypogonadal men receiving supplemental testosterone experience an increase in prostate growth that corresponds to their eugonadal age-matched counterparts,[17] but more recent evidence indicates that the volume and growth of the gland in those hypogonadal men is modulated by CAG polymorphism of the androgen receptor gene.[18] There is a majority consensus that testosterone administration does not cause prostate cancer. It is also commonly agreed that subclinical (not detectable by digital rectal examination and/or elevated prostatic specific antigen) prostatic adenocarcinoma may become manifest rapidly after androgen therapy. The recommendations on prostatic safety are based on a number of publications.[19,20] None has included a sufficient number of men or has adequate follow-up, therefore definitive answers are not yet available.

The Sexual Medicine Society of North America, adopted the following position statement at its annual meeting in April 2003:

> Testosterone supplementation is indicated for men who have signs and symptoms of hypogo-nadism accompanied by subnormal serum testosterone measurements. Testosterone supple-mentation can provide important health benefits to these hypogonadal men. Testosterone supplementation should be administered only under competent and careful medical surveil-lance in order to identify early signs of possible adverse effects. Although the benefits and risks of long-term testosterone supplementation have not yet been definitively established, the weight of current evidence does not suggest an increased risk of heart disease or prostate cancer with long-term use of testosterone. Testosterone is not medically indicated in men who do not have hypogonadism.

This is a reasonable position on the relevant issues of cardiovascular and prostate health, pending definitive studies.

Serum lipids

Androgens also have an effect on serum lipids. Men generally have a lower plasma con-centration of high-density lipoprotein (HDL) cholesterol and higher concentration of triglycerides, low-density lipoprotein (LDL) cholesterol, and very low-density lipopro-tein cholesterol than do pre-menopausal women. It also appears that hypoandro-genism is associated with coronary artery disease.[21] A definitive answer on the effect of androgens on the lipid profile in men is not yet available but the early evidence is reas-suring.[22,23] A lipid profile is recommended prior to the onset of ART.

Sexual function

Androgens are essential in the stimulation and maintenance sexual function in men (and probably in women too). Adequate T levels are necessary for adequate sexual interest, ejaculation, and both sleep and sexual penile erections. There is a threshold, with marked interindividual variation, below which sexual function is impaired.[24] It has been reported that androgens are important in the expression of neuronal nitric oxide synthase (NOS) and in the expression of the phosphodiesterase-5 (PDE-5) gene expression.[25] Recently a small number of studies have shown a significant enhance-ment in response to the administration of PDE-5 inhibitors in combination with T, clearly suggesting a therapeutic synergism between central and peripheral sexual response modulators[26] in all domains of male erectile function.

Body composition

Androgens increase nitrogen retention, lean body mass, and body weight. In the skeletal system, androgens have an impact both on bone formation and bone resorption. The amount of androgen required to maintain bone mass in men is not known, nor is it known whether the beneficial effect of androgen is due to androgen itself or to the oestrogen produced from it. Regardless, hypogonadism is a major cause of osteoporosis in men.[27]

Haematology

Marginal elevations in haemoglobin and haematocrit are commonly observed in patients receiving ART and do not carry clinical significance. Occasionally, significant increases are detected and they demand either dose adjustments, change of preparation, regular phlebotomies, or, rarely, discontinuation of therapy.

Fluid retention and gynaecomastia

These can occur, are usually modest, and do not require therapeutic adjustments.

Recommendations

The International Society for the Study of the Aging Male (ISSAM)[28] and the Consensus Conference sponsored by the World Health Organization produced a set of recommendations for the diagnosis, treatment, and monitoring of ART in the adult male. The latter focused primarily on those receiving ART for the treatment of sexual dysfunction. These recommendations are reproduced here (with permission) because they represent an updated consensus by experts in the field and cover the topic in a concise, practical and well-balanced manner.

Box 13.1 **Recommendations for the diagnosis, treatment, and monitoring of ART in the adult male**

1 Definition

Adult onset hypogonadism is a clinical and biochemical syndrome frequently associated with advancing age and characterized by a deficiency in serum androgen levels, with or without changes in receptor sensitivity to androgens. It may affect the function of multiple organ systems and result in significant detriment in the quality of life, including major alterations in sexual function.

2 Clinical diagnosis

The clinical manifestations of adult hypogonadism are not specific. Sexual dysfunction (decrease in sexual interest and quality of erections) is prominent and often the presenting symptom. Depression, irritability, cognition and sleep, as well as diminished strength and endurance, may also be present. The physical examination is frequently unhelpful, but alterations in testicular size and consistency, hair distribution, muscle mass, body shape and sequelae of osteoporosis may be detected. Not

Box 13.1 *(continued)*

all the manifestations need to be evident simultaneously and their intensity shows marked interindividual variability.

3 Biochemical diagnosis

In patients with sexual dysfunction, the following biochemical investigations are recommended: a blood sample for testosterone (T) determination between 8:00 and 11:00 a.m. The most accessible and reliable assays to establish the presence of hypogonadism are the measurement of bio-available T or the calculated free T (cFT). Assays for total testosterone, particularly in the elderly, may not reflect the man's true androgenic status. If T levels are below or at the lower limit of the accepted normal values it is prudent to confirm the results with a second determination together with assessment of luteinizing hormone (LH), follicle stimulating hormone (FSH), and prolactin.

4 Prolactin

Hyperprolactinemia is an uncommon cause of ED. However, determination of serum prolactin is recommended in cases associated with diminished sexual interest and when biochemical hypogonadism has been documented.

5 Other hormonal alterations besides sex hormones

It is recognized that significant alterations in other endocrine systems occur in association with aging but the significance of these changes is not well understood, particularly in relation to sexual function. In general terms, determinations of estradiol, DHEA, DHEAS [DHEA sulphate], melatonin, GH [growth hormone] and IGF-1 [insulin-like growth factor-1] are not indicated in the uncomplicated evaluation of hypogonadism. Under special circumstances or for well-defined clinical research, assessment of these and other hormones may be warranted.

6 Diabetes

Diabetes mellitus is a frequent endocrinological cause of erectile dysfunction. It should be ruled out in men complaining of sexual inadequacy. Appropriate glycemic control is fundamental before consideration of any other hormonal treatment in men with ED.

7 Lipids

A lipid profile should be considered as a relevant option in the initial assessment of men with erectile dysfunction.

Box 13.1 *(continued)*

8 Indications for therapy

A clear indication (a clinical picture together with biochemical evidence of hypogonadism) should exist prior to initiation of androgen therapy.

9 Age

In the absence of defined contraindications, age is not a limiting factor to the initiation of ART in aged men with hypoandrogenism.

10 Sexual function

Hypogonadal men with specific sexual dysfunctions (e.g. ED and/or diminished interest) are candidates for androgen therapy. Absence of an adequate response after appropriate testosterone treatment calls for further investigation to rule out associated co-morbidities.

11 Combined treatment for erectile dysfunction

Evidence is emerging suggesting therapeutic synergism with combined use of testosterone and phosphodiesterase-5 inhibitors in hypogonadal or borderline eugonadal men. These observations are very preliminary and require additional study. However, the combination treatment can be considered in patients failing adequate treatment with phosphodiesterase inhibitors alone. No credible evidence for or against exists with other drugs in combination with androgens.

12 Testosterone commercial formulations

Currently commercially available preparations of testosterone (with the exception of the alkylated ones) are safe and effective. The treating physician should have sufficient knowledge and adequate understanding of the advantages and drawbacks of each preparation. The patient should be given the opportunity to actively participate in the choice of androgen formulation.

13 Serum levels

The purpose of ART is to bring and maintain serum T levels within the physiological range. Supraphysiological levels are to be avoided. Although it may appear desirable, no evidence exists for or against the need to maintain a circadian rhythm of serum T levels.

14 Other androgens

The use of DHEA and DHT has not been proven to be effective specifically in male sexual dysfunction. Current evidence on DHT efficacy is also insufficient. There is

Box 13.1 *(continued)*

a need for additional studies aimed expressly at investigating the effects of these hormones on sexual function.

15 Androgen abuse

Androgens should be used only when specific indications exist. Their (ab)use for performance enhancement, in the absence of hypogonadism, is to be condemned in the strongest terms.

16 Monitoring—liver

Although currently available T preparations are largely free of hepatic toxicity (methylated forms are an exception), liver function studies are advisable prior to onset of therapy. Periodic assessment during treatment may be considered. Despite the lack of evidence, commercial manufacturers, for regulatory purposes, include warnings about hepatic risks in their product insert.

17 Monitoring—lipids

A fasting lipid profile prior to initiation of treatment, if not done as part of the initial evaluation (Recommendation 7) and re-assessment at 3 or 6 months after onset of testosterone administration, is also recommended.

18 Monitoring—prostate

In men over the age of 40 years, digital rectal examination (DRE) and determination of serum prostatic specific antigen (PSA) are mandatory as baseline measurements of prostatic health prior to therapy with androgens, every three (3) to six (6) months for the first 12 months, and yearly thereafter. Transrectal ultra-sound guided biopsies of the prostate are indicated only if the DRE or the PSA are abnormal.

19 Prostatic and breast safety—I

Androgen administration is absolutely contraindicated in men suspected of harbouring carcinoma of the prostate or breast.

20 Prostatic safety—II

Men successfully treated for prostate cancer and suffering from symptomatic hypogonadism may become candidates for androgen therapy, after a prudent interval, if there is no evidence of residual cancer. The risk and benefits must be clearly understood by the patient and the follow-up must be particularly careful. No reliable evidence exists in favor or against this recommendation. The clinician must

Box 13.1 *(continued)*

exercise good clinical judgment together with adequate knowledge of the advantages and drawbacks of androgen therapy in this situation.

21 Prostatic safety—III

Androgen supplementation is contraindicated in men with severe bladder outlet obstruction due to an enlarged, clinically benign prostate. Moderate obstruction represents a partial contraindication to ART. After successful treatment of the obstruction, the contraindication can be lifted.

22 Monitoring—mood

Androgen replacement therapy normally results in improvements in mood and well being. The development of negative behavioral patterns (aggressiveness, hypersexuality) during treatment calls for dose modifications or discontinuation of therapy.

23 Monitoring—hematology

Polycythemia may develop during ART. Periodic hematological assessment is indicated. Dose adjustments, change of preparation, periodic phlebotomies or discontinuation of treatment may be necessary.

24 Monitoring—sleep apnea

Exacerbation of sleep apnea may occur during testosterone supplementation therapy. Proper assessment and treatment of the sleep apnea are indicated during testosterone supplementation. Careful consideration should be given to the need for testosterone treatment if the sleep disturbances deteriorate.

25 Physician's responsibilities

Since androgen replacement therapy is for life, this demands a lifelong commitment for follow-up. The treating physician must be familiar with the diagnostic, therapeutic and monitoring aspects of androgen therapy. Good clinical judgment is equally important. Inadequate therapeutic response or the appearance of significant adverse effects call for re-assessment of treatment indications.

References

1 Vermeulen A, VerdonckL, Kaufman JM (1999). A critical evaluation of simple methods for the estimation of free testosterone in serum. *J. Clin. Endocrinol. Metab.* **84**: 3666–72.

2 Morley JE, Patrick P, Perry HM III (2002). Evaluation of assays to measure free testosterone. *Metabolism* **5**: 554–9.

3 Conway AJ, Boylan LM, Howe C, Ross G, Handelsman DJ (1998). Randomized clinical trial of testosterone replacement therapy in hypogonadal men. *Int. J. Androl.* **11**: 247–53.

4 Morales AJ, Haubrich RH, Hwang JY, Asakura H, Yen SS (1998). The effect of six months treatment with a 100 mg daily dose of dehydroepiandrosterone (DHEA) on circulating sex steroids, body composition and muscle strength in age-advanced men and women. *Clin. Endocrinol.* **49**: 421–6.

5 Flynn MA, Weaver-Osterholtz D, Sharpe-Timms KL, Allen S, Krause G (1999). Dehydroepiandrosterone replacement on aging humans. *J. Clin. Endocrinol. Metab.* **84**: 1527–32.

6 Artl W, Callies F, Koehler I (2001). Dehydroepiandrosterone supplementation in healthy men with an age-related decline of dehydroepiandrosterone secretion. *J. Clin. Endocrinol. Metab.* **86**: 4686–92.

7 Baulieu EE, Thomas G, Legrain S (2000). DHEA, DHEA sulfate and aging: contribution of the DHEA age study to a sociobiomedical issue. *Proc. Natl. Acad. Sci. USA* **97**: 4279–85.

8 Labrie F, Diamond P, Cusan L, Candes B (1997). Effect of 12 month dehydroepiandrosterone replacement therapy on bone, vagina, and endometrium in postmenopausal women. *J. Clin. Endocrinol. Metab.* **82**: 3498–504.

9 Schaison G, Couzinet B (1998). Percutaneous dihydrotestosterone (DHT) treatment. In: *Testosterone: Action, Deficiency, Substitution* (ed. E Nieschlag, HM Behre), pp. 423–36. Springer, Berlin.

10 de Lignieres B (1993). Transdermal dihydrotestosterone treatment of 'andropause'. *Ann. Med.* **25**: 235–9.

11 Ly LP, Jimenez M, Zhuang TN, Celermajer DS, Conway AJ, Handelsman DJ (2001). A double-blind, placebo-controlled, randomized clinical trial of transdermal dihydrotestosterone gel on muscular strength, mobility, and quality of life in older men with partial androgen deficiency. *J. Clin. Endocrinol. Metab.* **86**: 4078–84.

12 Kunelius P, Lukkarinen O, Hannuksela ML, Itkonen O, Tapanainen JS (2002). The effects of transdermal dihydrotestosterone in the aging male: a prospective, randomized, double blind study. *J. Clin. Endocrinol. Metab.* **87**: 1467–72.

13 Writing Group for the Women's Health Initiative Investigators (2002). Risks and benefits of estrogen plus progestin in healthy postmenopausal women. *J. Am. Med. Assoc.* **288**: 321–9.

14 Negro-Vilar A (1999). Selective androgen receptor modulators (SARMs). A novel approach to androgen therapy for the new millennium. *J. Clin. Endocrinol. Metab.* **84**: 3459–64.

15 Sundaram K, Kumar N, Bardin CW (1993). 7α-methyl-nortestosterone (MENT). The optimal androgen for male contraception. *Ann. Med.* **25**: 199–204.

16 Cummings DE, Kumar N, Bardin CW, Sundaram K, Bremner WJ (1998). Prostate-sparing effects in primates of the potent androgen 7alpha-methyl-19-nortestosterone: a potential alternative to testosterone for androgen replacement and male contraception. *J. Clin. Endocrinol. Metab.* **83**: 4212–17.

17 Jin B, Conway AJ, Handelsman AJ (2001). Effects of androgen deficiency and replacement on prostate zonal volumes. *Clin. Endocrinol.* **54**: 437–45.

18 Zitzmann M, Depenbusch M, Gromoll J, Nieschlag E (2003). Prostate volumes and growth in testosterone-substituted hypogonadal men are dependent on the CAG repeat polymorphism of the androgen receptor gene: a longitudinal pharmacogenetic study. *J. Clin. Endocrinol. Metab.* **88**: 2049–54.

19 Morales A (2002). Androgen replacement therapy and prostate safety. *Eur. Urol.* **41**: 113–17.

20 Bhasin S, Singh AB, Phong Mac R, Carter B, Lee MI, Cunningham GR (2003). Managing the risks of prostate disease during testosterone replacement therapy of older men: recommendations for a standardized monitoring plan. *J. Androl.* **24**: 299–311.

21 English KM, Mandour O, Steeds RP, Diver MJ, Jones TH, Channer KS (2000). Men with coronary artery disease have lower levels of androgens than men with normal coronary angiograms. *Eur. Heart J.* **21**: 890–6.

22 Muller M, van der Schouw YT, Thijssen JHH, Grobbee DE (2003). Endogenous sex hormones and cardiovascular disease. *J. Clin. Endocrinol. Metab.* **88**: 5076–86.

23 Hak AE, Witteman JCM, deJong FH, Geerlings MI, Hofman A, Pols HAP (2002). Low levels of endogenous androgens increase the risk of atherosclerosis in elderly men: the Rotterdam Study. *J. Clin. Endocrinol. Metab.* **87**: 3632–7.

24 Carani C, Bancroft J, Granata A, Del Rio G, Marrama P (1992). Testosterone and erectile function, nocturnal penile tumescence and rigidity and response to erotic stimuli in hypogonadal and eugonadal men. *Neuropsychoendocrinology* **17**: 647–52.

25 Traish AM, Park K, Dhir V, Kim NN, Moreland RB, Goldstein I (1999). Effects of castration and androgen replacement on erectile function in a rabbit model. *Endocrinology* **140**: 1861–6.

26 Aversa A, Isidori AM, Spera G, Lenzi A, Fabbri A (2003). Androgens improve cavernous dilatation and response to sildenafil in patients with erectile dysfunction. *Clin. Endocrinol.* **58**: 632–8.

27 Benito M, Gomberg B, Wehrli FW, Weening RH, Zemel B, Wright AC *et al.* (2003). Deterioration of trabecular architecture in hypogonadal men. *J. Clin. Endocrinol. Metab.* **88**: 1497–1502.

28 Morales A, Lunenfeld B (2002). Investigation, treatment and monitoring of late onset hypogonadism in males. Official Recommendations of the Society for the Study of the Aging Male. *Aging Male* **5**: 74–86.

Chapter 14

The patient presenting with requirements for a urinary diversion or reservoir

Zbigniew Wolski

Introduction

Urinary diversion is a form of urinary tract reconstruction designed to reroute the stream of urine after bladder resection (e.g. radical cystectomy) or loss of function. Temporary urinary diversions are often utilized in paediatric patients with congenital anomalies; permanent forms of urinary diversion are performed in adults and paediatric patients. The necessity for permanent urinary diversion arises after radical cystectomy for infiltrative bladder cancer, involvement of the bladder by other pelvic neoplasms, loss of bladder function due to radiation therapy, severe end-stage interstitial cystitis or tuberculosis, or, uncommonly, neurogenic dysfunction. Radical cystectomy in patients with muscle-invasive bladder cancer is the most frequent indication.[1]

Radical cystectomy in male patients includes the *en bloc* removal of the bladder with lower ureters, prostate with seminal vesicles, and pelvic lymph nodes plus the urethra in patients with invasion into the prostate and/or the urethra. In female patients, the procedure is also called anterior pelvic exenterioration and incudes removal of the bladder, uterus, fallopian tubes, ovaries, anterior vaginal wall, and pelvic lymph nodes plus the urethra when the cancer involves the bladder neck and/or urethra.[2,3]

Selection of patients for urinary diversion

The decision to perform a cystectomy always requires some form of urinary diversion. Loss of normal urination through the urethra can cause a considerable amount of anxiety in the patient and his or her family which can be quite disabling. Recent advances in urological techniques focus on restoration of urination to make it as natural and as socially acceptable as possible. However, the principles of oncology must be maintained when choosing the appropriate type of diversion. For example, the primary objective of radical cystectomy is cure of cancer.

Modern urology offers many methods of urinary diversion depending upon the type of disease and its staging and the general condition and preference of the patient.

There are three basic forms and choices which include non-continent or continent urinary diversion and orthotopic voiding diversion (i.e. a neobladder).[1,4–8] Each has its advantages and disadvantages and the patient should thoroughly understand them before the choice is made.

Non-continent urinary diversion

There are two alternative methods of non-continent urinary diversion: cutaneous ureterostomy and ileal conduit.

Cutaneous ureterostomy

Cutaneous ureterostomy is mentioned for historical completeness as it is now rarely performed.[4] The distal ends of the ureters are brought out individually on each side of the abdomen (i.e. bilateral ureterocutaneostomies) or together as a single stoma (i.e. transuretero-ureterocutaneostomy). The urine is collected in a special bag or external collecting appliance. Although this form of urinary diversion is the simplest because there is no need for bowel surgery, its major disadvantage is the stenosis of the stoma(s) secondary to ischaemic necrosis of the end of ureters which may occur in as many as 50% of patients. Another frequently encountered disadvantage is the erosion of skin surrounding the stoma(s).[4] This procedure is still occasionally offered to patients in very poor general condition after palliative or salvage cystectomy but construction of a bowel conduit is almost always the preferred method.

Ileal conduit

Another method of incontinent diversion which is used more frequently is the ileal conduit (Fig. 14.1). This involves diverting the urine into a short segment of isolated ileum (i.e. the ileal loop), which is directed to the anterior abdominal wall as a stoma. The ileal conduit is the most common form of urinary diversion and is used in more than 50% of patients who require cystectomy for bladder cancer. Since bowel continuity is interrupted patients require a pre-operative bowel preparation of full fluid diet (1–4 days), mechanical bowel cleansing, and antibiotic administration.[4]

Ileal conduits are particularly useful for patients whose poor health or co-morbid conditions make more invasive reconstructive surgery unrealistic, whose lifestyle is sedentary, or who have insufficient dexterity or motivation to catheterize a reservoir or learn micturition *de novo*. Cystectomies with urethrectomy or insufficient preservation of the urinary sphincter are other indications for ileal conduit.

Typically, the ileal segment is isolated 15–20 cm proximal to the ileo-caecal valve (Bricker procedure).[4] When the healthy ileum is unavailable (e.g. due to previous surgery or radiation), other bowel segments can be used such as the sigmoid or transverse colon (Mogg procedure).[4] An antirefluxing uretero-intestinal anastomosis is not necessary.

Selection of the stomal site should be decided following discussions with an enterostomal therapist. Its location must be free from fat creases and scars in both the standing

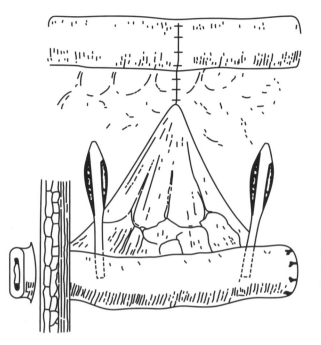

Fig. 14.1 Non-continent urinary diversion. Ileal conduit—a short ileal segment which directs the urine to the anterior abdominal wall (stoma). Bricker procedure.

and sitting positions so that the appliance can be properly used. The stoma is usually located in the right lower quadrant of the abdomen on the line extending between the umbilicus and anteriorsuperior iliac spine.[4] The collecting appliance is connected with the skin surrounding the stoma and emptied when it is full. Patients with multiple sclerosis, quadriplegia, or cognitive impairment may require that the appliance be cared for by family members or nurses.

Advantages of an ileal conduit include decreased operative time and lower rates of early and late post-operative complications than continent urinary diversion. The possibility of nighttime bedside drainage allows longer periods of uninterrupted sleep. The easier management of the stoma compared with a ureterocutaneostomy is an important benefit for the patient. Typically, the collecting urinary appliance must be changed after cleansing the peristomal area on a 4–7 day schedule. Special creams and liquids help in the care of the stoma and the surrounding skin. An enterostomal therapist or specially trained urology nurse is essential for teaching the patient daily care. In addition, when the patient is discharged from the hospital he or she is given the first set of external bags (e.g. collecting urinary appliances).

Since the mucosa of an ileal conduit has a very short contact time with urine, there is a low risk of absorption of urinary constituents. This allows it to be a reasonable alternative for patients with renal dysfunction. Because only a short intestinal segment is removed from the alimentary tract, patients are not at risk for metabolic disturbances or vitamin B_{12} malabsorption.[1,4] Those undergoing an ileal conduit may expect to return to full participation in all their pre-operative activities after a short time of training. One disadvantage of an ileal conduit includes the presence of an incontinent stoma and the requirement for an external appliance which may lead to a deterioration of body image; leakage of urine at the site surrounding the collecting appliance without warning due to device malformation is also a concern.[1,4]

Early, serious complications associated with ileal conduit surgery are associated with the bowel and include anastomic leaks, bowel obstruction, and enterocutaneous fistulae.[4] Long-term complications include ileo-ureteric and stoma stenosis, conduit prolapse, elongation of the ileal conduit, infection of the upper urinary tract, deterioration of renal function, and stone formation (5 to 10%).[1,4] Parastomal dermatitis often occurs and may be treated with special stomahesive creams and/or a change in the kind of collecting appliance.

Continent urinary diversion

Continent urinary diversion involves utilization of either the anal or urethral sphincter. One of the first described methods of continent urinary diversion was the ureterosigmoidostomy and its variations. Other methods include urinary pouches with a continent stoma or orthotopic voiding through the native urethra (i.e. neobladder).[1,4,6,7,9]

Ureterosigmoidostomy

Ureterosigmoidostomy is one of the oldest and simplest urinary diversions. The ureters are implanted into the sigmoid colon or rectum. Patients with an ureterosigmoidostomy excrete urine with stool. Since this type of urinary diversion leads to many long-term complications it is indicated only for very elderly patients. Mixture of urine with the faecal stream and exposure of urine to large bowel mucosa leads to a hyperchloraemic acidosis, hypokalaemia, pyelonephritis, nephropathy, and, potentially, colonic malignancy.[4,10] The incidence of adenocarcinoma of the colon is 6% to 29% under these circumstances, with mean of 11%; polypoid lesions may develop in up 40% of patients if followed long enough.[9,11,12]

New surgical techniques which partially separate urine and stool have been described as the Sigma Rectum Pouch (Mainz Pouch II), but late complications occur.[12] Patients must empty the rectum at intervals of no longer than 2 hours, particularly in the postoperative period; electrolytes and acidosis must be monitored carefully. Bicarbonate potassium citrate needs to be administered in the majority of cases. Routine insertion of a rectal tube (i.e. a special rectal catheter) each night is advocated in the long-term care of these patients in conjunction with oral antibacterial therapy (e.g. trimethoprim, nitrofurantoin). Due to the high probability of large bowel cancer after urinary diversion to the colon between 5 and 50 years after the procedure, it is advised that patients with this type of urinary diversion undergo annual colonoscopy and monitoring for blood in the stool.[4,9,11]

Continent cutaneous urinary diversion

Continent cutaneous urinary diversion is a modern alternative for patients and avoids some of the possible problems associated with ileal conduits. This procedure creates an intra-abdominal intestinal pouch or reservoir with a continent, self-catheterizable stoma. Patients selected for a continent cutaneous diversion must accept the presence of abdominal stoma and be motivated to catheterize the pouch every 4–6 hours during the day and at night. They must have sufficient manual dexterity and hand–eye coordination to perform this function. Quadriplegic patients and those with multiple sclerosis are not candidates for this type diversion.

The location of the stoma is similar to the ileal conduit but may be brought out through umbilicus for improved cosmesis. It is important that all continent cutaneous and orthotopic voiding pouches are created to allow low pressure and large volume. Both should collect up to 500 ml of urine without the need for an external collecting appliance or permission of volitional voiding through the native urethra. The objective is to allow the pouch to imitate the native bladder.

The principles of creating continent reservoirs developed over many years' experience. Kock was the first to report the functional continent reservoir in 1982.[4,6] The Kock pouch is made of a detubularized segment of ileum. The isolated segment is transsected on its antimesenteric border (i.e. detubularization) and transformed into a spheroidal reservoir. A short non-transsected part of ileal segment is anastomosed to the anterior abdominal wall. This ileal limb is specially duplicated for creation of the continent valve.

Most popular continent cutaneous diversions are created from ileum (Kock),[4] large bowel—ileo-caecal or colonic—segment (Indiana, Florida pouches).[4,6] A key part of the surgical procedure in all continent cutaneous reservoirs is to create the continent stoma. The success or failure of the procedure depends on the outlet which must have a leakage-prevention mechanism and be easily catheterizable. The Kock pouch is made of detubularized ileum with antirefluxing afferent and efferent nipple valves. Other pouches utilize different technologies for construction of the continence mechanism including intussuscepting, tapering, and/or plicating the external limb of ileum or appendix to create the continent stoma.[4,6,9]

Orthotopic voiding urinary diversion (neobladder)

An orthotopic voiding urinary diversion is the best reconstruction of the lower urinary tract because it attempts to preserve normal voluntary voiding. An orthotopic ileal neobladder is one of the most popular forms (Fig. 14.2).[4–6,13] The principles of surgery related to the creation of an orthotopic neobladder are similar to those of continent cutaneous pouches. The keys to success are detubularization and transformation of the bowel segment into a spheroidal reservoir which results in a large-volume, low-pressure pouch.[4,5,8] There must be a functional native urethra that can be preserved. Absolute contraindications for orthotopic neobladder substitution include tumour in

Fig. 14.2 Orthotopic volitional voiding urinary diversion (neobladder). The neobladder is an ileal reservoir which is connected with the patient's urethra. The Studer neobladder is created from 60 cm of specially transected and transformed ileal segment.

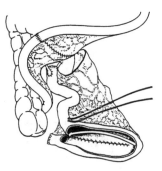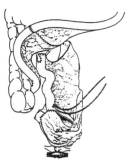

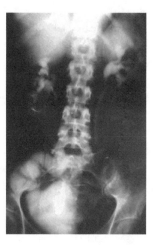

Fig. 14.3 Case 1: a 44-year-old woman with a neobladder 3 weeks after surgery. Intravenous pyelography—the upper urinary tract is normal, Studer neobladder.

the urethra, renal insufficiency, and poor mental or physical functioning.[4–6] Moreover, the patient must be able to accept the possibility of a relatively long period (e.g. several months) for the appropriate expansion to capacity of the new reservoir to occur and the possibility of day time and nocturnal incontinence.

There are many techniques for orthotopic neobladder construction, creation of which takes place after detubularization of the ileum or ileo-caecum or right or sigmoid colon segments. The Hautmann neobladder is constructed from 60 cm of ileum reconfigured as a 'W'. The Studer neobladder consists of 40 cm of detubularized ileum and 20 cm of an isoperistaltic limb to which the ureters are anastomosed to create an antirefluxing mechanism (Fig. 14.3).[4,8,14] The most cylindrical reservoir with antirefluxing implantation of ureters was described by Pagano (VIP –vesica ilealis Padovana. (4) Functional results can be achieved in other neobladders constructed from large bowel (Reddy, Le Bag, Mainz) (4,6).

In males an orthotopic neobladder is now almost the standard diversion. It has been used in male patients for more than two decades; in females neobladders are a more recent development because of a lack of data regarding the risk of recurrence of cancer in the urethra. Recently it has been concluded that the incidence of recurrent cancer in the urethra in females is lower than in males after radical cystectomy[2,3,6,13] but one of the contraindications for orthotopic neobladder in female patients is involvement of the bladder neck with cancer.[1,2,3,8]

Continence rates of 80–90 per cent are expected, but patients over the age of 70 have more difficulty with continence than younger patients. Female neobladder patients have the same risk of post-operative incontinence but in 10 to 30% of women impaired bladder emptying or complete retention of urine is observed.[1,2,13] The reason for this still remains unclear. Major early and long-term post-operative complications have been observed in 20 to 30% of patients including anastomotic ileo-urethral or uretero-ileal strictures, neobladder stones, and pyelonephritis.[4,5] Spontaneous rupture and malignancy of the neobladder have been reported rarely. The incidence of metabolic disturbances, especially hyperchloraemic acidosis with clinical symptoms, is low especially if pre-operative renal function is normal.[1,4,5,10] Deterioration of kidney function and upper urinary tract is uncommon.[10] Long-term observations report that about 70% of patients are satisfied with their neobladder.[1,3–5,13,14]

Follow-up and post-operative care of patients with urinary diversion

Long-term follow-up after all urinary diversion is advocated with particular regard to patients with orthotopic neobladder. The important points are:

- function of the stoma or neobladder
- function and drainage of the upper urinary tract
- metabolic disturbances
- development of malignancy.

Function of the neobladder is followed by ultrasonography with evaluation of residual urine and, when necessary, urodynamic examination (Fig. 14.4), especially in women since impaired emptying can develop many years after the surgery. Follow-up of the upper urinary tract is mandatory with ultrasonography and serum creatinine test to assess for evidence of satisfactory drainage, lack of stones, and function. Even if the neobladder or intra-abdominal pouch functions well, hyperchloraemic acidosis must be regularly ruled out because half of patients have mild acidosis requiring oral alkalinization. The high risk of late carcinoma appears related only to pouches constructed from large bowel. The incidence of cancer occurring at the uretero-intestinal anastomosis in patients with ureterosigmoidostomy varies between 6 and 29%. This is a 500-fold increase in the incidence of cancer; if the urinary diversion is performed before the age of 25 years, there is a 7000-fold increase.[9,10] The most common type of tumour is adenocarcinoma. Therefore, endoscopic and cytological reviews must occur annually from 5 years post-surgery for an indefinite time.[4,11]

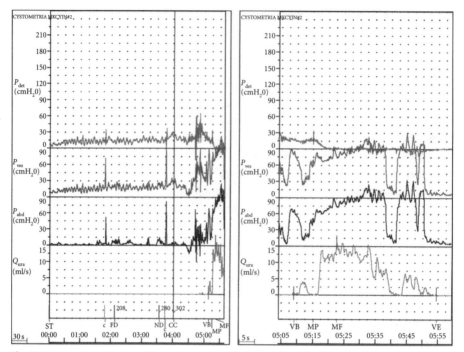

Fig. 14.4 Case 2: a 72-year-old woman with a Studer neobladder 6 years after surgery. Urinary continence during the day and night with nocturia twice. Urodynamic evaluation: neobladder capacity 300 ml, low intrareservoir pressure, no residual urine.

Post-operative care of continent cutaneous pouches

Care of the continent stoma is easier than that of incontinent one because there is less skin irritation, no trauma from the appliance, and a reduced need for protective creams. It is usually covered with gauze between catheterizations to avoid mucous drainage or soiling of clothing. Localization of the stoma at the umbilicus or right lower quadrant of the abdomen is simpler to catheterize than an orthotopic neobladder through the native urethra. The continent pouch is usually empted in a standing or sitting position by inserting the catheter deeply into the reservoir to allow complete emptying. Changes in position from lying supine or to one side may facilitate this. The technique of self-catheterization depends to some extent upon the type of continence arrangement. For example, an appendiceal stoma needs only a small-diameter catheter such as a 14 F[4] whereas a reservoir with a lot of mucus may need a larger 20–22 F one. Self-catheterization must be done with a clean catheter sized for the individual patient. Teaching is performed by an enterostomal nurse.

Post-operative complications occur in 20 to 30% of patients and include permanent or temporary leakage of urine from the continent stoma, strictures of ileo-ureteral anastomoses, stenosis of the stoma, stone formation in the reservoir, infection of the upper urinary tract, metabolic disturbances, and malignant transformation.[1,4,6,9] Most patients have a mild hyperchloraemic metabolic acidosis which does not result in substantial long-term complications. Those with renal dysfunction may have severe metabolic acidosis and problems with electrolyte abnormalities, bone demineralization, and vitamin B_{12} deficiency. Patients with an ileo-caecal reservoir may experience diarrhoea as a result of decreased transit time, loss of the ileo-caecal native valve, or lack of bile salt and water reabsorption.[9,10] Small and large bowel segments used in the urinary tract continue to produce mucus, and although it decreases over time, there are often problems with catheter plugging and struvite crystal; daily irrigations of the reservoir with saline and an antibacterial solution help.

Clinical outcomes of patients with continent reservoirs can be improved by careful selection of patients, especially those with very good renal function, and the appropriate part of the bowel for the reservoir. Post-operative teaching encourages increased fluid intake, balanced diet, appropriate medications, and proper technique of catheterization.[4,9,10] An external continent urinary diversion is more acceptable to patients compared with incontinent cutaneous urinary diversion.[1,4,6,9] It preserves body image, is more acceptable to patients, and obviates the necessity for an appliance.

Post-operative care of patients with neobladder

The ability to void using one's own urethra is the main advantage of an orthotopic ileal neobladder, but patients need to understand that the replacement bladder is not ideal and the achievement of full functioning might take several months.[1] During this time, patients will void more frequently (e.g. up to every 2 hours) with gradual increases in the interval over time. Voiding two to three times per night will always be necessary, including setting an alarm clock to ensure that it occurs, in order to reduce the absorption of urinary constituents.[1] Patients should be aware that there is no longer any neuro-feedback between the neobladder and the brain and, therefore, there is no automatic awakening from sleep when the neobladder is full. Voiding intervals longer than 6 hours may result in a neobladder capacity of greater than 500 ml but with increasing likelihood of high post-void residual urine.[1]

Most patients are able to empty their neobladder when they sit and generate intra-abdominal pressure (e.g. slight abdominal straining) and voluntarily relax their external urethral sphincter.[5] Partial or complete retention of urine requires self-catheterization. Drinking 2–3 l of fluids per 24 hours is advocated for prevention of mucous clots and metabolic and electrolytic disturbances. Metabolic acidosis can cause fatigue, mental depression, lack of appetite, nausea, and vomiting.[10] Venous blood gas and electrolyte analysis should be performed in these patients. Treatment requires supplementing 2–6 g of sodium bicarbonate every 24 hours for an ileal reservoir or titrated potassium citrate for a colonic reservoir when metabolic acidosis occurs (i.e. base excess below 2 mmol). Patients must be educated to realize that thorough lifelong follow-up is necessary in order to ensure proper reservoir function and to avoid long-term complications.[10,11]

Conclusions

The choice of urinary diversion after radical cystectomy depends upon many variables including location of the cancer, degree of renal function, presence of pre-existing intestinal disorders, status of general health and mental condition, extent of manual dexterity and patient age, preference, and motivation. Patients should be provided with pragmatic information regarding expected post-operative functioning with each type of urinary diversion. Realistic estimates of the rates of complications will allow the patient to make an informed choice. Many health-care professionals including urologists, nurses, and enterostomal therapists are important for comprehensive pre- and post-operative education and care.

References

1 Montie J, Matcovich R (2001). Selecting and counseling patients for cystectomy or cystoprostatectomy. In: *Office Urology* (ed. E Kursh, J Ulchaker), pp. 203–23. Humana Press, Totowa, NJ.

2 Stenzl A, Jarolim L, Coloby P, Golia S, Bartsch G, Babjuk M *et al.* (2001). Urethra-sparing cystectomy and orthotopic urinary diversion in women with malignant pelvic tumors. *Cancer* **92**: 1864–71.

3 Wolski Z, Siekiera J, Wronczewski A (1996). Functional orthotopic ileal neobladder following radical cystectomy in women. *Eur. Urol.* **30**:(2) 265.

4 Benson M, Olsson C (1992). Urinary diversion. In: *Compbell's Urology*, 6th edn (ed. P Walsh, A Retik, T Stamey, E Vaughan), pp. 2654–719. W. B. Saunders, Philadelphia, PA.

5 Freman J (1999). Construction of a Studer or Hautmann ileal neobladder. *Contemp. Urol.* April: 44–63.

6 Seigne J, Lockhard J (1999). Choosing a continent urinary diversion. *Contemp. Urol.* February: 19–32.

7 Studer U, Casanova G, Zingg E (1991). Historical aspects of continent urinary diversion. *Prob. Urol.* April–June: 197–202.

8 Studer U, Gerber E, Springer J, Zingg E (1992). Bladder reconstruction with bowel after radical cystectomy. *World J. Urol.* **10**: 11–19.

9 Kirsch A, Snyder H (1997). Trends in continent reconstruction of the lower urinary tract. *Contemp. Urol.* August: 61–9.

10 Craig Hall M, Koch M, McDougal W (1991). Metabolic consequences of urinary diversion through intestinal segments. *Urol. Clin. North Am.* **18**(4): 725–35.

11 McDougal WS (1992). Metabolic complications of urinary intestinal diversion. *J. Urol.* **147**: 1199–208.

12 Fisch M, Wammack R, Muller S, Hohenfellner R (1994). The Mainz Pouch II. *Eur. Urol.* **25**: 7–15.

13 Wolski Z, Siekiera J, Szymański A, Wronczewski A (2000). Reinforcement of the support of ileal neobladder by duplication of anterior vaginal wall—a method of prevention of hypercontinence after cystectomy in women. *Eur. Urol.* **37**(Suppl.): 567.

14 Hautmann R, Miller K, Steiner U, Wenderoth U (1993). The ileal neobladder 6 years of experience with more than 200 patients. *J. Urol.* **150**: 40–5.

Chapter 15

The patient presenting with recalcitrant urinary tract infections

Lindsay E. Nicolle

Introduction

In this chapter recalcitrant urinary tract infection is defined as frequent, recurrent symptomatic infection which is not adequately managed with standard therapeutic approaches. The discussion addresses only adult patients. Urinary infection is considered uncomplicated when it occurs in women with an otherwise normal genitourinary tract[1] and may include the less frequently encountered acute non-obstructive and non-refluxing pyelonephritis. Complicated urinary infection occurs in a patient with functional or structural abnormalities of the genitourinary tract.[2] A wide range of abnormalities may be associated with complicated urinary infection, but the consistent defect is failure of voiding to effectively clear organisms from the urinary tract. Recalcitrant urinary infection may occur in either of these groups, although it is more common with complicated urinary infection. Asymptomatic bacteriuria is bacteria in the urine with no signs or symptoms referable to infection.[3]

A number of factors may lead to recalcitrant urinary infection. Persistent symptomatic infection may occur because an individual has not received appropriate antimicrobial treatment, often because the infecting organism is resistant to the antimicrobial given for treatment. Occasionally, the organism may be susceptible but the antimicrobial chosen does not reach the site of infection, such as the kidney or prostate, in an appropriate drug level. An important differentiation in understanding recurrent urinary infection is whether it is reinfection or relapse. Reinfection is recurrent urinary infection with an organism arising from the colonizing flora of the gut or vagina. There is usually a new organism isolated from the urine compared with previous infecting strains. However, the same organism may be isolated if it has persisted in the host flora despite antimicrobial therapy. Relapse is recurrent infection with an organism which has persisted within the genitourinary tract and re-emerges in the urine following cessation of antimicrobial therapy. The organism isolated from recurrent episodes is the same, although increasing resistance may be observed with repeated courses of antimicrobials.

There is limited information describing the impact of recalcitrant urinary infection on the quality of life of individuals. While urinary infection seldom contributes directly to mortality, it may be associated with substantial morbidity. Clinicians who care for women with frequent acute uncomplicated urinary infection recognize the frustration these women experience with the repeated disruption of work or social life by these episodes.[4] Persons with recurrent complicated urinary infection may experience severe morbidity, particularly if they acquire infection with highly antimicrobial-resistant organisms. For any patient, repeated antimicrobial courses are costly, and may be associated with adverse effects of the antimicrobials themselves.

Diagnosis

Clinical presentation

The classical clinical presentations of urinary tract infection are straightforward. For bladder infection, or cystitis, these are irritative symptoms of the lower tract including dysuria, frequency, urgency, and suprapubic discomfort. Individuals with renal infection present with costovertebral angle pain or tenderness with or without associated fever or lower tract symptoms. Patients with neurological impairment, such as spinal cord injury or multiple sclerosis, may present with atypical symptoms including increased lower limb spasm or weakness, or exacerbation of neurological symptoms.[5,6] Spinal cord injured patients with high-level cervical lesions may experience autonomic dysreflexia including either fever or hypothermia, and hypertension with either upper or lower urinary infection.[7]

Patients who experience frequent recurrent urinary infection tend to have consistent symptoms with recurrent episodes. Young women with recurrent acute uncomplicated cystitis are 95% accurate in identifying the presence of urinary infection.[8,9] Spinal cord injured patients, as well, tend to report consistent symptoms, although the accuracy of self-diagnosis in this group has not been validated.

Microbiology

Recurrent acute uncomplicated urinary infection, either cystitis or pyelonephritis, has a consistent bacteriology. *Escherichia coli* is isolated from 80–85% of infections, *Staphylococcus saprophyticus* 5–10% of the time, and *Klebsiella pneumoniae, Proteus mirabilis*, or group B streptococci occasionally.[10] Women who have received recent antimicrobial therapy are more likely to have infection with *E. coli* of increased antimicrobial resistance.[11]

A wider spectrum of infecting organisms is isolated from patients with complicated urinary infection.[2] *E. coli* remains common, but other Enterobacteriaceae such as *K. pneumoniae, Enterobacter* species, *Serratia* species, *Citrobacter* species, *P. mirabilis, Morganella morganii* and *Providencia stuartii* are frequently isolated. Patients with repeated exposures to antimicrobial therapy or nosocomial acquisition following urological instrumentation are likely to have antimicrobial-resistant organisms. These may include *Pseudomonas aeruginosa* and other non-fermentors such as *Stenotrophomonas maltophilia* and *Acinetobacter* spp. Gram-positive organisms such as *Staphylococcus aureus* or Group B streptococcus are isolated occasionally. *Enterococcus* species and coagulase-negative staphylococci are common, but are less often isolated from patients with symptomatic infection.

Fungal urinary infections are increasing in frequency. Candiduria is usually identified in patients characterized by previous broad-spectrum antibacterial therapy, diabetes, and indwelling devices such as chronic urethral catheters or stents.[12] *Candida albicans* is the most common species, but other organisms including *C. glabrata, C. tropicalis, C. parapsilosis*, and *C. krusei* are also isolated. These non-albicans strains are more likely to be resistant to azole therapy, and may be increasing in prevalence.[13] A fungus ball leading to ureteric or intrarenal obstruction may increase the risk of invasive infection with candidaemia.

All chronic urological devices, including catheters, stents, and nephrostomy tubes, become coated with biofilm.[14] The biofilm consists of extracellular bacterial substances together with urinary salts and proteins. From two to five strains of microorganisms are generally present in the biofilm.[15] Even susceptible organisms growing in the biofilm contribute to post-therapy relapse, as they are relatively protected from both antimicrobials in the urine and the host immune and inflammatory response. A urine specimen obtained for culture through such a device reflects the microbiology of the biofilm as well as the urine.[15]

Pyuria

Pyuria is a virtually universal accompaniment of symptomatic urinary infection. Most individuals with asymptomatic bacteriuria, however, also have pyuria.[3,16,17] Neither the presence nor the degree of pyuria has been shown to have a negative prognostic value in patients with urinary infection.[18,19] The absence of pyuria in a urinalysis is useful to exclude urinary infection. However, the presence of pyuria is of limited clinical use, as it does not differentiate symptomatic from asymptomatic infection and, by itself, is not an indication for antimicrobial therapy.

Management

Clinical assessment

The initial assessment of any patient who may have recurrent urinary infection is a detailed and critical evaluation of symptoms. An important question is whether the symptoms are, in fact, attributable to urinary infection. Musculoskeletal back pain, yeast vulvovaginitis, sexually transmitted diseases, oestrogen deficiency, or prostatism may be misinterpreted as irritative symptoms attributable to urinary infection. Other patients may complain of non-localizing symptoms such as 'fatigue'. Assessing the contribution of urinary infection requires a careful review of the presence, location, duration, type, and severity of symptoms. Patients with voiding assisted by catheterization or with an ileal conduit may interpret cloudy or foul-smelling urine as infection. While these findings may be due to bacteriuria, other causes may also contribute, and they are not an indication for antimicrobial therapy. Other patients may have had urine cultures obtained which documented bacteriuria despite the absence of symptoms. These patients should be reassured that bacteriuria, by itself or associated with cloudiness or odour, is not an indication for antimicrobial treatment.

In addition to a critical evaluation of symptoms, the response to and tolerance of prior antimicrobial therapy should be characterized. If symptoms are present with microbiologically documented infection, absent when the urine culture is negative, and resolve or are substantially improved with antimicrobial therapy directed at the specific infecting organism, they are probably attributable to urinary infection. Patients with infections at non-urinary sites may, however, respond clinically to antimicrobials given for presumed urinary infection if the infecting organism at the other site is susceptible to the antimicrobial given. If symptoms persist despite negative urine cultures, or while effective antimicrobial therapy is being given, alternative explanations for the symptoms must be considered. The patient is either infected with a resistant organism, has an underlying genitourinary abnormality which requires intervention, or the symptoms are not due to urinary infection.

As patients often receive repeated courses of antimicrobials there may be a history of intolerance to one or more antimicrobial. The reaction experienced for each antimicrobial should be characterized. A hypersensitivity reaction characterized by rash, airway obstruction, or haemodynamic collapse must be differentiated from gastrointestinal intolerance. Immunological reactions usually preclude further use of any antimicrobial of the same class. If intolerance is not on the basis of an immunological reaction, other agents of the same class may be used, or the patient may be rechallenged with the same antimicrobial if necessary.

Urine culture

The definitive diagnosis of urinary infection requires microbiological confirmation by an appropriately collected urine specimen from which one or more uropathogens meeting established quantitative criteria are isolated. Detailed, comprehensive characterization of the urine microbiology is essential for the management of any patient with recalcitrant urinary infection. Essential information includes both current and previous infecting organisms and antimicrobial susceptibilities.

Only 50–70% of women with acute uncomplicated cystitis have quantitative counts $\geq 10^5$ colony-forming units (cfu)/ml.[10] About 30% will have a lower quantitative count of an isoloated uropathogen, usually *E. coli*, and 10–20% will have negative urine cultures. Isolation of a uropathogen from an appropriately collected urine specimen in a quantitative count of $\geq 10^2$ cfu/ml is consistent with urinary infection with this clinical presentation. As any quantitative count of a uropathogen, associated with pyuria, may be clinically significant, the laboratory should be alerted to identify potential uropathogens isolated in any quantitative count. The response to antimicrobial therapy is similar for women with negative or positive urine cultures. Women with negative cultures probably have urinary infection with a urine microbial count below the level of detection using standard semiquantitative laboratory methods. For women with acute uncomplicated urinary infection empirical treatment without obtaining a urine culture is a common practice.[20] However, a urine specimen for culture should be obtained for women with failure of therapy or early recurrence post-treatment. For acute uncomplicated pyelonephritis $\geq 10^4$ cfu/ml is the recommended quantitative level for organisms isolated from the urine.[1]

The accepted quantitative criteria for microbiological diagnosis of complicated urinary infection is $\geq 10^5$ cfu/ml.[1] Some symptomatic patients may have lower quantitative counts including patients experiencing diuresis, patients with renal failure, patients infected with selected organisms, or those receiving antimicrobials. For specimens obtained by catheterization, any quantitative count is consistent with infection.[16,17] The urine culture may be negative in patients already receiving antimicrobial therapy, when there is complete obstruction with infection proximal to the obstruction, or in rare cases of infection with fastidious organisms such as *Hemophilus influenzae* or *Ureaplasma urealyticum* which are not isolated with standard laboratory methods for urine specimens.

Patients with complicated urinary infection, especially with indwelling devices, often have multiple organisms isolated. The laboratory should be alerted that all organisms in any quantitative count should be identified and susceptibility testing performed for such patients. Individuals with chronic indwelling urethral catheters should have the catheter replaced immediately prior to institution of antimicrobial therapy, and urine for culture obtained through the newly placed catheter.[15] The specimen collected through the new catheter will reflect bladder rather than biofilm bacteriology, and is likely more relevant for clinical decisions.

In most cases, urine cultures should be obtained only if the patient is symptomatic. Documentation of microbiological cure post-therapy in asymptomatic patients is not recommended. Occasional exceptions to this may be valid for patients with frequent symptomatic relapse where the goal is to identify early relapse before symptoms recur. In addition, urine cultures are indicated for asymptomatic patients prior to undergoing an invasive genitourinary procedure. This allows optimal antimicrobial selection of pre-operative therapy to achieve sterile urine at the time of the procedure.

Other laboratory investigations

A urinalysis may document bacteriuria, crystals, casts, pyuria, nitrites, haematuria, or high pH, all of which may be associated with both infection and non-infectious renal or bladder abnormalities. Blood cultures should be obtained in patients presenting with systemic manifestations consistent with sepsis such as fever or haemodynamic instability, or in patients with urinary obstruction or other known anatomical abnormalities of the urinary tract. Renal function should be evaluated initially with serum creatinine. Knowledge of renal function assists in optimizing antimicrobial therapy as well as providing a potential explanation for suboptimal antimicrobial response for some patients.

Urological investigation

Women with a clinical presentation consistent with recurrent acute uncomplicated urinary infection seldom require urological investigation, even when recurrences are very frequent.[10] If symptoms consistent with acute cystitis respond promptly to antimicrobial therapy, especially when recurrences are associated with sexual activity, and there are no voiding symptoms between infections, an abnormality is unlikely and investigations are not indicated.[10] Women with relapsing pyelonephritis, failure to respond to therapy despite documented infection with a sensitive organism, recurrent infection despite receiving prophylaxis, or voiding symptoms between infections should have investigations to exclude abnormalities.

For other patients with recalcitrant urinary infection, it is essential to document the structural and functional status of the urinary tract. For some patients, the reason for recurrent infection is obvious, such as the patient using intermittent catheterization. In patients with previously characterized abnormalities, a change in frequency of infection may necessitate repeat investigations to identify any changes. For instance, a patient with voiding managed by intermittent catheterization may have developed bladder stones, leading to an increase in frequency of symptomatic episodes. A patient with a ureteric stent may have obstruction of the stent with hydronephrosis. The optimal approach to investigation will be determined by the clinical presentation of the individual patient and the results of any previous investigations. A renal ultrasound is a useful screening test to exclude obstruction. In some cases, measurement of post-void residual urine to document incomplete bladder emptying is sufficient. Urodynamic studies, voiding cystogram, computed tomography, cystourethroscopy, or retrograde pyelography may be appropriate for some patients. Where relapsing infection occurs in a person who appears to have a normal genitourinary tract, a renal scan to evaluate differential renal function may be informative as this may reveal unexpected renal dysfunction.

Treatment

Important considerations to be addressed in the management of any patient with recalcitrant urinary infection are listed in Table 15.1. Many antimicrobial agents are effective for the treatment of urinary infection.[21] The regimen selected for the individual patient with recalcitrant infection is determined by the results of urine culture, patient tolerance, renal function, whether recurrent infection is reinfection or relapse, and whether the clinical presentation or antimicrobial susceptibility requires parenteral

Table 15.1 Principles in the management of recalcitrant urinary infection

Management decisions are based on a critical evaluation of the clinical presentation

Antimicrobial selection is based on urine culture results

The urological status of the patient is known

Renal function is known

Whether infection is reinfection or relapse is assessed

Wherever possible, foreign bodies including stones, have been removed

Methods to ensure adequate voiding have been instituted

therapy. Clinicians must be aware of potential adverse effects of any antimicrobials used, as well as potential drug interactions with other therapies the patient is receiving.

Asymptomatic bacteriuria

Asymptomatic bacteriuria is a common finding in patients who also experience recurrent symptomatic urinary infection.[3] For pregnant women, asymptomatic bacteriuria is associated with an increased risk of acute pyelonephritis in late pregnancy, leading to premature labour and low-birth-weight infants.[3] Thus screening for and treatment of asymptomatic bacteriuria is recommended for pregnant women. If recurrent symptomatic or asymptomatic urinary infection occurs, prophylactic antimicrobial therapy continued until delivery is indicated, taking into consideration potential adverse fetal effects in selection of the antimicrobial.

Prospective, randomized clinical trials in other populations, including the elderly, diabetic women, and spinal cord injured patients, have consistently reported no benefits with antimicrobial treatment of asymptomatic bacteriuria.[3] Treatment of asymptomatic bacteriuria does not decrease the frequency of symptomatic episodes or other potential negative outcomes.[3] Treatment, however, is associated with increased adverse antimicrobial effects, and increased risk of reinfection with resistant organisms. Thus, non-pregnant populations should *not* be screened for asymptomatic bacteriuria nor treated if bacteriuria is identified.

Acute, uncomplicated urinary infection

The antimicrobial management of acute uncomplicated urinary infection is generally straightforward, and consistent for all patients.[20] Empirical therapy without prior urine culture is selected on the basis of patient tolerance and anticipated antimicrobial susceptibilities for the acute episode. The Infectious Diseases Society of America (IDSA) guidelines recommend empirical therapy with twice daily trimethoprim/sulfamethoxazole (TMP/SMX) 160/400 mg for 3 days or 100 mg TMP for sulfa allergic patients.[20] If the regional prevalence of resistance in community-acquired *E. coli* to these agents is over 20%, or if there is patient intolerance, alternative regimens should be used. Second-line therapy includes nitrofurantoin 50–100 mg q.i.d. for 7 days, a fluoroquinolone (norfloxacin 400 mg b.i.d., ciprofloxacin, 250 mg b.i.d., ofloxacin 500 mg o.d., gatifloxacin 400 mg o.d.) for 3 days, pivmecillinam 400 mg b.i.d. for 3 days or 200 mg b.i.d. for 7 days, or a single dose of fosfomycin tromethamine.

Women with frequent recurrences benefit from prophylactic antimicrobial therapy, given as either long-term low-dose or post-intercourse prophylaxis (Table 15.2). Prophylactic therapy will decrease symptomatic episodes by 95%, and is appropriate for women with symptomatic infection who are experiencing recurrences of sufficient frequency that there is a negative impact on their quality of life.[22] A general recommendation is to consider prophylactic therapy if there are two episodes within 6 months, or three within 1 year. Prophylactic therapy is initiated after treatment of a symptomatic episode, when the urine culture is sterile. Several antimicrobial regimens are suitable for prophylactic therapy (Table 15.2). The choice of post-intercourse or long-term low-dose prophylaxis is determined by patient preference. Nitrofurantoin, TMP/SMX, or TMP are recommended first-line agents. Cephalosporins are not usually first-line agents but are recommended for therapy of pregnant women because they are safe for the fetus.

Women who experience a symptomatic episode while receiving prophylactic antimicrobial therapy should have a urine specimen obtained for culture. For empirical treatment pending culture results, if necessary, an antimicrobial from a class different from the agent used for prophylaxis should be selected, as the infecting organism is likely to be resistant to the prophylactic antimicrobial. Patients with recurrent breakthrough symptomatic infections on first-line prophylactic agents should have compliance assessed and urine culture results reviewed to confirm antimicrobial susceptibility. If organisms resistant to the prophylactic agent are identified, persistent gut or vaginal

Table 15.2 Antimicrobial regimens effective for prophylaxis of recurrent acute, uncomplicated urinary infection

Agent	Regimen	
	Long-term, low-dose[a]	**Post-intercourse**
TMP/SMX	80 mg TMP/400 mg SMX daily or 3 × weekly	80 mg TMP/400 mg SMX
Trimethoprim	100 mg daily	100 mg
Nitrofurantoin	50 or 100 mg daily	50–100 mg
Cephalexin	125 mg daily	250 mg
Norfloxacin	200 mg 3 × weekly	200 mg
Ciprofloxacin	125 mg daily	125 mg
Ofloxacin		100 mg

TMP/SMX, trimethoprim/sulfamethoxazole.

[a] Recommended to be taken at night.

colonization with a resistant isolate may be a source of repeated infection. A fluoro-quinolone may be considered for subsequent prophylaxis, if the infecting organism is susceptible.

Complicated urinary infection

The management of recalcitrant complicated urinary infection is individualized for each patient based on genitourinary abnormalities, renal function, current and past urine microbiology, and antimicrobial tolerance. There is limited information from clinical trials to assist in developing management strategies in these cases. Recurrent relapsing infection may be attributable to resistant organisms, in which case selecting an agent to which the organism is susceptible should be effective. Another reason for relapse despite susceptible infecting organisms may be too short a duration of therapy, in which case a more prolonged course may cure the infection.[23–26] Wherever possible, indwelling devices should be removed or replaced prior to initiating antimicrobial therapy, to limit the biofilm burden.[15]

Two comparative studies evaluated the efficacy of a more prolonged duration of antimicrobial therapy for men with relapsing infection from a presumed prostatic source. Smith *et al.* reported that 12 weeks of TMP/SMX was more effective than 10 days' treatment,[23] and Gleckman *et al.* reported that 6 weeks of therapy was superi-or to 2 weeks.[24] In a more recent study of patients with severe urological conditions and chronic recurrent infections, Boerema and van Saene reported no benefit in sub-sequent recurrence if norfloxacin was continued for 3 months compared with 1 month.[25] Men with persistent or relapsing *P. aeruginosa* infection had similar outcomes with norfloxacin continued at full dose or half dose for a subsequent 2 months, follow-ing an initial 4 weeks of full-dose therapy.[26] These studies suggest that more prolonged therapy should be considered for men with recurrent or relapsing complicated urinary infection. The studies may be relevant only to men, where prostatic infection is a nidus for relapsing infection or requires more prolonged therapy because of limited antimi-crobial diffusion into the prostate. The applicability of these studies in the manage-ment of complicated infections in women is not clear.

For patients with persistent urological abnormalities and recurrent infection requir-ing repeated courses of antimicrobial therapy, reinfection with resistant organisms is common. In this situation, selection of a specific antimicrobial regimen must be based on culture results and susceptibilities. If the infecting organism is highly resistant, unique antimicrobial approaches may be required (see Case 1, Box 15.1). Occasionally, investigational antimicrobials may be considered, or antimicrobials not usually indic-ated for treatment of urinary infection. For patients with sulfonamide allergy, TMP by itself may be used for susceptible organisms. Nitrofurantoin is primarily used for treatment of acute uncomplicated cystitis, but is also effective for complicated urinary infection presenting as cystitis. It is not effective for *P. mirabilis, K. pneumoniae*, or *P. aeruginosa* infections, but is the oral agent of choice for cystitis with vancomycin-resistant

Box 15.1 **Case 1**

This 42-year-old female health-care professional had a right nephrectomy at age 20 for chronic pyelonephritis. Subsequently, she experienced infrequent, sporadic episodes of haematuria with left flank pain. Urine cultures obtained during these episodes were repeatedly negative. This was diagnosed at age 30 years, following urological and nephrology investigation, as haematuria loin pain syndrome. Approximately 5 years prior to infectious diseases referral, at age 37, recurrent left flank pain associated with new lower tract irritative symptoms without haematuria and which responded to antimicrobial therapy occurred. These symptoms uniformly recurred within a few weeks of discontinuing antimicrobial therapy, and urine cultures obtained during these episodes consistently grew *E. coli*. She received repeated courses of antimicrobials with symptomatic improvement. Infectious diseases referral was requested because of the increasing severity of symptoms not controlled with antimicrobial therapy and requiring parenteral morphine for pain control, with impaired ability to work or care for her family.

Evaluation

Her most recent antimicrobial course prior to evaluation had been prolonged (6 weeks) ciprofloxacin. The most recent urine culture, obtained after the ciprofloxacin, grew an *E. coli* susceptible only to imipenem and nitrofurantoin. Previous *E. coli* isolates had been susceptible to other oral antimicrobials, but repeated isolates collected over several years showed stepwise emergence of resistance to cephalosporins, TMP/SMX, fluoroquinolones, and aminoglycosides. She was receiving nitrofurantoin when initially evaluated, but her pain was still incapacitating. A urine culture obtained while on nitrofurantoin had *E. coli* isolated in low quantitative counts. This organism had the same susceptibility pattern as the previous isolate. Further testing demonstrated plasmid-mediated extended-spectrum beta-lactamase (ESBL) production and aminoglycoside resistance, and chromosomal resistance to fluoroquinolones. Urological reassessment within the prior year, including a CT scan, identified no abnormalities of the left kidney, ureter, or bladder. The serum creatinine was normal, but creatinine clearance was slightly reduced at 89. Following assessment by both infectious diseases and nephrology, the relative importance of infection or haematuria loin pain syndrome in contributing to her pain were not clear.

Management

The patient was initially treated with very high-dose oral ciprofloxacin, without clinical response. She then received a 6 week course of intravenous meropenem,

Box 15.1 *(continued)*

with resolution of her pain and negative urine cultures. This trial of therapy confirmed that her symptoms were primarily attributable to infection rather than haematuria loin pain syndrome, and could be managed with appropriate antimicrobial therapy. However, within 1 week of discontinuing meropenem she had a positive urine culture for the same highly resistant *E. coli*, followed by a prompt recurrence of symptoms. Additional testing of the isolate showed it was susceptible to pivmecillinam, and this antimicrobial was initiated at a dose of 400 mg orally twice daily. Her symptoms resolved with pivmecillinam and the urine culture remained negative. This therapy has been maintained at the same dose for over 1 year and she has remained pain free, apart from a single episode of pain with haematuria when the urine culture remained negative. She has returned to full time work and requires no continuing analgesia.

Commentary

This woman's relapsing *E. coli* infection progressed to a highly resistant ESBL-producing organism. Clinical assessment of the contribution of infection to symptoms was complicated by concurrent haematuria loin pain syndrome. The presence of a single kidney complicated management. Her lack of response to nitrofurantoin is consistent with the limited utility of this agent in treating upper tract infection. The clinical response to antibiotics to which the organism was susceptible was excellent, but required parenteral therapy. Early relapse after the carbapenem, and the previous history of relapse after appropriate antimicrobial therapy over several years, led to the decision to institute long-term suppressive therapy. As no abnormalities of the left kidney or bladder were identified, an explanation for the continuing relapse with this organism is not clear. However, it is speculated that the haematuria loin pain syndrome has some role. Pivmecillinam is not marketed in the United States but is available in Canada and northern Europe for the indication of treatment for acute cystitis. It has been widely used in some European countries for several decades, but there is little published experience with prolonged therapy. It was the only oral antimicrobial available for suppressive therapy for this woman. She elected to proceed with this agent after discussion of the limited availability of alternative therapy, and having been advised of the limited experience with long-term use. Should an oral carbapenem antimicrobial become available, this may provide an alternate option for oral suppressive therapy. There are no plans at present to discontinue suppressive therapy for this woman.

enterococci.[27] Patients with renal infection who receive nitrofurantoin may have symptoms suppressed but will invariably relapse once the nitrofurantoin is discontinued. Nitrofurantoin is contraindicated in patients with renal failure, as it does not achieve high enough levels in the urine for therapeutic efficacy, and toxic metabolites may accumulate. Some patients with resistant Enterobacteriaceae have organisms which remain susceptible to tetracyclines, and doxycycline may be an option for treatment. Many resistant organisms remain susceptible to pivmecillinam, an antimicrobial available in Canada and parts of Europe but not marketed in the United States.[28] While pivmecillinam is also indicated only for acute cystitis, it has some efficacy in treating renal infection, and may be considered where other oral options are not appropriate.

When infection with highly resistant organisms occurs, there may be no oral antimicrobial options available. Patients with severe sepsis, including haemodynamic instability, also require parenteral therapy. If renal function is normal, the aminoglycosides remain useful agents for parenteral therapy. They may be given once daily, which facilitates out-patient therapy. Ceftriaxone may also be given once daily as out-patient therapy but may not be as useful for treatment of resistant organisms. For highly resistant organisms, including those which produce extended beta-lactamases, or resistant *P. aeruginosa*, the carbapenems (imipenem, meropenem, eartapenem) may be effective. Out-patient parenteral therapy programmes, if available, are useful for treatment of clinically stable patients who require parenteral therapy for treatment of resistant organisms.

There are special considerations in treatment of urinary infection in patients with significant renal functional impairment. Antimicrobial levels may not be high enough at the site of infection because of the decreased renal blood flow which accompanies renal impairment. A more prolonged course of antimicrobial therapy may be required to achieve cure. Some antimicrobial agents, such as nitrofurantoin, are contraindicated in renal failure. Aminoglycosides are probably not as effective in treatment of patients with decreased renal function.[2] However, beta-lactam antimicrobials including ampicillin, piperacillin, and cephalosporins, as well as fluoroquinolones, have been used successfully in the treatment of patients with renal failure. In patients with end-stage renal disease, including renal transplant patients with infections in residual native kidneys, it may not be possible to eradicate bacteriuria.

There is no role for long-term antimicrobial prophylaxis in patients with recurrent complicated urinary infection. The continuing risk for infection in the face of persistent genitourinary abnormalities, together with antimicrobial pressure from continuing prophylactic therapy, invariably results in recurrent infection with more resistant organisms.[5,29] There may be an initial short-term benefit, but prophylaxis is ultimately limited by emergence of antimicrobial resistance. This is a particular concern for individuals with permanent or temporary indwelling devices with biofilm formation.[30–32] Short-term prophylaxis is indicated for bacteriuric patients prior to selected genitourinary procedures to prevent bacteraemia and sepsis resulting from mucosal trauma.[33–35] In this situation, antimicrobials are initiated only immediately prior to the procedure. Prophylaxis is not recommended for replacement of nephrostomy tubes, as this does not prevent bacteraemia,[36] or when replacing chronic indwelling urethral catheters because of the low risk of bacteraemia with this manipulation.[37,38]

Fungal urinary infection

Funguria is usually asymptomatic and does not require treatment.[39] There are several therapeutic options for treatment of symptomatic fungal infection (Table 15.3). Fluconazole is currently the treatment of choice for susceptible *Candida* species.[39,40] This azole antifungal is excreted in the urine, and can be given either parenterally or orally. For fluconazole-resistant *Candida* species, amphotericin B remains the treatment of choice. While amphotericin B bladder washout was a therapy previously recommended, it is costly and uncomfortable.[40,41] Systemic amphotericin B is an effective therapy, but has more adverse effects than fluconazole.[42] A single dose of parenteral amphotericin B was equivalent to a 5-day bladder washout in one study.[42] Newer antifungal agents such as caspofungin or voraconazole are not excreted in the urine, and their role in treatment of urinary infection is not yet clear.

Suppressive antimicrobial therapy

Suppressive antimicrobial therapy is long-term antimicrobial therapy given to prevent symptomatic episodes or other morbidity in patients with complicated urinary infection where cure is not feasible because of a persistent underlying abnormality. This approach is appropriate only for highly selected patients, such as those with recurrent symptomatic infection or with renal failure (see Case 1, Box 15.1, and Case 2, Box 15.2). Patients with asymptomatic infection and urolithiasis may also have stone enlargement prevented by suppressive therapy,[43] but this approach is now seldom indicated given the effectiveness of current stone removal strategies. The antimicrobial selected is individualized based on patient tolerance and the known infecting organisms and susceptibilities. Therapy is initiated at full dose, and the dose may be decreased to one-half after a few weeks if it is clinically effective.

Table 15.3 Treatment options for fungal urinary tract infection

Agent	Route	Dose
Fluconazole[24,25]	Oral or parenteral	400 mg once, then 200 mg IV. 200 mg daily orally
Amphotercin B[24–26]	Parenteral	15 mg/500 ml one dose
	Bladder irrigation, continuous	0.25 mg/500 mg 5% dextrose in water at 42 ml/h for 5 days
	Bladder irrigation, intermittent	1 mg/200 mg 5% dextrose in water 98 h for 3 days
Flucytosine	Oral	37.5 mg/kg every 6 h

Box 15.2 **Case 2**

This 70-year-old retired man presented with recurrent urinary infection complicating prostatic hypertrophy, with obstructive nephropathy and bladder stones. Carcinoma of the bladder was incidently diagnosed at prostate resection. He required axillo-bifemoral bypass for abdominal aortic aneurysm and bilateral iliac aneurysms at the same time as a radical cystectomy and ileal conduit. The right kidney was poorly functioning prior to surgery and, post-operatively, a left ureteric stent was left in place because of a small anastomotic leak. He was readmitted 2 months later with renal failure, left hydonephrosis, and urosepsis with *Citrobacter freundii* bacteraemia. He recovered from this episode with antibiotic therapy and placement of a left nephrostomy tube for urinary drainage, but deteriorated 1 week later with *Candida albicans* fungaemia and a fungus ball identified in the left renal collecting system.

   The subsequent clinical course was characterized by left ureteral stricture, repeated shunt reinsertion, and increasing renal failure despite drainage procedures. Two years after the cystectomy he required laparotomy for recurrent gross haematuria from the ileal conduit. A fistula between an external iliac artery aneurysm and the base of the ileal conduit was identified. The left distal ureter was excised and a permanent ureteric stent was placed, and the left ureter was reimplanted. Despite this, renal failure progressed and dialysis was instituted approximately 3 years after surgery. The patient died from an acute cardiac event 5 years after his surgery.

Management

Throughout this period urine cultures were persistently positive with a variety of organisms isolated. *Enterococcus* species and *P. aeruginosa* were most persistent, but *Klebsiella* species, *Citrobacter* species, and *C. albicans* were also occasionally grown. The patient experienced recurrent episodes of feeling 'generally unwell', usually with fevers, lethargy, and occasional chills, vomiting, and anorexia. These symptoms invariably responded to antimicrobial therapy selected to target organisms isolated from the urine culture. Because recurrent symptoms occurred whenever antimicrobials were discontinued, he was placed on suppressive therapy. Initially, the regimen was ciprofloxacin with fluconazole. When systemic symptoms possibly attributed to urine infection were experienced on this therapy, and *Enterococcus* species isolated, amoxicillin was added. He responded clinically to addition of amoxicillin, but when this was discontinued after 4 weeks of therapy there was prompt recurrence of his constitutional symptoms and repeat urine cultures continued to grow *Enterococcus* species. The amoxicillin was reinitiated with good clinical response and continued as suppressive therapy. Fluconazole was discontinued after 2 years, with no deterioration in clinical symptoms. Subsequently *P. aeruginosa* resistant to ciprofloxacin was

Box 15.2 *(continued)*

isolated when he had a further recurrence of systemic symptoms. He was treated with parenteral imipenem, as there was an allergy to cephalosporins, with improvement. Ultimately, he remained on continuous ciprofloxacin and amoxicillin as repeated efforts to discontinue either of these antimicrobials lead to deterioration in his symptoms.

Commentary

This patient with very complex underlying urological abnormalities and renal failure experienced recurrent episodes of systemic infection. Interpretation of urine culture results was complicated by the ileal conduit, ureteric stent, and, occasionally, nephrostomy tubes. Antimicrobial therapy targeted to organisms growing from urine or blood was always effective in ameliorating symptoms, but discontinuing these antibiotics was followed by recurrence of systemic symptoms. Failure to permanently eradicate infection was probably due to both renal failure and the presence of a foreign body. Continuous suppressive therapy maintained his quality of life, and superinfection was managed by additional antimicrobial therapy targeted to the new infecting organism. Trials of discontinuation of antimicrobials, other than the fluconazole, were unsuccessful. Frequent follow-up and repeated reassessment of clinical symptoms and urine cultures was necessary to maintain him free of symptoms.

Inappropriate use of suppressive therapy will lead to further resistance. The indication for suppressive therapy in an individual patient should be reviewed on a continuing basis. Patients maintained on suppressive therapy should be instructed to contact the physician should symptoms of urinary infection recur, or if they experience any adverse effects potentially attributable to antimicrobial therapy. A urine specimen for culture should always be obtained with recrudescence of symptoms, to assist in determining the reason for failure of suppressive therapy. This may be reinfection, with acquisition of a new infecting organism, often resistant to suppressive therapy. When this occurs, treatment with an effective antimicrobial for 7 to 10 days is indicated, and previous suppressive therapy should be continued. Recurrence due to development of resistance in the pre-infecting organism usually requires a change in suppressive therapy. If persistent bacteriuria with a resistant organism occurs, but the patient remains asymptomatic, it may be appropriate to continue suppressive therapy, as the goal is to prevent morbidity rather than bacteriuria.

Summary

Management of recalcitrant urinary infection is challenging. Successful therapeutic outcome requires careful clinical and microbiological evaluation and assessment by urology, infectious diseases, and, sometimes, nephrology. The majority of patients can be cured with appropriate urological intervention or antimicrobial therapy, or both. For some patients prolonged antimicrobial therapy will be necessary to maintain an acceptable clinical outcome.

References

1 Rubin RH, Shapiro ED, Andriole VT, Davis RJ, Stamm WE (1992). General guidelines for the evaluation of new anti-infective drugs for the treatment of urinary tract infection. *Clin. Infect. Dis.* **15**(Suppl. 1): S216–S227.

2 Nicolle LE (2001). A practical guide to the management of complicated urinary tract infection. *Drugs Aging* **18**: 243–54.

3 Nicolle LE (2003). Asymptomatic bacteriuria: when to screen and when to treat. *Infect. Dis. Clin. North Am.* **17**: 367–94.

4 Foxman B (2003). Epidemiology of urinary tract infections: incidence, morbidity, and economic costs. *Am. J. Med.* **113**(Suppl. 1A): 5S–13S.

5 Cardenas DD, Hooton TM (1995). Urinary tract infection in persons with spinal cord injury. *Arch. Phys. Med. Rehab.* **76**: 272–80.

6 Rapp NS, Gilroy J, Lerner AM (1995). Role of bacterial infection in exacerbation of multiple sclerosis. *Am. J. Phys. Med. Rehab.* **74**: 415–18.

7 Trop CS, Bennett CJ (1993). Autonomic dysreflexia and its urological implications: a review. *J. Urol.* **146**: 1461–9.

8 Gupta K, Hooton TM, Roberts PL, Stamm WE (2001). Patient-initiated treatment of uncomplicated recurrent urinary tract infections in young women. *Ann. Intern. Med.* **135**: 9–16.

9 Schaeffer JA, Stuppy BA (1999). Efficacy and safety of self-start therapy in women with recurrent urinary tract infections. *J. Urol.* **161**: 207–11.

10 Stamm WE, Hooton TM (1993). Management of urinary tract infections in adults. *N. Engl. J. Med.* **329**: 1328–34.

11 Brown PD, Freeman A, Foxman B (2002). Prevalence and predictors of trimethoprim-sulfamethoxazole resistance among uropathogenic *Escherichia coli* isolates in Michigan. *Clin. Infect. Dis.* **34**: 1061–6.

12 Kauffman CA, Vazquez JA, Sobel JD, Gallis HA, McKinsey DS, Karchmer AW *et al.* (2000). Prospective, multicenter surveillance study of funguria in hospitalized patients. *Clin. Infect. Dis.* **30**: 14–18.

13 Schwab U, Chernomas F, Larcom L, Weems J (1997). Molecular typing and fluconazole susceptibility of urinary *Candida glabrata* isolates from hospitalized patients. *Diagn. Microbiol. Infect. Dis.* **29**: 11–17.

14 Donlan RM, Costerton JW (2002). Biofilms: survival mechanisms of clinically relevant microorganisms. *Clin. Microbiol. Rev.* **15**: 167–93.

15 Raz R, Schiller D, Nicolle LE (2000). Chronic indwelling catheter replacement prior to antimicrobial therapy for symptomatic urinary infection. *J. Urol.* **164**: 1254–8.

16 Gribble MJ, McCallum NM, Schecter MT (1998). Evaluation of diagnostic criteria for bacteriuria in acutely spinal cord injured patients undergoing intermittent catheterization. *Diagn. Microbiol. Infect. Dis.* **9**: 197–206.

17 Stark RP, Maki DG (1984). Bacteriuria in the catheterized patient. What quantitative level of bacteriuria is relevant. *N. Engl. J. Med.* **311**: 560–4.

18 Nicolle LE, Duckworth H, Brunka J, Urias B, Kennedy J, Murray D *et al.* (1998). Urinary antibody level and survival in bacteriuric institutionalized older subjects. *J. Am. Geriatr. Soc.* **46**: 947–53.

19 Harding GKM, Zhanel GG, Nicolle LE, Cheang M, Manitoba Diabetic Urinary Infection Study Group (2002). Antimicrobial treatment in diabetic women with asymptomatic bacteriuria. *N. Engl. J. Med.* **347**: 1576–83.

20 Warren JW, Abrutyn E, Hebel JR, Johnson JR, Schaeffer AJ, Stamm WE (1999). Guidelines for antimicrobial treatment of uncomplicated acute bacterial cystitis and acute pyelonephritis in women. *Clin. Infect. Dis.* **29**: 745–58.

21 Nicolle LE (2003). Best pharmacological practice: urinary tract infections. *Expert Opin. Pharmacother.* **4**: 693–704.

22 Nicolle LE (2002). Urinary tract infections: traditional pharmacologic therapies. *Am. J. Med.* **113**(Suppl. 1A): 353–445.

23 Smith JW, Jones SR, Reed WP, Tice AD, Deupree RH, Kaijser B (1979). Recurrent urinary tract infections in men. *Ann. Intern. Med.* **91**: 544–8.

24 Gleckman R, Crowley M, Natsios GA (1979). Therapy of recurrent invasive urinary tract infections of men. *N. Engl. J. Med.* **301**: 878–80.

25 Boerema JB, van Saene HK (1986). Norfloxacin treatment in complicated urinary tract infection. *Scan. J. Infect. Dis.* **48**(Suppl.): 20–6.

26 Sheehan GJ, Harding GKM, Haase DA, Thomson MJ, Urias B, Kennedy JK *et al.* (1988). Double-blind, randomized comparison of 24 weeks of norfloxacin followed by 12 weeks of placebo in the therapy of complicated urinary tract infection. *Antimicrob. Agents Chemother.* **32**: 1292–3.

27 Zhanel GG, Laing NM, Nichol KA, Palatnick LP, Noreddin A, Hisanaga T *et al.* (2003). Antibiotic activity against urinary tract infection isolates of vancomycin-resistant enterococci: results from the 2002 North American vancomycin resistant enterococci susceptibility study. *J. Antimicrob. Chemother.* **52**: 382–8.

28 Nicolle LE (2000). Pivmecillinam in the treatment of urinary tract infections. *J. Antimicrob. Chemother.* **46**: 35–40.

29 Gribble MJ, Puterman ML (1993). Prophylaxis of urinary tract infection in persons with recent spinal cord injury: a prospective, randomized, double-blind, placebo controlled study of trimethoprim/sulfamethoxazole. *Am. J. Med.* **95**: 141–52.

30 Mountokalakis T, Skounakis M, Tselentis J (1985). Short-term versus prolonged systemic antibiotic prophylaxis in patients treated with indwelling catheters. *J. Urol.* **134**: 506–8.

31 Nyren P, Runeberg L, Kostiala AI, Renkonen D-V, Roine R (1981). Prophylactic methenamine hippurate or nitrofurantoin in patients with an indwelling urinary catheter. *Ann. Clin. Res.* **13**: 16–21.

32 Butler HK, Kunin CM (1968). Evaluation of specific systemic antimicrobial therapy in patients while on closed catheter drainage. *J. Urol.* **100**: 567–72.

33 Cafferky MT, Falkiner FR, Gillespie WA, Murphy PM (1982). Antibiotics for the prevention of septicemia in urology. *J. Antimicrob. Chemother.* **9**: 471–7.

34 Olson E, Cookson BD (2000). Do antimicrobials have a role in preventing septicemia following instrumentation of the urinary tract? *J. Hosp. Infect.* **45**: 85–97.

35 Grabe M (2001). Prospective antibiotic prophylaxis in urology. *Curr. Opin. Urol.* **11**: 81–5.

36 Cronan JJ, Horn DL, Marcello A, Robinson A, Paolella LP, Lambiase RE *et al.* (1989). Antibiotics and nephrostomy tube care: preliminary observations Part II. Bacteremia. *Radiology* **172**: 1043–5.

37 Jewes LA, Gillespie WA, Leadbetter A, Myers B, Simpson RA, Stower MJ *et al*. (1988). Bacteriuria and bacteremia in patients with long-term indwelling catheters—a domiciliary study. *J. Med. Microbiol.* **26**: 61–5.

38 Bregenzer T, Frei R, Widmer AF, Seiler W, Probst W, Mattarelli G *et al*. (1997). Low risk of bacteremia during catheter replacement in patients with long-term urinary catheters. *Arch. Intern. Med.* **157**: 521–5.

39 Sobel JD, Kauffman CA, McKinsey D, Zervos M, Vazquez JA, Karchmer AW *et al*. (2000). Candiduria: a randomized, double-blind study of treatment with fluconazole and placebo. *Clin. Infect. Dis.* **30**: 19–24.

40 Jacobs LG, Skidmore EA, Freeman K, Lipshultz D, Fox N (1996). Oral fluconazole compared with amphotericin B bladder irrigation for fungal urinary infection in the elderly. *Clin. Infect. Dis.* **22**: 30–5.

41 Fan-Havard P, O'Donovan C, Smith SM, Oh J, Bamberger M, Eng RHK (1995). Oral fluconazole versus amphotericin B bladder irrigation for treatment of candidal funguria. *Clin. Infect. Dis.* **21**: 960–5.

42 Leu HS, Huang CT (1995). Clearance of funguria with short course antifungal regimens: a prospective, randomized controlled study. *Clin. Infect. Dis.* **20**: 1152–7.

43 Chinn RH, Maskell R, Mead JA, Polak A (1976). Renal stones and urinary infection: a study of antibiotic treatment. *Br. Med. J.* **2**: 1411–13.

Chapter 16

The patient presenting with chronic prostatitis

Ashley McLellan and Peter A. M. Anderson

Background

Prostatitis is a condition of the prostate gland which occurs in 5–9% of men.[1,2] It is the most common chronic urological diagnosis made by physicians in men aged less than 50 years and the third most common in men aged over 50.[3] Taken literally, prostatitis means 'inflammation of the prostate gland'. As our knowledge of this condition expands, it has become apparent that such a traditional definition may be too simplified. Prostatitis represents a spectrum of conditions ranging from the sudden onset of urinary symptoms and fever due to bacterial infection of the prostate to chronic pelvic pain without evidence of prostatic inflammation or infection. The goal of this chapter is to describe the various forms of prostatitis, their presentations and appropriate investigations and to outline treatment and supportive care with an emphasis on chronic prostatitis.

History

Prostatitis was first recognized as a distinct entity during the 1800s. Physicians attributed the disease to events that might have irritated the prostate gland such as sexual activity, cold, alcohol, or violent exertion.[4] During the 1900s, physicians began to analyse secretions from the prostate and discovered that bacterial infection of the prostate was one of the causes of this condition. Massage of the prostate, with or without antibiotics, remained the major form of treatment until the middle of the twentieth century. Around the same time, it was discovered that a chronic form of prostatitis not due to bacterial infection existed and that this form of prostatitis was resistant to traditional therapies.[5] Like other forms of prostatitis, it was felt to be due to excessive masturbation or sexual gratification. The landmark work of Meares and Stamey[6] in 1968 led to the classification of prostatitis, based upon the presence or absence of bacteria and white blood cells in urine and prostate secretions. To utilize this classification, four specimens were required (four glass). The initial 10 ml of voided urine represents the urethral sample (VB1). The second sample consists of a clean-catch urine specimen (VB2), representing the bladder specimen, followed by a prostatic massage and examination of the expressed prostatic secretions (EPS). The fourth sample is the first 10 ml voided after prostatic massage (VB3). Using this system, prostatitis was defined as: acute bacterial prostatitis, chronic bacterial prostatitis, chronic non-bacterial prostatitis, and prostatodynia (non-specific pain from the prostate). This classification provided the framework for the diagnosis, treatment, and study of prostatitis in the modern era.

Causes

Prostatitis is recognized clinically as either an acute disease with the sudden onset of symptoms or, more commonly, a chronic condition. Acute prostatitis is easily recognizable and is distinct from the chronic forms of the disease, both in its cause and treatment. Chronic prostatitis and the chronic pelvic pain syndrome (CPPS) have less readily identifiable causes, and are the focus of this chapter. Various theories have arisen to describe the origins of chronic prostatitis and they will be discussed in the following section.

Bacteria

When EPS and VB3 specimens are examined, the Enterobacteriaceae family of Gram-negative bacteria are the most common agents implicated in both the acute and chronic bacterial forms of prostatitis. Within this family of bacteria, *Escherichia coli* is the most common and is identified in 65 to 80% of patients. Other bacteria which are often identified include *Pseudomonas aeruginosa, Serratia* species, *Klebsiella* species, and *Enterobacter aerogenes*.[7] Gram-positive bacteria are less commonly implicated, with enterococci species being the most common Gram-positive organisms. Staphylococci and streptococci have been postulated as causative agents, although their significance has been questioned. The role of anaerobic bacteria has not been clarified. *Cornyebacterium, Chlamydia trachomatis*, and *Ureaplasma urealyticum* have all been investigated as possible bacterial causes[8–10] without definitive results. It has been postulated that non-culturable organisms may also be responsible for chronic abacterial prostatitis/chronic pelvic pain syndrome (CPPS).[11]

Dysfunctional voiding

Dysfunctional voiding with high voiding pressures has been implicated as a cause of prostatitis. Barbalias *et al.* demonstrated that many patients with prostatitis have obstructive voiding patterns which may predispose them to chronic prostatitis.[12] In some men, anatomical abnormalities of the bladder outlet, prostate, and urethra may cause prostatitis,[13] although most men with this condition have no such anatomical abnormalities.

High-pressure dysfunctional voiding may lead to intraprostatic ductal reflux of urine and bacteria. The reflux of sterile urine into the prostatic ducts may induce a chemical inflammation within the prostate, causing the symptoms of chronic prostatitis. Support for the presence of intraprostatic ductal reflux in patients with chronic non-bacterial prostatitis has been demonstrated.[14] Urate has been implicated as an irritant responsible for prostatic inflammation and has been demonstrated in EPSs from patients with chronic prostatitis.[15]

Immunological dysfunction

There is little doubt that the immune system is activated during an episode of acute bacterial prostatitis. Serum antibody levels rise almost immediately and fall after the resolution of infection. In chronic bacterial prostatitis, serum antibody levels are not elevated, but increased antibody levels are detected in prostatic secretions.[16]

In non-bacterial chronic prostatitis, antibodies and complement are both present in prostate biopsies,[17] suggesting a role for the immune system in the origins or propagation of this condition.

Other causes

Other non-infectious causes of chronic prostatitis and CPPS have been evaluated. These include: abnormalities of the pelvic floor muscles and soft tissues ('myofascial pain'),[7] psychological origins,[18–20] pathophysiology similar to interstitial cystitis,[21] and impaired neural regulation of the urinary tract.[22]

It is clear that the cause of chronic prostatitis and CPPS has not been clearly elucidated. It is likely that this condition has more than a single cause, with some or all of the above mechanisms being responsible.

Modern classification

The work of Meares and Stamey[6] provided a classification scheme for prostatitis, guiding physicians in the diagnosis and treatment of this condition. Unfortunately, the placement of patients into a specific category of prostatitis according to this classification has led to disappointing treatment results, as well as inadequacies in research studies. These shortcomings were recognized at the National Institutes of Health (NIH) Consensus Conference on prostatitis in 1995. A new classification consisting of four categories was proposed, primarily for research purposes (Table 16.1). Category I represents acute bacterial prostatitis. Category II indicates chronic bacterial prostatitis. Category III consists of those patients who traditionally were classified as chronic non-bacterial prostatitis (category IIIA, white blood cells in EPS/VB3/semen) and prostatodynia (category IIIB, no white blood cells in EPS/VB3/semen), now collectively referred to as chronic prostatitis/CPPS. Category IV represents individuals with asymptomatic prostatic inflammation.

This classification is not without its own deficits. Using the Meares–Stamey bacterial localization procedure (four glass), Nickel et al.[23] demonstrated that 8% of males with

Table 16.1 Urine characteristics used to classify the various types of prostatitis using the traditional and updated NIH classification systems

Urine characteristics	Classic classification	NIH classification
Bacteria, WBC, ±RBC	Acute bacterial prostatitis	Acute bacterial prostatitis (I)
Bacteria, WBC (VB3/EPS)	Chronic bacterial prostatitis	Chronic bacterial prostatitis (II)
WBC (VB3/EPS)	Chronic non-bacterial prostatitis	Chronic pelvic pain syndrome, inflammatory (IIIA)
Normal	Prostatodynia	Chronic pelvic pain syndrome, non-inflammatory (IIIB)
Normal	NA	Asymptomatic (IV)

Abbreviations: EPS, expressed prostatic secretions; RBC, red blood cells; VB3, urine after prostatic massage; WBC, white blood cells; NA, not applicable.

the diagnosis of chronic prostatitis and 8% of asymptomatic controls had bacteria localized to the prostate. The value of separating category II and category III prostatitis, at least for clinical reasons, becomes even more questionable when one considers that patients in both categories have been shown to respond equally to antibiotic therapy.[24] The separation of category III prostatitis into categories A and B may not be necessary from a clinical standpoint. White blood cells can be found in the urine of normal, asymptomatic males.[23] In males with chronic prostatitis, the presence of white blood cells in EPS is intermittent.[25] Regardless of the shortcomings of the classification system in the clinical setting, it remains useful for research purposes, and will be used here to further consider the various categories of prostatitis. Acute bacterial prostatitis is discussed briefly for completeness, and to demonstrate the contrast that exists between the acute and chronic forms of this disease.

Category I (acute bacterial prostatitis)

A 35-year-old male presents to the local emergency department complaining of pain in the perineum (the area behind the scrotum) and penis, urinary frequency and urgency, painful urination, and decreased urinary flow for 24 hours. On physical exam, he appears unwell and has a fever. His bladder is distended. A gentle digital rectal examination reveals an exquisitely tender prostate gland. A complete blood count reveals an increased white blood cell count, and urinalysis demonstrates white blood cells and bacteriuria. He is treated with 4 weeks of ciprofloxacin and his symptoms resolve.

Although acute bacterial prostatitis is not a common diagnosis, it is one that is made easily by most physicians. Classically, patients present with the sudden onset of pain (perineum, above the pubic bone, genital, pelvic) associated with irritative (frequency, urgency, dysuria) and obstructive (decreased urinary flow, hesitancy, retention) voiding symptoms. Systemic symptoms such as fever, nausea, and vomiting are usually present, and hypotension and shock may be present in a few unfortunate patients.

Digital rectal examination reveals a 'swollen' prostate that is extremely tender on manipulation. Prostatic massage is not necessary in these patients, and may actually be dangerous, as harmful bacteria may be shed into the bloodstream. Microscopic examination of the urine reveals white blood cells and bacteriuria with variable amounts of blood. Urine and blood cultures should be sent before prompt implementation of antibiotic therapy.

Common uropathogens are responsible for most cases of acute bacterial prostatitis (*E. coli, Enterococcus, Pseudomonas*, etc.), making antimicrobial selection quite simple. Appropriate choices include: fluoroquinolones, trimethoprim/sulfamethoxazole, aminoglycosides, and cephalosporins, plus ampicillin if enterococci are suspected. Antibiotic penetration into the prostate is augmented by the prostatic inflammation that accompanies the disease. Patients who have severe symptoms, low blood pressure, diabetes, immunosuppression, renal failure, or other major health problems are candidates for intravenous antibiotic therapy. All other patients may be managed as outpatients with an oral fluoroquinolone or trimethoprim/sulfamethoxazole. A minimum of 4 weeks of antibiotics should be administered to decrease the risk of relapse and the development of chronic infection. Some patients may require a short period of opioid analgesia. Non-steroidal anti-inflammatory drugs, sitz baths, and stool softeners are addition treatments that may provide benefit to some patients. Patients with a pre-existing urological condition (e.g. obstruction) require urological consultation.

Prostatic abscess is a rare complication of acute bacterial prostatitis. Immuno-compromised patients, people with diabetes, and individuals with indwelling urinary catheters are at increased risk of abscess formation. It should be suspected in patients with symptoms resistant to culture-specific antibiotic therapy, persistent pain, or a fluctuant mass on digital rectal exam. The diagnosis is confirmed with transrectal ultrasound or computed tomography (CT) scanning. Drainage is required for definitive therapy.

Category II (chronic bacterial prostatitis)

> A 40-year-old male presents with a history of recurrent urinary tract infections with *E. coli* for 1 year. Between episodes of urinary tract infection, he describes perineal pain, pain with ejaculation, as well as urinary frequency and urgency. His symptoms worsen when he has a urinary tract infection, and improve after short term oral ciprofloxacin therapy. Examination of the penis, testes, and scrotum is normal. Digital rectal examination reveals a slightly enlarged, non-tender prostate. Renal ultrasound and routine blood work are normal. He is most frustrated by the symptoms he is experiencing daily between infections.

Chronic bacterial prostatitis represents 5–15% of all cases of chronic prostatitis.[26] A diagnostic clue to the presence of this condition is a history of recurrent urinary tract infections with common uropathogens. Patients may have no symptoms between infections or have longstanding symptoms similar to patients with category III prostatitis. The diagnostic work-up and management of these patients is similar to category III prostatitis.

Category III (chronic pelvic pain syndrome)

A 44-year-old healthy male presents to his physician with a history of testicular and perineal pain, urinary frequency, and pain with ejaculation for 9 months. He appears to be quite anxious. He has no history of documented urinary tract infection, but another physician has treated him twice with trimethoprim/sulfamethoxazole for a total of 6 weeks. This gave slight but temporary relief of his symptoms. His physical and digital rectal examinations are normal. Routine blood work was normal and urine culture revealed no bacterial growth. Urodynamics reveal slightly decreased uroflow but still within the normal range. His urologist performs a cystoscopy and renal ultrasound, both of which are normal. The patient is frustrated with the care he has received, and he feels that no one is taking his complaints seriously.

Clinical features

Chronic prostatitis is a common condition, affecting 5–9% of all men over many age groups.[1,2] Category III prostatitis is divided into category IIIA (white blood cells in EPS, VB3, or semen) and category IIIB (no white blood cells in EPS, VB3, or semen). This distinction is of academic and research interest only, as patients in either group cannot be distinguished from one another clinically,[27] nor does their therapy differ. It has been suggested that patients with inflammatory CPPS often have severe and frequently bothersome symptoms.[28]

The most common complaint of patients with CPPS is pain. This pain can be located in the perineum, penis, suprapubic area, testes, groin, and/or lower back. Patients have a variable number of urinary complaints. Sexual symptoms may include painful or delayed ejaculation, painful erections, or erectile dysfunction.[29] To confirm a diagnosis of CPPS, the symptoms must be present for at least 3 months. The symptoms tend to be of variable severity over time, with periods of remission and exacerbation characterizing the patient's disease.

CPPS has a marked negative impact on the quality of life of afflicted patients. In a landmark study, Wenninger et al.[30] demonstrated, using a sickness impact score, that patients with CPPS have scores similar to patients who have had a heart attack, angina, or Crohn's disease (inflammatory bowel disease). The severity of the impact of chronic prostatitis was confirmed in another study, where affected individuals were found to have mental health scores worse than patients with severe diabetes mellitus and congestive heart failure.[31] In one study of patients with prolonged symptoms of CPPS refractory to therapy, 80% were found to have some degree of psychiatric problems,[32] with anxiety, depression, and labile mood being most frequently encountered. The patients' level of anxiety increased with time, while social function declined. Up to 50% of patients with chronic prostatitis meet the criteria for depression and are often plagued by relationship and sexual problems.[20] In comparison with patients with this condition, patients with chronic prostatitis fare poorer on scales to measure hypochondriasis, hysteria, depression, and somatization.[19] It has been observed that patients with chronic prostatitis and CPPS often also have syndromes such as chronic headaches, fibromyalgia, chemical sensitivity, and atypical chest pain. Such syndromes were present in 65% of 89 patients studied with chronic prostatitis and CPPS.[33] These studies indicate that chronic prostatitis and CPPS can be associated with serious psychiatric problems as well as a range of other medical conditions. Patients and physicians should address these issues, as their presence may worsen a patient's symptoms, further impairing health and quality of life, and have a serious impact on outcome.

Clinical evaluation

All patients suspected of having chronic prostatitis and CPPS should undergo a thorough history and physical examination including digital rectal examination. History and physical examination should focus on, but not be limited to, the genitourinary system. There are few, if any, abnormal physical findings in most patients with chronic prostatitis and CPPS, but other conditions that may account for the patient's symptoms may be discovered. The prostate is classically described as 'boggy', although this is variable. All patients should have a routine urinalysis and urine culture to assess for blood in the urine and urinary tract infection. Other conditions which should be considered in the diagnosis and identified include: urethral stricutre, benign prostatic hyperplasia, urethritis, cystitis, prostate cancer, and bladder cancer.

Most urologists who subspecialize in chronic prostatitis would recommend bacterial localization studies for all patients with chronic prostatitis and CPPS, particularly in those with a history of recurrent urinary tract infection, previous response to antibiotic therapy, or abnormal results on urinalysis or culture.[34] The Meares–Stamey technique for bacterial localization was discussed previously. Its interpretation in relation to the NIH classification is summarized in Table 16.1. This method of localization has largely been abandoned as it is time-consuming, expensive, and does not alter antimicrobial use by urologists.[35] A simpler study was suggested by Nickel.[4] Collecting pre- and post-prostatic massage urine specimens allows accurate classification of patients within the NIH classification system (Table 16.1). In a review of this technique, it was found that both the sensitivity and the specificity of this test was 91% when compared with the traditional four-glass technique.[36]

Other recommended evaluations include: post-void residual urine measurement, uroflow, and urinary cytology.[34] Depending on the history and physical exam other evaluation may need to include cystoscopy, urodynamics, transrectal ultrasound, pelvic imaging, urethral swabs, semen culture and microscopy, and prostate specific antigen measurement.[34]

The assessment of symptom severity and response to therapy in patients with chronic prostatitis and CPPS is of utmost importance. It focuses on the impact the disease is having on a patient's quality of life, and allows physicians to monitor changes in a patient's disease status over time. Symptom severity indices have been developed to assist with this assessment,[37,38] although none has been considered completely satisfactory. This has led to the development of the NIH-Chronic Prostatitis Symptom

Table 16.2 NIH-Chronic Prostatitis Symptom Index (NIH-CPSI)

Pain or discomfort

1. In the last week, have you had pain or discomfort in any of the following areas?

(a) Area between rectum and testicles

(b) Testicles

(c) Tip of penis (not related to urination)

(d) Below your waist, in pubic or bladder area

2. In the past week, have you experienced:

(a) Pain or burning during urination?

(b) Pain or discomfort during or after sexual climax (ejaculation)?

For each, score 0 for 'No', 1 for 'Yes'

3. How often have you had pain or discomfort in any of these areas over the last week?

(a) Never (0)

(b) Rarely (1)

(c) Sometimes (2)

(d) Often (3)

(e) Usually (4)

(f) Always (5)

4. Which number best describes your AVERAGE pain or discomfort on the days that you had it, over the last week?

On a scale from 0 (no pain) to 10 (worst pain you can imagine)

Urination

5. How often have you had a sensation of not emptying your bladder completely after you finished urinating, over the last week?

(a) Not at all (0)

(b) Less than 1 time in 5 (1)

(c) Less than half the time (2)

(d) About half the time (3)

(e) More than half the time (4)

(f) Almost always (5)

6. How often have you had to urinate again less than 2 hours after you finished urinating, over the last week?

(a) Not at all (0)

(b) Less than 1 time in 5 (1)

(c) Less than half the time (2)

(d) About half the time (3)

(e) More than half the time (4)

(f) Almost always (5)

Impact of symptoms

7. How much have your symptoms kept you from doing the kinds of things you would usually do, over the last week?

(a) Not at all (0)

(b) Only a little (1)

(c) Some (2)

(d) A lot (3)

8. How much did you think about your symptoms, over the last week?

(a) Never (0)

(b) Only a little (1)

(c) Some (2)

(d) A lot (3)

Quality of life

9. If you were to spend the rest of your life with your symptoms just the way they have been during the last week, how would you feel about that?

(a) Delighted (0)

(b) Pleased (1)

(c) Mostly satisfied (2)

(d) Mixed (about equally satisfied and dissatisfied) (3)

(e) Mostly dissatisfied (4)

(f) Unhappy (5)

(g) Terrible (6)

Scoring the NIH-Chronic Prostatitis Symptom Index domains:

Pain: Total of items 1a, 1b, 1c,1d, 2a, 2b, 3, and 4

Urinary symptoms: Total of items 5 and 6

Quality of life impact: Total of items 7, 8, and 9

Index (NIH-CPSI) (Table 16.2). It is a validated tool in the research setting to measure patient symptom severity and changes in symptoms over time and with therapy.[39] It consists of nine questions that address the three major domains of chronic prostatitis/CPPS: pain, urinary problems, impact of symptoms, plus a statement about overall quality of life. Its usefulness in the clinical setting has yet to be validated, although it does appear to be a useful tool for following patients' clinical symptoms objectively.

Treatment

The treatment of chronic prostatitis/CPPS is often frustrating for both physicians and patients. Here we will review accepted therapies as well as those that have been investigated as potential therapies.

Antibiotic therapy

Acute bacterial prostatitis is easily recognized and its microbiological origins are evident. As noted previously, only 5–15% of patients with chronic prostatitis have a proven bacterial cause.[26] Despite the lack of proof of a bacterial basis for chronic prostatitis and CPPS in the majority of patients, antibiotic therapy remains the most common initial treatment.[1,35]

The prostate gland represents a challenging target for antimicrobial therapy. In order for an antibiotic to achieve therapeutic levels within the prostate gland it must be lipophilic, demonstrate minimal protein binding in serum, and be non-ionized.[40] The fluoroquinolones and trimethoprim are the antibiotics that best meet these requirements. They achieve adequate levels within the prostate gland while demonstrating good activity against the organisms most often responsible for chronic prostatitis and CPPS. It is, therefore, not surprising that the greatest clinical success in the treatment of chronic prostatitis has been achieved with these two agents.

In patients with NIH category II prostatitis, bacterial eradication rates of about 40% can be expected using trimethoprim/sulfamethoxazole (160/800 mg twice daily) for 12 weeks.[40] Therapy of 90 days' duration is felt to provide a better result than shorter courses of treatment.[7] The fluoroquinolones (ciprofloxacin, norfloxacin, ofloxacin) have been evaluated as therapy for chronic prostatitis. Bacterial eradication rates between 57 and 86% have been reported.[41] A 4 week course of fluoroquinolone therapy is superior to treatment with trimethoprim/sulfamethoxazole for 3 months.[7] There has been no proven benefit to prolonging fluoroquinolone therapy beyond 6 weeks. The fluoroquinolones can provide bacteriological cure in patients who have failed primary therapy with other antibiotics.[42,43] In patients who have repeated episodes of chronic bacterial prostatitis, low-dose suppressive therapy with an antibiotic that attains high urinary concentrations (e.g. nitrofurantoin, trimethoprim) is effective in reducing recurrences.[40]

Although no bacteriological origin has been discovered for category III prostatitis, antibiotic therapy remains the first-line therapy for these patients. Uncontrolled studies have demonstrated that approximately 40% of patients with category III prostatitis will experience clinical improvement with antibiotic therapy,[44,45] despite no proven bacterial cause. Nickel *et al.* demonstrated in a prospective study that, regardless of culture results or the presence of white blood cells in urine or EPS, the results of antimicrobial therapy measured by patient symptoms are equivalent.[24] Most physicians, therefore, will offer 4 to 6 weeks of antibiotic therapy as the first therapy for all patients with chronic prostatitis and CPPS, although this remains controversial.[33] A patient should not receive additional courses of antibiotic therapy if benefit was completely absent from the initial treatment and the patient has category III prostatitis.

Alpha-blockers

Many of the symptoms of category III prostatitis are similar to those found in patients with benign prostatic hyperplasia (BPH), a benign growth of the prostate gland. The clinical efficacy of alpha-blockers for BPH is known. With the overlap in symptoms observed in these two conditions, it is not surprising that alpha-blockers have been pursued as a therapeutic option for patients with category III prostatitis. The symptoms of category III prostatitis may be secondary to dysfunctional voiding with or without intraprostatic ductal reflux (see section on causes). By relaxing the bladder neck and prostate, which are dense in alpha-adrenergic receptors, alpha-blockers may improve dysfunctional voiding, subsequently decreasing intraprostatic ductal reflux.

Phenoxybenzamine was the first alpha-blocker to be studied for patients with category III prostatitis.[46–48] Although effective, side-effects limited its clinical usefulness. Other agents which have been studied include alfuzosin,[49] terazosin,[37,50] and tamsulosin.[51] Response rates of up to 76% have been reported after 1 month of therapy.[37] A recent placebo-controlled study assessing the effects of tamsulosin in category III prostatitis demonstrated significant symptom relief, particularly for patients with severe symptoms.[52] This effect increased with prolonged tamsulosin utilization (up to the study follow-up of 45 days). The combination of antibiotic therapy and alpha-blockers has been studied in patients with both category II and category III prostatitis.[53] The authors concluded that combination therapy reduced symptoms in both groups as well as recurrence in patients with category II prostatitis.

Anti-inflammatory agents

Category III prostatitis (particularly category IIIA prostatitis) is felt to be associated with prostatic inflammation. Non-steroidal anti-inflammatories have been studied in non-placebo-controlled studies with demonstrated symptom improvement.[54,55] Most recently, rofecoxib, a cyclo-oxygenase-2 inhibitor, has been studied in a placebo-controlled trial, with a trend towards superior symptom improvement with this agent.[56] Further study is needed, although this appears to be a promising therapy. Pentosan polysulfate, an agent used for the treatment of interstitial cystitis, is an anti-inflammatory drug that has been investigated in patients with chronic prostatitis and CPPS;[57] further trials are required to confirm efficacy.

Other medical therapies

When a disease lacks one specific reliable, reproducible, and high efficacy therapy, many different therapies are investigated. In chronic prostatitis and CPPS this has indeed been the case.

Allopurinol has been investigated as a potential therapy. It has been hypothesized that, since intraprostatic ductal reflux of urate is a potential cause of chronic prostatitis and CPPS, allopurinol, by reducing the production of uric acid, may have a potential role in improving the symptoms due to this disease. The results of one placebo-controlled study are controversial,[58] as reanalysis of the data with traditional statistical methods yielded results which conflicted with the authors' findings. Consequently, allopurinol is not considered standard therapy.

Finasteride, a 5-α-reductase inhibitor, has been investigated in chronic prostatitis and CPPS. A small, inadequately powered, pilot study revealed that finasteride was superior to placebo in decreasing the Prostatitis Symptom Severity Index and prostatism scores.[59] Although these initial results were promising, treatment with finasteride remains experimental.[60]

Smooth muscle relaxants have been studied as therapy in chronic prostatitis and CPPS. Baclofen demonstrated superiority to placebo in a small study of 27 patients who received either baclofen, phenoxybenzamine, or placebo[61] and is sometimes used as therapy. Diazepam is utilized as therapy[29] despite a lack of evidence to support its use.

With growing patient and physician frustration with 'traditional' medical therapies, phytotherapeutic agents have been explored as a therapeutic option for chronic prostatitis and CPPS patients. A bee pollen extract, Cernilton, has been assessed in non-placebo-controlled studies,[62,63] with patients experiencing subjective improvement. Another phytotherapeutic agent, Quercetin, a natural bioflavonoid, was studied in a small placebo-controlled study.[64] The authors concluded that this agent was effective in reducing symptoms in most patients. Saw palmetto, a herbal therapy often used to treat BPH, is currently being studied by the authors to determine its effectiveness in patients with chronic prostatitis and CPPS.

Physical and surgical therapies

Prostatic massage once comprised the major therapeutic modality for patients with chronic prostatitis and CPPS. Its use declined with the advent of antibiotics and the implementation of the Meares–Stamey localization test. Theoretically, prostatic massage is effective by clearing obstructed prostatic ducts. Recently this therapy has been revisited, undoubtedly due to the ineffectiveness of other therapies in many patients. Initial results in uncontrolled studies combining repetitive prostatic massage and antibiotic therapy are promising.[65,66]

Minimally invasive therapies have been investigated for use in patients who fail medical and more conservative treatments. Despite initial promising results[67,68] transurethral needle ablation of the prostate was equivalent to a sham operation in further studies.[69] Balloon dilatation of the prostate has been explored as therapy with initial results suggesting improvement in urinary symptoms.[70] Combining balloon dilatation with heat therapy did not improve patient symptoms, and had adverse effects in many.[71] Balloon dilatation is not currently used as therapy. Microwave thermotherapy, delivered via the transrectal or transurethral approach, has been investigated for use in patients with refractory symptoms.[38,72,73] Although initial results have been promising, this therapy remains a treatment of last resort.

Surgery does not play a role in the treatment of prostatitis and CPPS and should be avoided unless used to correct associated and clearly reversible conditions. There is currently no evidence to support the use of surgery for cure in this condition.

Supportive therapy

Until an effective medical or surgical cure is discovered for chronic prostatitis and CPPS, alternative forms of treatment will continue to be explored as therapeutic options. The variety of such therapies that exists is a testament to the frustration experienced by both patients with this condition and physicians who are trying to treat them. In this section, we will discuss some of the supportive therapies that are available to assist with treatment of this bothersome condition.

Biofeedback is a training technique in which people are taught to improve their health and certain behaviours by using signals from their own bodies, and then altering an action or behaviour based on these signals. In patients with CPPS, biofeedback and pelvic floor muscle re-education can provide an effective and durable decrease in symptoms.[74,75] Using urodynamic studies, patients with the diagnosis of category IIIB prostatitis (CPPS) who had failed antibiotic therapy were actually found to have non-relaxation of their urinary sphincter during urination. After 6 months, biofeedback and behavioural therapy was effective in decreasing symptoms in 83% of patients.[76]

A recent pilot study to assess the role of acupuncture in chronic prostatitis and CPPS demonstrated promising results, with no untoward effects.[77] Other modalities that may be explored include massage therapy, lifestyle modification, relaxation exercises, and sitting on soft or ringed cushions to remove perineal pressure.[4]

Treatment plans

The treatment of chronic prostatitis and CPPS requires patience and understanding by both the physician and patient. In the absence of a reliable single therapy, frustration can quickly develop and compromise the physician–patient relationship. Quite often, patients may require multimodal therapy to gain relief from their symptoms. This therapeutic approach has been demonstrated to be an effective treatment method using a step-wise approach based on current literature.[78] Using this study and the result of current literature discussed previously, a logical approach to the treatment of chronic prostatitis and CPPS can be formulated.

Category II prostatitis

Patient with category II prostatitis should receive antimicrobial therapy (trimethoprim/sulfamethoxazole 160/800 mg twice daily for 12 weeks or ciprofloxacin 500 mg twice daily for 4 to 6 weeks) as initial therapy. For patients with recurrent infections, daily, long-term prophylaxis as described previously can be instituted. These patients may benefit from the addition of an alpha-blocker to their antibiotic therapy.[53] Repetitive prostatic massage is an acceptable, yet unproven, adjunctive therapy.

Category IIIA/IIIB prostatitis

The overall goal of therapy in patients with chronic prostatitis/CPPS is to improve the quality of life experienced by the patient. Complete cure of symptoms is elusive, and the goals of therapy should be discussed and clarified between patient and physician to minimize frustration. Use of a questionnaire, such as the NIH-CPSI, to track a patient's symptoms after instituting a therapy is a valuable addition to a therapeutic regimen.

Most patients with chronic prostatitis/CPPS will receive antimicrobials as outlined for category II prostatitis as initial therapy, despite the absence of bacteria in localization studies. This seems reasonable based on the results discussed previously. Consideration can be given to antimicrobials that are effective for cryptic organisms such as *Chlamydia* and *Ureaplasma* at the discretion of the treating physician. If patients do not respond to antimicrobial therapy, further courses of antibiotics should not be utilized. In refractory cases, alpha-blockers, anti-inflammatory agents (including pentosan polysulfate), and a short course of analgesics can be utilized. Other medications, which may be considered in refractory patients, include finasteride, phytotherapy, baclofen, and diazepam. All of these medications may be utilized in conjunction with repetitive prostatic massage, biofeedback, pelvic floor massage, and lifestyle modification. Surgery should be avoided.

Conclusion

Chronic prostatitis and CPPS are common conditions manifested by urinary and sexual symptoms plus pelvic pain. The majority of cases are not caused by a proven infection. The origin of non-infectious cases has not been elucidated, although it is most likely caused by a combination of factors. It presents in men of all age groups and ethnicities, significantly decreasing the quality of life of afflicted individuals. This condition is frequently refractory to therapy, creating a challenge for physicians and causing frustration for patients and physicians. A multimodal approach to therapy is often necessary to alleviate a patient's symptoms; the goal of therapy is often 'cope', not 'cure'.

References

1 Moon TD (1997). Questionnaire survey of urologists and primary care physicians' diagnostic and treatment practices for prostatitis. *Urology* **50**(4): 543–7.

2 Roberts RO, Jacobson DJ, Girman CJ, Rhodes T, Lieber MM, Jacobsen SJ (2002). Prevalence of prostatitis-like symptoms in a community based cohort of older men. *J. Urol.* **168**(6): 2467–71.

3 Collins MM, Stafford RS, O'Leary MP, Barry MJ (1998). How common is prostatitis? A national survey of physician visits. *J. Urol.* **159**(4): 1224–8.

4 Nickel JC (1999). Prostatitis: evolving management strategies. *Urol. Clin. North Am.* **26**(4): 737–51.

5 Campbell MF (1957). *Principles of Urology: an Introductory Text to the Diseases of the Urogenital Tract.* W. B. Saunders, Philadelphia, PA.

6 Meares EM, Stamey TA (1968). Bacteriologic localization patterns in bacterial prostatitis and urethritis. *Invest. Urol.* **5**(5): 492–518.

7 Nickel J (2002). Prostatitis and related conditions. In: *Campbell's Urology*, 8th edn (ed. P Walsh), pp. 603–30. W. B. Saunders, Philadelphia, PA.

8 Riegel P, Ruimy R, de Briel D, Prevost G, Jehl F, Bimet F *et al.* (1995). *Corynebacterium seminale* sp. nov., a new species associated with genital infections in male patients. *J. Clin. Microbiol.* **33**(9): 2244–9.

9 Mardh P, Colleen S, Holmquist B (1972). Chlamydia in chronic prostatitis. *Br. Med. J.* **4**(836): 361.

10 Fish DN, Danziger LH (1993). Antimicrobial treatment for chronic prostatitis as a means of defining the role of *Ureaplasma urealyticum. Urol. Int.* **51**: 129–32.

11 Domingue GJ Sr, Hellstrom WJ (1998). Prostatitis. *Clin. Microbiol. Rev.* **11**(4): 604–13.

12 Barbalias GA, Meares EM Jr, Sant GR (1983). Prostatodynia: clinical and urodynamic characteristics. *J. Urol.* **130**(3): 514–17.

13 Blacklock NJ (91974). Anatomical factors in prostatitis. *Br. J. Urol.* **46**(1): 47–54.

14 Kirby RS, Lowe D, Bultitude MI, Shuttleworth KE (1982). Intra-prostatic urinary reflux: an aetiological factor in abacterial prostatitis. *Br. J. Urol.* **54**(6): 729–31.

15 Persson BE, Ronquist G (1996). Evidence for a mechanistic association between nonbacterial prostatitis and levels of urate and creatinine in expressed prostatic secretion. *J. Urol.* **155**(3): 958–60.

16 Kumon H (1992). Detection of a local prostatic immune response to bacterial prostatitis. *Infection* **20**(Suppl. 3): S236–S238.

17 Doble A, Walker MM, Harris JR, Taylor-Robinson D, Witherow RO (1990). Intraprostatic antibody deposition in chronic abacterial prostatitis. *Br. J. Urol.* **65**(6): 598–605.

18 de la Rosette JJ, Ruijgrok MC, Jeuken JM, Karthaus HF, Debruyne FM (1993). Personality variables involved in chronic prostatitis. *Urology* **42**(6): 654–62.

19 Berghuis JP, Heiman JR, Rothman I, Berger RE (1996). Psychological and physical factors involved in chronic idiopathic prostatitis. *J. Psychosom. Res.* **41**(4): 313–25.

20 Egan KJ, Krieger JN (1994). Psychological problems in chronic prostatitis patients with pain. *Clin. J. Pain* **10**(3): 218–26.

21 Sant GR, Nickel JC (1999). Interstitial cystitis in chronic prostatitis: the same syndrome? In: *Textbook of Prostatitis*, (ed. JC Nickel), pp. 169–76. ISIS Medical Media, Oxford.

22 Zermann DH, Ishigooka M, Doggweiler R, Schmidt RA (1999). Neurourological insights into the etiology of genitourinary pain in men. *J. Urol.* **161**(3): 903–8.

23 Nickel JC, Alexander RB, Schaeffer AJ, Landis JR, Knauss JS, Propert KJ (2003). Leukocytes and bacteria in men with chronic prostatitis/chronic pelvic pain syndrome compared to asymptomatic controls. *J. Urol.* **170**(3): 818–22.

24 Nickel JC, Downey J, Johnston B, Clark J, Group TC (2001). Predictors of patient response to antibiotic therapy for the chronic prostatitis/chronic pelvic pain syndrome: a prospective multicenter clinical trial. *J. Urol.* **165**(5): 1539–44.

25 Wright ET, Chmiel JS, Grayhack JT, Schaeffer AJ (1994). Prostatic fluid inflammation in prostatitis. *J. Urol.* **152**(6, Pt 2): 2300–3.

26 Weidner W, Ludwig M (1994). Diagnostic management of chronic prostatitis. In: *Prostatitis— Etiopathololgy, Diagnosis and Therapy* (ed. W Weidner, PO Madsen, HG Schiefer), pp. 158–74. Springer, Berlin.

27 Schaeffer AJ (2002). Classification (traditional and National Institutes of Health) and demographics of prostatitis. *Urology* **60**(6, Suppl.): 5–6; discussion 6–7.

28 Krieger JN, Ross SO, Penson DF, Riley DE (2002). Symptoms and inflammation in chronic prostatitis/chronic pelvic pain syndrome. *Urology* **60**(6): 959–63.

29 Lobel B, Rodriguez A (2003). Chronic prostatitis: what we know, what we do not know, and what we should do! *World J. Urol.* **21**(2): 57–63.

30 Wenninger K, Heiman JR, Rothman I, Berghuis JP, Berger RE (1996). Sickness impact of chronic nonbacterial prostatitis and its correlates. *J. Urol.* **155**(3): 965–8.

31 McNaughton Collins M, Pontari MA, O'Leary MP, Calhoun EA, Santanna J, Landis JR *et al.* (2001). Quality of life is impaired in men with chronic prostatitis: the Chronic Prostatitis Collaborative Research Network. *J. Gen. Intern. Med.* **16**(10): 656–62.

32 Keltikangas-Jarvinen L, Jarvinen H, Lehtonen T (1981). Psychic disturbances in patients with chronic prostatis. *Ann. Clin. Res.* **13**(1): 45–9.

33 Potts JM (2003). Chronic pelvic pain syndrome: a non-prostatocentric perspective. *World J. Urol.* **21**(2): 54–6.

34 Nickel JC (2002). Clinical evaluation of the man with chronic prostatitis/chronic pelvic pain syndrome. *Urology* **60**(6, Suppl.): 20–2; discussion 22–3.

35 McNaughton Collins M, Fowler FJ Jr, Elliott DB, Albertsen PC, Barry MJ (2000). Diagnosing and treating chronic prostatitis: do urologists use the four-glass test? *Urology* **55**(3): 403–7.

36 Nickel JC (1997). The Pre and Post Massage Test (PPMT): a simple screen for prostatitis. *Tech. Urol.* **3**(1): 38–43.

37 Neal DE Jr, Moon TD (1994). Use of terazosin in prostatodynia and validation of a symptom score questionnaire. *Urology* **43**(4): 460–5.

38 Nickel JC, Sorensen R (1996). Transurethral microwave thermotherapy for nonbacterial prostatitis: a randomized double-blind sham controlled study using new prostatitis specific assessment questionnaires. *J. Urol.* **155**(6): 1950–4; discussion 1954–5.

39 Litwin MS, McNaughton-Collins M, Fowler FJ Jr, Nickel JC, Calhoun EA, Pontari MA *et al.* (1999). The National Institutes of Health chronic prostatitis symptom index: development and validation of a new outcome measure. Chronic Prostatitis Collaborative Research Network. *J. Urol.* **162**(2): 369–75.

40 Fowler JE Jr (2002). Antimicrobial therapy for bacterial and nonbacterial prostatitis. *Urology* **60**(6, Suppl.): 24–6; discussion 26.

41 Naber KJ (1999). Antibiotic treatment of chronic bacterial prostatitis. In: *Textbook of Prostatitis* (ed. JC Nickel), pp. 283–92. ISIS Medical Media, Oxford.

42 Weidner W, Schiefer HG, Brahler E (1991). Refractory chronic bacterial prostatitis: a re-evaluation of ciprofloxacin treatment after a median followup of 30 months. *J. Urol.* **146**(2): 350–2.

43 Schaeffer AJ, Darras FS (1990). The efficacy of norfloxacin in the treatment of chronic bacterial prostatitis refractory to trimethoprim-sulfamethoxazole and/or carbenicillin. *J. Urol.* **144**(3): 690–3.

44 de la Rosette JJ, Hubregtse MR, Meuleman EJ, Stolk-Engelaar MV, Debruyne FM (1993). Diagnosis and treatment of 409 patients with prostatitis syndromes. *Urology* **41**(4): 301–7.

45 Ohkawa M, Yamaguchi K, Tokunaga S, Nakashima T, Shoda R (1993). Antimicrobial treatment for chronic prostatitis as a means of defining the role of *Ureaplasma urealyticum*. *Urol. Int.* **51**(3): 129–32.

46 Dunzendorfer U, Kruschwitz K, Letzel H (1983). Effects of phenoxybenzamine on clinical picture. laboratory test results and spermatogram in chronic abacterial prostatitis. *Therapiewoche* **33**: 4694–705.

47 Dunzendorfer U (1981). Alpha-difluoromethylornithine (alpha DFMO) and phenoxybenzamine hydrochloride in the treatment of chronic non-suppurative prostatitis. *Arzneimittelforschung* **31**(2): 382–5.

48 Kaneko S, Minami K, Yachiku S, Kurita T (1980). Bladder neck dysfunction: the effect of the alpha-adrenergic blocking agent phentolamine on bladder neck dysfunction and a fluorescent histochemical study of bladder neck smooth muscle. *Invest. Urol.* **18**(3): 212–18.

49 de la Rosette JJ, Karthaus HF, van Kerrebroeck PE, de Boo T, Debruyne FM (1992). Research in 'prostatitis syndromes': the use of alfuzosin (a new alpha 1-receptor-blocking agent) in patients mainly presenting with micturition complaints of an irritative nature and confirmed urodynamic abnormalities. *Eur. Urol.* **22**(3): 222–7.

50 Cheah PY, Liong ML, Yuen KH, Teh CL, Khor T, Yang JR *et al.* (2003). Terazosin therapy for chronic prostatitis/chronic pelvic pain syndrome: a randomized, placebo controlled trial. *J. Urol.* **169**(2): 592–6.

51 Lacquaniti S, Destito A, Servello C, Candidi MO, Weir JM, Brisinda G *et al.* (1999). Terazosine and tamsulosin in non bacterial prostatitis: a randomized placebo-controlled study. *Arch. Ital. Urol. Androl.* **71**(5): 283–5.

52 Nickel JC, Narayan P, McKay J, Doyle C (2004). Treatment of chronic prostatitis/chronic pelvic pain syndrome with tamsulosin: a randomized double blind trial. *J. Urol.* **171**(4): 1594–7.

53 Barbalias GA, Nikiforidis G, Liatsikos EN (1998). Alpha-blockers for the treatment of chronic prostatitis in combination with antibiotics. *J. Urol.* **159**(3): 883–7.

54 Canale D, Turchi P, Giorgi PM, Scaricabarozzi I, Menchini-Fabris GF (1993). Treatment of abacterial prostato-vesiculitis with nimesulide. *Drugs* **46**(Suppl. 1): 147–50.

55 Canale D, Scaricabarozzi I, Giorgi P, Turchi P, Ducci M, Menchini-Fabris GF (1993). Use of a novel non-steroidal anti-inflammatory drug, nimesulide, in the treatment of abacterial prostatovesiculitis. *Andrologia* **25**(3): 163–6.

56 Nickel JC, Pontari M, Moon T, Gittelman M, Malek G, Farrington J *et al.* (2003). A randomized, placebo controlled, multicenter study to evaluate the safety and efficacy of rofecoxib in the treatment of chronic nonbacterial prostatitis. *J. Urol.* **169**(4): 1401–5.

57 Wedren H (1987). Effects of sodium pentosanpolysulphate on symptoms related to chronic non-bacterial prostatitis. A double-blind randomized study. *Scand. J. Urol. Nephrol.* **21**(2): 81–8.

58 Persson BE, Ronquist G, Ekblom M (1996). Ameliorative effect of allopurinol on nonbacterial prostatitis: a parallel double-blind controlled study. *J. Urol.* **155**(3): 961–4.

59 Leskinen M, Lukkarinen O, Marttila T (1999). Effects of finasteride in patients with inflammatory chronic pelvic pain syndrome: a double-blind, placebo-controlled, pilot study. *Urology* **53**(3): 502–5.

60 Batstone GR, Doble A, Batstone D (2003). Chronic prostatitis. *Curr. Opin. Urol.* **13**(1): 23–9.

61 Osborn DE, George NJ, Rao PN, Barnard RJ, Reading C, Marklow C *et al.* (1981). Prostatodynia—physiological characteristics and rational management with muscle relaxants. *Br. J. Urol.* **53**(6): 621–3.

62 Buck AC, Rees RW, Ebeling L (1989). Treatment of chronic prostatitis and prostatodynia with pollen extract. *Br. J. Urol.* **64**(5): 496–9.

63 Rugendorff EW, Weidner W, Ebeling L, Buck AC (1993). Results of treatment with pollen extract (Cernilton N) in chronic prostatitis and prostatodynia. *Br. J. Urol.* **71**(4): 433–8.

64 Shoskes DA, Zeitlin SI, Shahed A, Rajfer J (1999). Quercetin in men with category III chronic prostatitis: a preliminary prospective, double-blind, placebo-controlled trial. *Urology* **54**(6): 960–3.

65 Nickel JC, Downey J, Feliciano AE Jr, Hennenfent B (1999). Repetitive prostatic massage therapy for chronic refractory prostatitis: the Philippine experience. *Tech. Urol.* **5**(3): 146–51.

66 Shoskes DA, Zeitlin SI (1999). Use of prostatic massage in combination with antibiotics in the treatment of chronic prostatitis. *Prostate Cancer Prostatic Dis.* **2**(3): 159–62.

67 Chiang PH, Tsai EM, Chiang CP (1997). Pilot study of transurethral needle ablation (TUNA) in treatment of nonbacterial prostatitis. *J. Endourol.* **11**(5): 367–70.

68 Lee KC, Jung PB, Park HS, Whang JH, Lee JG (2002). Transurethral needle ablation for chronic nonbacterial prostatitis. *BJU Int.* **89**(3): 226–9.

69 Leskinen MJ, Kilponen A, Lukkarinen O, Tammela TL (2002). Transurethral needle ablation for the treatment of chronic pelvic pain syndrome (category III prostatitis): a randomized, sham-controlled study. *Urology* **60**(2): 300–4.

70 Lopatin WB, Martynik M, Hickey DP, Vivas C, Hakala TR (1990). Retrograde transurethral balloon dilation of prostate: innovative management of abacterial chronic prostatitis and prostatodynia. *Urology* **36**(6): 508–10.

71 Nickel JC, Siemens DR, Johnston B (1998). Transurethral radiofrequency hot balloon thermal therapy in chronic nonbacterial prostatitis. *Tech. Urol.* **4**(3): 128–30.

72 Liatsikos EN, Dinlenc CZ, Kapoor R, Smith AD (2000). Transurethral microwave thermotherapy for the treatment of prostatitis. *J. Endourol.* **14**(8): 689–92.

73 Choi NG, Soh SH, Yoon TH, Song MH (1994). Clinical experience with transurethral microwave thermotherapy for chronic nonbacterial prostatitis and prostatodynia. *J. Endourol.* **8**(1): 61–4.

74 Clemens JQ, Nadler RB, Schaeffer AJ, Belani J, Albaugh J, Bushman W (2000). Biofeedback, pelvic floor re-education, and bladder training for male chronic pelvic pain syndrome. *Urology* **56**(6): 951–5.

75 Nadler RB (2002). Bladder training biofeedback and pelvic floor myalgia. *Urology* **60**(6, Suppl.):42–3; discussion 44.

76 Kaplan SA, Santarosa RP, D'Alisera PM, Fay BJ, Ikeguchi EF, Hendricks J *et al.* (1997). Pseudodyssynergia (contraction of the external sphincter during voiding) misdiagnosed as chronic nonbacterial prostatitis and the role of biofeedback as a therapeutic option. *J. Urol.* **157**(6): 2234–7.

77 Chen R, Nickel JC (2003). Acupuncture ameliorates symptoms in men with chronic prostatitis/chronic pelvic pain syndrome. *Urology* **61**(6): 1156–9; discussion 1159.

78 Shoskes DA, Hakim L, Ghoniem G, Jackson CL (2003). Long-term results of multimodal therapy for chronic prostatitis/chronic pelvic pain syndrome. *J. Urol.* **169**(4): 1406–10.

Chapter 17

The patient presenting with genitourinary AIDS

Paul Toren and Wendy Wobeser

Introduction

Care for the HIV/AIDS patient is a rapidly evolving area of medicine, with guidelines and drugs frequently being updated as knowledge of the disease progresses. With the success of highly active antiretroviral therapy (HAART), care for HIV-infected persons has become increasingly long-term. Yet, despite many advances, AIDS is still without a cure. To the health-care professional, care for an HIV/AIDS patient presents many challenges because:

- living with HIV/AIDS is difficult
- atypical presentations of disease are common
- co-morbid illness can be masked by immunosuppression
- the severity of illness is often greater than expected
- increasingly, drug interactions and side-effects of antiretroviral therapy are being recognized.

A team approach to management, with involvement of multiple other physicians and health-care professionals, is essential for the highest quality of care. This chapter will focus on several long-term conditions which may exist in the course of treatment of HIV/AIDS including genitourinary infections and neoplasms and androgen deficiency, as well issues of incontinence, erectile dysfunction, stones, and nephropathy related to the HIV virus and its various treatments.

Epidemiology

Traditionally, care for the HIV-infected patient tended to include several different sociodemographic groups, varying widely according to region: men who have sex with men (MSM), intravenous drug users, persons originating from countries with a high rate of HIV, and heterosexual contacts with other high-risk groups. Increasingly, HIV is less confined to certain segments of the population, with the largest relative increase occurring in women and heterosexuals.[1]

Worldwide, approximately 40 million people are infected with HIV, with 5 million new cases in 2003. An estimated 60–70% of cases occur in sub-Saharan Africa.[1] The transmission of HIV mainly occurs through sexual transmission or sharing of contaminated needles. Contact with infected blood also poses a risk for transmission, although the risk in the developed world is exceedingly low. The generally accepted rate of seroconversion in a needlestick injury is 0.3%.[2] The strain of the virus, co-infection with sexually transmitted diseases (STDs), barrier protection, viral load, sexual practices, and treatment with HAART all affect the risk of transmission.[3–5]

Diagnosis

A seroconversion illness occurs in about a third to a half of persons infected with HIV. This typically occurs within 3–4 weeks of infection and manifests as a severe febrile illness with or without lympadenopathy, skin rash, and aseptic meningitis. Early in the infection (<3 months), HIV is diagnosed by the presence of HIV-1 RNA in the blood. Later in the disease, antibody levels to virus antigens may be measured more reliably.[6] Testing for HIV infection requires pre- and post-test counselling. Clinical presentation or risk factors cannot reliably predict HIV infection; however, certain illnesses may raise a flag, such as oral thrush, shingles in persons less than 50 years of age, and other sexually transmitted diseases.

Receiving the diagnosis of HIV is understandably very difficult for patients. As well as the possibility of a shortened lifespan, all HIV patients are faced with the adaptive challenges of coping with a stigmatizing illness, adopting strategies for maintaining physical and emotional health, and initiating behavioural changes to prevent transmission of HIV to others.[7] Research has shown that older patients diagnosed with HIV, in contrast to the typical reaction for other chronic diseases, are more prone to maladaptive coping strategies.[8] Therefore, referral of patients to proper counselling services is very important in the management of HIV-infected patients. The availability of HIV-oriented supportive services varies with hospital and sociogeographical factors. Counselling is important both for the quality of life of the individual and prevention of further spread of the disease. Intensive HIV prevention interventions, drug abuse counselling, safe sex education, mental health services, or social services referral may be appropriate, according to the patient's circumstances and motivation. The positive impact of appropriate social, psychological, and spiritual care on quality of life in HIV patients has been well established.[8]

Management

Clinical manifestations of HIV infection include susceptibility to opportunistic infections, certain associated cancers, cachexia and muscle wasting, and HIV-associated dementia. The impact of advanced AIDS on lowering quality of life has been shown to be greater than other chronic diseases such as depression and cancer.[8]

Antiretroviral therapy has increased the life expectancy and quality of life for HIV-infected patients significantly. HAART drastically reduces HIV levels in the blood and slows progression of the disease. It typically consists of various combinations of three

Box 17.1 **Case study 1**

A 39-year-old male presents to your office complaining of a persistent chancre on his penis. History reveals that he had been travelling in southeast Asia for the last 3 months. He admits to having had unprotected intercourse on several occasion with sex-workers there. He also admits a long history of using intravenous drugs. Following his return to Canada, he describes being sick with the flu for a week. The physical exam reveals a hard, well-defined painless chancre on the dorsal penis suggestive of primary syphilis. An IgA fluorescent treponemal antibody (FTA) absorption test is performed as well as Venereal Disease Research Laboratory (VDRL) and rapid plasmin reagin (RPR) titres. He is treated empirically with intramuscular benzathine pencillin.

You ask him if he has ever been tested for HIV. He responds that he prefers to be ignorant, even though he realizes he might have HIV. After listening to his concerns and past experiences with friends who died of AIDS, you discuss with him that there have been many advances in the management of HIV infection so that the life expectancy and quality of life for HIV patients has significantly improved. Further, you explain that you will be available to follow-up his care, regardless of test results. You discuss with him the ramifications of a positive result. He agrees for testing to be done.

Results for both syphilis and HIV tests return positive. Treatment for syphilis successfully resolves his initial symptoms. Repeat enzyme-linked immunosorbent assay (ELISA) testing and a Western blot confirm the HIV diagnosis. He is devastated by the diagnosis and becomes depressed and suicidal. You refer him to a psychiatrist with experience with AIDS patients. His depression improves, and he subsequently undergoes a concentrated drug rehabilitation course.

---

antiviral classes: protease inhibitors, nucleoside transcription inhibitors, and non-nucleotide transcription inhibitors. Fusion inhibitors may also be used. Improvements in pharmacokinetics have considerably reduced the number of pills that need to be taken per day.

Genitourinary infections

Screening for STDs

Sexually transmitted diseases are very common in HIV-infected persons. Current American recommendations[9] for the initial visit of a patient who has tested positive for HIV recommend screening for syphilis in men and women, *Trichomonas* in women, and cervical chlamydia in women ≤ 25 years old. Consideration for screening for chlamydia and gonorrhoea should also be given for both men and women, taking into account the prevalence of the infection, availability of the test, cost, as well as patient factors. Some

Table 17.1 Laboratory tests and their indications for selected sexually transmitted diseases[7,12]

STD	Indication	Test
Syphilis	Screening	VDRL, RPR, *Treponema pallidum* haemagglutionation (TPHA)
	Diagnosis/confirmation	Dark field examination. IgA fluorescence Treponema antibody absorption test (IgA FTA-Abs) or 19-S IgM FTA-Abs test
	Follow-up	VDRL or 19-S IgM FTA-Abs-test at 3, 6, 12 months and annually for 4 years
Herpes	Diagnosis	Viral culture. Type analysis by immunofluorescence
Trichomoniasis	Diagnosis	Microscopic examination of wet mount or culture of vaginal secretions
Gonorrhoea	Screening	Microscopic examination and Gram stain
	Diagnosis/confirmation	Culture of intraurethral/endocervical swab. NAAT of swab or urine (less sensitive)
	Follow-up	Unnecessary; culture for resistance organisms in patients with persistent symptoms
Chancroid	Diagnosis	Gram stain and culture; PCR available
Donovanosis	Diagnosis	Gram stain; culture difficult
Lymphogranuloma venereum	Diagnosis	Fluorescence antibody test (FTA); special culture needed
Chlamydia (less sensitive)	Screening/diagnosis	NAAT of intraurethral/endocervical swab or urine

Abbreviations: VDRL, Venereal Disease Research Laboratory; RPR, rapid plasmin reagin; NAAT, nucleic acid amplification test; PCR, polymerase chain reaction.

specialists also recommend screening for Herpes simplex virus 2. Testing should be repeated periodically (e.g. once a year) in patients who are sexually active, and more frequently (e.g. every 3–6 months) in patients whose lifestyle puts them at greater risk (Table 17.1).

Sexually transmitted diseases which cause genital ulceration or mucosal inflammation have clearly been shown to increase rates of transmissions of HIV.[10,11] The physiological mechanisms by which STDs enhance HIV transmission include increased concentration of HIV in genital secretions, number of cells receptive to HIV, and number of receptors per cell.[4]

Genital ulcers

Herpes simplex virus (HSV) is a very common, and unfortunately incurable, cause of genital ulcers. HSV-2 represents approximately 70% of cases, HSV-1 the remaining 30%.[12] HIV-infected persons have a considerably higher seroprevalence of HSV-2.[13]

HSV-2 tends to be more recurrent and tends to account for more genital ulcers than HSV-1, which predominantly manifests as oral ulcers but is increasingly found in genital ulcers.[12]

In HIV-infected patients the ulcers tend to recur more frequently and severely as the immune system becomes weakened. The frequency of HSV shedding and ulceration is increased in HIV-infected patients, but varies considerably among patients with similar CD4+ cell counts.[13] Diagnosis can be confirmed with fluorescence staining and culture of swabs or biopsy specimens.

Treatment is aimed at symptom relief, as even in healthy people herpes is incurable. In persons with HIV the recurrence rate of herpes and the possibility that recurrences may induce HIV replication and disease progression justifies the utilization of chronic suppressive therapy. The usual dose of acyclovir is 400 mg b.i.d., although higher doses are sometimes required. New generation antiherpes therapies (e.g. valacyclovir and famcyclovir) may reduce tablet burden in those requiring higher doses. Resistance of the herpes virus to these drugs is uncommon but is most likely to occur in persons with HIV.

Other STDs may also present with genitourinary ulcers, although these are uncommon in North America. Chancroid (*Hemophilus ducreyi*) presents with painful ulcers and bubo formation. 'Pseudobubo' formation, lymphoedema, and local fibrosis herald donovanosis (*Calymmatobacterium granulomatis*). Lymphogranuloma venereum (L1,2,3 serovars of *Chlamydia trachomatis*) is very rare in the developed world and tends to mimic other STDs and occur in small outbreaks.

Genital warts

Genital warts are the most common sexually transmitted disease in the world,[12] and are most commonly caused by human papilloma virus (HPV). HIV-infected patients are more likely to be infected with HPV than the general population.[14,15] The estimated prevalence of HPV in HIV-infected MSM is >85%, 57–70% in HIV-infected women[13] and 26–60% in HIV-infected heterosexual men.[16]

Treatment is difficult, as recurrence is common, and is aimed at improving cosmesis and symptoms.[17] Medical management includes podophyllin or podophylotoxin. Imiquimod as a 5% cream has the advantage that it is self-administered three times a week for a couple of months. Its efficacy is reduced substantially in HIV patients not treated by HAART.[18] Although very toxic, cidofovir may be useful in resistant and recurrent cases.[16] The mechanism of action of cidofovir is not specific for HPV, and thus it has the added benefit that it also acts against other DNA viruses, including cytomegalovirus (CMV), HSV, and molluscum contagiosum.[16]

Cryotherapy is the preferred non-medical treatment option. Application of 5% acetic acid can be topically applied to facilitate visualization of warts on mucosal surfaces.[17] CO_2 laser can be used, although there is concern that this form of therapy may spread microscopic droplets of virus.

Human papilloma virus is of concern because of its oncogenic properties. Common, low-risk strains include 6 and 11, whereas 16, 18, 31 and 33 are associated with higher rates of malignancy.[17] HPV may induce transformation of epithelial cells to squamous cell carcinoma (SCC) *in situ* (Bowen's disease) or invasive SCC in both men and women. The incidence of penile or labial Bowen's disease is increased in HIV-infected patients.[19] Bowen's papulosis is a benign tumour than can be difficult to differentiate clinically and pathologically from Bowen's disease. It is also strongly associated with HPV.[20] Treatments for benign and malignant lesions are comparable to genital warts, ranging from excision, cryotherapy, to topical application of fluorouracil (5-FU) or cidofovir.[20]

Urinary tract infections

Overall, urinary tract infections (UTIs) are reported to occur more commonly in HIV-infected patients.[3,21] As expected, the frequency increases with severity of the disease, but even asymptomatic HIV-infected patients have a higher incidence than the general population.[21] HAART has decreased this incidence.[22] The aetiological bacteria are more commonly *Enterococcus* spp. in HIV-infected patients than the ubiquitous *Escherichia coli* in the general population. *Pseudomonas aeruginosa* is found in approximately 15–30% of HIV-infected patients with UTIs.[21,23] *Gardnerella vaginalis* and *Trichomonas* spp. are two sexually transmitted organisms that tend to only be symptomatic in women.[12] Patients on prophylactic antibiotics due to low CD4+ cell counts should be assumed to have bacteria resistant to drugs similar to the prophylactic antibiotics.

Chlamydia trachomatis and *Neisseria gonorrhea* cause similar symptoms in the HIV-infected patient as in the general population with dysuria and urethral discharge, varying in purulence. Their prevalence in the HIV-positive population has been found to be comparable to a sociodemographically similar community sample.[12] Evidence supports empirical treatment of both organisms, as concomitant infection is found in 20–40% of cases.[7,24] Evaluation and treatment of sexual partners is also indicated. Recommended treatment consists of 1 g azithromycin by mouth as a single dose to cover chlamydia and 1 g intramuscular ceftriaxone for gonorrhoea.[7] A microbiological test of cure is not needed unless the patient's symptoms persist.[19]

A correlation between Reiter's syndrome and HIV has been noted.[25,26] Its prevalence in HIV-positive patients has been estimated at 1.7–11.2%.[26] Reiter's syndrome is a seronegative spondyloarthropathy that consists of the triad of urethritis, arthritis, and haemorrhagic conjunctivitis, as well as other features such as balanitis circinata. The severity and progression are both increased in AIDS patients, and it is often refractory to treatment. It is commonly associated with *C. trachomatis* infection, but other organisms may also be responsible. Diagnosis of the causative organism is the same as for isolated urethritis with the addition of a rheumatological work-up. Ophthalmological referral may also be needed. Treatment with tetracyclines shows improvement in cases

Box 17.2 **Case study 2 (modified from Studmeister[28])**

A 43-year-old female presents with gross haematuria, urinary urgency, and suprapubic pain. She has a mild fever. Twelve years ago she was diagnosed with HIV and she has been on HAART since 1997. Her most recent CD4+ cell count was 190 cells/μl. AIDS was diagnosed 6 months ago following diagnosis of non-Hodgkin's lymphoma for which she finished her third cycle of chemotherapy 6 days ago.

Protein, leucocytes, and red blood cells are seen on urinalysis. Ultrasound shows kidneys that are normal, with no calculi observed. Blood and urine cultures return negative. A computed tomography (CT) scan of the abdomen reveals thickening of the bladder mucosa. Cystoscopy is performed showing an inflamed bladder mucosa. Biopsy shows acute inflammation and eosinophilic intranuclear inclusions within the endothelium and stroma characteristic of CMV cystitis.

She is initiated on intravenous gancyclovir and symptoms resolve in a few days. Following resolution of symptoms, she is maintained on valgancyclovir until the chemotherapy is finished.

due to *C. trachomatis*, especially where persistent antigen is fuelling the systemic inflammation, such as in the onset of HAART following persistent chlamydial infection.[27]

Viral haemorrhagic cystitis has been reported to occur occasionally in AIDS patients. Presenting symptoms are haematuria, bladder pain, fever, and urinary urgency. Aetiological agents include cytomegalovirus,[28] and to a lesser extent adenovirus[29] and JC and BK viruses.[30] These infections tend to appear to be associated with severe immunosuppression, and patients who develop these rare infections often are undergoing chemotherapy for AIDS-related lymphoma.

Prostatitis can be the result of urinary stasis and tends to occur acutely in HIV patients with very low CD4+ cell counts. Enterobacteriaceae and other Gram-negative organisms are the most common identified aetiological microorganisms.[23] Treatment with antibiotics is usually sufficient to resolve symptoms, although some infections may require surgery.

Fungal infections

Weakened cellular immunity in HIV infection results in increased susceptibility to fungal and viral infections, and typically heralds the onset of AIDS. While respiratory infections are often the most serious, genitourinary infections can also be very serious, leading to septicaemia and death. Abscesses may affect the kidneys, testes, prostate, and epididymis.

In particular, atypical aetiological organisms are more common (Fig. 17.1). Immunosuppression also results in more atypical symptoms, such as non-specific

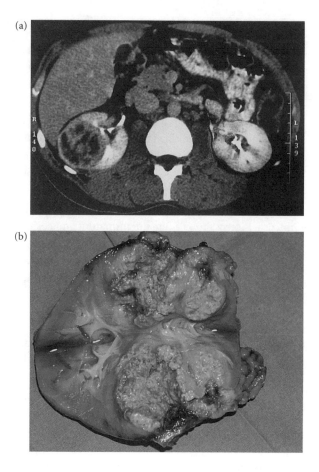

Fig. 17.1 (a) Abdominal CT scan showing a 5.5 cm heterogeneous mass in the middle of the right kidney. *Asperigillus fumigus* was identified by urine culture. This 29-year-old HIV-infected patient with normal CD4+ cell counts had recently started HAART. (b) Macroscopic specimen following right nephrectomy. (From Figs 1 and 2 in Rey D, de Mautort E, Saussine C, *et al.* (1999) *Eur. J. Clin. Microbiol. Infect. Dis.* 1 8:138–9. Copyright Springer-Verlag, with permission.)

constitutional symptoms that are difficult to distinguish from the effects of HIV and treatment. A high level of suspicion is required. Opportunistic fungal organisms that occur in the genitourinary system include *Candida*, *Aspergillus*, and *Cryptococcus*, as well as others according to locality. Fungal abscesses are usually secondary manifestations of primary infection.[23]

Treatment is challenging, as eradication of the organism can be difficult to achieve. Its success will depend upon immunological recovery. Insufficient treatment leads to persistent fungal colonization that may result in disseminated infection. On the other hand, prophylaxis with fluconazole may result in the development of resistance.[31] Thus, a careful balance between success with azoles and development of resistance must be maintained. Surgery is a good option in suitable patients when medical therapy fails.

Vulvovaginal candidiasis is a common problem in women with HIV and may be the presenting illness leading to an HIV diagnosis. However, given the incidence of recurrent vulvovaginal candidiasis in the general population, it is not a sentinel sign on which to justify HIV testing.[7] Prophylactic antibiotic use exacerbates its occurrence in HIV-infected patients. Topical therapy can be used for mild disease, whereas systemic azole therapy is required for more serious cases or in more severely immunocompromised patients.

Re-emergent infections

Once thought to be a disease of the past, syphilis is now found to be re-emerging in North America and Europe. The majority of these cases occur in men who have sex with men.[13] The most common presentation of syphilis in HIV-infected patients is that of condylomata lata, a form of secondary syphilis.[5] However, HIV-infected patients are also more likely to present with atypical presentations of syphilis, such as persistent chancres, skin ulcers, early ocular involvement, and gummatous disease.[13] It is unclear how commonly these atypical presentations of syphilis occur in the HIV population, but with HAART it seems likely that their incidence has declined. Serological tests (VDRL and RPR) are considered less reliable in persons co-infected with HIV, with significantly lower specificity.[13]

Standard treatment against *Treponema pallidum*, the causative organism, is a single dose of 2.4×10^6 units of intramuscular benzathine penicillin G for primary, secondary, and early latent syphilis (<1 year). For syphilis of unknown duration or late syphilis, three weekly doses of 2.4×10^6 units of intramuscular benzathine penicillin G are given.[13] For persons with HIV, most experts agree that early syphilis should also be treated for three successive weeks with benzathine penicillin. As with other HIV co-infections, close follow-up to monitor treatment efficacy is important.

TB is another disease that has experienced a resurgence associated with AIDS. Worldwide, one-third of all AIDS-related deaths are due to TB. HIV increases the risk of active TB by 15–30 times.[5] TB tends to develop earlier in the course of HIV disease than other opportunistic organisms. Disseminated TB disease occurs in 30–40% of cases.[5] Notably, rifampin interacts with certain protease inhibitors and non-nucleoside reverse transcriptase inhibitors (NNRTIs) and dosage needs to be adjusted.[32] TB does not commonly cause genitourinary manifestations, but should be considered, especially in patients with active TB or from countries where it is endemic.

Genitourinary neoplasms

Epidemiology

Patients with HIV are more likely to develop certain cancers. Kaposi's sarcoma (KS), intermediate or high-grade non-Hodgkin's lymphoma, and invasive cervical cancer are all currently considered AIDS-defining cancers.[33] Other cancers implicated in HIV infection are Hodgkin's disease, lung cancer, anal cancer, skin cancer, body cavity lymphoma, and testicular cancer.[34-37] Spindle cell tumours, such as leiomyosarcomas and leimyomas, occur more frequently in HIV-infected children, but not adults.[38,39] Studies do not strongly suggest an increased rate of bladder, prostate, or kidney cancer.[36,40,41]

The advent of HAART has reduced the incidence of KS and non-Hodgkin's lymphoma.[33] However, studies do not appear to support the notion that HAART also decreases incidence of non-AIDS-defining cancer.[33,36] Epidemiological studies have suggested that mild immunosuppression does not significantly increase the risk of developing cancer.[41]

Aetiology

It is difficult to correlate cancers with HIV infection or immunosuppression due to other risk factors that may be present more frequently in HIV infection, such as smoking or sexual practices. The biological mechanism by which cancers occur more frequently in HIV patients is also unclear. Several contributing theories have been proposed, including direct and indirect effects of HIV.[34,37] A role for concomitant viruses has been established in certain tumours: Epstein–Barr virus (EBV) in lymphoma, KS-associated herpesvirus (KSHV) in KS, and certain HPV strains in invasive cervical and rectal cancer, among others.[34,37] Evidence suggests that leiomyomas in HIV-infected children are due to direct infection by EBV.[39]

Kaposi's sarcoma

The AIDS-related variant of KS appears predominantly in men who have sex with men, and is associated with a more severe prognosis than other less common variants. At the outset of the AIDS epidemic KS was a common index diagnosis; now with HAART, it is often a late manifestation of AIDS.[42] Antiretroviral therapy and protease inhibitors in particular have significantly decreased the incidence of Kaposi's sarcoma in HIV-infected patients.[33,34,38,43] KSHV co-infection has been indicated as necessary, but not sufficient by itself to induce KS in HIV-infected persons.[43]

Patients may be asymptomatic for a long time. HIV-associated KS tends to be more aggressive and occur at certain body sites (e.g. the nose, mouth, and genitalia).[34] Clinically, it appears as macules or papules and progresses to small plaques or nodular lesions with a purple-brownish colour. These may spontaneously disappear as new lesions appear. Lymphoedema may also be present.[42]

Treatment must take into account the rate of tumour growth, patient symptoms, concurrent illnesses, and status of HIV infection. Kaposi's sarcoma has no definite cure. Intralesional chemotherapy is a simple and effective option. Surgical excision is not a good option, as Kaposi's sarcoma appears to be a neoplasm of vascular origin.[34] For more advanced illness, systemic chemotherapy may be considered as a palliative measure.

Testicular cancer

There is good evidence that HIV infection infers a greater risk of developing testicular cancer, particularly seminomas.[38,40,41,44,45] It is still unclear if advanced immuno-suppression is a risk factor for development of seminomas.[38,44] A recent study reports an increased incidence in Whites and men who have sex with men.[38] The odds ratio for HIV-related testicular cancer has been estimated at two to nine times that of the general population.[40]

Aggressive chemotherapy lowers mean CD4+ cell counts, necessitating prophylactic antibiotics in some cases. Nonetheless, standard treatment should be followed, given that survival rates can be the same as the HIV-negative population.[42,45] The continued use of HAART is recommended as it improves long-term survival, an important consideration given that most patients can be cured of their malignancy.[45] Special consideration needs to be given to overlapping drug toxicities and drug interactions.

Lymphoma also may originate in the testes. In particular, non-Hodgkin's lymphoma is more common, more aggressive, and more likely to be bilateral than in the general population.[23] Lymphoma may also be present in the kidneys, ureter, or urethra, causing obstructive symptoms or urinary retention. Treatment is evolving, and typically involves radiotherapy and/or chemotherapy.

Andrology

Androgen deficiency

Endocrine abnormalities are common in HIV infection. Their aetiology is often multifactorial, and may be related to opportunistic infections, HIV-associated malignancies, the virus itself, side-effects of therapy, and nutritional deficiencies.[46]

Hypogonadism is a common sequela of HIV infection, reported to occur in 29–50% of AIDS patients[47,48] and 21% of patients receiving HAART.[47] It results in a significantly compromised quality of life.[8] HIV-infected men with AIDS wasting syndrome should be screened for hypogonadism.[46] Wasting syndrome consists of loss of weight, loss of appetite, associated metabolic abnormalities, and nutritional deficiencies. With the advent of HAART, wasting syndrome appears to have declined in prevalence. Total testosterone and free or bioavailable testosterone should be measured, with bioavailable testosterone yielding the most reliable marker. Diagnosis can be made by comparing free or bioavailable testosterone levels with standard age-adjusted values. Borderline free testosterone values can be repeated to obtain an overall idea of testosterone levels.

Androgen deficiency resulting in weight loss and muscle atrophy can also occur in HIV-infected women with wasting syndrome. Clinical recognition is more difficult in women than in men. Furthermore, with insensitive assays and laboratory values not yet standardized for women, treatment is very difficult. Nevertheless, some advocate that androgen supplementation can be successfully given in women.[49,50]

Box 17.3 **Case study 3**

A 51-year-old male has been HIV positive for 12 years. In the last year he describes being very tired, amotivated, and depressed. He has also lost 15 lbs (6.8 kg) in that time. He appears cachexic and has some gynaecomastia. A complete blood count shows normal haemoglobin. Serum testosterone shows free testosterone values well below normal for his age. Luteinizing hormone (LH) and follicle-stimulating hormone (FSH) levels are increased. You discuss with him the pros and cons of testosterone therapy including the effect it will have on his libido. He is agreeable to try an intramuscular injection of testosterone and return in 2 weeks. You also encourage good nutrition and exercise to help improve his muscle mass.

Testosterone replacement therapy has been used successfully to improve symptoms of cachexia, loss of appetite, and weight loss.[46,51] In particular, lean body mass and quality of life were noted to improve significantly in a randomized, double-blind controlled study of patients with AIDS wasting syndrome.[52] A meta-analysis of six trials found that testosterone was more effective than placebo in increasing lean body mass.[53]

Some have advocated that patients with normal or borderline testosterone values should not be treated to avoid potential iatrogenic problems.[46] Concern exists over the long-term use of testosterone, but long-term studies have yet to be done in HIV-infected patients. Other recent data suggest that treatment of eugonadal persons with low body weight with testosterone may be beneficial with respect to muscle strength and quality of life[50,54] (see Chapter 13 for details on treatment options). As testosterone increases libido, safe sex education and counselling must accompany treatment to prevent sexual transmission of the disease. This is especially important, as many studies have shown that sexual risk-taking may not decline when patients are diagnosed as HIV positive.[4]

Erectile dysfunction

Sexual dysfunction has been reported to occur in approximately 30% of HIV-positive patients.[48,55,56] Studies prior to the advent of HAART suggest that advanced immunosuppression and its sequelae result in a high prevalence of sexual problems and that this may be related to declining testosterone levels.[51,57] Symptoms include difficulty maintaining erections and achieving ejaculation. Impotence may be related to psychological circumstances associated with HIV diagnosis, such as depression.[56] Studies suggest that use of protease inhibitors, especially ritonavir and saquinavir, is an independent risk factor for development of sexual dysfunction.[55,58] Protease inhibitors are metabolized by the same enzyme system as sildenafil, increasing its blood concentration. Therefore it is recommended that sildenafil should be started at 25 mg for patients on protease inhibitors and not be taken more than once in a 48-hour period.[23,56]

Micturition

Micturition problems in AIDS patients can be particularly challenging given the many complications of AIDS that are often present. Few studies have been done in this area, with most of them reporting on men who have sex with men with severely progressed AIDS.[59–61] Indeed, in one study, 43% of the patients died within 2 years (mean 8 months).[60] As the disease is increasingly representing all demographics, the proportion of women presenting with HIV-related incontinence may be expected to rise. Also, with HIV-infected patients living longer and remaining healthier than before, aetiologies identical to the general population are more likely to be seen.

Voiding dysfunction appears to become more common as the AIDS progresses. The prevalence is controversial, with estimates up to 27%.[23] Common voiding symptoms are incontinence, frequency or urgency, and acute urinary retention. Dysuria and frequency or low flow rates are less common presentations.[60]

Neurological causes are much more common than non-neurological causes.[59–61] A hyper- or hypoactive detrusor may be the first sign of opportunistic CNS infections such as cerebral toxoplasmosis and progressive multifocal leucoencephalopathy. HIV-associated dementia may also be responsible for voiding difficulties.[60,61] Peripheral demyelinating HIV-associated diseases have also been reported to cause a neurogenic bladder.[60] CMV polyradiculopathy is a rare cause of urinary retention. Clinically, it presents with back pain, proximal leg weakness, and bowel dysfunction.[62] Lumbar puncture shows polymorphonuclear pleocytosis and polymerase chain reaction (PCR) can identify CMV in the cerebrospinal fluid. This condition can be treated successfully with gancyclovir or valgancyclovir. The lack of impotence in men suggests that the cause is not neurological.

Non-neurological aetiological agents to consider are abscesses, prostatitis, stones, and urethral stricture secondary to urethritis, especially where long-standing sexually transmitted infections are present.[60] Infectious and oncological aetiologies tend to occur in cases where the CD4+ cell count is severely diminished.[23]

Urodynamics may be performed to confirm neurological involvement in complex cases. Post-void urinary volume (PVR) and flow rate studies may help identify obstructive aetiologies. Urinalysis and urine cultures should be done in all patients.

Treatment should be appropriate to the severity of symptoms. Anticholinergics are effective treatment for symptoms of hyperreflexia. Antispasmodics can also be helpful. Obstructive symptoms may be treated with alpha-1 blockers. Areflexia is best treated with clean intermittent catheterization,[23] but Foley catheterization or suprapubic cystostomy may also be necessary.

Kidney stones

A well-known side-effect of the protease inhibitor indinavir sulphate is nephrolithiasis. Taken orally, the drug is rapidly absorbed and mainly metabolized by the liver with less than 20% excreted unchanged in the urine.[63] The incidence of nephrolithiasis in patients receiving indinavir has been estimated to be between 3 and 13%.[63–67] Patients who have a low body mass index are thought to be at increased risk for nephrolithiasis due to higher drug levels that are not adjusted for body weight.[64,65]

Patients usually present with acute renal colic, haematuria, and fever, with a severity generally worse than patients with conventional stones.[68] Symptoms of back or flank pain, dysuria, and urgency have also been reported with indinavir crystalluria.[69] The stones are radiolucent and are not visualized on non-contrast CT. Magnetic resonance imaging (MRI) may image the stones, but ultrasound is the modality of choice.[63] An intravenous pyelogram (IVP) may also image the stones. On gross observation, the stones appear yellow, friable, and soft. This relative pliability allows the calculi to conform to ureteral walls and induce obstruction.[68]

Treatment and prevention remain largely conservative. Increased fluid intake is the only practical method of prevention.[68] Despite universal hypocitraturia, oral citrate is currently not recommended as alkalinization decreases the solubility of indinavir.[68] When clinical severity necessitates procedural intervention, an endoscopic approach is usually the method of choice.

Persistent pyuria is another complication of indinavir therapy. This may be due to an interstitial nephritis or inflammation of the uroepithelium.[70] Kidney biopsy will show normal glomeruli, prominent interstitial fibrosis, and tubular atrophy accompanied by inflammation.[71] In the majority of patients, serum creatinine will not continue to rise and therapy can be continued.[67] A study of 781 patients noted that 7.3% experienced renal complications with indinavir.[67] The median time to development of symptoms has been reported at 21–53 weeks. Symptoms resolve promptly with cessation of therapy.[67,70]

Despite these complications, most patients continue to take indinavir. Studies report that only 5–12% of patients experiencing renal complications discontinue therapy with indinavir.[63,64,67] Indinavir stones will become a less common occurrence as indinavir becomes less popular in the treatment of HIV.[32]

Nephropathy

HIV-associated nephropathy (HIVAN), prior to HAART, rapidly progressed to end-stage renal disease. Its prevalence in HIV-infected persons is estimated at 4–7% (7–12% in the African-American population).[72] It typically consists of a focal segmental glomerulosclerosis that manifests predominantly as proteinuria.[73] Oedema and hypertension may also be seen. Treatment standards are not yet clear, but it is clear that antiretroviral therapy is effective in reducing the incidence of HIVAN. ACE inhibitors and steroid use are being investigated as treatment options, although steroids increase the problem of opportunistic infections.[73] Kidney transplants have been done in a limited number of HIV-infected patients.[72]

None of the antiretrovirals currently used are listed as directly causing nephrotoxicity.[32] However, nephrotoxicity has been reported to occur with protease inhibitors, for example ritonavir and indinavir.[71,74] Tenofovir, a new nucleoside reverse transcriptase inhibitor, has been associated with Fanconi's syndrome.[75] Several drugs commonly used in the treatment of opportunistic infections are also nephrotoxic, these include trimethoprim/sulfamethoxazole (TMP/SMX), acyclovir, foscarnet, and amphotericin B.[32] In particular, concomitant acyclovir doubles the risk of renal complications with indinavir.[67]

Summary

HIV/AIDS presents a variety of issues related to the diagnosis itself as well as the individual body systems involved. It is often not recognized how often the genitourinary tract is involved. Many of the effects have a very negative impact on quality of life. This chapter has emphasized the major areas of concern and outlined ways to provide supportive care in a compassionate and practical manner.

References

1 **UNAIDS and WHO** (2003). *AIDS Epidemic Update.* UNAIDS, Geneva.

2 **Cardo D, Culver D, Ciesielski C, Srivastava PU, Marcus R, Abiteboul D** *et al.* (1997). A case-control study of HIV seroconversion in health care workers after percutaneous exposure. Centers for Disease Control and Prevention Needlestick Surveillance Group. *N Engl J Med* **337**: 1485–90.

3 **Kwan D, Lowe F** (1995). Genitourinary manifestations of the acquired immunodeficiency syndrome. *Urology* **45**: 13–27.

4 **DiClemente R, Wingwood G, Rio C, Crosby R** (2002). Prevention interventions for HIV positive individuals. *Sex. Transm. Infect.* **78**: 393–5.

5 **Fauci A, Lane H** (2004). Human Immunodeficiency Virus (HIV) disease: AIDS and related disorders. In: *Harrison's Online* [www.harrisonsonline.com] (ed. E Braunwald, A Fauci, K Isselbacher, L Kasper, S Hauser, D Longo *et al.*) McGraw-Hill, New York.

6 **Hecht F, Busch M, Rawal B, Webb M, Rosenberg E, Swanson M** *et al.* (2002). Use of laboratory tests and clinical symptoms for identification of primary HIV infection. *AIDS* **16**: 1119–29.

7 **Centers for Disease Control and Prevention** (2002). Sexually transmitted diseases treatment guidelines 2002. *Morbidity and Mortality Weekly Report* **51** (RR06): 7–10.

8 **Douaihy A, Singh N** (2001). Factors affecting quality of life in patients with HIV infection. *AIDS Read.* **11**: 450–61.

9 **Centers for Disease Control and Prevention and the HIV Prevention in Clinical Care Working Group** (2004). Recommendation for incorporating human immunodeficiency virus (HIV) prevention into the medical care of persons living with HIV. *Clin. Infect. Dis.* **38**: 104–21.

10 **Fleming D, Wasserheit J** (1999). From epidemiological synergy to public health policy and practice: the contribution of other sexually transmitted diseases to sexual transmission of HIV infection. *Sex. Transm. Infect.* **75**: 3–17.

11 **Wald A, Link K** (2002). Risk of human immunodeficiency virus infection in herpes simplex virus type 2 seropositive persons: a meta-analysis. *J. Infect. Dis.* **185**: 45–52.

12 **Schneede P, Tenke P, Hofstetter A** (2003). Sexually transmitted disease (STDs)—a synoptic overview for urologists. *Eur. Urol.* **44**: 1–7.

13 **Collis T, Celum C** (2001). The clinical manifestations and treatment of sexually transmitted diseases in human immunodeficiency virus-positive men. *Clin. Infect. Dis.* **32**: 611–22.

14 Sobel J (2000). Gynecologic infections in human immunodeficiency virus-infected women. *Clin. Infect. Dis.* **31**: 1225–33.

15 Smith K, Skelton H, Yeager J (1994). Cutaneous findings in HIV-1 positive patients: a 42-month prospective study. *J. Am. Acad. Dermatol.* **31**: 746–54.

16 Toro J, Sanchez S, Turiansky G, Blauvelt A (2003). Topical cidofovir for the treatment of dermatologic conditions: verruca, condyloma, intraepithelial neoplasia, herpes simplex and its potential use in smallpox. *Dermatol. Clin.* **21**: 301–9.

17 Fitzpatrick T, Johnson R, Wolff K, Suurmond D (2001). *Color Atlas and Synopsis of Clinical Dermatology*, 4th edn. McGraw-Hill, New York.

18 Gilson R, Shupack J, Friedman-Kien AE (1999). A randomised, controlled, safety study using imiquimod for topical treatment of anogenital warts in HIV-infected patients. *AIDS* **13**: 2397–404.

19 Lee L, Dinneen M, Ahmad S (2001). The urologist and the patient infected with human immunodeficiency syndrome. *BJU Int.* **88**: 500–10.

20 Snoeck R, Van Laethem Y, De Clercq E, De Mauberge J, Clumeck N (2001). Treatment of a Bowenoid papulosis of the penis with local applications of cidofovir in a patient with acquired immunodeficiency syndrome. *Arch. Intern. Med.* **161**: 2382–4.

21 Schonwald S, Begovac J, Skerk V (1999). Urinary tract infections in HIV disease. *Int. J. Antimicrob. Agents* **1**: 309–11.

22 de Gaetano Donati K, Tumbarello M, Tacconelli E, Bertagnolio S, Rabagliati R, Scoppettuolo G *et al.* (2003). Impact of highly active antiretroviral therapy (HAART) on the incidence of bacterial infections in HIV-infected subjects. *J. Chemother.* **15**: 60–5.

23 Hyun G, Lowe F (2003). AIDS and the urologist. *Urol. Clin. North Am.* **30**: 101–9.

24 Lyss SB, Kamb ML, Peterman TA, Moran JS, Newman DR, Bolan G *et al.* (2003). Chlamydia trachomatis among patients infected with and treated for Neisseria gonorrhea in sexually transmitted disease clinics in the United States. *Ann. Intern. Med.* **139**: 178–85.

25 Altman E, Centeno L, Mahal M, Bielory L (1994). AIDS-associated Reiter's syndrome. *Ann. Allergy* **72**: 307–16.

26 Cuellar M, Espinoza L (2000). Rheumatic manifestations of HIV-AIDS. *Baillieres Best Pract. Res. Clin. Rhematol.* **14**: 579–93.

27 Neumann S, Kreth F, Schubert S, Mossner J, Caca K (2003). Reiter's syndrome as a manifestation of an immune reconstitution syndrome in an HIV-infected patient: successful treatment with doxycycline. *Clin. Infect. Dis.* **36**: 1628–9.

28 Studmeister A (2002). Cytomegalovirus-induced hemorrhagic cystitis in AIDS patient treated successfully with valgancyclovir. *AIDS* **16**: 1437–8.

29 Murphy G, Wood DJ, McRoberts J, Henslee-Downey P (1993). Adenovirus-associated hemorrhagic cystitis treated with intravenous ribavirin. *J. Urol.* **149**: 565–6.

30 Ghez D, Oksenhendler E, Scleux C, Lassoued K (2000). Haemorrhagic cystitis associated with adenovirus in a patient with AIDS treated for a non-Hodgkin's lymphoma. *Am. J. Hematol.* **63**: 32–4.

31 Wise G (2001). Genitourinary fungal infections: a therapeutic conundrum. *Expert Opin. Pharmacother.* **2**: 1211–26.

32 Panel on Clinical Practices for Treatment of HIV Infection (2004). *Guidelines for the Use of Antiretroviral Agents in HIV-1 Infected Adults and Adolescents.* US Department of Health and Human Services.

33 International Collaboration of HIV and Cancer (2000). Highly active antiretroviral therapy and incidence of cancer in human immunodeficiency virus-infected adults. *J. Natl. Cancer Inst.* **92**: 1823–30.

34 Boshoff C, Weiss R (2002). AIDS-related malignancies. *Nature Rev. Cancer* **2**: 373–82.

35 Grulich A, Xinan W, Law M, Coates M, Kaldor J (1999). Risk of cancer in people with AIDS. *AIDS* **13**: 839–43.

36 Herida M, Mary-Krause M, Kaphan R, Cadranel J, Poizot-Martin I, Rabaud C *et al.* (2003). Incidence of non-AIDS-defining cancers before and during the highly active antiretroviral therapy era in a cohort of human immunodeficiency virus-infected patients. *J. Clin. Oncol.* **21**: 3447–53.

37 Blattner W (1999). Human retroviruses: their role in cancer. *Proc. Assoc. Am. Physicians* **111**: 563–72.

38 Frisch M, Biggar R, Engels E, Goedart J (2001). Association of cancer with AIDS-related immunosuppression in adults. *J. Am. Med. Assoc.* **285**: 1736–45.

39 Zinn H, Haller J (1999). Renal manifestations of AIDS in children. *Pediatr. Radiol.* **29**: 558–61.

40 Goedert JJ, Cote TR, Virgo P, Scoppa SM, Kingma DW, Gail MH *et al.* (1998). Spectrum of AIDS-associated malignant disorders. *Lancet* **351**: 1833–9.

41 Grulich A, Li Y, McDonald A, Correl P, Law M, Kaldor J (2002). Rates of non-AIDS-defining cancers in people with HIV infection before and after AIDS diagnosis. *AIDS* **16**: 115–61.

42 Spina M, Vaccher E, Carbone A, Tirelli U (1999). Neoplastic complications of HIV infection. *Ann. Oncol.* **10**: 1271–86.

43 Sgadari C, Monini P, Barillari G, Ensoli B (2003). Use of HIV protease inhibitors to block Kaposi's sarcoma and tumour growth. *Lancet Oncol.* **4**: 537–47.

44 Bernardi D, Salvioni R, Vaccher E, Repetto L, Piersantelli N, Marini B *et al.* (1995). Testicular germ cell tumours and human immunodeficiency virus infection: a report of 26 cases. Italian Cooperative Group of AIDS and Tumors. *J. Clin. Oncol.* **13**: 2705–11.

45 Powles T, Bower M, Daugaard G, Shamash J, De Ruiter A, Johnson M *et al.* (2003). Multicenter study of human immunodeficiency virus-related germ cell tumours. *J. Clin. Oncol.* **21**: 1922–7.

46 Mylonakis E, Koutkia P, Grinspoon S (2001). Diagnosis and treatment of androgen deficiency in human immunodeficiency virus-infected men and women. *Clin. Infect. Dis.* **33**: 857–64.

47 Rietschel P, Corcoran C, Stanley T, Basgoz N, Klibanski A, Grinspoon S (2000). Prevalence of hypogonadism among men with weight loss related to human immunodeficiency virus infection who were receiving highly active antiretroviral therapy. *Clin. Infect. Dis.* **31**: 1240–4.

48 Dobs A, Dempsey M, Ladenson P, Polk B (1988). Endocrine disorders in men infected with human immunodeficiency virus. *Am. J. Med.* **84**: 611–16.

49 Guay A, Davis S (2002). Testosterone insufficiency in women: fact or fiction? *World J. Urol.* **20**: 106–10.

50 Dolan S, Wilkie S, Alibadi N, Sullivan MP, Basgoz N, Davis B *et al.* (2004). Effects of testosterone administration in human immunodeficiency virus-infected women with low weight: a randomized placebo controlled study. *Arch. Intern. Med.* **164**: 897–904.

51 Hofbauer L, Heufelder A (1996). Endocrine implications of human immunodeficiency virus infection. *Medicine* **75**: 262–78.

52 Grinspoon S, Corcoran C, Askari H, Schoenfeld D, Wof L, Burrows B *et al.* (1998). Effects of androgen administration in men with AIDS wasting syndrome: a randomized, double-blind, placebo-controlled trial. *Ann. Intern. Med.* **129**: 18–26.

53 Kong A, Edmonds P (2002). Testosterone therapy in HIV wasting syndrome: systematic review and meta-analysis. *Lancet Infect. Dis.* **2**: 692–9.

54 Fotheringham J, Wobeser W, Liu T, Tenzif S, Ross R, Ford P (2002). Effect of exogenous testosterone (ET) on quality of life (QOL) among HIV-infected males on HAART. *Antivir. Ther.* **7**: 63.

55 Colson A, Keller M, Sax P, Pettus P, Platt R, Choo P (2002). Male sexual dysfunction associated with antiretroviral therapy. *J. Acquired Immune Defic. Syndr.* **30**: 27–32.

56 Hijazi L, Nandwani R, Kell P (2002). Medical management of sexual difficulties in HIV-positive individuals. *Int. J. STD AIDS* **13**: 587–92.

57 Tindall B, Forde S, Goldstein D, Ross M, Cooper D (1994). Sexual dysfunction in advanced HIV disease. *AIDS Care* **6**: 105–7.

58 Sollima S, Osio M, Muscia F, Gambaro P, Alciati A, Zucconi M *et al.* (2001). Protease inhibitors and erectile dysfunction. *AIDS* **15**: 2331–3.

59 Gyrtrup H, Kristiansen V, Zachariae C, Krogsgaard K, Colstrup H, Jensen K (1995). Voiding problems in patients with HIV-infection and AIDS. *Scand. J. Urol. Nephrol.* **29**: 295–8.

60 Hermieu J, Delmas V, Boccon-Gibod L (1996). Micturition disturbances and human immunodeficiency virus infection. *J. Urol.* **156**: 157–9.

61 Khan Z, Singh V, Yang W (1992). Neurogenic bladder in acquired-immune-deficiency-syndrome (AIDS). *Urology* **40**: 289–91.

62 So Y, Olney R (1994). Acute lumbosacral polyradiculopathy in acquired immunodeficiency syndrome: experience with 23 patients. *Ann. Neurol.* **35**: 53–8.

63 Wu D, Stoller M (2000). Indinavir urolithiasis. *Curr. Opin. Urol.* **10**: 557–61.

64 Meraviglia P, Angeli E, Del Sorbo F, Rombola G, Vigano P, Orlando G *et al.* (2002). Risk factors for indinavir-related renal colic in HIV patients: predictive value of indinavir dose/body mass index. *AIDS* **16**: 2089–93.

65 Saltel E, Angel J, Futter N, Walsh W, O'Rourke K, Mahoney J (2000). Increased prevalence and analysis of risk factors for indinavir nephrolithiasis. *J. Urol.* **164**: 1895–7.

66 Reiter W, Schon-Pemerstorfer H, Dorfinger K, Hofbauer J, Marberer M (1999). Frequency of urolithiasis in individuals seropositive for human immunodeficiency virus treated with indinavir is higher than previously assumed. *J. Urol.* **161**: 1082–4.

67 Herman J, Ives N, Nelson M, Gazzard B, Esterbrook P (2001). Incidence and risk factors for the development of indinavir-associated renal complications. *J. Antimicrob. Chemother.* **48**: 355–60.

68 Kohan A, Armenakas N, Fracchia J (1999). Indinavir urolithiasis: an emerging cause of renal colic in patients with human immunodeficiency virus. *J. Urol.* **161**: 1765–8.

69 Kopp JB, Miller KD, Mican JA, Feuerstein IM, Vaughan E, Baker C *et al.* (1997). Crystalluria and urinary tract abnormalities associated with indinavir. *Ann. Intern. Med.* **127**: 119–25.

70 Kopp JB, Falloon J, Filie A, Abati A, King C, Hortin GL *et al.* (2002). Indinavir-associated interstitial nephritis and uroepithelial inflammation: clinical and cytologic findings. *Clin. Infect. Dis.* **34**: 1122–8.

71 Tashima K (1997). Indinavir nephropathy. *N. Engl. J. Med.* **336**: 138–40.

72 Roland M, Stock P (2003). Review of solid-organ transplantation in HIV-infected patients. *Transplantation* **75**: 425–9.

73 Ross M, Klotman P (2002). Recent progress in HIV-associated nephropathy. *J. Am. Soc. Nephrol.* **13**: 2997–3004.

74 Chugh S, Bird R, Alexander E (1997). Ritonavir and renal failure. *N. Engl. J. Med.* **336**: 138.

75 Verhelst D, Monge M, Meynard JL, Fouqueray B, Mougenot B, Girard PM *et al.* (2002). Fanconi syndrome and renal failure induced by tenofovir: a first case report. *Am. J. Kidney Dis.* **40**: 1331–3.

Chapter 18

The patient presenting with painful bladder syndrome

Jerzy B. Gajewski

Interstitial cystitis (IC) was first described as a Hunner ulcer in 1915.[1] Ever since, the disease has continued to elude researchers and clinicians and, even today, the pathogenesis, diagnosis, and treatment remain controversial. Several attempts have been made to standardize the diagnosis and evaluation of the patient with IC[2] but initial attempts were focused mainly on research variables. In the USA, the National Institute of Diabetes and Digestive and Kidney Diseases (NIDDK) criteria were introduced in 1987 and further refined in 1988[3] and were quickly adopted into general urological practice. With time, however, it became apparent that this definition was too strict and a broader definition was introduced in the 1990s. NIDDK formed the Interstitial Cystitis Data Base (ICDB) and the Interstitial Cystitis Clinical Trial Group (ICCTG) introduced more inclusive criteria[4] based on clinical symptoms and by exclusion. Controversy remains, however, regarding the diagnostic criteria and extent of investigations required to confirm a diagnosis.

The term 'interstitial cystitis' is being replaced slowly by 'painful bladder syndrome' (PBS) to accentuate the diversity of clinical presentations.

It is safe to define IC/PBS as chronic symptoms of pain associated with the bladder and/or urgency and frequency unexplained by other causes. There are two clinical subtypes of IC/PBS:

1 Classical—destructive, progressive inflammatory disease of the bladder eventually causing small-capacity fibrotic bladder (accounts for 5–50% of IC/PBS cases[2,5,6]).

2 Non-ulcerative disease which is more stable and non-progressive.

How common is this disease in the population?

Because there is no standardized definition of IC/PBS, it is difficult to assess the prevalence and incidence of this disease. Generally, it can be stated that it is more frequently diagnosed in the developed countries in comparison with developing ones. Early reports from Finland[7] and The Netherlands[8] estimated the prevalence at 18.1 women per 100 000 with 10% of cases being severe. More recently, the reported prevalence of urinary symptoms corresponding to probable interstitial cystitis in Finland is

450/100 000—an order of magnitude higher than previously reported.[9] In the USA, based on symptoms alone, the estimated prevalence is 36.6 per 100 000.[10]. Although most commonly seen in middle age, IC/PBS has been diagnosed in very young and very old patients. Another survey from the USA showed a higher prevalence of 0.51–0.67% among the adult population,[11,12] and it may be as high as 1 out of 4.5 women.[13] A slightly lower prevalence was reported in Japan at 4.5 per 100 000.[14] Data on physician-made diagnoses of IC/PBS showed lower figures. The overall age- and sex-adjusted prevalence rate was 1.1 (0.6–1.5) per 100 000 population. The age-adjusted prevalence rates were 1.6 per 100 000 in women and 0.6 per 100 000 in men. The median age at initial diagnosis was 44.5 (27–76) years in women and 71.5 (23–79) years in men.[15] It appears that the prevalence of IC/PBS is higher than previously esti-mated. Furthermore, adult female first-degree relatives of patients with IC may have a prevalence of IC 17 times that found in the general population.[16] There is general agreement that the disease is 8–10 times more common in women than in men[7] and is often confused with prostatitis and benign prostatic hyperplasia (BPH).[17]

What is the cause of interstitial cystitis/painful bladder syndrome?

No single aetiology can explain IC/PBS. Most likely we are dealing with a heteroge-neous clinical syndrome and several different factors may initiate the common patho-logical pathway responsible for IC/PBS. The initial insult may be caused by a bladder infection (e.g. bacterial, viral, fungal) or bladder injury due to chemical or physical fac-tors. The main component of the urothelium is the glycosaminoglycan (GAG) layer which is defective in most patients with IC/PBS. This mucosal defect leads to excessive absorption of potassium and other urinary toxins which causes disruption to blood and lymphatic vessels. Almost 80% of patients with the clinical picture of IC/PBS have increased permeability to KCl.[18] Secondary changes in bladder mucosal permeability lead to increased activity of mast cells and trigger pathological neural-immune responses. It has been shown that mast cell activation further increases epithelial per-meability[19] and interacts with sensory nerves. The release of vasoactive, nociceptive, and inflammatory transmitters triggers pain and other sensory neurons causing up-regulation of the nervous system.[20] There is also evidence that mast cells are intimately involved in the interaction with the intrinsic nerves in the bladder.[21] Chronic inflammation also stimulates normally quiet afferent C-fibres from the bladder and subsequently leads to chronic pain from the affected area similar to reflex sympathetic dystrophy. This may be initiated by injury (e.g. infection, pelvic, surgery, childbirth, etc.) to the sympathetic bladder nerves causing a compensatory increase in adrenoreceptors and remodelling of afferent receptors causing up-regulation of sensory output from the bladder (Fig. 18.1).[22]

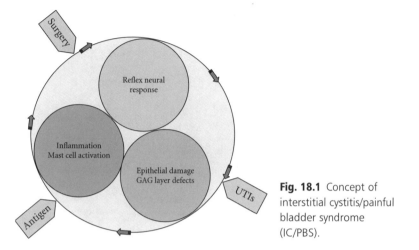

Fig. 18.1 Concept of interstitial cystitis/painful bladder syndrome (IC/PBS).

What are the most common symptoms of IC/PBS?

The most common symptoms are pain from the bladder area, i.e. suprapubic pain, urgency, and/or frequency.

Lower abdominal pain is present in 75–80% of patients with IC/PBS.[23] It is aggravated by stress, constrictive clothing, and sexual intercourse. Certain foods, particularly acid and carbonated beverages, alcohol, coffee, and spices, may also aggravate the discomfort. Pain is usually improved or relieved by emptying the bladder. In one study, using the overall pain–urgency–frequency score, 7% of patients presented with mild, 44% with moderate and 49% with severe symptoms. Severe urgency in 41% of cases and severe 24-h frequency in 41% were more common than severe pain in 29%. Fifty-one per cent reported nocturia of two or more voids.[24] Other symptoms may include dyspareunia (painful sexual intercourse) or lower back pain.

Urgency is the complaint of a sudden compelling desire to pass urine, which is difficult to defer.[25] Urgency in IC/PBS may or may not be associated with urge incontinence (overactive bladder).

Increased daytime frequency can be the only initial symptom, and is defined as voiding what the patient considers to be too often,[25] usually more than every 2 hours. Some patients urinate up to 60 times in 24 hours. Some patients also have have nocturia, defined as waking up at night one or more times to void. In the later stages, patients also often complain of hesitancy, decreased stream, and incomplete voiding.

Early interstitial cystitis presents variably and usually with only a single symptom of urgency/frequency, nocturia, or pain.[26] Very often symptoms resemble overactive bladder or bacterial cystitis (Fig. 18.2). Some patients initially present with symptoms of recurrent bacterial urinary tract infections (UTIs); however, urine cultures are usually

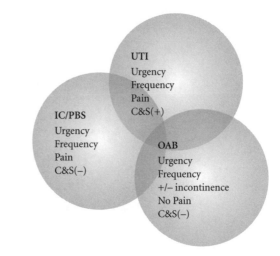

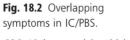

Fig. 18.2 Overlapping symptoms in IC/PBS.

C&S: 'Culture and Sensitivity'

negative although the urinanalysis may show microhaematuria. Patients may benefit initially from antibiotic treatment, but this benefit doesn't last long. Bacterial cystiti, endometriosis, vulvodynia, irritable bowel syndrome (IBS), and chronic prostatitis in men are common initial misdiagnoses.

The median duration of interstitial cystitis symptoms at diagnosis is 2–8 years.[24] Although all symptoms fluctuate, there is no evidence of significant long-term change in overall disease severity. Since oestrogen receptors are expressed on mast cells symptoms may get worse during ovulation.[27] Patients with interstitial cystitis may complain of pelvic discomfort, backache, dizziness, chest pain, aches in joints, abdominal cramps, nausea, heart pounding, and headache.[28]

Quality of life

The quality of life of patients with IC/PBS is significantly affected. Women with interstitial cystitis experience less decrease in physical function compared with women with rheumatoid arthritis but more compared with women with hypertension. In addition, they experience greater differences in vitality and mental health than women with rheumatoid arthritis, hypertension,[29] and even kidney dialysis patients.[30] IC/BPS accentuates all domains of depression and correlates with disease severity.[31] Suicidal thoughts are three to four times more frequent than in the general population.[30] It has also been shown that misdiagnosed patients have more IC/PBS symptoms[32] and have poorer coping strategies and lower self-esteem than properly diagnosed patients.[33] Sexual interest and satisfaction decline significantly, in part due to dyspareunia. It has been shown there are gaps in clinical practice regarding sexual well-being of the patient requiring further education of health professionals.[34] Even if the diagnosis of IC is made and the patient feels relief that it is not 'all in her head', the feelings of hopelessness and despair may prevail.[30] The most devastating fact for patients is that they may be given only very vague explanations of the disease and little support in management.[35,36] The disease affects entire families because of sleep interruption, increased household and child care responsibilities, financial hardship[37] and isolation. Stress exacerbates symptoms in interstitial cystitis patients.[38,39]

How are patients initially investigated?

The initial evaluation includes history and physical examination. Patients are asked specifically about voiding symptoms. Several symptoms questionnaires have been developed to standardize the process.

The O'Leary–Sant Interstitial Cystitis Symptom Index (ICSI) (Fig. 18.3) has been proposed as a treatment outcome measure in IC/PBS.[40,41] Recently Parsons developed and validated the pelvic pain and urgency/frequency (PUF) patient symptoms scale (Fig. 18.4).[42] A 3-day voiding diary is also an important instrument in evaluation of patients with IC/PBS and lower urinary tract symptoms (LUTS).[43]

It is important to document past history and concomitant disease. Some patients have multiple drug and environmental allergies.[44] The Interstitial Cystitis Association

Interstitial Cystitis Symptom Index

Q1. *During the past month*, how often have you felt the strong need to urinate with little or no warning?

- 0. ＿＿ not at all
- 1. ＿＿ less than 1 time in 5
- 2. ＿＿ lessthan half the time
- 3. ＿＿ about half the time
- 4. ＿＿ more than half the time
- 5. ＿＿ almost always

Q2. *During the past month*, have you had to urinate less than 2 hours after you finished urinating?

- 0. ＿＿ not at all
- 1. ＿＿ less than 1 time in 5
- 2. ＿＿ less than half the time
- 3. ＿＿ about half the time
- 4. ＿＿ more than half the time
- 5. ＿＿ almost always

Q3. *During the past month*, how often did you most typically get up at night to urinate?

- 0. ＿＿ none
- 1. ＿＿ once
- 2. ＿＿ 2 times
- 3. ＿＿ 3 times
- 4. ＿＿ 4 times
- 5. ＿＿ 5 or more times

Q4. *During the past month*, have you experienced pain or burning in your bladder?

- 0. ＿＿ not at all
- 2. ＿＿ a few times
- 3. ＿＿ almost always
- 4. ＿＿ fairly often
- 5. ＿＿ usually

Add the numerical values of the checked entries: total score: ＿＿＿＿＿

Interstitial Cystitis Symptom Index

During the past month, how much has each of the following been a problem for you?

Q1. Frequent urination during the day?

- 0. ＿＿ no problem
- 1. ＿＿ very small problem
- 2. ＿＿ small problem
- 3. ＿＿ medium problem
- 4. ＿＿ big problem

Q2. Getting up at night to urinate?

- 0. ＿＿ no problem
- 1. ＿＿ very small problem
- 2. ＿＿ small problem
- 3. ＿＿ medium problem
- 4. ＿＿ big problem

Q3. Need to urinate with little warning?

- 0. ＿＿ no problem
- 1. ＿＿ very small problem
- 2. ＿＿ small problem
- 3. ＿＿ medium problem
- 4. ＿＿ big problem

Q4. Burning, pain, discomfort, or pressure in your bladder?

- 0. ＿＿ no problem
- 1. ＿＿ very small problem
- 2. ＿＿ small problem
- 3. ＿＿ medium problem
- 4. ＿＿ big problem

Add the numerical values of the checked entries: total score: ＿＿＿＿＿

Fig. 18.3 The O'Leary–Sant Interstitial Cystitis Symptom Index.

PELVIC PAIN and URGENCY/FREQUENCY
PATIENT SYMPTOM SCALE

Please circle the answer that best describes how you feel for each question.

		0	1	2	3	4	SYMPTOM SCORE	BOTHER SCORE
1	How many times do you go to the bathroom during the day?	3–6	7–10	11–14	15–19	20+		
2	a. How many times do you go to the bathroom at night?	0	1	2	3	4+		
	b. If you get up at night to go to the bathroom does it bother you?	Never	Mildly	Moderate	Severe			
3	Are you currently sexually active YES _____ No _____							
4	a. IF YOU ARE SEXUALLY ACTIVE, do you now or have you ever had pain or symptoms during or after sexualy intercourse?	Never	Occassionally	Usually	Always			
	b. If you have pain, does it make you avoid sexual intercourse?	Never	Occassionally	Usually	Always			
5	Do you have pain associated with your bladder or in your pelvis (vagina, lower abdomen, urethra, perineum, testes, or scrotum)?	Never	Occassionally	Usually	Always			
6	Do you have urgency after going to the bathroom?	Never	Occassionally	Usually	Always			
7	a. If you have pain, is it usually		Mild	Moderate	Severe			
	b. Does your pain bother you?	Never	Occassionally	Usually	Always			
8	a. If you have urgency, is it usually		Mild	Moderate	Severe			
	b. Does your urgency bother you?	Never	Occassionally	Usually	Always			

SYMPTOM SCORE = (1, 2a, 4a, 5, 6, 7a, 8a)	
BOTHER SCORE = (2b, 4b, 7b, 8b)	
TOTAL SCORE (Symptom Score + Bother Score) =	

Fig. 18.4 Pelvic pain and urgency/frequency (PUF) patient symptoms scale.

survey (ICA Study Group) reported a higher prevalence of fibromyalgia, Crohn's disease, irritable bowel syndrome, colitis, and lupus in IC/PBS patients than in the general population. Many have psychological problems which may be related to the debilitating symptoms. The disease has often been reported to start after pelvic or abdominal surgery; however, no definite correlation has been reported. Some medications such as Surgam and methotrexate can cause similar diseases in the bladder. Bladder cancer in the form of carcinoma *in situ* (CIS) may mimic IC/PBS.

Urinalysis typically shows microhaematuria. Urine culture should be done to confirm urine sterility. Cystoscopy will help rule out malignancy and confirm the presence of bladder abnormalities consistent with IC/PBS as reported by Messing.[45] Cystoscopy under anaesthesia will:

- document inflammation (e.g. glomerulations, submucosal haemorrhages, ulcers)
- assess the degree of inflammation
- determine bladder capacity
- exclude other diseases
- allow biopsy if necessary
- permit therapeutic hydrodistention
- permit coagulation of the Hunner's ulcers.

Diagnostic hydrodistention is done under general anaesthesia at 80 cmH$_2$O for 1 minute. The presence of glomerulations and submucosal haemorrhages may indicate IC/PBS (Fig. 18.5) although these are not pathognomic of IC. Some studies have shown the presence of glomerulations in apparently 'normal' women undergoing tubal ligation. Subjects were never asked specifically about voiding problems.[46] Therapeutic hydrodistention benefits 20–45% of women and the improvement in symptoms usually lasts 3–12 months. Reported treatment efficacy in a prospective study was 60% at 6 months and 43% at 1 year. Good response correlates to a maximal cystometric capacity $\geq$150 ml.[47] Typically patients complain of increased symptoms for a day or two after the dilatation. Bladder stretching increases heparin-binding epidermal growth factor (HB-EGF) and reduces antiproliferative factor activity in urine from patients with interstitial cystitis.[48]

Bladder biopsy may be useful to exclude other diseases but is not essential to make the diagnosis. Some European studies rely on biopsy for confirmation of diagnosis.[49,50]

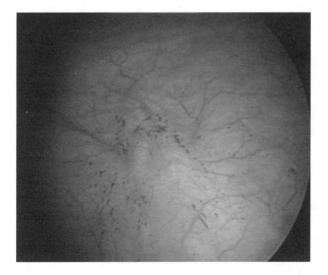

Fig. 18.5 Glomerulations at cystoscopy.

The severity of cystoscopic findings observed during hydrodistention under anaesthesia does not correlate with the degree of inflammation.[51] Cystoscopic findings are not associated with most IC symptoms, although the increased urinary frequency may be suggestive of the presence of Hunner's ulcers. Nocturia and urgency are related to some histological findings but not the presence or severity of glomerulations.[52]

Urodynamic studies are not essential for the diagnosis of IC/PBS; however, they play an important role in the evaluation of bladder dysfunction in these patients and add to a better understanding of the disease.[53] Patients with IC/PBS often have symptoms overlapping with those of an overactive bladder. Urodynamics may be helpful in detecting detrusor overactivity. The incidence of instability in patients with IC/PBS ranges between 5 and 26%.[54,55] Maximal cystometric capacity appears to be greater than the functional capacity obtained by diary.[56] Only 10–25% of patients with IC/PBS have detrusor failure based on low flow, large residual volume, and lack of bladder outlet obstruction.[53,57] Some reports suggest an element of increased bladder outlet resistance.[53] There is no correlation between urodynamic and cystoscopic findings.[53] Urodynamics may be indicated in male patients with IC/PBS to rule out possible concomitant bladder outlet obstruction and as another diagnostic tool when initial treatment strategies fail.

The potassium test has been recommended by some clinicians, mostly in North America (Fig. 18.6). It is asserted that intravesical potassium reproduces pain related to IC/BPS and indicates the presence of the disease. This test was introduced by Parsons et al.[18,58] and showed marked sensitivity to intravesical potassium in 75% of patients with interstitial cystitis versus only 4% of controls.[58] Other investigators showed less

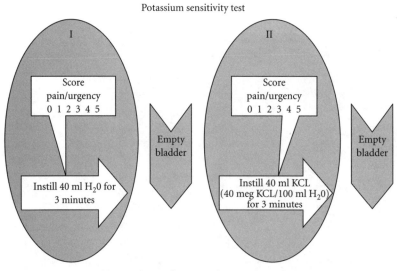

Potassium sensitivity test

Positive test = score from I < II by two or more points

Fig. 18.6 Potassium test protocol.

impressive characteristics with a sensitivity of 70% and a specificity of 50%. Likelihood ratios (positive 1.39, negative 0.61) indicated poor inclusion and exclusion capabilities.[59,60] The potassium test should not be taken as diagnostic of IC/PBS but as an additional tool in management of the disease.

What is the initial treatment for IC/PBS?

Lifestyle adjustment and IC/PBS

Since IC/PBS has such a tremendous impact on a patient's quality of life, management should involve a holistic approach. This includes:

* quick diagnosis;
* information on the disease;
* support groups;
* psychological counselling: reassurance, self validation—disease not 'all in the head', distraction techniques, family involvement, and comparison and acceptance;
* involvement in self-management of disease: information seeking, choosing diagnosis, and monitoring compliance;
* flexible treatment protocols (timing, dosage).

Certain foods are detrimental and aggravate symptoms. These may include acidic and carbonated beverages, alcohol and coffee, and foods high in potassium. Dietary suggestions for an IC/PBS diet are shown in Fig. 18.7. Several herbal remedies have been reported by patients to be helpful but there is no good scientific evidence of their beneficial activity.

Prelief® (calcium glycerophosphate), a food-grade mineral classified as a dietary supplement for use with acidic foods and beverages, was found to reduce food-related symptoms in patients with IC/PBS.[61] It 'takes the acid out' of foods and beverages, such as tomato sauce, coffee, wine, beer, colas, and orange juice. Recommended dosage is two tablets three times a day with meals and two tablets at bedtime as necessary.

Cysta-Q® and Prosta-Q® are special formulations designed for IC patients and non-bacterial prostatitis patients. Cysta-Q® consists of a patented, extracted blend of quercetin, bromelain, papain, cranberry powder (non-acidic), black cohosh (non-acidic), skullcap, wood betony, passionflower, and valerian. Prosta-Q® is an over-the-counter quercetin dietary supplement for chronic pelvic pain syndrome in men.[62]

Bladder retraining

Patients who experience bladder pain have tendency to urinate more frequently and establish pattern of frequent voiding. The goal of bladder retraining is to break this pattern and achieve longer periods between urination. The patient slowly forces herself or himself to void less frequently and subsequently improve functional bladder capacity.

OK ✓ Allowed	Products	STOP ✗ Avoid
• Bottled or spring water • Acid-free coffee or tea • Some herbal teas	Beverages	• Alkohol such as beer or wine • Carbonated drinks • Coffee or tea • Cranberry, Apple, and all citrus juices
• Melon • Blueberries	Fruits	• Most fruits
• Potatoes • Organic tomato	Vegetables	• Fava beans • All varieties of onions • Rhubarb • Tofu • Tomato
• Almonds • Pine nuts • Cashew	Nuts	• Most nuts
• White and milk? chocolate • Cottage cheese • Milk	Dairy	• Aged cheeses • Sour cream • Eggs • Yogurt • Dark chocolate
• Pasta • Rice • Light bread	Grains	• Rye breads • Sourdough breads
• Poultry • Fish • Light meats	Meat/Fish	• Aged, cured, smoked meats • Liver
• Garlic	Garnishes/ Spices	• Mayonnaise • Spicy food
• None	Preservatives	• Benzol alcohol • Citric acid • Monosodium glutamate • Aspartame • Saccharin • Artificial ingredience and colours

Fig. 18.7 Dietary suggestions for IC/PBS diet.

It is indicated in early and mild to moderate disease. Steps in bladder retraining with a target goal of voiding every 2–4 hours include:

◆ completion of a 3-day voiding diary;

◆ calculation of voiding frequency (e.g. every hour);

- increasing the time between voiding gradually at weekly intervals;
- employ 'distraction' techniques to increase intervals.

Oral medications: pharmacological treatment

Pentosan polysulphate sodium (PPS) (Elmiron) is considered as a first-line pharmacological therapy and is the only oral agent approved by health regulatory bodies for treatment of IC/PBS. PPS is a weak anticoagulant (only 1/15 the activity of heparin) and has been used in prevention of thrombotic disease. The drug action is based on improving GAG layer pathophysiology. Reports have shown wide rates of improvement in IC symptoms—10% up to 63%.[63–65] PPS also appears to be a potent inhibitor of allergic and non-immune mast cell stimulation.[66] Patients undergoing invasive procedures or having signs/symptoms of underlying coagulopathy or who are otherwise at increased risk of bleeding (due to other therapies such as Coumadin, heparin, tissue plasminogen activator (tPA), streptokinase, high-dose aspirin) should be evaluated for increased haemorrhagic risk when taking this drug. The usual dosage is 100 mg three times per day. Occasionally, because of compliance problems, some patients take the medication twice a day with double dosing in the morning or evening. Increased dosages of up to 900 mg/day have been evaluated but without significant advantages and with more side-effects.[67] It usually takes 4–6 months to appreciate effectiveness of the medication. The most common side-effect is diarrhoea in 15% of subjects. Other side-effects include headache, GI discomfort, nausea, and alopecia (reversible after stopping medication). Some patients have an adverse reaction to the drug capsule and instructing patients to take only the active powder from inside the capsule may eliminate some of the GI side-effects. Although PPS should be taken on an empty stomach, some patients cannot tolerate the medication that way and have to take it with meals, leading to reduced absorption.

Some studies have shown decreased nitric oxide synthesis in the urine of patients with IC/PBS and, as a result, L-arginine, a substrate for nitric oxide synthesis, has been tried in patients with IC/PBS with variable results.[68–70]

Antihistamines (i.e. H1-receptor blockers) are indicated in patients with coexisting allergies. The premise is that mast cell degranulation releases histamine which is responsible for the pain. The most widely used compound is hydroxyzine[71] which has an effect on mast cell degranulation as well as analgesic and sedative qualities. Histamine H2 blockers (e.g. cimetidine, ranitidine, nizatidine, famotidine, etc.) have been found in preliminary studies to be beneficial in some patients.[72,73]

Suplatast tosilatedouble is a new oral immunoregulator that suppresses helper T cell-mediated allergic responses, including IgE production and eosinophilic inflammation, and has been suggested as a treatment for IC/PBS. One year of therapy resulted in a significantly increased bladder capacity and decreased symptoms, such as urinary urgency, frequency, and lower abdominal pain, in patients with non-ulcerative IC/PBS.

These effects also correlated with a reduction in blood eosinophils, CD20-positive cells and IgE and urine CD45RO positive memory T cells. No major side-effects were observed.[74]

Antibiotics alone or in combination may sometimes be associated with decreased symptoms in some patients but they do not represent a major advance in therapy.[75]

Anticholinergics are not indicated as an initial treatment; however, they may be useful in patients with coexisting overactive bladder (OAB). Intravesical oxybutynin in combination with bladder training improved bladder capacity and frequency but not pain.[76]

What if initial treatments fail?

Intravesical instillations

Dimethyl sulphoxide (DMSO), first synthesized in 1866, has been available as a by-product of the pulp and paper industry for many years. In 1962, Jacob et al. described the remarkable medicinal properties of DMSO.[77] They teamed up with a urologist to use DMSO intravesically, instilling a mixture referred to as a 'cocktail' of heparin, cortisone, bicarbonate, and DMSO (15%) into the bladder. Initial reports of the use of DMSO in IC/PBS patients were encouraging and led to the approval of the drug by the FDA.[78,79]

DMSO has anti-inflammatory, analgesic, muscle relaxant, and collagen dissolution properties. Different protocols have been utilized, but most typically the drug is instilled weekly or bi-weekly for 3–4 months followed by monthly maintenance doses. Relief of symptoms has been reported in 50% or more of patients.[80,81] The medication is absorbed into the blood within 10 minutes of instillation into the bladder and, although associated with very few side-effects,[81] a garlic-like taste may be noted by the patient. This may last several hours and, because of the presence of metabolites, an odour on the breath and from the skin may remain for 72 hours; it is obvious to others. Some patients experience moderate discomfort on administration but this usually becomes less prominent with repeated administrations. DMSO can interfere with liver function tests and give falsely elevated enzyme readings that return to normal on stopping the drug.

Changes in the refractive index and lens opacities have been seen in animals with chronic administration. No ophthalmic changes attributable to intravesical instillation have been reported in patients carefully followed for up to 17 months; however, full eye evaluations, including slit-lamp examinations are recommended periodically.

Heparin can be instilled alone or in combination with DMSO in dosages of 5000 to 20 000 units in 20–50 ml sterile water or saline. Heparin has anti-inflammatory and surface protective properties by restoring the GAG layer. Most protocols initially suggest frequent instillations (e.g. once a day) and then two to three times per week and then once a week for 4–8 months. Sometimes the treatment must be indefinite. Patients are encouraged to hold the heparin solution in the bladder for at least 20 minutes. Some patients are able to do self-instillations at home. Reported success rates are 50–60%[82] and no significant side-effects have been reported.

Hyaluronic acid instillation also restores defective mucosal lining of the bladder by replacing the defective GAG layer. One report indicated a success rate of 56%.[83] although the author's experience is less favourable. It is also expensive, and beneficial results require long-term treatment.[84] Hyaluronic acid (40 mg) is instilled weekly for 4 weeks and then monthly. No significant side-effects have been reported.

Chondroitin sulphate is a major component of the uroepithelial GAG layer.[85] Forty millilitres of 0.2% sterile sodium chondroitin sulphate once a week and then monthly led to 67% patient improvement.[86,87] A Canadian study showed 73% improvement in symptom score with initial instillation twice a week followed by weekly and then monthly instillations.[88] No significant side-effects have been reported.

Oxychlorosene sodium is only available in some countries. Instillation is painful and requires general anaesthesia. It is rarely used.

Several anecdotal 'bladder cocktails' have been used for instillation, but no publications have been reported on this topic.

Experimental treatments which are not yet widely approved for treatment of IC/PBS

BCG (bacille Calmette–Guérin) treatment was introduced recently[89] and a large randomized, prospective trial confirmed promising results[90] with long-term follow-up.[91] Approximately 60% of the patients responded to BCG in comparison to 27% treated with placebo; 89% continued to have a good response up to 27 months. Side-effects were mostly irritative voiding symptoms, and no systemic adverse effects were reported. BCG instillation boosts the local immune response in the bladder.[92] These favourable results were not confirmed when compared with DMSO treatment.[93]

RTX (resiniferatoxin) is a potent analogue of capsaicin and vanilloid receptor agonists. The compound produces prolonged desensitization of sensory C fibres from the bladder responsible for some symptoms in IC/PBS. A small study showed beneficial results in patients with IC.[94,95]

Botulinum toxin (BTX-A) is a very experimental treatment requiring intravesical injections under general anaesthesia. Botulinum works by paralysing smooth muscle activity and increases functional capacity.

Electromotive drug administration (EMDA) is a new medical delivery system used in combination with intravesical instillations. An electrical current accelerates directional movement of the medication and improves deep tissue penetration of the bladder wall.[96]

Minimally invasive treatments

Transurethral resection and coagulation and Nd:YAG laser ablation of Hunner's ulcers is an excellent, minimally invasive, and safe method of treating focal bladder lesions in

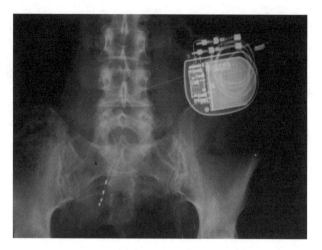

Fig. 18.8 Sacral nerve neuromodulator.

interstitial cystitis. While it is not a cure, and there are frequent relapses, it offers patients an opportunity to have decreased symptoms for an extended period of time and it may be repeated as necessary.[97,98]

Sacral nerve neuromodulation (Fig. 18.8) consists of temporary percutaneous sacral root stimulation and permanent implantation for those who responded well to the temporary one. Temporary stimulation was effective in 73% of women with refractory IC/PBS.[99] In this study the mean voided volume during treatment increased significantly and mean daytime frequency, nocturia, and pain decreased significantly. As indicated by the Short Urinary Distress Inventory and SF-36 Health Survey, the quality of life parameters of social functioning, bodily pain and general health significantly improved during the stimulation period. Percutaneous sacral third nerve root neurostimulation not only improves symptoms but also normalizes urinary HB-EGF levels and antiproliferative activity.[100]

Zermann *et al.*[101] reported significant improvement in 60-year-old woman treated for severe interstitial cystitis pain using a sacral nerve stimulator implant. Pain and accompanying bladder dysfunction were improved by temporary and permanent sacral nerve stimulation. Six months after implantation of the sacral neuromodulator the patient was pain free and significantly improved on bladder dysfunction.

Comiter[102] reported a series of 25 patients with a mean age of 47 years and refractory interstitial cystitis who were prospectively evaluated with a trial of sacral nerve stimulation. Patients who demonstrated a 50% improvement in frequency, nocturia, voided volume, and average pain qualified for permanent sacral nerve stimulator implantation. Of the 25 patients 17 qualified for permanent sacral nerve stimulator implantation. At an average of 14 months' follow-up mean daytime frequency, nocturia, and voided volumes improved significantly. Average pain decreased from 5.8 to 1.6 points on a scale of 0 to 10 and Interstitial Cystitis Symptom and Problem Index scores decreased from 16.5 to 6.8 and 14.5 to 5.4, respectively. Of the

17 patients, 16 (94%) with a permanent stimulator demonstrated sustained improvement in all parameters at the last post-operative visit. Neuromodulation remains an investigational treatment but it appears likely that it will have a long-term role in the management of these patients.

What can be considered as the last resort?

Neurosurgery

Cystolysis—peripheral denervation

The first report of bladder denervation was from Hunner in 1918.[103] He simply dissected the bladder from surrounding tissues. Initial results were encouraging; however, after 3 years of follow-up the symptoms recurred. Further attempts to do more formal cystolysis by Worth and Turner-Warwick[104] were more successful in regard to symptom control for up to 7 years. Bladder areflexia was a significant complication of this procedure.[105,106] Patients had to empty their bladders by the Credé technique or self-catheterization. Another attempt to revive the procedure also failed since most of the patients had recurrence after 4 years.[107] This procedure is very rarely performed today.

Sympathetic denervation

Visceral pain is transmitted in most of the patients by the sympathetic nervous system. Using this principle, Gino Pieri in 1926 applied it to the bladder pathology and suggested resection of the superior hypogastric plexus (presacral nerves), paravertebral sympathetic chain, and grey rami from the S1–3 ganglia.[108] This was repeated by Douglas few years later.[109] Immediate results were very good; however, further attempts with longer follow-ups showed that the long-term results were short lived.[110,111] This procedure is not used currently.

Parasympathetic denervation

Based on the presumption that S2–S4 segments contribute to bladder innervation Moulder and Meirowsky[112] used S3 neurectomy in three patients. All three patients responded well to S3 sacral block with procaine. Long-term follow-up was very good.[113] More patient data were reported by Milner and Garlick[114] and Mason.[115] Results after 5 years, however, were not encouraging.[116] In an attempt to improve results, selective dorsal sacral roots, either unilateral or bilateral, were approached by Bohm and Franksson.[117] The outcomes of this procedure were unclear. Overall, parasympathetic denervation has some undesirable side-effects such as atonic bladder, numbness, and some motor neuron paresis. The procedure is used very seldomly.

Bladder surgery involving the bowel

Bladder augmentation—cystoplasty

This procedure has been commonly used for refractory IC/PBS since 1958 when the first reports of ileocystoplasty appeared promising.[118] Later publications were less clear—some reporting good responses of up to 100%[119,120] and others poor with only 25%.[121,122] There is a general consensus that the intestinal segment used for bladder augmentation should be detubularized.[123] Several studies also indicate that cystoplasty with a subtrigonal cystectomy offers better results[119,124] compared with that without subtrigonal cystectomy.[125,126] There is generally no difference in outcome regardless of what segment of intestine is used—ileum[119,122], ileo-caecum[120,121,127], caecum[119,126], colon,[119,126] or sigmoid[119,125]. Patients with low cystoscopic capacity (<200 ml) under general anaesthesia achieved better results.[118,120,121,125,128] Long-term results are also good with fewer than 10% failures.[129] In summary, bladder augmentation can achieve good results (70–80% of cases) by using a detubularized intestinal segment, performing supratrigonal bladder resection, and selecting patients with low cystoscopic bladder capacity.

Urinary diversion is the most invasive solution to intractable IC/BPS and should be used as a last therapeutic procedure in selected patients. Some small studies have reported relatively good response to diversion with or without cystectomy.[121,131] Initially, for patients with IC/PBS, diversion is recommended without cystectomy, and only when the bladder pain persists after surgery is cystectomy indicated. Unfortunately, cystectomy rarely abolishes the pain.[131] Very often diversion is performed as a next step after unsuccessful bladder augmentation, and to prevent loss of further bowel the segment used for cystoplasty can often be converted to the conduit. In some patients, chronic inflammatory changes have been seen in the cystoplasty pouch resembling interstitial cystitis.[2,122] Similar changes have been noticed with other pathologies as well.[132] Bladder substitution is not recommended since most patients develop secondary changes resembling IC/PBS and causing severe symptoms, mostly pain.

Consequences of using bowel in bladder surgery

The decision to put part of the bowel into the urinary tract and expose it to urine should not be taken lightly, as there many potential metabolic abnormalities which may ensue such as:

1 Hyperchloraemic metabolic acidosis is caused by secretion of sodium and bicarbonate and absorption of hydrogen, chloride, and ammonium by ilel and colonic mucosa.[133] Most patients with good hepatic or renal function will not experience these metabolic changes but those without are at risk. Treatment of hyperchloraemic metabolic acidosis includes alkalinizing agents.[134]

2 Loss of distal ileum may result in decreased absorption of fat, bile salts, and fat-soluble vitamins (i.e. A, D, E, K).[135] Unabsorbed bile salts cause secondary diarrhoea by secretion of chloride and water into the colon.[136] Treatment includes cholestyramine resin which adsorbs and combines with the bile acids in the intestine to form an insoluble complex which is excreted in the faeces. This results in a partial removal of bile acids from the enterohepatic circulation by preventing their absorption.

3 Resection of the terminal ileum may also result in vitamin B_{12} deficiency and subsequently in megaloblastic anaemia and peripheral neuropathy.[137] Monthly injections of vitamin B_{12} are recommended to prevent this complication when more than 50 cm of terminal ileum has been removed.

4 Patients with urinary diversion tend to be chronically dehydrated and, therefore, susceptible to increased risk of stone formation. They may also have hyperoxaluria and hypercalciuria as a result of the acidosis. Urea-splitting organisms colonizing the intestinal segment further increase the risk of stone formation. Adequate hydration and calcium citrate is often used to prevent nephrolithiasis.[138]

5 Long-term consequences include the development of osteoporosis and osteomalacia, especially for post-menopausal women.[139] Oral alkalinizing agents, vitamin D, and calcium supplementation are often recommended in this situation.

6 Patients with cystoplasty should be followed annually with cystoscopies because of the possibility of developing neoplastic changes at the site of bowel and bladder anastomosis.

How can pain be controlled in IC/PBS?

Pain is an integral part of IC/PBS symptomatology and its pathophysiology includes neuropathic pain and inflammatory pathways. Inflammatory pain usually responds well to narcotic therapy and non-steroidal anti-inflammatory drugs (NSAIDs). Treatment with long-acting opiates is a very important component of this pain management when it is refractory to the other options discussed previously. Although the long-acting morphines oxycodone, levorphanol, methadone, or fentanyl may be necessary, narcotics should be only used in those exceptional cases when all alternative treatments have failed, and under close surveillance. There are few clinical data on the use NSAIDs in IC/PBS, although there is a theoretical basis for their use. It is suggested that non-selective less potent NSAIDs are used first and COX-2 selective drugs should be reserved for resistant patients. Some neuropathic pain, however, is more poorly responsive to opiates but may improve on antidepressant and anti-epileptic agents. Gabapentin is an anti-epileptic agent used in the adjunctive treatment of other causes of neuropathic pain such as post-therapeutic neuralgia and diabetic neuropathy and the pain of reflex sympathetic dystrophy. It has been suggested for use as an adjunctive agent in IC/PBS patients.[140,141] Tricyclic antidepressants such as amitriptyline, desipramine, doxepin, and imipramine are often useful. Amitriptyline has been used most extensively with high 'success' rates in patients with significant pain. The starting dosage is 25 mg at bed time with gradual increases to 75 mg. Frequency and urgency are usually improved minimally.[142]

Physical therapy treats viscero-somatic and somatic–visceral reflexes and involves approaching pelvic floor myofascial trigger points with manual physiotherapy.[143]

Other lifestyle-related pain relief strategies include:

* hot baths or heating pads
* relaxation strategies
* distraction techniques (e.g. involvement in absorbing activities)
* alternatives or modifications to sexual activities (e.g. different positions)
* loose clothing.

IC/PBS is a complex disease, not yet fully understood. Management should be tailored to the patient's needs and must be very compassionate. There will be many ups and downs, trials and errors, and successes and failures throughout the treatment course.

Self-help in IC/PBS

Since the final answers on many issues related to IC/PBS are still unknown, there is a large body of research under way. Methods to disseminate new findings and share knowledge and coping skills have flourished. These allow the individual patient to maintain some ownership of her or his treatment strategy through a variety of self-help options including support groups and internet websites. Some of the more popular are listed below.

IC support groups

1 The Interstitial Cystitis Association, 110 North Washington Street, Suite 340, Rockville, MD 20850, USA. Tel: 301.610.5300. Fax: 301.610.5308. Toll-free: 1–800-HELP-ICS. E-mail: ICAmail@ichelp.org

2 The Interstitial Cystitis Network, 4983 Sonoma Highway, Suite L Santa Rosa, CA 95409, USA. Tel: (707)538–9442. Fax: (707)538–9444

3 National Kidney and Urologic Diseases Information Clearinghouse, 3 Information Way, Bethesda, MD 20892–3580, USA. Tel: 1–800–891–5390 or (301) 654–4415. Fax: (301) 907–8906. E-mail: nkudic@info.niddk.nih.gov

4 The Cystitis and Overactive Bladder Foundation, 76 High Street, Stony Stratford, Buckinghamshire, MK11 1AH. Tel: +44 (0) 1908 569169. Fax: +44 (0) 1908 565665. E-mail: info@cobfoundation.org

Web pages

http://www.ichelp.org
http://www.ic-network.com
http://www.interstitial-cystitis.org
http://www.urologychannel.com/interstitialcystitis
http://www.kidney.niddk.nih.gov/kudiseases/pubs/interstitialcystitis
http://www.intercyst.org
http://www.interstitialcystitis.co.uk

References

1 Hunner GL (1915). A rare type of bladder ulcer in women; report of cases. *Boston Med. Surg. J.* **172**: 660–5.

2 Messing EM, Stamey TA (1978). Interstitial cystitis. Early diagnosis, pathology, and treatment. *Urology* **12**: 381–92.

3 Gillenwater JY, Wein AJ (1988). Summary of the National Institute of Arthritis, Diabetes, Digestive and Kidney Diseases workshop on interstitial cystitis, National Institutes of Health, Bethesda, Maryland, August 28–29. *J. Urol.* **140**: 203–6.

4 Simon LJ, Landis JR, Tomaszewski JE, Nyberg LM and the ICDB Study Group (1997). The Interstitial Cystitis Data Base Study. In: *Interstitial Cystitis* (ed. RS Grannum), pp. 17–24. Lippincott-Raven, Philadelphia, PA.

5 Peeker R, Fall M (2002). Toward a precise definition of interstitial cystitis: further evidence of differences in classic and nonucler disease. *J. Urol.* **167**: 2470–2.

6 Koziol JA, Adams HP, Frutus A (1996). Discrimination between the ulcerous and the nonulcerous forms of interstitial cystitis by noninvasive findings. *J. Urol.* **155**: 87–90.

7 Oravisto KJ (1975). Epidemiology of interstitial cystitis. *Ann. Chir. Gynaecol. Fenn.* **64**: 75–7.

8 Bade JJ, Rijcken B, Mensink HJA (1995). Interstitial cystitis in the Netherlands. Prevalance, diagnostic criteria and therapeutic preferences. *J. Urol.* **154**: 2035–8.

9 Leppilahti M, Tammela TL, Huhtala H, Auvinen A (2002). Prevalence of symptoms related to interstitial cystitis in women: a population based study in Finland. J. Urol. **168**: 139–43.

10 Held PJ, Hanno PM, Wein AJ, Pauly MV, Cann MA (1990). Epidemiology of interstitial Cystitis. In: *Interstitial Cystitis* (ed. PM Hanno, DR Staskin, RJ Krane, AJ Wein), pp. 29–48. Springer, New York.

11 Jones CA, Harris M, Nyberg L (1994). Prevalence of interstitial cystitis in the United States. *J. Urol.* **151**: 423A.

12 Curhan GC, Speizer FE, Hunter DJ, Curhan SG, Stampfer MJ (1999). Epidemiology of interstitial cystitis: a population based study. *J. Urol.* **161**: 549–52.

13 Parsons CL, Dell J, Stanford EJ, Bullen M, Kahn BS, Waxell T *et al.* (2002). Increased prevalence of interstitial cystitis: previously unrecognized urological and gynecologic cases identified using a new symptom questionnaire and intravesical potassium sensitivity. *Urology* **60**: 573–8.

14 Ito T, Miki M, Yamada T (2000). Interstitial cystitis in Japan. *BJU Int.* **86**(6): 634–7.

15 Roberts RO, Bergstralh EJ, Bass SE, Lightner DJ, Lieber MM, Jacobsen SJ (2003). Incidence of physician-diagnosed interstitial cystitis in Olmsted County: a community-based study *BJU Int.* **91**: 181–5.

16 Warren JW, Jackson TL, Langenberg P, Meyers DJ, Xu J (2004). Prevalence of interstitial cystitis in first-degree relatives of patients with interstitial cystitis. *Urology* **63**(1): 17–2

17 Forrest J, Vo Q (2001). Observations on the management of interstitial cystitis in men. *Urology* **57**: 107.

18 Parsons CL, Zupkas P, Parsons JK (2001). Intravesical potassium sensitivity in patient with interstitial cystitis and urethral syndrome. *Urology* **57**: 428–32.

19 Saban R, Christensen M, Keith I, Graziano FM, Undem BJ, Aagaard J *et al.* (1991). Experimental model for the study of bladder mast cells degranulation and smooth muscle contraction. *Semin. Urol.* **9**: 88–101.

20 Theoharides TC, Sant GR (1991). Bladder mast cell activation in interstitial cystitis. *Semin. Urol.* **9**: 74–87.

21 Elbadawi A (1997). Interstitial cystitis: a critique of current concepts with a new proposal for pathologic diagnosis and pathogenesis. *Urology* **49**(Suppl.): 14–40.

22 Galloway NTM, Gabale DR, Irwin PP (1991). Interstitial cystitis or reflex sympathetic dystrophy of the bladder. *Semin. Urol.* **9:** 148–53.

23 Simon LJ, Landis JR, Erickson DR, Nyberg LM and the ICDB Study Group (1997). The Interstitial Cystitis Data Base (ICDB) Study: concepts and preliminary baseline descriptive statistics. *Urology* **49**(Suppl. 5A): 64–75.

24 Propert KJ, Schaeffer AJ, Brensinger CM, Kusek J, Nyberg LM, Landis JR and the Interstitial Cystitis Data Base Study Group (2000). A prospective study of interstitial cystitis: results of longitudinal follow-up of the interstitial cystitis data base cohort. *J. Urol.* **163**: 1434–9.

25 Abrams P, Cardozo L, Fall M, Griffiths D, Rosier P, Ulmsten U *et al.* (2002). The standardisation of terminology of lower urinary tract function: report from the Standardisation Sub-committee of the International Continence Society. *Neurourol. Urodyn.* **21**: 167–78.

26 Driscoll A, Teichman JM (2001). How do patients with interstitial cystitis present? *J. Urol.* **166**: 2118–20.

27 Theoharides TC, Pang X, Letourneau R, Sant GR (1998). Interstitial Cystitis: a neuroimmunoendocrine disorder. *Ann. N. Y. Acad. Sci.* **840**: 619–34.

28 Erickson DR, Morgan KC, Ordille S, Keay SK, Xie SX (2001). Nonbladder related symptoms in patients with interstitial cystitis. *J. Urol.* **166**: 557–61.

29 Michael YL, Kawachi I, Stampfer MJ, Colditz GA, Curhan GC (2000). Quality of life among women with interstitial cystitis. *J. Urol.* **164**: 423–7.

30 Slade D, Ratner V, Chalker R (1997). A collaborative approach to managing interstitial cystitis. *Urology* **49**: 10–13.

31 Rothrock NE, Lutgendorf SK, Hoffman A, Kreder KJ (2002). Depressive symptoms and quality of life in patients with interstitial cystitis. *J. Urol.* **167**: 1763–7.

32 McCormick NB, Vinson RK (1989). Interstitial cystitis: how women cope. Urol. Nurs. **9:** 11–17.

33 Draucker CB (1991). Coping with a difficult-to-diagnose illness. The example of interstitial cystitis *Health Care Women Int.* **12**: 191–8.

34 Butler LJ, Conner LL, Marsh SM (2003). The meaning of quality of life and relationships for women living with interstitial cystitis. *J. Sex. Reprod. Med.* **1**: 9–14.

35 McCormick NB (1999). When pleasure causes pain: living with interstitial cystitis. *Sexual. Disab.* **17**: 7–18.

36 Webster DC, Brennan T (1995). Use and effectiveness of psychological self-care strategies for interstitial cystitis. *Health Care Women Int.* **16**: 463–75.

37 Azevedo K, Payne CK (2001). The psychosocial economic impact of invisible chronic disease: examining the experience of patients with interstitial cystitis. *Urology* **57**: 118.

38 Rothrock NE, Lutgendorf SK, Kreder KJ, Ratliff T, Zimmerman B (2001). Stress and symptoms in patients with interstitial cystitis: a life stress model. *Urology* **57**: 422–7.

39 Rothrock NE, Lutgendorf SK, Kreder KJ, Ratliff TL, Zimmerman B (2001). Daily stress and symptom exacerbation in interstitial cystitis patients. *Urology* **57**: 122.

40 O'Leary MP, Sant GR, Fowler FJ, Whitmore KE, Spolarich-Kroll J (1997). The interstitial cystitis symptoms and index and problem index. *Urology* **49**: 58–63.

41 Lubeck DP, Whitmore K, Sant GR, Alvarez-Horine S, Lai C (2001). Psychometric validation of the O'Leary–Sant interstitial cystitis symptom index in a clinical trial of pentosan polysulfate sodium. *Urology* **57**: 62–6.

42 Parsons CL, Dell J, Stanford EJ, Bullen M, Kahn BS, Waxell T *et al.* (2002). Increased prevalence of interstitial cystitis: previous unrecognized urologic and gynecologic cases identified using a new symptom questionnaire and intravesical potassium sensitivity. *Urology* **60**: 573–8.

43 Mazurick CA, Landis JR (2000). Evaluation of repeat daily voiding measures in the National Intersticial Cystitis Data Base Study. *J. Urol.* **163**: 1208–11.

44 Clauw DJ, Schmidt M, Radulovic D, Singer A, Katz P, Bresette J (1997). The relationship between fibromyalgia and interstitial cystitis. *J. Psychiatr. Res.* **31**: 125–31.

45 Messing EM (1987). The diagnosis of interstitial cystitis. *Urology* **29**(Suppl. 4): 4–7.

46 Waxman JA, Sulak PJ, Kuchl TJ (1998). Cystoscopic findings consistant with interstitial cystitis in normal women undergoing tubal ligation. *J. Urol.* **160**: 1663–7.

47 Glemain P, Riviere C, Lenormand L, Karam G, Bouchot O, Buzelin JM (2002). Prolonged hydrodistention of the bladder for symptomatic treatment of interstitial cystitis: efficacy at 6 months and 1 year. *Eur. Urol.* **41**: 79–84.

48 Chai TC, Zhang CO, Shoenfelt JL, Johnson HW, Warren JW, Keay S (2000). Bladder stretch alters urinary heparin-binding epidermal growth factor and antiproliferative factor in patients with interstitial cystitis. *J. Urol.* **163**: 1440–4.

49 Toozs-Hobson P, Gleeson C, Cardozo L (1996). Interstitial cystitis: still an enigma after 80 years. *Br. J. Obstet. Gynaecol.* **103**: 621–4.

50 Ito T, Miki M, Yamada T (2000). Interstitial cystitis in Japan. *BJU Int.* **86**: 634–7.

51 Denson MA, Griebling TL, Cohen MB, Kreder KJ (2000). Comparison of cystoscopic and histological findings in patients with suspected interstitial cystitis. *J. Urol.* **164**: 1908–11.

52 Tomaszewski JE, Landis JR, Russack V, Williams TM, Wang LP, Hardy C *et al.* (2001). Biopsy features are associated with primary symptoms in interstitial cystitis: results from the interstitial cystitis database study. *Urology* **57**: 67–81.

53 Gajewski JB, Awad SA (1997). Urodynamic evaluation in interstitial cystitis. In: *Interstitial Cystitis* (ed. GR Sant), pp. 169–72. Lippincott-Raven, Philadelphia PA.

54 Parsons CL (1990). Interstitial cystitis: clinical manifestations and diagnostic criteria in over 200 cases. Neurourol. Urodyn. **9**: 241–50.

55 Awad SA, Gajewski JB, Katz NO, Acker-Roy K (1992). Final diagnosis and therapeutic implications of mixed symptoms of urinary incontinence in women. *Urology* **39**: 352–7.

56 Awad SA, MacDiarmid S, Gajewski JB, Gupta R (1992). Idiopathic bladder storage versus interstitial cystitis. *J. Urol.* **148**: 1409–12.

57 Holm-Bentzen M, Larsen S, Hainanau B, Hald T (1985). Nonobstructive detrusor myopathy in a group of patients with chronic abacterial cystitis. *Scan. J. Urol. Nephrol.* **19**: 21–6.

58 Parsons CL, Greenberger M, Gabal L, Bidair M, Barme G (1998). The role of urinary potassium in the pathogenesis and diagnosis of interstitial cystitis. *J. Urol.* **159**: 1862–6.

59 Chambers GK, Fenster HN, Cripps S, Jens M, Taylor D (1999). An assessment of the use of intravesical potassium in the diagnosis of interstitial cystitis. *J. Urol.* **162**: 699–701.

60 Gregoire M, Liandier F, Naud A, Lacombe L, Fradet Y (2002). Does the potassium stimulation test predict cystometric, cystoscopic outcome in interstitial cystitis?. *J. Urol.* **168**: 556–7.

61 Bologna RA, Gomelsky A, Lukban JC, Tu LM, Holzberg AS, Whitmore KE (2001). The efficacy of calcium glycerophosphate in the prevention of food-related flares in interstitial cystitis. *Urology* **57**: 119–20.

62 Katske F, Shoskes DA, Sender M, Poliakin R, Gagliano K, Raifer J (2001). Treatment of interstitial with a quercetin supplement. *Tech. Urol.* **7**: 44–6.

63 Waters MG, Suleskey JF, Finkelstein LJ, Van Overbeke ME, Zizza VJ, Stommel M (2000). Interstitial cystitis: a retrospective analysis of treatment with pentosan polysulfate and follow-up patient survey. *J. Am. Osteopath. Assoc.* **100**(Suppl. 3): S13–S18.

64 Mulholland SG, Hanno P, Parsons CL, Sant GR, Staskin DR (1990). Pentosan polysulfate sodium for therapy of interstitial cystitis: a double-blind placebo-controlled clinical study. *Urology* **35**: 552–8.

65 Hwang P, Auclair B, Beechinor D, Diment M, Einarson TR (1997). Efficacy of pentosan polysulfate in treatment of interstitial cystitis: a meta-analysis. *Urology* **50**: 39–43.

66 Chiang G, Patra P, Letourneau R, Jeudy S, Boucher W, Green M *et al.* (2000). Pentosanpolysulfate inhibits mast cell histamine secretion and intracellular calcium ion levels: an alternative explanation of its beneficial effect in interstitial cystitis. *J. Urol.* **164**: 2119–25.

67 Nickel JC, Forrest J, Barkin J, Payne C, Mosbaugh P (2001). Safety and efficacy of up to 900 mg/day polysulfate sodium (elmiron) in patients with interstitial cystitis *Urology* **57**: 122–3.

68 Korting GE, Smith SD, Wheeler MA, Weiss RM, Foster HE Jr (1999). A randomized double-blind trial of oral l-arginine for treatment of interstitial cystitis. *J. Urol.* **161**: 558–65.

69 Wheeler MA, Smith SD, Saito N, Foster HE Jr, Weiss RM (1997). Effect of long-term oral L-arginine on the nitric oxide synthase pathway in the urine from patients with interstitial cystitis. *J. Urol.* **158**: 2045–50.

70 Ehren I, Lundberg JO, Adolfsson J, Wiklund NP (1998). Effects of L-arginine treatment on symptoms and bladder nitric oxide levels in patients with interstitial cystitis. *Urology* **52**: 1026–9.

71 Theoharides TC (1994). Hydroxizine in treatment of interstitial cystitis. *Urol. Clin. North Am.* **21**: 113–19.

72 Dasgupta P, Sharma SD, Womack C, Blackford HN, Dennis P (2001). Cimetidine in painful bladder syndrome: a histopathological study. *BJU Int.* **88**: 183–6.

73 Thilagarajah R, Witherow RO, Walker MM (2001). Oral cimetidine gives effective symptoms relief in painful bladder disease: a prospective, randomized double-blind placebo controlled trial. *BJU Int.* **87**: 207–12.

74 Ueda T, Tamaki M, Ogawa O, Yamauchi T, Yoshimura N (2000). Improvement of interstitial cystitis symptoms and problems that developed during treatment with oral IPD-1151T. *J. Urol.* **164**: 1917–20.

75 Warren JW, Horne LM, Hebel JR, Marvel RP, Keay SK, Chai TC (2000). Pilot study of sequential oral antibiotics for the treatment of interstitial cystitis. *J. Urol.* **163**: 1685–8.

76 Barbalias GA, Liatsikos EN, Athanasopoulos A, Nikiforidis G (2000). Interstitial cystitis: bladder training with intravesical oxybutynin. *J. Urol.* **163**: 1818–22.

77 Jacob SW, Bischel M, Herschler RJ (1964). Dimethyl sulfoxide (DMSO): a new concept in pharmacotherapy. *Curr. Ther. Res.* **6**: 134.

78 Stewart BH, Branson AC, Hewitt CB, Kiser WS, Straffon RA (1971). The treatment or patients with interstitial cystitis with special reference to intravesical DMSO. *Trans. Am. Assoc. Genitourin. Surg.* **63**: 69.

79 Stewart BH, Shirley SW (1976). Further experience with intravesical DMSO in the treatment of interstitial cystitis. *J. Urol.* **116**: 36.

80 Sant GR (1987). Intravesical 50% dimethyl sulfoxide (Rimso-50) in treatment of interstitial cystitis. *Urology* **29**(Suppl. 4): 17–21.

81 Stewart BH, Persky L, Kiser WS (1967). The use of dimethyl sulfoxide (DMSO) in the treatment of interstitial cystitis. *J. Urol.* **98**: 671–2.

82 Parsons CL, Housley T, Schmidt JD, Lebow D (1994). Treatment of interstitial cystitis with intravesical heparin. *Br. J. Urol.* **73**: 504–7.

83 Morales A, Emerson L, Nickel JC, Lundie M (1996). Intravesical hyaluronic acid in the treatment of refractory interstitial cystitis. *J. Urol.* **156**: 45–8.

84 Nordling J, Jorgenson S, Kallestrup E (2001). Cystistat for the treatment of interstitial cystitis: a 3-year follow up study. *Urology* **57**(Suppl. 1): 123.

85 Hurst RE, Roy JB, Min KW, Veltri RW, Marley G, Patton K *et al.* (1996). A deficit of chondroitin sulfate proteoglycans on the bladder urothelium in interstitial cystitis. *Urology* **48**: 817–21.

86 Steinhoff G, Ittah B, Rowan S (2002). The efficacy of chondroitin sulfate 0.2% in treating interstitial cystitis. *Can. J. Urol.* **9**: 1454–8.

87 Steinhoff G (2003). The efficacy of chondroitin sulphate in treating interstitial cystitis. *Eur. Urol.* **2**(Suppl. 2): 14–16.

88 Sorensen RB (2003). Chondroitin sulphate in the treatment of interstitial cystitis and chronic inflammatory disease of the urinary bladder. *Eur. Urol.* **2**(Suppl. 2): 16–18.

89 Zeidman EJ, Helfrick B, Pollard C, Thompson IM (1994). Bacillus Calmette–Guerin immunotherapy for refractory interstitial cystitis. *Urology* **43**: 121–4.

90 Peters K, Diokno A, Steinert B, Yuhico M, Mitchell B, Krohta S *et al.* (1997). The efficacy of intravesical Tice strain bacillus Calmette–Guerin in treatment of interstitial cystitis: a double-blind, prospective, placebo controlled trial. *J. Urol.* **157**: 2090–4.

91 Peters K, Diokno A, Steinert B, Gonzalez JA (1998). The efficacy of intravesical bacillus Calmette–Guerin in the treatment of interstitial cystitis: long-term follow-up. *J. Urol.* **159**: 1483–6.

92 Peters K, Diokno A, Steinert B (1999). Preliminary study on urinary cytokine levels in interstitial cystitis: does intravesical bacille Calmette–Guerin treat interstitial cystitis by altering the immune profile of the bladder? *Urology* **54**: 450–3.

93 Peeker R, Haghsheno MA, Holmang S, Fall M (2000). Intravesical bacillus Calmette–Guerin and dimethyl sulfoxiade for treatment of classic and nonuclear interstitial cystitis: a prospective, randomized double-blind study. *J. Urol.* **164**: 1912–15.

94 Lazzeri M, Beneforati P, Spinelli M, Zanollo A, Barbagli G, Turini D (2000). Intravesical resiniferatoxin for the treatment of hypersensitive disorder: a randomized placebo controlled study. *J. Urol.* **164**: 676–9.

95 Lazzeri M, Spinelli M, Beneforti P, Malaguti S, Giardiello G, Turini D (2004). Intravesical infusion of resiniferatoxin by temporary in situ drug delivery system to treat interstitial cystitis: a pilot study. *Eur. Urol.* **45**: 98–102.

96 Rosamilia A, Dwyer PL, Gibson J (1997). Electromotive drug administration of lidocaine and dexamethasone followed by cystodistantion in women with interstitial cystitis. *Int. Urogynecol. J. Pelvic Floor Dysfunct.* **8**: 142–5.

97 Peeker R, Aldenborg F, Fall M (2000). Complete transurethral resection of ulcers in classic interstitial cystitis. *Int. Urogynecol. J. Pelvic Floor Dysfunct.* **11**: 290–5.

98 Rofeim O, Hom D, Freid RM, Moldwin RM (2001). Use of the neodymium:YAG laser for interstitial cystitis: a prospective study. *J. Urol.* **166**: 134–6.

99 Maher CF, Carey MP, Dwyer PL, Schluter PL (2001). Percutaneous sacral nerve root neuromodulation for intractable interstitial cystitis. *J. Urol.* **165**: 884–6.

100 Zermann DH, Ishigooka M, Schubert J (2001). Percutaneous sacral third nerve root neurostimulation improves symptoms and normalizes urinary HB-EGF levels and antiproliferative activity in patients with interstitial cystitis. *Urology* **57**: 207.

101 Zermann DH, Weirich T, Wunderlich H, Reichelt O, Schubert J (2000). Sacral nerve stimulation for pain relief in interstitial cystitis. *Urol. Int.* **65**: 120–1.

102 Comiter CV (2003). Sacral neuromodulation for the symptomatic treatment of refractory interstitial cystitis: a prospective study. *J. Urol.* **169**: 1369–73.

103 Hunner GL (1918). Elusive ulcer of the bladder. Further notes on rare type of bladder ulcer, with a report of twenty-five cases. *Am. J. Obstet.* **78**: 374–95.

104 Worth PL, Turner-Warwick R (1973). The treatment of interstitial cystitis by cystolysis with observations on cystoplasty. *Br. J. Urol.* **45**: 65–71.

105 Worth PHL (1980). The treatment of interstitial cystitis by cystolysis with observations on cystoscopy. A review after 7 years. *Br. J. Urol.* **52**: 232.

106 Freiha FS, Stamey TA (1980). Cystolysis: a procedure for selective denervation of the bladder. *J. Urol.* **123**: 360–3.

107 Albers DD, Geyer JR (1988). Long-term results of cystolysis (supratrigonal denervation) of the bladder for intractable interstitial cystitis. *J. Urol.* **139**: 1205–6.

108 Pieri G (1926). Enervation ou ramisection? *Presse Méd* **34**: 1141–2.

109 Douglass HL (1934). Excision of the superior hypogastric plexus in the treatment of intractable interstitial cystitis. *Am. J. Surg.* **25**: 249–57.

110 Nesbit RM (1947). Anterolateral chordotomy for refractory interstitial cystitis with intractable pain. *J. Urol.* **57**: 741–5.

111 Jacobson CE, Braasch WF, Love JG (1944). Presacral neurectomy for intractable vesical pain and neurogenic vesical dysfunction. *Surg. Gynecol. Obstet.* **79**: 21–6.

112 Moulder MK, Meirowsky AM (1956). The management of Hunner's ulcer by differential sacral neurotomy:preliminary report. *J. Urol.* **75**: 261–2.

113 Meirowsky AM (1969). The management of chronic interstitial cystitis by differential sacral neurotomy. *J. Neurosurg.* **30**: 604–7.

114 Milner WA, Garlick WB (1957). Selective sacral neurectomy in interstitial cystitis. *J. Urol.* **78**: 600–4.

115 Mason TH, Heines GL, Leversee BW (1960). Selective sacral neurotomy for Hunner's ulcer. *J. Neurosurg.* **17**: 22–6.

116 Saris SC, Silver JM, Vieira JFS, Nashold BS (1986). Sacrococcygeal rhizotomy for perineal pain. *Neurosurgery* **19**: 789–93.

117 Bohm E, Franksson C (1957). Interstitial cystitis and sacral rhizotomy. *Acta Chir. Scand.* **113**: 63–7.

118 Goodwin WE, Turner RD, Winter CC (1958). Results of ileocystoplasty. *J. Urol.* **80**: 461–6.

119 von Garrelts B (1966). Interstitial cystitis: thirteen patients treated operatively with intestinal bladder substitutes *Acta Chir. Scand.* **132**: 436–43.

120 Webster GD, Maggio MI (1989). The management of chronic interstitial cystitis by substitution cystoplasty. *J. Urol.* **141**: 287–91.

121 Nielsen KK, Kromann-Andersen B, Steven K, Hald T (1990). Failure of combine subtrigonal cystectomy and Mainz ileocystoplasty in intractable interstitial cystitis: is histology and mast cells count a reliable predictor for the outcome of surgery. *J. Urol.* **144**: 255–9.

122 Badenoch AW (1971). Chronic interstitial cystitis. *J. Urol.* **43**: 718–21.

123 Hinman FJ (1988). Selection of intestinal segments for bladder substitution: physical and physiological characteristics. *J. Urol.* **139**: 519–23.

124 Bruce PT, Buckham GJ, Carden ABG, Salvaris M (1977). The surgical treatment of chronic interstitial cystitis. *Med. J. Aust.* **1**: 581–2.

125 Kontturi MJ, Hellström PA, Tammela TLJ, Lukkarinen OA (1991). Colocystoplasty for the treatment of severe interstitial cystitis. *Urol. Int.* **46**: 50–4.

126 Holm-Bentzen M, Klarskov P, Opsomer R, Hald T (1986). Coecocystoplasty: an evaluation of operative results. *Urol. Int.* **41**: 21–5.

127 de Juana CP, Everett JC (1977). Interstitial cystitis. *Urology* **10**: 325–9.

128 Hohenfellner M, Black P, Linn JF, Dahms SE, Thuroff JW (2000). Surgical treatment of interstitial cystitis in women. *Int. Urogynecol. J. Pelvic Floor Dysfunct.* **11**: 113–19.

129 van Ophoven A, Oberpenning F, Hertle L (2002). Long-term results of trigone-preserving orthotopic substitution enterocystoplasty for interstitial cystitis. *J. Urol.* **167**: 603–7.

130 Webster GD, Galloway N (1987). Surgical treatment of interstitial cystitis. Indications, techniques and results. *Urology* **29**(Suppl. 4): 34–9.

131 Baskin LS, Tanagho EA (1992). Pelvic pain without pelvic organs. *J. Urol.* **147**: 683–6.

132 MacDermott JP, Charpied GL, Tesluk H, Stone AR (1990). Recurrent interstitial cystitis following cystoplasty: fact or fiction? *J. Urol.* **144**: 37–40.

133 Mills RD, Studer UE (1999). Metabolic consequences of continent urinary diversion. *J. Urol.* **161**: 1057–66.

134 McDougal WS (1992). Metabolic complications of urinary intestinal diversion. *J. Urol.* **147**: 1199–207.

135 Hoffman AF (1972). Bile acid malabsorbtion caused by ileal resection. *Arch. Intern. Med.* **130**: 597–605.

136 Durrans D, Wujanto R, Carrol RN, Torrance HB (1989) Bile acid malabsorbtion: a complication of ileal conduit surgery. *Br. J. Urol.* **64**: 485–8.

137 Babior BM, Bunn HF (1994). Megaloblastic anemias. In: *Harrison's Principles of Internal Medicine* 13th edn (ed. KJ Isselbacher, E Braunwald, JD Wilson, JB Martin, AS Fauci, DL Kasper), ch. 304. McGraw-Hill, New York.

138 Cohen TD, Streem SB, Lammbert G (1996). Long-term incidence and risks for recurrent stones following contemporary management of upper tract lculi in patients with urinary diversion. *J. Urol.* **155**: 62–5.

139 Mundy AR, Nurse DE (1992). Calcium balance, growth and skeletal mineralization in patient with cystoplasties. *Br. J. Urol.* **69**: 257–9.

140 Hansen HC (2000). Interstitial cystitis and the potential role of gabapentin. *South. Med. J.* **93**: 238–42.

141 Lutgendorf SK, Kreder KJ, Rothrock NE, Ratliff TL, Zimmerman B (2000). Stress and symptomatology in patients with interstitial cystitis: a laboratory stress model. *J. Urol.* **164**: 1265–9.

142 Hanno PM (1994). Amitriptyline in the treatment of interstitial cystitis. *Urol. Clin. North Am.* **21**: 89–91.

143 Weiss JM (2001). Pelvic floor myofascial trigger points: manual therapy for interstitial cystitis and the urgency-frequency syndrome. *J. Urol.* **166**(6): 2226–31.

Chapter 19

Supportive care for the renal transplant patient

David Nicol and Catherine Martin

Introduction

Renal transplantation has now become an extremely successful treatment for end-stage renal disease (ESRD). In virtually all groups of patients with ESRD it confers a very significant survival advantage over long-term dialysis.[1,2] Individual stories abound about lives being extended and improved. The International Transplant Olympics movement is a testimony to the high level of health, fitness and normality achievable through transplantation.

Current graft survival rates at 1 and 10 years are approximately 90% and 60% for cadaver donors and 95% and 70% with living donors.[2] Rejection rates have dropped significantly over the past two decades, and rejection is now an uncommon cause of early loss of a graft. Organ supply is a major limiting factor in the availability of this treatment option. The incidence of ESRD in our ageing population is increasing, and as a result many more patients are being considered for transplantation.[1,3] However, in most countries the number of available cadaveric organs is limited and increasing discrepancies have occurred between the number of patients awaiting transplantation and available organs. As a consequence, living donor transplantation is increasingly being utilized.

Transplantation involves a period of acute management immediately following surgery. This is usually undertaken within a specialized hospital unit. Longer-term management and care in many cases will not be in the context of a specialized unit. However, in their care, patients with renal transplants require specific consideration as a consequence of their medications including immunosuppressives, chronic co-morbidities which may have contributed to or caused their ESRD, as well as consequences and complications of the transplant including loss of the graft.

Supportive care of renal transplant patients is also influenced by multiple psycho-social factors which can arise as a consequence of these medical issues as well as the unique circumstances of organ transplantation.

Immunosuppression

Long-term immunosuppression is required in all renal transplant recipients to prevent rejection of the graft.[4,5] Most centres utilize combinations therapy comprising a calcineurin inhibitor, an antiproliferative agent, and corticosteroids.

1 Calcineurin inhibitors (cyclosporin, tacrolimus) are fungal derivatives which inactivate calcineurin, a key enzyme in T-lymphocyte receptor signalling and cytokine (IL-2) production.[6] Both drugs are potentially nephrotoxic, and hence monitoring of blood levels is used to determine individual doses to minimize toxicity and maintain adequate immunosuppression.[7,8] Glucose intolerance and diabetes can emerge with the use of both these drugs, occurring in approximately 15% of patients with tacrolimus and 10% with cyclosporin.[9] Both drugs can be associated with hypertension and dyslipidaemias.[3,6] Hirsuitism and gingival hyperplasia are seen with cyclosporin, particularly in the paediatric population.[3]

2 Antiproliferative agents (azathioprine, mycophenolic acid) inhibit DNA synthesis and limit the proliferation of activated B and T lymphocytes.[4,5] Azathioprine is a purine analogue whereas MPA inhibits purine synthesis. Both are associated with bone marrow suppression. MPA is a more potent agent but can be associated with gastrointestinal side-effects and an increased risk of infection.

3 Corticosteroids are non-specific anti-inflammatory agents inhibiting cytokine production by lymphocytes and macrophage function. These have numerous well-known side-effects including glucose intolerance, hypertension, dyslipidaemia, and osteoporosis.[10] Steroid withdrawal is attempted in selected cases although this can be complicated by the risk of rejection.[5]

A number of newer agents have also been trialled and may confer advantages in specific cases. Of these sirolimus is now the only one widely available for long-term use. Sirolimus is also a fungal derivative and inhibits T-lymphocyte responses to cytokine stimulation.[4,8,11] Hyperlipidaemia and thrombocytopenia are its main side-effects.[11]

These medications are associated with a number of potential complications and side-effects discussed below.

Complications and side-effects of immunosuppressants

Risks of infection

Transplant recipients are at increased risk of infection as a consequence of immunosuppression. Approximately 20% of deaths in renal transplant recipients are due to infection.[2] In many cases these relate to opportunistic pathogens including cytomegalovirus, fungi, and atypical bacteria.[12] Infections tend to occur from approximately the second month following transplantation with treatment of rejection, long-term over-immunosuppression, diabetes, and older age as specific risk factors.[13]

Cosmetic changes

Immunosuppressive medications can produce a number of cosmetic changes. These include the Cushingoid effects of corticosteroids and hirsuitism and gingival hyperplasia with cyclosporin.[5] This can contribute to problems with compliance, particularly in adolescence and young adults. Simple cosmetic measures such as use of bleach for facial hair and dental attention should be recommended early.

Osteoporosis

This occurs in many patients after renal transplantation. Most bone loss seems to occur in the first year after transplantation. The risk of fracture depends on pre- and post-transplant variables, with the risk highest in post-menopausal women.[14] Steroid-sparing immunosuppression may be important in improving the long-term outcome of bone mineral density in transplant patients. Avascular necrosis of the hips can also occur related to the effects of steroids.[10]

Malignancy

Transplant recipients are at increased risk of malignancy as a consequence of immuno-suppression although the incidence of some tumours including prostate and colorectal appear similar to the general population.[2,15] Lymphoproliferative disorders and skin are specific cancers which are dramatically increased.[16,17] With the latter, multiple dermato-logical and surgical interventions may be necessary with close surveillance recommended for individuals at particular risk (i.e. significant sun exposure, red hair, pale skin).[17]

Co-morbidities

Diabetes

This can be present and may have contributed to the patient's renal failure or it can arise following transplantation secondary to medications (e.g. calcineurin inhibitors and steroids). The consequences of this disease exacerbate the multiple co-morbidities associated with renal transplantation.[9]

Cardiovascular disease

This contributes significantly to the long-term morbidity and mortality following renal transplantation. Patients often have multiple risk factors relating to prior chronic renal failure, hypertension, dyslipidaemias, and diabetes all of which may be exacerbated by immunosuppressive medications.[18] Management of patients with renal disease, including the post-transplant patient, should include reduction of cardiovascular risk factors. The target for blood pressure control in many transplant units is below the 145/85 mmHg recommended for the general population. Inhibitors of the renin–angiotensin system appear to be of specific benefit and are often combined with calcium channel blockers which reduce both the doses of cyclosporin required as well as some of its intra-renal effects. Hyperlipidaemias should also be aggressively treated. Despite these measures ischaemic heart disease, cerebrovascular events, and the consequences of peripheral vascular disease will need to be managed in many transplant recipients.

Impotence and infertility

Erectile dysfunction (ED) is present in up to 50% of patients with chronic renal failure.[19] Multiple factors have been implicated, including the effects of chronic illness.

The hypothalamic–pituitary axis is affected with a decrease in testosterone production, possibly as a direct effect of uraemia on the testes.[20] Hyperprolactinaemia caused by an increased production or a reduced metabolism of prolactin, or induced by drugs, is often present.[21] Autonomic neuropathy can arise from uraemia and secondary hyperparathyroidism. Due to associated risk factors (e.g. diabetes, hypertension, and hyperlipidaemia) atherosclerosis is commonly present, with eventual severe involvement of the venous corporo-occlusive mechanism caused by fibrosis of the trabeculae. Pharmacological factors including antihypertensives may also be implicated. Psychological factors can also contribute, including the effects of chronic illness, loss of self-esteem, and depression. With renal transplantation erectile function improves in up to 75% of cases.[19] An additional risk factor for erectile dysfunction is the use of the internal iliac artery as well as patients who undergo a second transplant. In transplant recipients oral agents including sildenafil citrate appear to have similar efficacy to that seen in other patients with ED.[22] Sildenafil is mainly degraded by the cytochrome P-450 system. Although this enzyme system also degrades cyclosporin and FK506, neither drug appears affected by the use of sildenafil. Where oral agents fail, intracavernosal drugs and penile prostheses can be considered as they would be in other patients. Uraemic hypogonadism is a common feature of end-stage renal disease associated with loss of libido and infertility.[21,23,24] These features reflect impaired Leydig cell function as well as markedly depressed spermatogenesis with severe oligospermia or azoospermia. Whilst transplantation may improve libido, potency, and fertility, it does not appear to reverse uraemic hypogonadism completely.[20] Defects in pituitary luteinizing hormone secretion and seminiferous tubule function may persist. It has also been suggested that in transplant recipients, better sperm motility is required to achieve fertility compared with the general population.[25] Division of the vas with renal transplantation or subsequent allograft nephrectomy can also have an impact on fertility.

Chronic allograft nephropathy

Despite an early successful outcome following renal transplantation progressive deterioration of function and eventual loss of the graft occurs in many patients. This principally relates to what is referred to as chronic allograft nephropathy which is characterized by progressive renal dysfunction associated with chronic interstitial fibrosis, tubular atrophy, vascular occlusive changes, and glomerulosclerosis.[26,27] The pathophysiology of chronic allograft nephropathy remains poorly understood. Early rejection episodes are a risk factor. Reperfusion injury, calcineurin inhibitor toxicity, hypertension, other risk factors for vascular disease, and possibly hyperfiltration injury also contribute. Previously termed chronic rejection, it does not respond to changes in immunosuppressives. Reduction of risk factors for vascular disease (smoking, lipids, and hypertension) can limit the progression of chronic allograft nephropathy and at the present time is the main therapeutic strategy.[27,28] Other causes of late graft loss include non-compliance and recurrent glomerulonephritis.

Psychosocial implications of renal transplant

As a consequence of the implications of long-term immunosuppression and numerous potential co-morbidities as outlined above, renal transplant recipients continue to have complex long-term health issues. This can have significant psychosocial implications for patients and their families despite their relief from the disruption associated with the diagnosis of renal failure and the consequences of dialysis. The following scenarios illustrate the types of situations that may be encountered.

- 58-year-old male retired veteran who has endured many years of dialysis, but without a transplant, would soon be facing death due to deteriorating vascular access. Peritoneal dialysis is medically untenable.

- 44-year-old mother of three with a failing second transplant, facing the prospect of a third transplant. She describes a sense of ongoing heartache associated with the donor families' grief at losing loved ones.

- 51-year-old female, sole caregiver for two small grandchildren, who for dialysis purposes has relocated from her remote aboriginal home community to a regional town 700 kilometres away, is on the cadaveric transplant waiting list for transplant at the nearest transplant centre, which is another 1500 kilometres away.

- 36-year-old disability pensioner on home haemodialysis 180 kilometres from the transplant centre, who has been contending with ESRD since his early twenties, struggling to comply with diet and fluid recommendations. His reported self-hatred of his 'distorted' body, and of the 'foreign nature' of transplanted organs, were phenomena that contributed to non-compliance and associated loss of a previous graft.

- 25-year-old female, professionally employed, recently diagnosed with ESRD, otherwise in good health, with plans to accept a live donor kidney from her mother.

- 53-year-old male truck driver whose transplant of 18 years failed, necessitating a return to peritoneal dialysis. His wife died unexpectedly 6 months ago, the day before their 30th wedding anniversary.

- 73-year-old female, with a functioning graft transplanted 26 years ago, mid-stage dementia, and recently diagnosed with malignancy.

- 18-year-old female with a long history of ESRD, childhood abuse, self-harm behaviours, and foster care placements, facing imminent graft loss due to non-compliance with medication.

- 58-year-old female near ESRD secondary to diabetes, described as depressed, under consideration for a live related transplant from her healthy 30-year-old single (non-diabetic) daughter. The potential donor's sister (patient's daughter) was killed 3 years previously in a motor vehicle accident.

- 28-year-old female, married, with a 15-year history of ESRD, haemodialysing in-centre, under consideration for a live related transplant from her 21-year-old sister. The sister has expressed ambivalence about donation yet is the only available live related donor.

Collectively, these scenarios exemplify a raft of actual or prospective renal transplant experiences, from which distinctive features can be identified:

- Patients present for renal transplantation with a vast range of treatment backgrounds and illness histories.
- ESRD is demographically, ethnically, and socioeconomically non-discriminatory yet is over-represented in cohorts including the elderly and diabetic.
- Prospective or actual recipients all have ESRD, which as a chronic and incurable illness is experienced and interpreted differently by every patient, depending upon the patient's psychosocial background, functioning, and infrastructure.
- Transplantation in our society is based on the notion of 'gift of life', irrespective of whether the 'gift' emanates from a cadaveric or live donor; and that the gift relationship carries certain connotations of gratitude, reciprocity, and obligation.
- Cadaveric transplantation assumes no prior relationship between donor and recipient. The reverse is usually true for live transplantation. Both live and cadaveric donations convey themes of loss and gain.
- Transplantation frequently occurs within the context of a large institution. This may be geographically remote from patients' social support systems and primary care physicians who are responsible for the patient's pre-transplant management, their referral to the transplant unit, and the patient's long-term post-transplant management.
- In addition to the surgical procedure and associated care, a period of follow-up with daily medical review is usually required at the transplant centre. In many cases, the patient has had minimal or no prior contact with the transplant centre, at a time when they are negotiating significant new processes and issues associated with transplantation.
- The interaction, communication, and relationships between the patient's primary clinicians and the speciality transplant unit clinicians, can significantly influence the flow of relevant information, the interpretation of specific care needs, and the subsequent application of specialized support.
- Quality and quantity of life can be either enhanced or diminished by transplantation. The presence of co-morbidities, particularly other chronic diseases such as diabetes, significantly influences both.
- Transplant patient non-compliance (with immunosuppressive medication) can cause acute or chronic rejection, loss of graft, or patient death.
- Transplant failure—acute and chronic—is generally accompanied by disappointment and grief, and has implications for patients considering return to dialysis and the transplant waiting list and integration into supportive care.

◆ Demand for relatively scarce transplantable organs is occurring at a time when the community is simultaneously ageing *and* experiencing an expansion of recipient and donor selection criteria. This is broadening the scope, opportunity, burden, and consequence of live and cadaveric organ transplantation/retransplantation, on an individual, family, and community level.

◆ Transplantation is contraindicated or not considered in some ESRD patients.

Amidst the historically unparalleled success of transplantation, are many confronting practice and ethical issues which need to be considered by clinicians in providing appropriate care and support to kidney transplant patients and families. The identified and distinctive transplant-related features noted above have implications for clinical practice; most notably with regard to: psychological implications and obligations arising from organ donation, chronic illness and care need, compliance, and the failing transplant.

Psychological implications and obligations arising from organ donation

Any illness can elicit anxiety and uncertainty relating to treatment processes and outcomes. Transplantation potentially carries additional psychological implications for recipients, stemming from the relationship between the recipient, donor (whether live or cadaveric), the partners and families of each, and the clinicians. These in turn can influence the recipient's transplant experience and support needs.

Donor source

An inherent feature of cadaveric renal transplantation is that the donor kidney is from a person unknown to the recipient, who died following an unexpected, often traumatic event, and with whom there has been no past relationship. In most countries, donor anonymity is a legislative requisite of cadaveric organ donation. This restricts personal contact between the cadaveric transplant recipient and the donor family.

Recently transplanted cadaveric transplant recipients, and often their families, are in a highly emotional situation, which may include anxiety and concerns about the death of a stranger. Joy at receiving the transplant can be intermingled with sadness that an unknown family is grieving a premature and sudden death. Many recipients describe feeling guilty, even grief-stricken, that someone 'had to die' despite reassurance that the person's death would have occurred irrespective of organ donation and that the donor family had opportunity to proceed or not, with donation. Not uncommonly, recipients suppress information and thoughts about the donor. Such suppression is not always successful, and spontaneous feelings of gratitude toward the donor emerge. The defensive strategies against anxiety associated with the donor tend to be most intensive in the first 6 months, reducing over 2 years. One noted coping strategy is for recipients to identify with the randomness of organ allocation matching, thus enabling them to feel innocent in relation to the death of the donor. Depersonalizing the donor kidney to a spare body part or viewing the donor as a supply of material necessary to repair the body can act as another coping strategy. It is unknown whether this assists the patient to any extent in complying with post-transplant regimens.[29] Recipients are more likely to overidentify with the loss of the donor family, if already grieving actual, feared, or anticipated losses of their own—including losses pertaining to the transplant, past transplants, loved ones, quality of life, or other life loss.

Recipients usually want to acknowledge their donor family's 'gift of life'. Recipients, in thoughts about their cadaveric donor, know that they are unable to 'repay' the gift received. As alternatives, recipients may write a letter of thanks to the donor family, establish rituals (such as lighting candles), commit to an enjoyable and productive life, undertake a 'special' act each year around the time of the anniversary of the transplant—which may include attendance at a remembrance thanksgiving ceremony, in honour of the donor and donor family. Some recipients justify that they would donate if they could, or perceive themselves as 'helpful people too'. Many consider the donor 'a fellow-being like me', recognizing or creating similarities between themselves and the donors, interpreting this in a positive way. Implied, is that the donation was a good deed, allowing feelings of guilt and inequity to be dealt with by the recipient. In the event of acute or chronic transplant failure compliant recipients often wish for the donor family to know that despite the organ's failure, they appreciate being given a transplant opportunity. There is often anxiety however, about compounding the donor family's grief.[29]

Concern has been expressed that the concept of 'gift of life' is fallacious, because its very nature does not enable cadaveric transplant recipients to properly reciprocate to the source of the gift (the deceased donor), and that the associated psychological and moral burden felt by recipients toward donors (or their families) is unhelpful. It has been identified that if the repayment characteristic of gift exchange is removed from the equation, then donor families can acknowledge that neither their loss nor the act of organ donation is an act of 'exchange'. It is unknown whether the incapacity for complete reciprocation, indirectly affects graft or patient survival.[30,31]

Recipients may believe their behaviour and attitude are affected by receiving a 'foreign' organ.[19,32–34] Personalities are considered, and some feel that if an important organ is added to one's body, the new composition would affect both one's body and one's mind. The transplant can be perceived as a segment of the whole donor, expressing the donor in his or her totality. Many recipients are reluctant, or are not encouraged, to discuss their feelings about the 'foreign organ' with their physicians, yet refer to their transplant with tenderness and admiration, perceiving it as a 'friend' or 'rescuer'.[29] Recipients' explanations of post-transplant personality change include 'transmission' and 'geneticalization'. Transmission refers to contamination through an unspecified 'essence' from the donor to the recipient via the transplant, whereas geneticalization refers to differences and similarities between living beings, as explained by genetic factors. Thereby, that 'some genes would slip over', places strange feelings of vicissitude into a scientific and current context.[35] The intuitive observation that a mixed substance usually shows traits from the constituent components further confirms for some recipients the reality of the two concepts. It is known for a small minority of ESRD patients not to accept a transplant for fear of becoming another person or because it is 'distasteful' having a foreign organ in one's body.[29,36] We have seen instances of renal transplant recipients requesting transplant nephrectomy, months or even years after the procedure, as they are haunted by the 'foreign nature' of the transplanted organ. Some patients have been known to prefer a donor of their own sex, because 'it feels more natural'.[29] These under-researched areas have been noted more specifically in patients with a pre-morbid mental illness, highlighting the importance of thoroughly assessing prospective transplant recipients.

Recipients of live donor organs do not seem to experience the same cognition and reaction as cadaveric transplant recipients, regarding influence and identification, through receiving a transplanted kidney. Whilst live related transplant recipients describe (genetic) similarities between them and the donor, they do not necessarily view these similarities as being strengthened after transplantation.[29] It seems possible that identification and influence are of lesser consequence for live donor recipients than for cadaveric recipients, for whom there is more donor mystique.

Waiting times generally allow potential recipients a period of time to prepare for cadaveric renal transplantation. Countering this, the 'not knowing' when or if a transplant will eventuate, the 'shock' of receiving the call, compounded by the 'anonymity' of the donor, all potentially contribute to recipient anxiety, in the immediate post-transplant stage. Pre- and post-transplant education needs to consider these issues. Individual/family counselling and group work may be required on occasion to help dispel myths associated with cadaveric donation, to acknowledge the ambivalent feelings recipients and families might experience given the circumstances of their 'gift' of life, and to assist recipients to consider their responsibilities toward the donated organ, donor family, themselves, and their own family and community (employment/social/other). Such support can also assist recipients to process their grief within their own life context and history, whilst successfully integrating the transplant and new medical regimen into their domain.

Relationships and obligations—live donors

'I never liked my sister much, but once the request was made, it was impossible to refuse—sort of family and moral duty . . . I don't mind too much . . .'

'I have no regrets about donating my kidney—wish I had a dozen to give . . .'

'Our life has never been better, since I gave my wife a kidney . . .'

'She would do it for me, if I needed a kidney . . .'

'No-one really asked me—it just happened. . . . Afterwards, I hated the idea of having his kidney inside me . . . I would not mind if it rejected and I could receive a kidney from a stranger . . .'

'I feel I can never be grateful enough . . . and he never lets me forget that he gave me his kidney . . .'

'All will be well, if I donate a kidney to my sister . . . my family had banished me, but this will bring me back into favour . . .'

'Mum is so sad these days. If I give her a kidney, she will feel much better, and we will all be happier . . .'

In Australia, live related and known unrelated donors provide 39% of all donor kidneys, with 69% of the live unrelated donations, being spousal.[2] With a similar and significant worldwide increase in live organ donation during the last decade, the psychological and social meaning of live organ donation is increasingly relevant for all clinicians interacting with families of potential renal transplant recipients and donors. By its very nature, kidney donation from a live, known donor assumes a pre-established, and in all probability an ongoing, relationship between donor and recipient. The pool of potential donors has expanded from that of immediate kin, to include distant relatives and known, unrelated individuals. Fundamentally, clinicians have an obligation to ensure the donor's medical and psychological suitability, competency, willingness, autonomy, awareness of risks and benefits to themselves and the recipient, and awareness of recipient's options. The relationship between the clinician and the donor brings a mutual responsibility, which should not be abrogated by the donor claim of autonomy, nor the obligation fostered by the recipient's needs. Ultimately, the transplant surgeon must ensure that informed consent can be provided before reaching a decision about whether to perform the procedure.[37–39]

Furthermore, clinicians have a major responsibility to assist the donor and recipient identify how they perceive overt or covert obligations which might exist between them, by virtue of their relationship. This can assist with the identification of the complex motives behind an individual donation, which can have an impact on either the decision or the outcome of the transplant. The clinician must therefore identify the meaning of the donation and legitimacy of the motives, for each donor, within the context of that donor's and recipient's life and the donor's and recipient's relationship.[37,38] Reasons for donation include:

- a desire to help
- increased self-esteem
- a feeling of moral duty
- self- and family benefit (from relative's improved health)
- external pressure or coercion
- identification with and love for patient
- logic (I can, so I shall)
- recognition within family
- the only option (no-one else available)
- cultural and religious beliefs.

Numerous studies exploring a donor's motives, feelings, and experience, demonstrate that, overall, most donors do not suffer from any lasting negative physical or psychological consequences of donation but rather experience significant psychological gain from helping another person. Donors frequently attained higher quality of life scores than those in the general community.[29,40–46] Investigations into the ethical, social, and psychological dynamics of the family process related to live kidney transplant have examined families' decision-making processes, levels of stress/conflict, and communication patterns related to live organ donation. Consistently, positive feelings about donation and the relationship between donor and recipient give rise to intensely forged ties of closeness, increased self-esteem, and appreciation of life, whilst donor ambivalence and negative self-esteem tend toward negative feelings about donation.[45]

The extent to which the donation is experienced by donors as a positive one varies. This depends on factors such as donor and recipient recovery rate, post-donation attitude of the recipient, and degree of donor aggression/depression experienced. The importance of maintaining an encouraging and pleasing environment for donors cannot be overestimated, given the growing reliance on live organ donors; within the context of a consumerist society. It is particularly important to ensure that clinical protocols and pathways regarding pre-donation assessment and education, along with post-nephrectomy care are reviewed regularly, and are highly responsive to patient needs.[47–50]

Live organ donation is essentially supererogatory, yet clinicians can assist potential recipients and donors make sense of their feelings about mutual responsibility and obligation; to understand the moral significance of their intrinsic value as autonomous persons, and as an extension of the patient. If an ethical 'pull' exists between agents in social relationships, then the strength of associated obligations is intricately bound with the quality of the relationship between the potential recipient and the live donor. The more disjointed, fragmented, unequal, or exploitative; the less autonomous and less respectful is the relationship.[51] The duty to consider donation is arguably weaker, and proceeding with donation holds far greater potential for harm to the exploited person, either donor or recipient.

ESRD can interfere with the patient's and family members' employment, economic security, career plans, and future hopes. The offer of a live kidney is a practical way in which the needs and vulnerabilities of those associated with a patient with ESRD can be considered, enabling a family to problem solve a situation which could have entailed a far greater loss for all of its members. It is valuable to take into account treatment options that afford maximum benefit to all members, this way ensuring that patients and family members mutually consider their obligations.[52,53]

The clinician is well placed to assess the situation, and to identify the moral issues associated with the patient's illness, severity, and life stage and the roles, relationships, and history of both the donor and the recipient, as independents and in relation to one another. Understanding the specific meaning of the donation for the potential recipient and donor, being aware that there might be psychological risks and benefits involved in the donor's act of giving or refusing, and recognition of patterns of ambivalence, altruism, coercion, avoidance, denial, and depression are key factors. Patient and family priorities may be quite different from the typical risk–benefit information that clinicians emphasize.[54]

The obligation that a recipient, the clinicians, and the community might have towards supporting in turn the live donor has been little investigated. Whilst the transaction is non-commercial in nature, recipients often express their gratitude in ways commensurate with their means—spending extra time with the donor, organizing a 'special' event, or giving the donor a vacation. The community has an obligation to ensure that the donor incurs minimal personal financial cost associated with the donation, is comfortable about the donation process, and is provided with a regular, free of charge, medical and psychological review.

Chronic illness and care needs

Transplantation occurs in the context of ESRD, in turn characterized as a chronic illness due to its long-term debilitating sequence. Chronic illness can be life-threatening, early, or late onset. Its uneven, unpredictable features result in it being neither fully arrested nor compensated. It carries burdens and opportunities for family and social relationships, the health-care system and welfare services. Its challenge is defined around the notion that chronic illness defies the normal moral boundaries of caring and conventional expectations about the care-giving duties of the family *vis-à-vis* the obligations of society.[55] Whilst treatments, including transplantation, vary, chronic illness is not eliminated. Transplantation overcomes many of the lifestyle and medical problems associated with dialysis. Chronic illness persists as a result of the need for long-term medical treatment, with patient compliance a necessary requirement for a long-term successful outcome. Problems which may be encountered include the consequences of long-term immunosuppressive drugs including steroids, ongoing hypertension, emergence of treatment-related diabetes, as well as the subsequent development of chronic renal impairment with decline in graft function due to chronic rejection or disease recurrence.

The ESRD patient is thus required to work within the particular limitations that the illness or its treatments might impose, whilst finding ways to maintain a meaningful and purposeful life. Treatment for ESRD often becomes a process of negotiation incorporating the various forms of dialysis and transplantation, which may be used in sequential fashion. As a result, it may become a long-standing and permanent feature of the person. The relationship between chronic illness and self-identity is a dynamic one, which is affected by many variables including current disease symptoms, the reactions of family, friends, and caregivers; and the various strategies individuals use to sustain themselves.[55]

All transplant or prospective transplant patients share the need for supportive care as a result of their chronic illness. Different care needs exist, yet 'supportive care' is the mantle, the means, and the outcome by which patient support needs must be evaluated. Supportive care within the chronic illness arena takes on a moral significance, in that it raises questions about the nature of self and the continuity—or discontinuity—of self-identity over time amid changes in physical capacity, social circumstances, and ability/inability to shape and direct one's life. People experiment, innovate, and reorganize to maintain control over themselves and their lives.[56]

In considering this type of care, there are two important principles:

1 Taking care of the sick person, which is largely the description for providing objective and competent care.

2 Caring for or caring about the sick person, which suggests a virtue of devotion or concern for the other as a person.[57,58]

Supportive care of the transplant patient must commence well before the transplant, given that there is a pre-transplant illness and treatment context already requiring multilevel care. Acts of caring include listening to patients with personal attentiveness, enabling patients to relate their experiences in terms of their own values and concerns, being attentive to the physical and emotional aspects of illness, and offering maximum understanding, freedom, and support to the individual patient.[58] Given that transplantation is demanding for cadaveric and live organ recipients, pre-transplant assessment can elucidate the context and manner in which the patient is living with their ESRD and their experience of care. Necessary insight into the patient's past and present life experiences, thought patterns, and associated behaviours, is highlighted.[59] Assessment of care-needs is not simple and must consider the following:

◆ age, life stage, gender, ethnicity, and socioeconomic and educational level of patient;

◆ experience of employment or other life activity, particularly in relation to managing ESRD/treatments;

◆ ESRD treatment history;

◆ income levels and whether ESRD has eroded the patient's capacity for income generation and access to care;

◆ length of illness, its course, and the patient's interpretation of illness meaning and sense of hope;

◆ treatment history—short or long term;

◆ responsibilities (family, employment, other) outside the ESRD context;

◆ psychosocial/familial history, network function, support, maturity, and context;

◆ self-perception/self-esteem;

◆ history [or not] of abuse (e.g. substance, physical, emotional, sexual, domestic violence);

◆ individual physical and mental health history;

◆ whether the patient has a 'caregiver' or whether the patient him/herself is a caregiver for children, aged relatives, spouse, or others;

- if on dialysis

    how the patient copes with his/her dialysis treatment,

    relationship between patient to clinicians and other patients,

    degree of compliance,

    interpretation of dialysis, for example, does the patient have full working and family life around which dialysis is fitted or does the patient 'live' for dialysis and the companionship of staff and fellow patients?

- patient's perception of his/her quality of life;
- whether loss and grief have featured in pre-transplant times and whether the patient has addressed or incorporated these losses into everyday living. Losses include those of loved ones, migratory or refugee experiences, war or other international trauma, childhood abuses and associated loss of bodily and emotional integrity;
- cultural, religious, or personal beliefs, values and frameworks which could influence the patient's attitude toward and capacity for transplant.

Further to this, recipients with one or more of the following characteristics are often at higher risk for poor coping with their ESRD as a chronic illness indicating a need for even greater support than recipients without these characteristics:

- must temporarily relocate a significant geographical distance to access the transplant and aftercare;
- belong to a cultural minority;
- express feeling severe dislocation in leaving the dialysis centre;
- have limited language skills ;
- have poor body image and low self-esteem;
- have reduced capacity to negotiate with their environment;
- have experienced abuses or are currently in a domestically violent situation;
- have a fear of 'foreign' organs;
- have significant other responsibilities affected by transplantation and the post-transplant routine;
- have identified financial difficulties;
- have a poor/non-functioning new transplant;
- have expressed fear, depression, insomnia, or mood swings;
- have a significant history of loss.

In considering care that clinicians need to provide in the long term to post-transplant recipients, it is relevant to note that transplant recipients of all types, show long-term quality of life (QOL) advantages over similarly ill patients who have not received transplants. In explaining why the global QOL so consistently changed, even in the face of modest changes in specific health-related QOL domains, it is proposed that in receipt of the gift of life, transplant patients commonly redefine 'normal' life, so that despite living with medication and side-effects life holds particular value. Suggestively, there is a more spiritual, philosophical, and existential domain than has been addressed in standard transplant QOL studies.[59]

Rates of post-transplant employment—a QOL indicator—vary, from an estimated 18% to 86%.[60] Social rehabilitation and perceived 'wellness' might not be synonymous with the improved medical outcomes of transplantation, but rather based on the belief system of the patient and the associated behaviours. The physician's expectation, regarding the patient's capacity to work, significantly influences whether or not the patient engages in employment post-transplant. Clinicians have a significant responsibility for endorsing or liberating the patient from the 'sick role', which symbolically, is a crucial care component.

Organ transplant recipients in the USA are increasingly among the patients for whom ongoing 'life care planning' by certified life care planners occurs, enabling identification of medical, physical, social, and emotional and rehabilitation needs.[61] The support of rehabilitation consultants, as a way of enhancing patient QOL and reinforcing capacity for productivity, is highly relevant in the renal transplant area.

Age does not appear to affect QOL outcomes. Despite additional co-morbidities, older patients achieve significant improvement in QOL with transplantation. Their additional medical risk factors do, however, reduce long-term outcomes compared with younger age groups. In the context of ageing communities and disability rates, including those with ESRD in the 60–79 year age group markedly higher than those of younger age cohorts, a greater number of older patients with associated co-morbidities are joining the transplant queue and will continue to challenge clinicians with their specific care needs.[62–64]

Compliance

The main negotiation and process adaptation processes for ESRD patients include acceptance, adjustment, coping, and adaptation. Acceptance is the recognition and understanding of the limitations imposed by illness; adjustment is the change required to address problems that occur; coping is the capacity for toleration, reduction, or minimization of environmental and external demands; and adaptation is the dealing with change, without the loss of long-term goals which involve family, religious, cultural, or environmental elements.[55,64]

Compliance in the health-care setting has been defined as the extent to which patient behaviour conforms to clinical needs. The implication is that the greater the patient's adaptation processes the stronger the compliance.[65] Patient's clinical outcomes are often used as an index of compliance, despite the fact that patients may improve or deteriorate for a number of reasons unrelated to treatment adherence. Inability to or difficulty in accepting, adjusting, coping, or adapting to the rigours associated with transplantation, results in varying degrees of non-compliance. Even though non-compliance has emerged as a significant problem in clinical practice, there is scant empirical literature on non-compliance in renal and transplant patients. There is no adequate theoretical framework to account for or to consistently predict non-complaint behaviour in the ESRD setting. There have been efforts to examine the role of attitudes, environmental influences, treatment characteristics, demographic factors, and the clinician–patient relationship with the majority of studies relying completely on outcome-related dependent variables (e.g. graft loss/patient morbidity/cyclosporin A levels).[65, 66] The ability to carry out complex, lengthy regimens may be more important than the will to do so, and recipients who complain of medication side-effects, show fatalism towards the health of their graft, and are relatively young; are more likely to be non-compliant. Four broad patterns of non-compliance, associated with length, frequency, complexity, and focus, whether the prescribed regimen is for prophylactic or curative purposes, have been identified as part of reactance theory.[67] An increase in any of these four characteristics increases the likelihood that valued freedoms will be threatened, and therefore have an impact on compliance. The locus of control (LOC) model and the five factor model of personality examine control, responsibility, and conscientiousness in relation to levels of compliance with health and therapies.[68–69] Given the threat to perceived freedoms that any aspect of ESRD treatments present to some patients, and given the varying degrees of conscientiousness and responsibility with which recipients present, further research is required into the interplay between their roles and actions upon decision-making processes and compliance with transplant regimens.

It has been estimated that renal transplant non-compliance runs at 34%.[65] Whilst it is well recognized that non-compliance in the transplant population is problematic, it is relevant to note, that ANZDATA 2002 reported that of the 305 grafts lost in 2001, 144 were due to death of the patient, of which seven were identified as having occurred as a result of non-compliant behaviours.[2] Of relevance, however, is the fact that non-compliance manifests not only in graft failure but also in poorly controlled diabetes, hypertension, and skin lesions—all of which affect patient care, QOL, the health system, and the clinician–recipient relationship. There are some key points for clinicians. Not all non-adherences to medication are active defiance, but can be reflective of dishevelment or dislocation, poor treatment negotiation skills in the patient or family network, or culturally determined factors such as time orientation or cultural activity which prescribes priorities other than those associated with ESRD treatment. Specific indicators risking greater non-compliance include:

◆ youth/adolescence,

◆ underdeveloped emotional maturity and poorer LOC and conscientiousness,

- poor self-esteem and/or history of abuse or self-harm/mutilation,
- fatalism toward graft,
- unstable social support,
- poor health-care provider/patient relationship,
- unemployment or lack of meaningful life activity,
- poor post-transplant life planning/rehabilitation,
- mental illness,
- clinic non-attenders,
- diabetics.

Strategies to reduce the likelihood of non-compliance include:

1 Pre-transplant psychosocial assessment of all prospective live or cadaveric transplant recipients, identifying and working with the strengths and deficits inherent within each individual's situation. Establish a transplant contract, whereby prospective recipients commit to learning as much as possible about the responsibilities and consequences of consenting to become a 'partner in transplantation'. This would involve a multipronged and multidisciplinary approach—booklets, education seminars, video, and pre-/post-transplant 'life planning'.

2 Pre- and early post-transplant education regarding the seriousness of non-compliance in renal transplantation and identification of the patient's options if tempted to non-compliance. Educate patients and families about long-term risks and consequences of even occasional non-adherence to medication. Enhance patient's self-efficacy by providing role models/mentors.[65, 70]

3 Establishment of a transplant support network (e.g. face-to-face/virtual/ telephone/newsletter), as a means of reducing isolation and providing support amongst patients, especially for those 2–3 months post-transplant, including those who have returned to their home regions.[71–76]

4 Encourage recipients to consider their responsibilities to donors and donor families and to seek early counselling if they are distressed by any associated issues.

The failing transplant

In Australia in 2001 there were 5466 functioning renal transplant grafts, which represented 42% of all kidney transplants performed since 1962. Of the functioning grafts, 32% had been functioning for over 10 years and 6% had been functioning for over 20 years. There were 46 recipients still alive who received their grafts over 30 years ago. During 1992–2001, 2739 patients died or lost their grafts through either non-compliance (60, 2%), chronic rejection (885, 32%), or acute rejection (150, 6%).[2] Recipients are well aware that there is a risk of morbidity and mortality associated with transplantation. The potential prospects of graft rejection, infection, and development of malignancy are realistic fears harboured by most patients, although these may not be verbalized to family or clinicians involved in their care.

Acute rejection occurs within the first 4–6 weeks following transplantation.[4] Occasionally, it may be seen at much later stages, although this is often triggered by intercurrent illness such as infection or non-compliant behaviour. If unresponsive to antirejection treatment, the patient is likely to return to dialysis and possibly undergo a nephrectomy. Such an episode can be tumultuous for the patient. The loss, after anticipation of the transplant, can be deep and overwhelming for some patients, although it is not uncommon for justification to set in quite early, with comments such as '. . . it was not meant to be', '. . . there must be a more suited kidney around the corner', '. . . it doesn't really matter, as I can easily return to dialysis', '. . . at least I did not die'. Factors that seem to determine how a patient copes with the acute loss include:

- the degree of identified and understood risk associated with this particular transplant;
- pre-surgical transplant and general surgical history;
- the patient's chances for retransplant;
- how well the patient was managing the pre-transplant dialysis regimen;
- how sick the patient is post-surgically;
- personality and social factors.

It is important that the patient and family have the opportunity to discuss in detail with the physicians the reasons for the acute loss of graft, and what treatment options remain. The patient's greatest fear might be removal from the transplant waiting list altogether, and, if this fear is confirmed, counselling is indicated. The key to the patient's recovery from the experience is an early assessment of the patient's responses, support needs, and past experiences, allowing for implementation of a support plan relevant to that patient's needs.

The course of chronic allograft nephropathy can occur over several months or a number of years.[27] Many recipients experiencing chronic rejection describe feeling never completely well, nor extremely ill. There can be a sense of abiding disappointment and grief that the transplant did not deliver the good health which had been hoped for. Commensurately, there can be gratitude for the opportunity to have had time out from dialysis, enabling travel, employment, or other meaningful activities. There could be guilt that recipient non-compliance contributed to graft loss (i.e. threat/actual). There is the underlying awareness that dialysis might be required again in the future. The patient's prior experience with dialysis can determine their responses to this. Patients who have not had recent dialysis experiences (e.g. for over 15 years) commonly carry ambivalent or even traumatic feelings about dialysis, remembering the older styles of dialysis technique and the impact it had on them. This can add weight to their anxiety about recommencement of dialysis, particularly as the patient has aged in the meantime and might have a changed set of psychosocial circumstances. The patient's general medical circumstances will determine whether retransplant is a possibility, and if it is not then there are three treatment options when the transplant fails altogether—return to dialysis, return to the transplant waiting list, or commencement of conservative treatment which implies palliative care. If compounding health issues have arisen, which are likely to result in the patient's death, irrespective of the level of graft function, or if a return to dialysis would fail to enhance or maintain the patient's QOL, it is recommended that the conservative care option be explored with the patient and their family. For many patients and families the fear and process of dying are barriers to consideration of conservative treatments. Talking specifically about patient and family concerns of pain and suffering and about the emotional and physiological aspects of dying, will help allay fears. Of great significance is the pre-existing relationship that usually exists between the clinician and the patient/family, as this provides a framework of trust regarding the patient's best interest.[77]

There must be a concerted and integrated approach to the management of ESRD when the technological treatments are no longer viable. There is compulsion to ask how medicine, no less in the treatment of ESRD, should conduct itself to promote both a good life and a peaceful death. Rather than death being 'what happens' when ESRD treatments fail, palliation must be acknowledged as legitimate a treatment as dialysis and transplantation. That the hospice movement is a separate system of caring for the dying has been described as a 'specially constructed sideshow, out of sight of the main tent'.[78] That renal and transplant units are generally designed to manage acute care needs, rather than palliative ones, confirms that management of the dying renal transplant patient has traditionally been a 'side show' rather than a significant component of core business. Whilst there is generally a high level of care, commitment, and compassion shown by clinicians toward patients who withdraw from dialysis or do not resume dialysis post-transplant-failure, the increasing numbers of older, sicker, co-morbid ESRD patients, all of whom are ageing, are challenging the treatment providers to more pro-actively consider the implications of 'when a chronic illness becomes terminal'. Integration of palliative care on acute care renal and transplant wards, and providing patients with full and early choices regarding home palliative or hospice care, are becoming crucial components of the 'main tent'. Hospice facilities are, in fact, well placed to care for conservatively treated ESRD patients and can provide an excellent alternative to the acute ward environment which is the reality of renal medicine. End-of-life care needs to be comprehensive, encompassing the physical social, emotional, and spiritual needs of the patient. The needs of the palliative patient and his/her family, in the general and the renal and renal transplant context, are now being seriously considered.[77, 79–83] Care must focus upon the quality of remaining life and, importantly, encompass the family, which has often provided years of care for the ESRD patient. Bereavement care for the family, particularly for those with long-standing relationships with the transplant centre, should include supportive counselling; a condolence card, information package about bereavement in the renal setting, and opportunity for attendance at a remembrance ceremony or religious service.

Conclusions

Care of renal transplant patients can span from weeks to decades, presenting specific challenges to the range of clinicians who may become involved in their care. The challenge extends from the complex medical and psychological care of the patient to that of their families, who increasingly are being recognized for their role as caregivers and as active components in the treatment process. The ultimate responsibility of clinicians is in assisting transplant recipients, donors, and families by considering their needs and subsequent responsibilities within this process. The ultimate aim is to enable renal transplant recipients and their families to achieve a meaningful and productive life and eventual death, within the context of a long-term chronic illness which has occurred as a consequence of previous or recurrent ESRD.

References

1 Johnson DW, Herzig K, Purdie D, Brown AM, Rigby RJ, Nicol DL *et al.* (2000). A comparison of the effects of dialysis and renal transplantation on the survival of older uremic patients. *Transplantation* **69**: 794–9.

2 Australia and New Zealand Dialysis and Transplant Registry (2002). *25th Annual Report*, data to 2001 (http:www.anzdata.org.au)

3 French CG, Belitsky P, Lawen JG (2000). Progress in renal transplantation. *Can. J. Urol.* **7**: 1030–7.

4 Chan L, Gaston R, Hariharan S (2001). Evolution of immunosuppression and continued importance of acute rejection in renal transplantation. *Am. J. Kidney Dis.* **38**(6, Suppl. 6): S2–S9.

5 Gaston RS (2001). Maintenance immunosuppression in the renal transplant recipient: an overview. *Am. J. Kidney Dis.* **38**(6, Suppl. 6): S25–S35.

6 Luke PP, Jordan ML (2001). Contemporary immunosuppression in renal transplantation. *Urol. Clin. North Am.* **28**: 733–50.

7 de Mattos AM, Olyaei AJ, Bennett WM (2000). Nephrotoxicity of immunosuppressive drugs: long-term consequences and challenges for the future. *Am. J. Kidney Dis.* **35**(2): 333–46.

8 Kreis H (2001). New strategies to reduce nephrotoxicity. *Transplantation* **72**(12, Suppl.): S99–S104.

9 First MR, Gerber DA, Hariharan S, Kaufman DB, Shapiro R (2002). Posttransplant diabetes mellitus in kidney allograft recipients: incidence, risk factors, and management. *Transplantation* **73**: 379–86.

10 Veenstra DL, Best JH, Hornberger J, Sullivan SD, Hricik DE (1999). Incidence and long-term cost of steroid-related side effects after renal transplantation. *Am. J. Kidney Dis.* **33**: 829–39.

11 Kahan BD (2000). Efficacy of sirolimus compared with azathioprine for reduction of acute renal allograft rejection: a randomised multicentre study. The Rapamune US Study Group. *Lancet* **356**: 194–202.

12 Tanphaichitr NT, Brennan DC (2000). Infectious complications in renal transplant recipients. *Adv. Renal Replace. Ther.* **7**: 131–46.

13 Schmidt A, Oberbauer R (1999). Bacterial and fungal infections after kidney transplantation. *Curr. Opin. Urol.* **9**: 45–9.

14 Patel S, Kwan JT, McCloskey E, McGee G, Thomas G, Johnson D *et al.* (2001). Prevalence and causes of low bone density and fractures in kidney transplant patients. *J. Bone Miner. Res.* **16**: 1863–70.

15 London NJ, Farmery SM, Will EJ, Davison AM, Lodge JPA (1995). Risk of neoplasia in renal transplant patients. *Lancet* **346**: 403–6.

16 Carroll RP, Ramsay HM, Fryer AA, Hawley CM, Nicol DL, Harden PN (2003). Incidence and prediction of nonmelanoma skin cancer post-renal transplantation: a prospective study in Queensland, Australia. *Am. J. Kidney Dis.* **41**: 676–83.

17 Ramsay HM, Fryer AA, Hawley CM, Smith AG, Nicol DL, Harden PN (2003). Factors associated with nonmelanoma skin cancer following renal transplantation in Queensland, Australia. *J. Am. Acad. Dermatol.* **49**: 397–406.

18 Pascual M, Theruvath T, Kawai T, Tolkoff-Rubin N, Cosimi AB (2002). Strategies to improve long-term outcomes after renal transplantation. *N. Engl. J. Med.* **346**: 580–90.

19 Palmer BF (2003). Sexual dysfunction in men and women with chronic kidney disease and end-stage kidney disease. *Adv. Renal Replace. Ther.* **10**: 48–60.

20 Handelsman DJ, Dong Q (1993). Hypothalamo-pituitary gonadal axis in chronic renal failure. *Endocrinol. Metab. Clin. North Am.* **22**: 145–61.

21 Saha MT, Saha HH, Niskanen LK, Salmela KT, Pasternack AI (2002). Time course of serum prolactin and sex hormones following successful renal transplantation. *Nephron* **92**: 735–7.

22 Prieto Castro RM, Anglada Curado FJ, Regueiro Lopez JC, Leva Vallejo ME, Molina Sanchez J, Saceda Lopez JL *et al.* (2001). Treatment with sildenafil citrate in renal transplant patients with erectile dysfunction. *BJU Int.* **88**: 241–3.

23 Diez JJ, Iglesias P, Selgas R (1995). Pituitary dysfunctions in uremic patients undergoing peritoneal dialysis: a cross sectional descriptive study. *Adv. Perit. Dial.* **11**: 218–24.

24 Veldhuis JD, Iranmanesh A, Wilkowski MJ, Samojlik E (1994). Neuroendocrine alterations in the somatotropic and lactotropic axes in uremic men. *Eur. J. Endocrinol.* **131**: 489–98.

25 Eid MM, Abdel-Hamid IA, Sobh MA, el-Saied MA (1996). Assessment of sperm motion characteristics in infertile renal transplant recipients using computerized analysis. *Int. J. Androl.* **19**: 338–44.

26 Vazquez MA (2000). Chronic rejection of renal transplants: new clinical insights. *Am. J. Med. Sci.* **320**: 43–58.

27 Nankivell BJ, Borrows RJ, Fung CL, O'Connell PJ, Allen RD, Chapman JR (2003). The natural history of chronic allograft nephropathy. *N. Engl. J. Med.* **349**: 2326–33.

28 Womer KL, Vella JP, Sayegh MH (2000). Chronic allograft dysfunction: mechanisms and new approaches to therapy. *Semin. Nephrol.* **20**: 126–47.

29 Sanner MA (2003). Transplant recipients' conceptions of three key phenomena in transplantation: the organ donation, the organ donor, and the organ transplant. *Clin. Transplant.* **17**: 391–400.

30 Siminoff LA, Chillag K (1999). The fallacy of the 'gift of life'. *Hastings Cent Rep.* **29**: 34–41.

31 Fox R. Swazey JP (1979). *The courage to fail: a social view of organ transplants and dialysis.* University of Chicago Press, Chicago.

32 Adler ML (1972). Kidney transplantation and coping mechanisms. *Psychosomatics.* **13**: 337: 41.

33 Bunzel B, Schmidl-Mohl B, Grundbock A, Wollenek G (1992). Does changing the heart mean changing personality? A retrospective inquiry on 47 heart transplant patients. *Qual. Life Res.* **1**: 251–6.

34 Mai FM (1986). Graft and donor denial in heart transplant recipients. *Am. J. Psychiatry.* **143**: 1159–61.

35 Castelnuovo-Tedesco P (1981). Transplantation: psychological implications of changes in body image. In B. Levy (ed.) *Psychonephrology: psychological factors in hemodialysis and transplantation* Springer.

36 Cramond W, Fraenkel M, Barratt L (1990). On letting go: the patient, haemodialysis and opting out. *Aust. N. Z. J. Psychiatry* **24**: 268–75.

37 Franklin PM, Crombie AK (2003). Live related renal transplantation: psychological, social, and cultural issues. *Transplantation* **76**: 1247–52.

38 Lennerling A, Forsberg A, Nyberg G (2003). Becoming a living kidney donor. *Transplantation* **76**: 1243–7.

39 Delmonico FL, Surman OS (2003). Is this live-organ donor your patient? *Transplantation* **76**:1257–60.

40 Sharma VK, Enoch MD (1987). Psychological sequelae of kidney donation. A 5–10 year follow up study. *Acta Psychiatr. Scand.* **75**: 264–7.

41 Hirvas J, Enckell M, Kuhlback B, Pasternack A (1976). Psychological and social problems encountered in active treatment of chronic uraemia. II. The living donor. *Acta Med. Scand.* **200**: 17–20.

42 Corley MC, Elswick RK, Sargeant CC, Scott S (2000). Attitude, self-image, and quality of life of living kidney donors. *Nephrol. Nurs. J.* **27**: 43–50.

43 Johnson EM, Anderson JK, Jacobs C, Suh G, Humar A, Suhr BD *et al.* (1999). Long-term follow-up of living kidney donors: quality of life after donation. *Transplantation* **67**: 717–21.

44 Gouge F, Moore J Jr, Bremer BA, McCauly CR, Johnson JP (1990). The quality of life of donors, potential donors, and recipients of living-related donor renal transplantation. *Transplant Proc.* **22**: 2409–13.

45 Simmons RG, Marine SK, Simmons RL (1987). Gift of life: the effect of organ transplantation on individual, family, and societal dynamics. *Transaction Publishers*, New Brunswick NJ.

46 Fehrman-Ekholm I, Brink B, Ericsson C, Elinder CG, Duner F, Lundgren G (2000). Kidney donors don't regret: follow-up of 370 donors in Stockholm since 1964. *Transplantation* **69**: 2067–71.

47 Swizer GE, Dew MA, Twillman RK (2000). Psychosocial issues in living organ donation. In PT Trzepacz, AF DiMartini (eds.) *The transplant patient*. Cambridge University Press, Cambridge.

48 Conrad NE, Murray LR (1999). The psychosocial meanings of living related kidney organ donation: recipient and donor perspectives-literature review. *ANNA J.* **26**: 485–90.

49 Russell S, Jacob RG (1993). Living-related organ donation: the donor's dilemma. *Patient Educ. Couns.* **21**: 89–99.

50 Siddins M, Hart G, He B, Kanchanabat B, Mohan Rao M (2003). Laparoscopic donor nephrectomy: meeting the challenge of consumerism? *ANZ J. Surg.* **73**: 912–5.

51 Sommers CH (1986). Filial morality. *Journal of Philosophy* **83**: 439–56.

52 Hardwig J (1990). What about the family? *Hastings Cent. Rep.* **20**: 5–10.

53 Mappes TA, Zembaty JS (1994). Patient choices, family interests, and physician obligations. *Kennedy Inst. Ethics J.* **4**: 27–46.

54 Martin CJ (1997). *A Renal Quandary: considerations and guidelines for patients, families and healthcare professionals involved in the treatment of end-stage renal failure*. Unpublished Thesis. Centre for Human Bioethics. Monash University.

55 Jennings B, Callahan D, Caplan AL (1988). Ethical challenges of chronic illness. *Hastings Cent. Rep.* **18**: S1–16.

56 Charmaz K (1983). Loss of self: a fundamental form of suffering in the chronically ill. *Sociol. Health Illn.* **5**: 168–95.

57 Peabody FW (1987). The care of the patient in encounters between patients and doctors. In JM Stockie (ed.) *An Anthology*. MIT Press, Cambridge Mass.

58 Reich WT (1995). *Encyclopedia of Bioethics*. Macmillan Library Reference, New York.

59 Dew MA, Goycoole A, Swizer GE, Allen AS (2000). Quality of life in organ transplantation: effects on adult recipients and their families. In PT Trzepacz, AF DiMartini (eds.) *The transplant patient*. Cambridge University Press, Cambridge.

60 Newton SE (1999). Renal transplant recipients' and their physicians' expectations regarding return to work posttransplant. *ANNA J.* **26**: 227–32.

61 Rice J, Hicks PB, Wiehe V (2000). Life care planning: a role for social workers. *Soc. Work Health Care* **31**: 85–94.

62 Gonzalez MP, Sudilovsky A, Dimartini A (2000). Quality of life in geriatric patients following transplanation: short and long term outcomes. In PT Trzepacz, AF DiMartini (eds.) *The transplant patient*. Cambridge University Press, Cambridge.

63 Goss J (2003). *Population ageing and its impact on health expenditure to 2031*. Paper presented to Australian Institute of Health and Welfare Seminar Canberra. http://www.abs.gov.au.

64 Keogh AM, Feehally J (1999). A quantitative study comparing adjustment and acceptance of illness in adults on renal replacement therapy. *ANNA J.* **26**: 471–7.

65 Rudman LA, Gonzales MH, Borgida E (1999). Mishandling the gift of life: noncompliance in renal transplant patients. *Journal of Applied Social Psychology* **4**: 835–852.

66 DiMatteo MR (1982). Social psychology and medicine. Oelgeschlager, Gunn & Hain. Cambridge, Mass.

67 Fogarty J, Youngs Jr G (2000). Psychological reactance as a factor in patient noncompliance with medication taking: a field experiment. *Journal of Applied Social Psychology* **30**: 2365–91.

68 Strickland BR (1978). Internal-external expectancies and health-related behaviors. *J Consult. Clin. Psychol.* **46**: 1192–1211.

69 McCrae RR, John OP (1992). An introduction to the five-factor model and its applications. *J. Pers.* **60**: 175–215.

70 Moran PJ, Christensen AJ, Lawton WJ (1997). Social support and conscientiousness in hemodialysis adherence. *Ann. Behav. Med.* **19**: 333–8.

71 Heap K (1985). *Practice of social work with groups: systematic approach*. Unwin Hyman, London.

72 Mann LM (1985). A group approach to teaching and support in a renal transplant unit. *ANNA J.* **12**: 102–5.

73 Sarnoff Schiff H (1996). *The support group manual: a session-by-session guide*. Penguin Books, New York.

74 Roy CA, Atcherson E (1983). Peer support for renal patients: the Patient Visitor Program. *Health Soc. Work* **8**: 52–6.

75 Russell CL, Brown K (1986). The effects of information and support on individuals awaiting cadaveric kidney transplantation. *Prog. Transplant.* **12**: 201–7.

76 Suszycki LH (1986). Social work groups on a heart transplant program. *J. Heart Transplant.* **5**: 166–70.

77 Loftin LP, Beumer C (1998). Collaborative end-of-life decision making in end stage renal disease. *ANNA J.* **25**: 615–7.

78 Callahan D (1993). Pursuing a peaceful death. *Hastings Cent. Rep.* **23**: 32–8.

79 Germino BB (1998). When a chronic illness becomes terminal. *ANNA J.* **25**: 579–82.

80 Soltys FG, Brookins M, Seney J (1998). Why hospice? The case for ESRD patients and their families. *ANNA J.* **25**: 619–24.

81 Berns R, Colvin ER (1998). The final story: events at the bedside of dying patients as told by survivors. *ANNA J.* **25**: 583–7.

82 Cooper MC (1998). Ethical decision making in nephrology nursing for end-of-life care: a responsibility and opportunity. *ANNA J.* **25**: 603–8.

83 Jennings B, Ryndes T, D'Onofrio C, Baily MA (2003). Access to hospice care. Expanding boundaries, overcoming barriers. *Hastings Cent. Rep.* Suppl: S3–7, S9–13, S15–21.

Chapter 20

The patient presenting with a genitourinary prosthesis

Gregory G. Bailly

Introduction

The genitourinary (GU) system can be the target of a variety of pathological insults that may result in chronic conditions with lifelong affects on quality of life. Whether it is an advanced pelvic or abdominal malignancy causing ureteric obstruction or pain, or a benign functional condition such as overactive bladder and urge incontinence, symptoms can be devastating to a patient's overall health and emotional well-being. In an attempt to alleviate pain, suffering, or other symptoms of chronic disease, health-care professionals try to reverse those processes as best they can, and alter the course of others with the goal of restoring some normality of function. Not all patients respond to medical therapy, and many are not candidates for radical surgery, but often there are treatment modalities available which can provide supportive care and aim to improve quality of life. Using the same philosophy as in the development of a functional prosthesis for those who have suffered an amputation of a limb, many chronic conditions affecting the genitourinary system can be successfully treated with prostheses. Although each device does not simulate 'normal function' perfectly, in most cases they do provide an attractive alternative for both the patient and physician.

This chapter is intended to educate health-care professionals about the common urological conditions in which prostheses have been used in past and current practice. It will also provide an understanding of what impact a GU prosthesis might have on other aspects of patient care in a supportive or palliative care setting. These conditions include erectile dysfunction, urinary incontinence, bladder outlet obstruction, urethral stricture disease, ureteric obstruction, and testicular loss. Various types of prostheses, along with their indications for use, effectiveness, complications, and troubleshooting will be discussed.

Erectile dysfunction: penile implants

The availability of effective oral medications for the treatment of erectile dysfunction (ED) has dramatically increased awareness of this common problem and encouraged many people to seek treatment. Regardless of the type of treatment chosen, the majority of patients experience ED as a chronic condition for the rest of their lives. The treatment options available are not considered curative, but are directed toward supportive care to improve overall quality of life. In the current environment, penile implants have played a secondary role in the treatment of erectile difficulties but they are still useful when medical therapy such as oral phosphodiesterase-5 (PDE-5) inhibitors, intraurethral alprostadil, and intracorporeal injection with vasoactive agents or vacuum erection devices are ineffective or contraindicated. Unlike their medical counterparts, implants generally provide a predictable and reliable way of restoring erectile function.

Penile implants were introduced over 30 years ago with the three-piece inflatable and the semirigid rod.[1,2] In 2003, projected implant sales have approached the pre-sildenafil numbers of approximately 18 000. In the USA, the three-piece inflatable model represents 70% of the market, the two-piece 20% and the semirigid 10%; elsewhere, about 60% are inflatable with the remaining 40% semirigid (Mulcahy JJ, unpublished).

Today's three classes of implants include hydraulic, semirigid, and soft silicone ones. The hydraulic consists of the three- and two-piece inflatable models. The three-piece type is more commonly used than the two-piece. It consists of a pump in the scrotum, two cylinders, one in each erectile body, and a reservoir placed behind the rectus muscles in the prevesical space (Fig. 20.1). The three-piece provides the best rigidity and flaccidity since the fluid can completely fill the corporal cylinders or be completely drained when the non-erect state is desired. The two-piece inflatable consists of a resipump in the scrotum and two cylinders in the penis. The pumping mechanism of either type is located in the scrotum and requires some manual dexterity to use. The two-piece is the

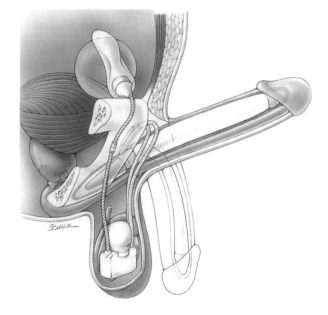

Fig. 20.1 Three-piece inflatable penile prosthesis. The main components include the scrotal pump, two cylinders, one for each corporal body, and the fluid reservoir (with permission from American Medical Systems, Minnetonka, MN).

safer choice if the implantation of the abdominal reservoir is met with anticipated surgical complexity as is sometimes seen in patients who have had previous abdominal procedures such as kidney transplants or neobladders. The three-piece version is not absolutely contraindicated but its insertion might be more challenging.

The semirigid rod and soft silicone implants are easy to insert and manipulate. The tubes are especially bendable and can be easily positioned in the upward or downward position. This type of implant is more often chosen in someone with poor manual dexterity, or if cost is an issue, since they are much less expensive than their inflatable counterparts.

Indications for penile implants

Patients who have failed medical therapy, or when medical therapy is contraindicated, are generally candidates for penile implants. They must be highly motivated to continue with sexual activity and each should be given the option of an inflatable or semi-rigid device. Patients with larger penises are best served by a three-piece inflatable which gives the best rigidity in the longer phallus. Patients with limited manual dexterity or those who cannot understand or be taught to use the scrotal pump should be advised to have a semirigid or soft silicone implant. The patient should be given realistic expectations—the erection will not be perfect and will be shorter (by 1–2 cm) than the original erection. Sensitivity of the penis, ejaculatory ability, and sexual drive are usually unchanged. In the event that the implant has to be removed (e.g. if it becomes infected), the penis will not respond to other treatments such as medications or the vacuum erection device because of scar tissue.

Surgery

As with the insertion of any prosthesis, one of the most important aspects of the surgery is to limit the risk of bacterial contamination and infection. Antibiotics are administered 1 hour prior to making the incision. The choice varies from centre to centre but usually includes one for Gram-positive bacteria such as vancomycin or a first-generation cephalosporin and one for Gram-negative coverage such as gentamicin or a fluoroquinolone. Antibiotics to cover skin contaminants are continued for at least a week post-operatively. Pre-operatively, the genital area is shaved. The procedure can be done under general or regional anaesthesia. The skin is scrubbed with betadine-based soap for 10–15 minutes and, subsequently, prepped with an antiseptic solution, such as betadine, and dried. A urethral catheter is inserted and urine should be sterile. The surgery is performed by an experienced prosthetic surgeon through an infrapubic or peno-scrotal incision. Post-operatively, the patient stays in hospital for 1 to 2 days. The implant should not be used for a further 6 to 12 weeks until follow-up by the surgeon.

Efficacy

Patient and partner satisfaction with penile prostheses ranges from 60 to 80%.[3–5] The major dissatisfaction is usually with the shorter length of the erection. For patients who have primary placement of a modern penile prosthesis, reoperation for mechanical failure can be expected in 5% of the cases when the device has been in place for 5 to 10 years.[3] The chance of mechanical failure is greater in patients who have experienced previous prosthetic problems. Patients requiring secondary placement also have a more significant risk for infection.

In North America, all penile prostheses sold now have a lifetime warranty. If a malfunction occurs within 2 years, consideration should be given to replacing only those parts which are defective and leaving the others, in particular the corporal cylinders. Some reports have indicated that infection rates are higher when doing revisions and that positive cultures taken from the wound during repair are common even in the absence of clinical infection.[6,7] This has led to the choice of replacing the entire prosthesis in some centres whenever a component malfunctions.[7]

Complications

Infection associated with a penile prosthesis can be a devastating problem. The incidence of implant-associated infection is only 1 to 3%, although it is higher with secondary or tertiary procedures.[6,7] The usual source of contamination is the operative wound and the most common organism is *Staphylococcus epidermidis*. Persistent pain over parts of the implant is a common sign that infection may be brewing. If pain is associated with fever or chills and signs of cellulitis then infection is suspected. Increasing fixation of parts, especially the pump to the scrotal wall, is further evidence of infection. Any purulent drainage from the wound, especially if it is increased upon pressing on prosthesis parts, necessitates exploration of the wound. If an infection is associated with a penile prosthesis, use of systemic antibacterials alone will not eradicate it. The formation of a capsule and biofilm or slime layer surrounding the prosthesis limits diffusion of nutrients and antibacterials to the area.[8]

When infection is suspected, the wound must be explored and all the implant parts and foreign materials removed. Traditionally, a new prosthesis is replaced in 2–6 months. Recently, however, there has been a move toward performing salvage or rescue procedures.[9–11] This involves removing all implant and foreign material, cleansing the wound with a series of antiseptic solutions, and replacing the prosthesis at the same procedure.[9] The advantage of this is to maintain most of the penile length and make it easier to place the new cylinders.[12] Waiting several months allows corporofibrosis to set in and makes reinsertion more difficult. Success rates have been reported in the range of 85%.[13,14]

Erosion of the prosthetic cylinder through the end of the corporal body is not uncommon. It may be due to over zealous dilation or aggressive use of the device and generally occurs in two locations—into the glans where it appears that the cylinder is going to wear through the end of the penis or into the fossa navicularis—although it can also erode laterally. Suspected erosion should be evaluated by an experienced prosthetic surgeon because it can usually be fixed using special surgical techniques. It is rare that a cylinder erodes far enough that it penetrates the skin and, under these circumstances, it should be removed. Urethral erosion is a more difficult problem to manage and requires removal of the eroded cylinder and replacement at a later date after the urethra has completely healed.

Caring for a patient with a penile implant in place should be considered no different than someone without one. Insertion of a urethral catheter is not contraindicated. Rigid cystoscopy is more difficult when a semi-rigid implant is in place and use of a flexible cystoscope is recommended.

Urinary incontinence: the artificial urinary sphincter (AUS)

Urinary incontinence is a major health concern across the world. It affects adults of all ages, with an estimated prevalence of 17–55% of community-dwelling people and up to 50% of nursing home residents, making it one of the most prevalent and costly diseases.[15] Incontinence carries a physical, psychological, and economic toll for affected individuals as well as their caregivers.[16] In the USA, direct costs related to urinary incontinence have been estimated at more than US$16 billion, and with the addition of costs to society, the total cost is greater than $26 billion.[15,17]

It can be treated successfully in many patients with medication or anti-incontinence surgery. Despite our advances in treatment, there are some patients who experience severe chronic urinary incontinence who require a mechanical prosthesis. Health-care professionals should have a thorough understanding of urinary incontinence prostheses and how to manage them in the supportive care setting so as to limit any potential complications that might arise.

Although many anecdotal reports of urethral compression devices were reported earlier, the first reliable artificial sphincter (AS-721) was implanted in 1972.[18] It consisted of an occlusive inflatable cuff, an abdominal reservoir and separate inflation and deflation bulbs. After many modifications, the AMS 800 (American Medical Systems, Minnetonka, MN) was introduced in 1983 and continues to be used today. This device consists of a scrotal or labial pump, an abdominal reservoir, and urethral cuff. The pump includes a deactivation button permitting simple deactivation by the physician.

Indications

Any patient with urinary incontinence secondary to urethral sphincteric deficiency can be considered a candidate for AUS implantation. The number of men receiving AUS exceeds the number of women, and its role in children has diminished since the increased use of bladder augmentation and continent diversion. Instead of using limits on severity of leakage, most believe that a patient's bother and lifestyle issues should determine whether incontinence is severe enough to warrant AUS insertion. More common patient groups that that may require an AUS include those who had a previous radical prostatectomy, bladder, or urethral surgery, traumatic injuries to the urethra or pelvic floor, radiotherapy, and neurogenic causes such as myelodysplasia and spinal cord injury. The most common indication for placement of an AUS is post-radical prostatectomy incontinence.[19]

Surgery

As with the implantation of any prosthesis, careful attention must be paid to reducing the risk of peri-operative bacterial contamination. Urine must be sterile before surgery, and pre-operative antibiotics are administered intravenously to cover Gram-positive and enteric Gram-negative organisms. Unless there is significant urethral disease present, most men have the cuff placed around the bulbar portion of the urethra; women, and traditionally children, have the cuff placed around the bladder neck. The reservoir is placed in the retropubic space next to the bladder when it is present. In men, the pump is situated in the scrotum and in women in one of the labia.

Efficacy

Experience with the AMS 800 now exceeds two decades. Outcomes in post-prostatectomy incontinence are excellent. A 3-year social continence rate of 96% in 28 patients has been reported.[20] In a review of 323 patients from the Mayo Clinic, where 70% of patients underwent device insertion for post-prostatectomy incontinence, with a mean follow-up of 68.8 months, 88% of the prostheses were functioning at a mean of 6.5 years.[21] The reoperation rate was 17% and only 7.6% had mechanical failure. It was concluded that improvements over previous models related to modifications in the cuff design (i.e. a narrow back) were meaningful.[21] The mean time to first operation was 26.2 months.[21] In a recent review, the outcome of 100 patients in whom an artificial urinary sphincter was implanted more than 10 years before was reported.[22] The bulbar cuff, as compared to the bladder neck cuff, provided a slightly better continence rate at 10 years of 92% and 84%, respectively.[22] Thirty-six per cent had their original sphincter and were continent at a mean follow-up of 11 years. No other treatment for this devastating condition approaches these success rates.

Complications

If a patient with an AUS develops recurrent incontinence, several possible causes must be considered either alone or in combination—alteration in bladder function, urethral atrophy, or mechanical failure.

Alterations in bladder function occur principally in children with neurogenic bladders. These changes can include involuntary detrusor contractions, decrease in bladder compliance, and the development of a high-pressure system with its incontinence, hydronephrosis, and ultimately renal failure if not recognized and treated properly. When identified, it should be treated with anticholinergic medication, but if ineffective it may require bladder autoaugmentation or enterocystoplasty. In fact, enterocystoplasty can be performed together with the placement of an AUS, but it may carry increased risk of infection.[23]

Atrophy of the urethra requiring revision occurs in 3 to 9.3% of patients and is the result of long-term compression of urethral tissues at the cuff site.[24] Increasing cuff pressure via a 71–80 cm balloon reservoir has had limited success due to further pressure atrophy and erosion.[25] The same concern holds true for decreasing the cuff size. However, down-sizing the cuff size of 4.5 cm to 4.0 cm in 17 patients with urethral atrophy yielded 80% patient satisfaction at a 22-month mean follow-up.[26] Placing a second urethral cuff has also gained popularity recently (Fig. 20.2). The concept of tandem urethral cuff placement is to disperse effective urethral cuff pressure over a larger surface area to achieve urethral coaptation. In a study on the use of tandem cuffs in 18 patients, daily pad use decreased from 4.3 to 1.6; 10 of the 18 patients (56%) needed one pad or less daily, 16 (88%) said they would have the tandem cuff placed again and 17 (94%) would recommend the procedure.[27]

As with any prosthesis, mechanical failure can lead to incontinence. It can occur as a result of a leak in any of the components of the device, but the most common site is at the urethral cuff. The exact site of leakage is often identified only at the time of a salvage surgery. Treatment involves surgical replacement of the failed component and reconnecting the device.

Infection and erosion require removal of the AUS device. Infection occurs in 1 to 3% of patients. Traditionally, reinsertion is delayed at least 3 months, but recently several

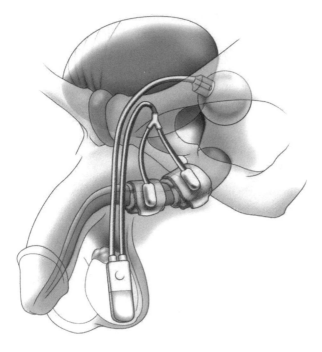

Fig. 20.2 Artificial urinary sphincter (AMS-800 model) with tandem cuff. Despite having two urethral cuffs present, there is still only one scrotal pump and one fluid reservoir (with permission from American Medical Systems, Minnetonka, MN).

authors have described their results with salvage AUS procedures.[13,28] In one study, there was an 87% success rate in eight patients who underwent a salvage AUS.[28] More experience is being gained at present, but this new approach is still under investigation.

Erosion can occur at any time, but the highest incidence (i.e. two-thirds) is seen within the first year. Previous surgery at the site of cuff placement increases the risk of erosion. Other common risk factors occurring, sometimes unnecessarily, in the hospital are urethral catheterization and urethral endoscopic manipulations with an activated sphincter in place. Therefore, when a patient with an AUS requires a catheter, we recommend deactivating the device and inserting a small (12–14 F) urethral catheter for several days only. If prolonged catheterization is required, the patient is best managed with a suprapubic catheter. Cuff erosion usually presents with incontinence, and sometimes clinical infection. It is diagnosed cystoscopically and requires removal of the cuff. Most urologists leave a small catheter in the urethra to aid in healing. A new cuff can be replaced several months later once the urethra is healthy and no stricture is identified. The cuff must be positioned away from the erosion site. An alternative is to place a larger cuff around the urethra and one of the corporeal bodies. Transcorporeal cuff placement reinforces the artificial sphincter with corporeal tissue to decrease focal pressure on the attenuated urethra. Of 31 men undergoing this technique, 84% required 0 to 1 pad daily and 25 of the 26 (96%) were satisfied on a survey at a mean follow-up of 17 months.[29]

Long-term follow-up of the AUS

Patients with AUS devices should be followed long-term by a urologist. Most of the information regarding incontinence, possible infection, and voiding symptom alterations can be gathered from a patient history on each visit. New signs or symptoms are best evaluated with cystourethroscopy and, sometimes, urodynamics. When managing patients requiring supportive or palliative care, it is imperative that the caregiver be aware of the AUS, how to activate and deactivate the device, and when to call for help from the urologist. Avoiding infection and erosion should be a priority in patients who have serious co-morbidities and are poor surgical candidates for revision or replacement.

How to use the AUS: directions for the caregiver

The AUS 800 device requires between one and three pumps to fully decompress the cuff depending upon its size. Patients have 2 to 3 minutes within which to empty the bladder until the cuff automatically reinflates. They are instructed to depress the scrotal pump again if complete bladder emptying did not occur before the reocclusion by the cuff. All patients should be instructed that the AUS can and should be deactivated by medical personnel familiar with the device prior to any urethral catheterization or manipulation. As stated previously, it must be emphasized that if a patient who has an AUS requires a urethral catheter, the device must be deactivated and the catheter inserted must be small (i.e. 12–14 F) and used for a short period of time only (e.g. for several days). Intermittent catheterization can be performed but it is imperative to ensure that the cuff is deflated during catheterization. If uncertainty exists, a health-care professional experienced with the AUS should be consulted. If prolonged catheterization is required, the patient is best managed with a suprapubic catheter. Patients are instructed to notify their physicians immediately with symptoms of urinary tract infection, haematuria, or increased pain or swelling around any of the components.

Box 20.1 Case study

A 63-year-old man underwent a radical prostatectomy for localized prostate cancer. His peri-operative course was complicated by an anastomotic urine leak which resolved spontaneously after 7 days of observation. When the catheter was removed at day 20, he experienced severe urinary incontinence initially, with slight improvement over the following 9 months after doing daily Kegel exercises. His employment involved heavy lifting and strenuous activity. During the day he used five to seven pads. He voided small volumes infrequently (three to four times) during the day and did not complain of urgency. He experienced incontinence on a continuous basis with minimal activity. He was incontinent during the night and leaked in the supine position requiring a diaper while he slept. Non-video urodynamics revealed a maximum cystometric capacity of 435 cm^3 with no evidence of uninhibited contractions or instability. At a volume of 250 cm^3 he leaked very little in the sitting position and leak point pressure was 67 cmH$_2$O. With Valsalva, in the upright position, he leaked considerably. He was felt to be a good candidate for an AUS. He also had significant erectile dysfunction and did not respond to sildenafil; he had a good response to intracorporeal injections and did not wish to have a penile implant. Three months after receiving an AUS he reported a significant improvement in his incontinence. He wore only one to two pads during the day while at work and none at night.

Four years later, he sustained a myocardial infarction and a 16 F urethral catheter was inserted with the AUS deactivated by the patient. He remained in intensive care for 28 days and had the catheter for 32 days. When the catheter was removed, he experienced significant incontinence. Urology was consulted and cystoscopy was performed, showing urethral cuff erosion. The AUS and all components were removed. Six months later he underwent simultaneous insertion of a new AUS and a three-piece inflatable penile prosthesis. Both devices work well and he was satisfied.

Comment

Unfortunately, this case is not an uncommon scenario. The patient was mismanaged with long-term urethral catheterization despite the presence and awareness that he had an AUS. In his case, he was not aware that long-term urethral

Box 20.1 *(continued)*

catheterization could cause erosion and neither was the cardiology team. The urologist may be to blame, as well, since he did not ensure that the patient and his family were aware of the risks of urethral catheterization in the presence of an AUS. Proper management would have included consulting the urology service initially, with deactivation of the AUS, and insertion of a small (12 F) catheter. If the catheter was to be left in long term (>5 days), the patient should have received a suprapubic catheter with removal of the urethral one. In the end, he was still able to undergo successful reinsertion of an AUS.

Urinary urge lincontinence: sacral neuromodulation

Considered a chronic condition, urge incontinence has a significant impact on daily living and quality of life.[30] Approximately 65% of men and women with incontinence report that their symptoms have a negative impact on daily living, of whom 60% found their symptoms bothersome enough to consult a medical practitioner.[31] Ninety per cent of Canadians experiencing urinary incontinence report that it has an effect on their overall feeling of well-being and over 80% report feelings of embarrassment and frustration.[32] In 8–10%, this results in social isolation.[33,34] Urinary urge incontinence has been shown to be independently associated with falls and fractures among community-dwelling elderly women. In one study, women with weekly urge incontinence have a 26% greater risk of sustaining a fall and a 34% risk of fracture adjusting for other causes.[35] Depression is also strongly associated with incontinence.[35]

The mainstay of treatment of urge incontinence caused by detrusor overactivity is antimuscarinic therapy with oxybutynin or tolterodine. Despite the improvements in their clinical profiles and extended-release formulations, there are still many people who have a poor response to or cannot tolerate these medications; these patients have refractory urge incontinence. Sacral nerve stimulation, often referred to as sacral neuromodulation, is becoming the standard of care for treatment of refractory overactive bladder and urge incontinence. Neuromodulation using the InterStim Continence Control System (Medtronic, Minneapolis, MN) is a less invasive therapy that has been available for commercial use in Europe, Canada, and Australia since 1994 and in the USA since 1997. To date, it has been performed on over 8000 patients.[36]

The concept of neuromodulation is based on the understanding that urge incontinence results from an imbalance of facilitatory and excitatory control systems, often causing a hyperexcitable detrusor, leading to incontinence in the filling phase.[37] Although not fully understood, neuromodulation is felt to correct this imbalance via direct or indirect actions on the sacral nerves.[38] Used initially for the treatment of refractory urge incontinence only, its use has extended to other chronic pelvic conditions including idiopathic chronic urinary retention, pelvic pain, and interstitial cystitis.[39]

Indications

Sacral neuromodulation should be considered in patients with refractory urge incontinence before contemplating more invasive surgical procedures such as ileo-cystoplasty, detrusor myectomy, or urinary diversion. It should also be considered before committing patients to a lifetime of absorbent products and their associated problems. For idiopathic urinary retention and refractory interstitial cystitis, it is still considered investigational, but results are promising.

Surgery

Technically, the treatment is introduced in two steps. The first involves a screening test known as percutaneous nerve evaluation (PNE), in which a temporary electrode is inserted into the S3 foramen and an external pulse generator is used to identify which patients may benefit from therapy. The second step involves permanent neuroprosthesis implantation in those who respond favourably to the PNE.

Efficacy

Outcomes of sacral neuromodulation come from multicentre trials initiated in 1992 across 22 centres.[40–42] At 6 months almost half (47%) of the group of 125 women and 30 men were dry, compared with none in the control group.[40] Defining clinical benefit as being dry or a reduction in incontinent episodes by 50%, over three-quarters (76%) achieved this level of improvement.[40] There was also improvement in quality of life as assessed by the Short Form-36. The response was durable, with a consistent benefit noted up to 18 months.[42] In a 3-year follow-up study, 59% of urge incontinent patients showed greater than 50% reduction in leaking episodes.[43] The response in patients over the age of 55 years has been shown to be less that in younger patients.[44] The procedure is being performed using a percutaneous technique at many centres today, reducing its surgical complications even more.

Complications

Sacral neuromodulation is a safe treatment option. In a large prospective multicentre trial the most common adverse events included pain at the neurostimulator site (15%), suspected lead migration (8%), infection (6%), transient electrical shock (5%), adverse change in bowel function (3%), and adverse change in voiding function (0.6%).[43] Of the 219 patients receiving the device, the overall surgical revision rate was 33%, usually for relocation of the neurostimulator because of pain or/and revision of the lead system because of suspected lead migration. There were no reports of serious injury. Despite the high revision rate, 84% of the patients said they would have the surgery again.[43]

Bladder outlet and urethral obstruction: urethral stents

Bladder outlet obstruction is a common urological condition in men. Benign prostatic hyperplasia (BPH) is its most common cause, although it can occur secondary to pelvic trauma, urethral stricture disease, and detrusor–sphincter dyssynergia (DSD). BPH is often managed initially with drugs, but when they fail or are not tolerated various endoscopic or open surgical procedures are performed. Strictures of the anterior urethra are usually treated with optical internal urethrotomy or urethroplasty, the latter providing superior results in carefully selected patients. Internal urethrotomy has poor long-term efficacy, especially in those patients with long, dense strictures who tend to have frequent recurrences. Not all patients are good candidates for urethroplasty, usually due to co-morbid conditions. In those patients with spinal cord injuries with neurogenic bladder and DSD, routine management has relied on endoscopic sphincterotomy or formal urinary diversion. Sphincterotomy has poor long-term efficacy and a significant complication profile. Each of these groups might be better treated with an endoscopically placed urethral stent.

The Urolume endoprosthesis was introduced in 1988, and at that time its primary indication was to treat bulbous urethral strictures.[45] Soon its role was extended to the treatment of BPH and DSD in select patients.

BPH and intraprostatic stents

Although transurethral resection of the prostate (TURP) is considered the gold standard for the treatment for BPH, up to 10–15% of patients are not candidates for such surgery because of significant co-morbidities. Hence, many less-invasive surgical options have been developed, one of which has been the intraprostatic stent introduced in 1980. Initially it had broad indications, but eventually its role became better defined for the management of patients who were unfit for surgery and where the alternative would have been a long-term indwelling urethral catheter. Although intraprostatic stents have been demonstrated to be safe and effective for the treatment of symptomatic BPH, their use is still not as widely accepted as many of the other forms of minimally invasive techniques.[46]

Temporary stents

Intraprostatic stenting can serve as a temporary or permanent solution for obstruction caused by BPH. Temporary stents are tubular devices that are made of either non-absorbable or biodegradable material. They remain in the prostatic urethra for a limited period of time and do not become covered with urothelium. They are easily removed every 6 to 36 months and can be replaced without difficulty using topical anaesthesia.[47] Designed for short-term use to relieve bladder obstruction, this type of stent acts as an alternative to urethral catheterization in a patient who is unfit for surgery. They are also used occasionally following laser or transurethral microwave therapy when secondary or temporary obstruction is expected. They allow normal micturition, with success rates in the range of 50 to 90%.[46] The side-effects include encrustation, migration, breakage, incontinence, and infection.[46] Several different types of non-absorbable stents exist including spiral and polyurethane ones.

Unlike the non-absorbable stents, biodegradable stents do not need to be removed. They are typically used after a laser procedure but are still considered experimental. They may have greater applicability in the future.

Permanent stents

In BPH, the permanent stent has been used as a definitive treatment for obstruction. Initially, there was great interest in this non-invasive form of treatment, but recently their use in BPH has become idle. The Urolume endourethral prosthesis (American Medical Systems, Minnetonka, MN) is a woven tubular steel mesh that maintains its position in the urethra by outward external pressure. Soon after it is deployed, it becomes epithelialized and incorporated into the urethral mucosa. The stent can be removed endoscopically using grasping forceps to pull it into a resectoscope sheath. The main indication for use has been in men who are unfit for a TURP. It has shown a significant reduction in the symptom score and an increase in peak flow rate.[47] Complications including irritative voiding, infection, encrustation, and migration have not been well tolerated.[47] Given the improvements in other less invasive forms of prostate surgery, the popularity of the Urolume has declined significantly and it is not frequently used for BPH today.

Detrusor–sphincter dyssynergia and Urolume stents

The ideal form of bladder management in patients with detrusor–sphincter dyssynergia maintains a low intravesical pressure and often involves the use of anticholinergic medications and clean intermittent catheterization. Patients who cannot tolerate these medications, who have difficulty performing catheterization, or who continue to have high bladder pressures despite doing both, often need other forms of management including sphincterotomy, suprapubic catheter, bladder augmentation, or urinary diversion. Sphincterotomy has been the initial treatment of choice in many of these men; however, complications include erectile dysfunction (2.8–64%), haemorrhage (5–23%), and technical failure requiring reoperation (12–26%).[48] Suprapubic or indwelling urethral catheters are not considered good long-term options either.

Urethral sphincter stents are an acceptable alternative to sphincterotomy, and have several advantages including potential reversibility, no significant effect on erectile function, minimal invasiveness, and short hospital stay.[49] The Urolume Wallstent (American Medical Systems, Minnetonka, MN) was first used for the treatment of DSD in 1988.[49] The North American Study Group reported the long term data in 160 men, showing a significant decrease in detrusor leak point pressure and residual urine. More than half experienced an improvement or resolution of their autonomic dysreflexia symptoms. Twenty-four patients (15%) required stent removal.[49] Stent migration occurred in 12.4% of patients after 3 months of implantation and in 5% at 6 months.[49] Forty-seven patients (26.3%) were diagnosed with bladder neck obstruction subsequent to stent placement which required treatment in 38 men.[49] In another study the Urolume was compared with sphincterotomy in a randomized trial and it was concluded that stent placement was as safe and effective as sphincterotomy and that the simplicity and minimal morbidity associated with stent placement made it an attractive alternative for the treatment of DSD.[50]

Urethral strictures and the Urolume

Historically, treatment options for urethral stricture disease included urethral dilation, internal urethrotomy, and urethroplasty. The long-term results of dilation or urethrotomy are similar, giving stricture-free rates of approximately 50–60%.[51] As an alternative to the other treatment options, urethral stenting was introduced in the late 1980s (Fig. 20.3). The Urolume endoprosthesis has a reported long-term efficacy of 63% in patients with recurrent urethral strictures.[52] Two-year follow-up from the Urolume clinical trial in North America reported that mean urinary peak flows increased from 9.0 to 23.6 ml/s and symptom scores decreased by almost 75%.[53] Eighty-five per cent of men required no further treatment. Most recently, the 11-year follow-up of 24 patients by the North American group showed mean flow rates of 9.5 and 20.8 ml/s before and after stent implantation, respectively; mean urinary symptom scores were 11.3 before and 3.0 after the stent.[53] Eight patients underwent nine retreatment procedures within the stented area during the follow-up.[53]

The Urolume stent offers a safe and effective minimally invasive approach to the management of recurrent bulbar urethral stricture disease with few complications, low retreatment rates, and the uncommon need for explantation (i.e. removal).[54] Its advantages include short operating time, minimal blood loss, ease of insertion, short

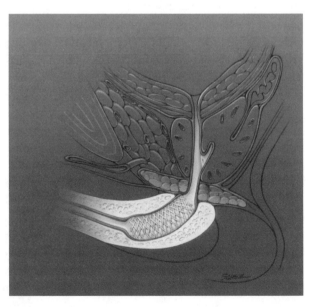

Fig. 20.3 Urolume endoprosthesis. The primary indication for a Urolume positioned in the bulbous urethra is urethral stricture disease (with permission from American Medical Systems, Minnetonka, MN).

hospitalization, and most notably minimal anaesthesia, which makes it suitable for even the most medically compromised patient. It has been advocated for use in patients with bulbar urethral strictures less than 3 cm in length after at least two recurrences with a minimal distance of 7 to 10 mm from the external sphincter and who are not candidates for urethroplasty.[53] Patients with strictures longer than 3 cm, or those who have had previous urethroplasties should be made aware of the higher retreatment rates. In addition, those with post-traumatic urethral strictures are not good candidates because of the massive peri-urethral scarring frequently associated with these cases. Similarly, patients with severe bladder neck contractures after prostatectomy are not good candidates because of the poor tissue quality in this area.

Urolume stent explantation

Early experience with the Urolume showed a high rate of explantation during years 1 and 2 after insertion. Recently the North American Study Group reported the factors relating to 69 men (14.8%) who required stent explantation of the 465 patients enrolled in the study over 7 years.[54] In patients treated for BPH, 23% of the stents were removed, as were 5% of those implanted for bulbar urethral strictures and 22% of those patients with DSD.[54] Of the explantations, 44% were done within 1 year.[54] Migration or incorrect placement were the most common reasons for removal. The most important factor identified which related to success was correct placement. When stenting the prostate, it should be placed more distal than the bladder neck. In DSD, it is essential that the stent extends at least 5 mm into the bulbar urethra. The proximal half should cover the caudal half of the verumontanum. For bulbous urethral strictures, the stent end should be at least 5 mm beyond the strictured area. If multiple stents are needed, their ends should overlap at least 5 mm to prevent overgrowth of tissue with repeated stenosis in the junctional area. Stenting should be avoided in irradiated urethras because epithelialization is likely to be poor. Previous urethroplasty is also a relative contraindication.

Ureteric obstruction

Ureteric obstruction may occur secondary to a variety of benign and malignant conditions, both extrinsic and intrinsic. Such instances can arise in those patients with advanced pelvic or abdominal malignancies such as lymphoma and colorectal, genitourinary, or gynaecological cancers. Benign conditions such as retroperitoneal fibrosis or iatrogenic ureteric strictures can also cause significant ureteric obstruction which can become chronic and difficult to manage. Major reconstructive surgery to relieve the obstruction is not appropriate in all patients. This may be the case in those who have extrinsic ureteric obstruction secondary to an inoperable malignancy or in patients with significant co-morbidities. Management options are either external or internal drainage.

Percutaneous nephrostomy tubes

The most common form of external drainage involves urinary diversion by percutaneous insertion of nephrostomy tubes. The other is cutaneous ureterostomy but this is rarely used today. For many patients, as a form of long-term or supportive urinary drainage, nephrostomy tubes are uncomfortable for the patient and often require supportive nursing care and frequent dressing changes. They can become dislodged or obstructed necessitating a visit to the urologist or interventional radiologist for exchange or unplugging. In an attempt to reduce their complications, several subcutaneous tunnelling techniques have been developed (Fig. 20.4).[55] Advantages include larger-calibre lumens and an exit site on the anterior abdominal wall which reduces the risk of displacement and makes it more comfortable and easier to manage for the patient.

Double-J ureteric stents

Because of the problems associated with external drainage, internal drainage using double-J (double pigtail) ureteric stents has become the conventional way of managing both acute and chronic ureteric obstruction. The concept was first introduced in the nineteenth century and the current pigtail stents in the late 1970s. Intrinsic stents have several advantages including ease of insertion, familiarity by urologists, maintenance of voiding, and cosmetic acceptability. They may be associated with several problems including encrustation (thus requiring 3–6 monthly changes), stone formation, infection, haematuria, irritative voiding symptoms including urgency and dysuria, painful ureteric reflux, decreased ureteric peristalsis, and stent migration. Despite their

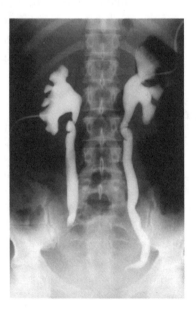

Fig. 20.4 Bilateral percutaneous nephrostomy tubes. This woman presented with bilateral hydronephrosis and obstructive renal failure secondary to locally invasive cancer of the cervix. Bilateral percutaneous nephrostomy tubes were inserted. This delayed antegrade nephrostogram shows both left and right nephrostomy tubes and bilateral ureteric obstruction.

disadvantages, double-J stents continue to be the most common form of management of chronic ureteric obstruction when open surgery is not a good option.

Metallic ureteral stents

In an attempt to improve upon the problems associated with double-J stents, metallic ureteric stents have been developed such as similar ones used successfully in the biliary tract, coronary arteries, and urethra. Since 1990, when the first metallic stent was introduced, a variety of similar versions have been used. Most use the self-expandable wall-stent system made from meshed steel wire that is inserted through a special endoscopic device into the ureter. They vary in length from approximately 3 to 20 cm and have diameter of approximately 10 F.[56]

Metallic stents are usually only considered for ureteric obstruction caused by malignant disease. Wallstents were placed across 54 malignant ureteric stenoses in 40 patients and, with a mean follow-up of 10.5 months, 41 ureters were patent.[57] It was concluded that the insertion of a self-expandable metallic stent was a safe and effective palliative treatment for malignant ureteric strictures.[57] Several reports regarding their use in benign disease have also been published.[58–60] Several complications can occur including infection, encrustation, obstruction, and migration.[59,60] Because they incorporate into the wall of the ureteric lumen, their removal is almost impossible.

Compared to our experience with double-J stents and nephrostomy tubes, the role of metallic stents for benign or malignant ureteric obstruction is still poorly defined among urologists. The lack of randomized studies and the few patients involved make interpretation of their usefulness difficult. At present, they appear to be best suited for patients with malignant ureteric obstruction with a reasonable life expectancy if the quality of life is significantly altered by the side-effects of a double-J stent. Concerted efforts are being made to improve the design and to better define which patients may benefit from these minimally invasive therapeutic stents.

Testicular loss: the testicular prostheses

Surgical castration, genital trauma, and testicular agenesis are the most common reasons to consider insertion of a testicular prosthesis. The only real indication for a testicular implant is patient preference and cosmesis. Being left without one or both testicles may produce psychological sexual dysfunction and loss of body image, especially in young men.[61] As a result, many men today have testicular implants inserted early in life and often maintain them for years. Therefore, it is important to have an understanding of managing the man who needs or has a testicular implant.

Testicular implants come in either saline-filled or silicone versions. The saline implants are the only ones sold in the USA at present, mainly because of the concerns about potential side-effects of silicone, as extrapolated from breast implants. Implants come in small, medium, and large sizes to match the other testicle and they have securing regions at the lower pole for suture fixation. Surgical implantation is usually performed with regional or general anaesthesia, and preferably at the time of orchiectomy. Complications are rare.[62] The risk of infection has been reported to be 4% in one large study of 2533 prosthesis patients.[62] When infection is suspected, the prosthesis must be removed, but a new one can be inserted at a later date.

It is important for health-care professionals to be aware of some of the issues relating to patient satisfaction in men with testicular implants. Of 234 men who completed a questionnaire after orchiectomy for testicular cancer, only two-thirds were offered a prosthesis whereas 91% felt it was important to have been offered one.[63] Most men (73%) were satisfied with their implant. Of the 71 who received an implant, 19 (27%) were dissatisfied and felt they had an average or poor cosmetic result. The reasons for dissatisfaction were: shape, most commenting that the prostheses was too round; position, the implant was too high and especially noticeable in warm weather when the dartos muscle is relaxed; comfort, the prosthesis was too uncomfortable; and weight, some declaring it too heavy and some too light. As a result of this study, it is recommended that men be offered the chance to physically examine and choose their implant and be adequately counselled on the possible outcomes.

Conclusion

The use of prostheses in patients with chronic urological conditions is intended to provide them with improved quality of life when curative treatment measures are not possible. From a supportive care point of view, these interventions can have a major impact on body image and social function. An understanding of the underlying condition specific to each prosthesis is an important aspect of patient management. Because all prostheses have potential complications, some of which can lead to very serious illness, it is imperative that health-care providers are comfortable with recognizing signs of prosthetic malfunction and infection. It is that individual who must take steps to notify the urologist of any potential problem which might arise. Equally important, health-care providers should know enough about these prostheses to avoid iatrogenic complications which might lead to unfortunate and irreversible consequences, and ultimate prosthetic failure.

References

1 Scott FB, Bradley WE, Timm GW (1974). Management of erectile impotence. Use of implantable inflatable prostheses. *Urology* 2: 80–2.

2 Small MP, Carrion HM, Gordon JA (1975). Small Carrion penile prostheses: new management of impotence. *Urology* 5: 479–86.

3 Lewis RW, Jordan GH (2002). Surgery for erectile dysfunction. In: *Campbell's Urology*, 8th edn, Vol. 2 (ed. PC Walsh, AB Retik, ED Vaughan Jr, AJ Wein), pp. 1673–709. Philadelphia: WB Saunders.

4 Chiang HS, Wu CC, Wen TC (2000). Ten years experience with penile implant prosthesis implantation in Taiwanese patients. *J. Urol.* 163: 476–80.

5   Montorsi F, Guazzoni G, Barbieri L, Maga T, Rigatti P, Graziottin A *et al.* (1996). AMS 700 CX inflatable penile implants for Peyronie's disease: functional results, morbidity, and patient-partner satisfaction. *Int. J. Impot. Res.* **8**: 81–6.

6   Jarrow JP (1996). Risk factors for penile prosthetic infection. *J. Urol.* **156**: 402–4.

7   Wilson SK, Henry GD, Delk JR, Cleves MA (2003). Prevention of infection in revision of penile prosthesis using antibiotic coated prostheses and Mulcahy salvage protocol. *J. Urol.* **163**: 225–7.

8   Nickel JC, Heaton J, Morales A, Costerton JW (1986). Bacterial biofilm in persistent penile prosthesis-associated infection. *J. Urol.* **135**: 586–8.

9   Mulcahy JJ (2000). Long-term experience with salvage of infected penile implants. *J. Urol.* **163**: 481–2.

10 Fishman IJ, Scott FB, Selim A, Nguyen TA (1997). The rescue procedure: an alternative to for managing an infected penile prosthesis. *Contemp. Urol.* **11**: 73–80.

11 Kaufman JM, Kaufman JL, Borges FD (1998). Immediate salvage procedure for infected penile prosthesis. *J. Urol.* **159**: 816–18.

12 Carson CC (2003). Diagnosis, treatment and prevention of penile prosthesis infection. *Int. J. Impot. Res.* **15**(Suppl. 5): S139–S146.

13 Mulcahy JJ (2003). Treatment alternatives for the infected penile implant. *Int. J. Impot. Res.* **15**(Suppl. 5): S147–S149.

14 Steven K, Wilson L (2003). Reimplantation of inflatable penile prosthesis into scarred corporeal bodies. *Int. J. Impot. Res.* **15**(Suppl. 5): S125–S128.

15 Wilson L, Brown JS, Shin GP, Luc KO, Subak LL (2001). Annual direct cost of urinary incontinence. *Obstet. Gynecol.* **98**: 398–406.

16 Kobelt G (1997). Economic considerations and outcome measurement in urge incontinence. *Urology.* **50**(6A, Suppl.): 100–7, discussion 108–10.

17 Wagner TH, Hu TW (1998). Economic costs of urinary incontinence in 1995. *Urology* **51**: 355–61.

18 Scott FB, Bradley WE, Timm GW (1973). Treatment of urinary incontinence by an implantable prosthetic sphincter. *Urology* **1**: 252–9.

19 Carlson KV, Nitti VW (2001). Prevention and management of incontinence following radical prostatectomy. *Urol. Clin. North Am.* **28**: 595–612.

20 Singh G, Thomas DG (1996). Artificial urinary sphincter for post-prostatectomy incontinence. *Br. J. Urol.* **77**: 248–50.

21 Elliott DS, Barrett DM (1998). Mayo Clinic long-term analysis of the functional durability of the AMS 800 artificial urinary sphincter: a review of 323 cases. *J. Urol.* **159**: 1206–8.

22 Venn SN, Greenwell TJ, Mundy AR (2000). The long-term outcome of artificial urinary sphincters. *J. Urol.* **164**: 702–7.

23 Furness PD 3rd, Franzoni DF, Decter RM (1999). Bladder augmentation: does it predispose to prosthetic infection of simultaneously placed artificial genitourinary sphincters or *in situ* ventriculoperitoneal shunts? *BJU Int.* **84**: 25–9.

24 Herschorn S, Bosch R, Bruschini H, Hanus T, Low A, Schick E (2002). Surgical treatment of urinary incontinence in men. In: *Second International Consultation on Urinary Incontinence* (ed. P Abrams, L Cardozo, S Khoury, A Wein), pp. 785–821. Plymouth, UK: Health Publication.

25 Brito CG, Mulcahy JJ, Mitchell ME, Adams MC (1993). Use of a double cuff AMS800 urinary sphincter for severe stress incontinence. *J. Urol.* **149**: 283–5.

26 Saffarian A, Walsh K, Walsh IK, Stone AR (2003). Urethral atrophy after artificial urinary sphincter placement: is cuff downsizing effective? *J. Urol.* **169**: 567–9.

27 Dimarco DS, Elliott DS (2003). Tandem cuff artificial urinary sphincter as a salvage procedure following failed primary sphincter placement for the treatment of post-prostatectomy incontinence. *J. Urol.* **170**: 1252–4.

28 Bryan DE, Mulcahy JJ, Simmon GR (2002). Salvage procedure for infected noneroded artificial urinary sphincters. *J. Urol.* **168**: 2464–6.

29 Guralnick ML, Miller E, Toh KL, Webster GD (2002). Transcorporal artificial urinary sphincter cuff placement in cases requiring revision for erosion and urethral atrophy. *J. Urol.* **167**: 2075–7.

30 Wein AJ, Rovner ES (2002). Definition and epidemiology of overactive bladder. *Urology* **60**(5, Suppl. 1): 7–12.

31 Milsom I, Stewart W, Thuroff J (2000). The prevalence of overactive bladder. *Am. J. Manag. Care* **6**(11, Suppl.): S565–S573.

32 Klag M (1998). *Experiences, Perceptions and Needs Among a Large-scale Canadian Population Experiencing Incontinence in the Community. Report for the Canadian Continence Foundation.* Toronto, Canada.

33 Angus Reid Group (1997). *Urinary Incontinence in the Canadian Adult Population.* Toronto, Canada: Augus Reid Group.

34 Klag M and the Canadian Continence Foundation (1999). *Experiences, Perceptions and Needs Among a Large-scale Canadian Population Experiencing Incontinence: a Quantitative Study Summary Report.* Toronto, Canada.

35 Brown JS, McGhan WF, Chokroverty S (2000). Comorbidities associated with overactive bladder. *Am. J. Manag. Care* **6**(11, Suppl.): S574–S579.

36 Abrams P, Blavais JG, Fowler CJ, Fourcroy JL, Macdiarmid SA, Siegel SW *et al.* (2003). The role of neuromodulation in the management of urinary urge incontinence. *BJU Int.* **91**: 355–9.

37 Fall M, Lindstrom S (1991). Electrical stimulation. A physiologic approach to the treatment of urinary incontinence. *Urol. Clin. North Am.* **18**: 393–400.

38 Schmidt RA, Senn E, Tanagho EA (1990). Functional evaluation of sacral nerve root integrity. Report on the technique. *Urology* **35**: 388–92.

39 Payne CK (2002). Urinary incontinence: nonsurgical management. In: *Campbell's Urology*, 8th edn, Vol. 2 (ed. PC Walsh, AB Retik, ED Vaughan Jr, AJ Wein), pp. 1069–91. Philadelphia: WB Saunders.

40 Schmidt RA, Jonas U, Oleson KA (1999). Sacral nerve stimulation for the treatment of refractory urge incontinence. *J. Urol.* **162**: 352–7.

41 Hassouna MM, Siegel SW, Nyeholt AA, Elhilali MM, van Kerrebroeck PE, Das AK *et al.* (2000). Sacral neuromodulation in the treatment of urgency-frequency symptoms: a multicentre study on efficacy and safety. *J. Urol.* **163**: 1849–54.

42 Jonas U, Fowlker CJ, Grunewald V (2001). Efficacy of sacral nerve stimulation for urinary retention: results of up to 18 months after implantation. *J. Urol.* **165**: 15–19.

43 Siegel SW, Catanzaro F, Dijkema HE, Elhilali MM, Fowler CJ, Gajewski JB *et al.* (2000). Long-term results of a multicenter study on sacral nerve stimulation for treatment of urinary urge incontinence, urgency-frequency, and retention. *Urology* **56**(6, Suppl 1): 87–91.

44 Amundsen CL, Webster GD (2003). Sacral neuromodulation in an older, urge-incontinent population. *Am. J. Obstet. Gynecol.* **187**: 1462–5.

45 Milroy EJ, Chapple C, Eldin A, Wallsten H (1989). A new treatment for urethral stictures: a permanently implanted urethral stent. *J. Urol.* **141**: 1120–4.

46 Fitzpatrick JM, Mebust WK (2002). Minimally invasive and endoscopic management of benign prostatic hyperplasia. In: *Campbell's Urology*, 8th edn, Vol. 2 (ed. PC Walsh, AB Retik, ED Vaughan, AJ Wein), pp.1379–422. Philadelphia: WB Saunders.

47 Wilson TS, Lemack GE, Dmochowski RR (2002). Urolume stents: lessons learned. *J. Urol.* **167**: 2477–80.

48 Hamid R, Arya M, Patel HRH, Shah PJR (2003). The mesh wallstent in the treatment of detrusor external sphincter dyssynergia in men with spinal cord injury: a 12-year follow-up. *BJU Int.* **91**: 51–3.

49 Chancellor MB, Bennett C, Simoneau AR, Finocchiaro MV, Kline C, Bennett JK *et al.* (1999). Sphincteric stent versus external sphincterotomy in spinal cord injured men: prospective randomized multicenter trial. *J. Urol.* **161**: 1893–8.

50 Chancellor MB, Gajewski J, Ackman CF, Appell RA, Bennett J, Binard J *et al.* (1999). Long-term follow-up of the North American multicenter Urolume trial for the treatment of external detrusor-sphincter dyssynergia. *J. Urol.* **161**: 1545–50.

51 Heyns CF, Steenkamp JW, DeKock M LS, Whitaker P (1998). Treatment of male urethral strictures: is repeated dilation or internal urethrotomy useful? *J. Urol.* **160**: 356–68.

52 Milroy E, Allen A (1996). Long-term results of Urolume urethral stent for recurrent urethral strictures. *J. Urol.* **155**: 904–6.

53 Shah DK, Paul EM, Badlani GH and the North American Study Group (2003). 11-year outcome analysis of endourethral prosthesis for the treatment of recurrent bulbar urethral stricture. *J. Urol.* **170**: 1255–8.

54 Shah DK, Kapoor R, Badlani GH and the North American Study Group (2003). Experience with urethral stent explantation. *J. Urol.* **169**: 1398–400.

55 Bell DG, Fischer MA (2002). Palliative subcutaneous tunneled nephrostomy tube (PSTN): a simple and effective technique for management of malignant extrinsic ureteral obstruction. *Can. J. Urol.* **9**: 1470–4.

56 Lugmayr H, Pauer W (1992). Self expanding metal stents for palliative treatment of malignant ureteral obstruction. *Am. J. Roentgenol.* **159**: 1091–4.

57 Lugmayr H, Pauer W (1996). Wallstents for the treatment of extrinsic malignant obstruction: midterm results. *Radiology* **198**: 105–8.

58 Arya M, Mostafid H, Patel HR, Kellett MJ, Philp T (2001). The self-expanding metallic ureteric stent in the long-term management of benign ureteric strictures. *BJU Int.* **88**: 339–42.

59 Kulkarni RP, Bellamy EA (1999). A new thermo-expandable shape memory nickel-titanium alloy stent for the management of ureteric strictures. *BJU Int.* **83**: 755–9.

60 Kulkarni R (2003). Metallic stents: the current situation. *BJU Int.* **92**: 188–9.

61 Incrocci L, Bosch JLHR, Slob AK (1999). Testicular prostheses: body image and sexual functioning. *BJU Int.* **84**: 1043–5.

62 Marshall S (1986). Potential problems with testicular prostheses. *Urology* **28**: 388–90.

63 Adshead J, Khoubehi B, Wood J, Rustin G (2001). Testicular implants and patient satisfaction: a questionnaire-based study of men after orchiectomy for testicular cancer. *BJU Int.* **88**: 559–62.

Chapter 21

The patient presenting with benign genitourinary pain

Allan B. Patrick

In all areas of medicine, including urology, an increasing number of patients present with pain as their primary complaint. It may be acute or chronic or a combination. Proper pain evaluation can be challenging and requires a thorough, organized diagnostic approach. Patients are often very uncomfortable during the physical exam and may be afraid or embarrassed to discuss their symptoms with family, friends, and physicians. Patients may have suffered for years and seen a variety of health-care providers. Anger, frustration, and depression can colour the interview. Stresses from substance abuse as well as occupational, relationship, and sexual issues may be significant. It is imperative to remove the 'blinders of prior misdiagnosis' and approach the patient as a clean slate. Despite these cautions, we are faced with many cases in which the diagnosis is unclear.

The history starts with a review of referral records and ideally a patient-completed questionnaire detailing prior illnesses, surgery, trauma, and current medications. Quality of life and pain severity questions expand on the impact of pain on level of function.[1] The chief complaint is evaluated along with aggravating and relieving factors. Location, timing, quality, and severity of pain are reviewed. An understanding of relevant neuroanatomy is helpful in deciphering referred pain. We will review the salient points in history taking, patient physical examination, diagnostic testing, and treatment for a variety of genitourinary pain presentations, namely:

- flank pain
- pelvic pain
- bladder pain
- penile pain
- orchalgia.

Flank pain

Neuroanatomy

Pain fibres from the kidney, renal pelvis, and ureter travel along the sympathetic nerves, from segments T12–L2, primarily near the renal artery. Afferents from the renal

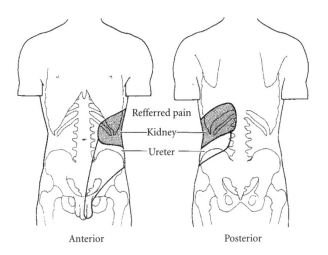

Anterior　　　　　　　Posterior

Fig. 21.1 Renal colic pain distribution.

capsule enter here as well and branches to the celiac and aortic plexi and lower thoracic and lumbar splanchnic nerves arise in the kidney. Afferents travel along the vagus nerve and contribute to the nausea, vomiting, and ileus associated with renal colic. Afferents from the ureter vary according to the level of the ureter. The upper one-third gives afferents to the renal plexus, the middle third to the superior hypogastric plexus, and the lower third to the inferior hypogastric plexus and hypogastric nerves.

Pain of renal origin is primarily produced by distention of the renal capsule and collecting system. Inflammation of the upper tract, as in pyelonephritis, can produce renal pain, but often a dull aching type less severe than true calculous renal colic. Figure 21.1 shows the typical location of flank pain based on the site of pathology.

Renal colic

The most frequent cause of flank pain is ureteral colic from passage of a urinary calculus. The prevalence of urinary stones in the adult population is 2–5% and the likelihood that a white male in the USA will have a stone in his lifetime is one in eight. Fifty per cent will have another stone within 10 years.[2] Colic is produced by the acute distention and spasm of the collecting system from a stone in the ureter; less commonly the sudden ureteric obstruction is due to a blood clot, sloughed renal papilla, or a fungus ball. Occasionally the colic is a result of a stone in a renal infundibulum or calyx or an intermittently obstructing stone in the renal pelvis. Pain is described as sharp, knife-like, stabbing, nauseating—'the worst pain of my life'. As a patient explanation, renal colic is similar to biliary colic or having food stuck in the oesophagus; there is an overwhelming sensation as the muscular tube attempts to propel the stone along. However, hyperperistalsis fails to completely explain this severe pain. Patients typically roll about the bed or floor trying to get comfortable, as opposed to other pains of abdominal visceral origin such as diverticulitis or appendicitis where patients lie still to avoid peritoneal irritation. Blood pressure, pulse, and respiratory rate are often elevated due to pain. Patients may have a reduced tolerance to pain in the referral area for up to 8 months after the acute event.[3]

Pain may also arise from passage of a blood clot (e.g. from a renal cell carcinoma) or tissue fragments in papillary necrosis (e.g. in diabetics). On examination, there may be moderate tenderness to deep palpation over the stone location and sharp pain to palpation or gentle percussion of the ipsilateral costovertebral angle is typical.

Urinalysis displays microscopic haematuria or gross blood, but as many as 10% of patients show no haematuria.[4] Pyuria may be seen in the absence of infection, but significant pus cells mandate antibiotics covering typical Gram-negative pathogens until urine culture reports are available. Infection in an obstructed renal collecting system is extremely serious and must be treated aggressively as an undrained abscess until proven otherwise.

Imaging of patients with renal colic has changed dramatically in recent years. Historically, the first image obtained on a patient with suspected renal colic was a plain abdominal X-ray or KUB (i.e. kidneys, ureters, and bladder). The sensitivity and specificity of this film can be limited due to overlying stool and gas and the presence of pelvic phleboliths. Currently, the KUB has its greatest utility in following a patient with a previously identified stone.

The intravenous pyelogram or urogram (IVP or IVU) was the gold standard imaging modality until recently when it was replaced by computed tomography (CT), specifically the spiral CT scan. Unenhanced CT scans are fast, safe (i.e. without intravenous contrast), and can reliably detect stones as small as 1 mm in size. The degree of collecting system dilatation and perinephric stranding are reliably assessed as indicators of obstruction. With non-contrast CT, the drug-seeking patient can be reliably screened.

CT does not assess function, however, and uncommon causes of flank pain such as a renal pedicle injury or artery embolus may be missed in the acute setting.[5]

Ultrasonography is a non-invasive imaging technique increasingly used in the emergency room as a general screening tool in the evaluation of patients with abdominal pain. Wider use of ultrasonography has led to much earlier detection of renal tumours and can reliably detect renal and proximal and distal ureteric calculi; those in the mid-ureter are far more difficult to image unless they reside at the end of a dilated ureteric segment. Ultrasound is very user dependent and most urologists now prefer CT as the definitive imaging modality in renal colic.

Patients with renal colic require prompt supportive treatment with analgesics, anti-emetics, and fluids while definitive interventions are planned; all urine should be strained in an attempt to capture a passed stone. Intravenous or intramuscular injections of an opioid should be given in sufficient quantities and at sufficient intervals to keep the patient comfortable. Adding an antihistamine or phenothiazine to the narcotic gives synergy, is sedating, and helps control associated nausea. Non-steroid anti-inflammatory medications including ketorolac given intramuscularly or

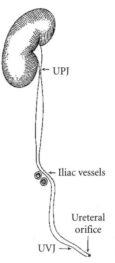

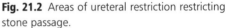

Fig. 21.2 Areas of ureteral restriction restricting stone passage.

indomethacin suppositories can often be surprisingly effective in renal colic, perhaps due to an antispasmodic effect.[6] Use of an antispasmodics such as hyoscine butylbromide potentially may also help reduce ureteric spasm.

Treatment of a particular stone is tailored to the individual patient and the stone size and location. There are three common sites in the ureter where stones tend to get stuck—the ureteropelvic junction (UPJ), where the ureter crosses the iliac vessels, and the ureterovesical junction (UVJ) (Fig. 21.2).

The decision to hospitalize and/or intervene early is based on inability to control pain, the presence of fever or signs of urinary tract infection, the presence of diabetes, or impaired renal function. Stones greater than 5 mm are less likely to pass spontaneously. Patients settling quickly who have no complicating factors and a small stone can be safely discharged home with strainers and a prescription for oral analgesics. They are instructed to bring the stone to their doctor for analysis or to return to the hospital if recurrent pain is not relieved by their prescription medication or if fever develops. Arrangements are made to reassess the patient in roughly 2 weeks with plain films if the stone is radio-opaque or with a renal ultrasound if it is not. Patients are reassured that obstruction to their kidney is unlikely to produce damage in the short term.[7] Patients are instructed to maintain a high fluid intake and strain their urine continuously, as passage of a small calculus from the bladder may go unnoticed.

Not surprisingly, patients may report changes in the type and location of pain as the stone moves through the urinary tract. Pain in the flank may progress to the groin as the stone moves to the pelvic ureter; a stone at the UVJ can produce irritative voiding symptoms such as frequency, urgency, and dysuria.

Specific urological intervention will vary with stone size and location, as well as the availability of local modalities of therapy. Extracorporeal shock wave lithotripsy

(ESWL) is often used as a first-line treatment for stones less than 1 cm in the kidney or upper ureter. Temporary ureteric stenting is usually used for larger stones or if there is associated infection or severe pain. Renal stones larger than 2 cm are best treated by percutaneous approaches. Flexible and rigid ureteroscopy with or without intracorporeal lithotripsy (e.g. holmium–YAG laser) has advanced dramatically in recent years and is used with increasing frequency to manage stones throughout the entire urinary tract.

Musculoskeletal pain

Musculoskeletal pain can sometimes mimic renal colic very closely. Typically the pain is chronic and can be associated with a repetitive physical acts or back strain/injury. Strenuous activity or certain motions will aggravate the pain. Tenderness and spasm in the paravertebral muscles quickly suggests a musculoskeletal cause. Point tenderness of a trigger point along an intercostal nerve followed by relief from a nerve block confirms the diagnosis of intercostal neuralgia. Patients are reassured of no sinister pathology and conservative measures or referral to a physiotherapist are indicated.

Ureteropelvic junction (UPJ) obstruction

UPJ obstruction is the most common cause of dilatation of the fetal kidney.[8] As a congenital anomaly, it is more common in males and more common on the left; it can present at any time of life.[9] Occasionally painless, UPJ obstruction can cause crampy abdominal pain usually not as severe as stone colic. Episodes of pain tend to occur during episodes of diuresis, known as Dietl's crisis, after high fluid intake. The urine output overwhelms the outflow through the UPJ, causing distention of the renal pelvis and pain. A dilated collecting system with a normal ureter in the absence of stones suggests this diagnosis. A diuretic renal scan will confirm the diagnosis and degree of renal function. Surgical correction options include open or laparoscopic pyeloplasty and retrograde or antegrade endopyelotomy.

Renal cystic disease

Ten per cent of the population will develop one or more simple benign cysts in their kidney; most remain asymptomatic. However, large cysts can stretch the renal capsule and cause a constant dull ache. Ultrasound and CT imaging readily make the diagnosis. Relief of pain following percutaneous aspiration, although usually temporary, will confirm the cyst as the cause of the discomfort. Laparoscopic marsupialization is the treatment of choice if the discomfort from the cyst is significant enough to interfere with daily activities.

Patients with autosomal dominant polycystic kidney disease (ADPCKD) have kidneys virtually replaced by cysts and go on to develop renal failure in the middle decades of life. Fifty to 70% will present at some time with abdominal, flank, or low back pain, due to the cysts, passage of stones or clots, or infection. Unroofing these cysts laparoscopically may offer some hope for these patients.[10]

Pyelonephritis

Acute pyelonephritis presents a toxic, ill patient with fever, chills, and flank pain. Lower tract symptoms may or may not precede the acute illness. Pain is usually less severe than stone colic, but patients are acutely ill and often dehydrated. Urine shows pyuria and bacteriuria; there is an elevated white blood cell count with a left shift. Immediate upper tract imaging with a renal ultrasound is required to rule out associated ureteric obstruction which would require prompt decompression by ureteric stenting or percutaneous nephrostomy drainage.

Infection can extend into the perinephric space and lead to abscess formation without prompt treatment of infection and obstruction. Irritation of the adjacent psoas muscle can produce pain on leg movement. Ultrasound and CT are highly sensitive for dilatation or calculi that may complicate the infection. Rapid diagnosis, broad spectrum antibiotics, and effective upper tract decompression have combined to dramatically reduce the morbidity and mortality of acute pyelonephritis.

Renal vein thrombosis

Renal vein thrombosis is a rare cause of flank pain with haematuria. In the adult, it is usually seen in the face of nephrotic syndrome, combined with haematuria, elevated blood pressure, and fever. Pain is related initially to stretching of the renal capsule and, later, from renal ischaemia; pain is severe and constant. The affected kidney can appear swollen on imaging and nuclear radiography is needed to assess the degree of renal damage. Treatment with fibrinolytics is controversial and carries significant risk.[11]

Renal artery embolus

Renal artery embolus is to be suspected in a patient presenting with flank pain and a history of a mechanical heart valve or atrial fibrillation with or without adequate anticoagulation. The clinical picture may be varied, but sudden onset of flank pain, fever, and vomiting are commonly seen; it is seen more frequently on the left side.[12] Urinalysis is often normal and anuria implies bilateral disease. A contrast study will show areas of non-perfusion, and prompt angiography and thrombolytic therapy is essential to preserve renal function. Renal revascularization may be required when thrombolytic therapy fails, especially with a solitary kidney.

Calyceal diverticulae

Calyceal diverticulae are usually asymptomatic unless the obstruction is associated with infection or a stone. Difficult to treat, methods employed include partial nephrectomy, open unroofing and excision and, more recently, percutaneous access to remove stones and incise the obstructing infundibulum.

Loin pain haematuria syndrome

This term refers to a diagnosis of absolute exclusion and is highly controversial. Patients present with chronic flank pain and macro- or microscopic haematuria, and no other explanation for their flank pain is found.[13] There is no reliable test for the loin pain haematuria syndrome. Drastic measures to treat this rare cause of flank pain have included renal denervation, autotransplantation, and even nephrectomy.

Pelvic pain

Pelvic pain represents a distressing condition for the patient and a diagnostic challenge for the clinician. The gynaecologist is clearly the first referral source for females with pelvic pain and links with the menstrual cycle and sexual function are explored. Clinical history, pelvic exam, and imaging in the form of a pelvic ultrasound are the basics to the work-up. Female patients are often referred to a urologist if their pain has a relationship to bladder function. It is important to rule out a urinary tract infection as a cause and, if recurrent, a period of low-dose antibiotic suppression with a sulfonamide or nitrofurantoin will remove that factor from the equation. Any history suggestive of interstitial cystitis (see Chapter 18) would warrant a diagnostic bladder hydrodistention under anaesthesia. A normal cystoscopy and absence of an imaging abnormality, stone, or recurrent infections effectively rules out a urological cause to the patient's pain.

Roughly 25% of out-patient visits for genitourinary problems in the USA are diagnosed as prostatitis.[14] Patients are often tense and anxious and, at times, obsessed with their symptoms, even if mild. Men often bring journals and internet references documenting in elaborate detail the duration, timing, and nature of their symptoms. Pain may be felt 'anywhere from the nipples to the knees', involving the penis, testicles, perineum, lower back, pelvis, and suprapubic area. Voiding and ejaculatory functions may be disturbed. Patients may have seen several other urologists or health-care workers in the area and beyond; many are worried and frustrated. It is important for the patient to receive and perceive a thorough work-up; no issues should be dismissed or the cycle is likely to continue with other consultants.

The vast majority of these men will be classified as one of the prostatitis syndromes (see Chapter 16). Regardless, in the male with pelvic pain and a tender prostate on digital rectal exam, a full therapeutic trial of an appropriate antibiotic for a minimum of 6 weeks is required. Such a treatment course with sulfonamides or quinolones will confirm or deny any possible infectious component to their disease. Numerous trials have failed to show a consistent response to antibiotics in these unfortunate men.[15] A strong placebo response hampers good statistical analysis of any review of antibiotics in prostatitis, but lack of a clear response to a full therapeutic trial should be a clear message that further prescriptions will be of no value. Thus the majority of patients, by definition,

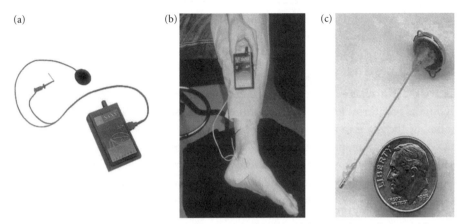

Fig. 21.3 (A) Stoller afferent nerve stimulator (SANS) device. (B) SANS electrode in position during treatment. (C) Implantable permanent SANS electrode (in development).

will have non-bacterial prostatitis or prostatodynia. If bowel symptoms colour the clinical picture, a gastroenterological referral is warranted. If voiding symptoms suggest interstitial cystitis, a diagnostic hydrodistention is recommended to avoid missing a treatable cause of the patient's symptoms. General guidelines regarding heat, non-steroidal anti-inflammatory medications, and avoidance of stress, caffeine, and alcohol are given along with reassurance.

Neuromodulation has been utilized for many years for overactive bladder symptoms; however, in recent years it has been shown effective in pelvic pain syndromes in both genders (see Chapters 18 and 20).[16] The exact mechanism of neuromodulation is unclear, but appears to involve inhibition of sacral nerve roots and reduction of pelvic floor spasticity. Stimulation of the S3 root with an implanted electrode and 'pacemaker' involves several surgical procedures and significant cost. Recently, direct percutaneous stimulation of the posterior tibial nerve above the ankle with an acupuncture needle has been described (see Fig. 21.3).[17] In several series, a course of weekly half-hour sessions leading to monthly maintenance therapy reduced frequency, urgency, and pelvic pain when pain was the dominant feature; 71% of patients were judged treatment successes using a pelvic pain intensity score.[18] In the author's experience, one-third of patients achieve a significant response, another third are improved and continue on treatment, and one-third see no significant improvement and discontinue therapy. A small implant is under development that will allow responders to perform their own treatments with an external stimulator.

Bladder pain

Most patients with bladder or suprapubic pain will eventually be referred to the urologist (see Chapter 18). Pain is related to bladder filling and is partly or completely relieved by voiding. Possible causes include bacterial and viral cystitis, interstitial cystitis, bladder cancer, and bladder stones.

Bacterial cystitis

Bacterial cystitis has a typical acute presentation with irritative symptoms including dysuria as prominent features. Urine culture is diagnostic, and response to appropriate antibiotic therapy is rapid. Irritative symptoms may persist for days to weeks following bacterial eradication, prompting repeated prescriptions instead of repeat cultures and reassurance. Phenazopyridine can be very helpful in reducing the pain and pressure, though not all patients find it helpful. Haematuria or fever in the face of urinary tract infection mandates upper tract imaging and cystoscopy.

Interstitial cystitis

Interstitial cystitis refers to a symptom complex of bladder pain, haematuria, frequency, urgency, and nocturia without dysuria or infection. Females outnumber males by a factor of 10 and the peak incidence is in the fourth decade of life. While the mechanism is unclear, association with migraine headache, irritable bowel, fibromyalgia, and chronic fatigue are often noted. Prevalence has been estimated as high as 1–2% of the adult population, though many urologists have a high index of suspicion despite typical symptoms.[19] While the cause of interstitial cystitis is uncertain, the most prevalent theory centres around a 'leaky' mucosal barrier of the bladder epithelium, allowing irritants in urine to diffuse into the bladder wall, years of which lead to the inflammation and scarring seen on biopsy. Spontaneous resolution of symptoms is common for unknown reasons. Patients are frequently misdiagnosed with urinary tract infections and often describe 3 to 5 years of progressive symptoms before proper diagnosis. While many health-care professionals include virtually any variant of pelvic pain as interstitial cystitis, this is an oversimplification. A suspicious history followed by improvement with diagnostic hydrodistention secures the diagnosis. These patients will be much more likely to respond to any given modality of treatment for interstitial cystitis. While beyond the scope of this chapter, therapy may involve dietary modification, use of oral pentosan polysulphate to augment the bladder's mucosal barrier, antihistamines, and a variety of solutions instilled into the bladder. As long as strict diagnostic criteria are met, most patients will respond favourably to treatment.

Bladder cancer

Bladder cancer is the fourth most common tumour in men after prostate, lung, and colorectal cancer and represents approximately 6.2% of all cancers; in females, it is the eighth most common tumour, representing 2.5% of all cancers.[20] Cigarette smoking is the most important risk factor and gross painless haematuria is the most common presentation. Bladder pain in this setting is an ominous symptom, suggesting more than superficial disease and a much poorer prognosis. Upper tract imaging and cystoscopy are required to evaluate haematuria, regardless of presentation.

Viral cystitis

Viral cystitis presents with sudden onset of severe frequency, urgency (with or without dysuria), and, at times, even gross haematuria. Adenovirus is the most common causative organism, though viral cultures of urine are rarely performed.[21] Often a viral upper respiratory or gastroenterological illness precedes the bladder illness by days to weeks. Irritative bladder symptoms may take several months to slowly resolve and reassurance is essential. Anticholinergic drugs such as oxybutinin may be required if frequency interferes with day to day living. Follow-up urinalysis shows resolution of haematuria and a further urological assessment is not required. It is more common in children than in adults.

Bladder stones

Bladder stones represent fewer than 5% of urinary calculi in North America, as they are most often associated with severe bladder outflow obstruction and impaired emptying.[22] Benign prostatic hyperplasia and urethral strictures are common causes of incomplete bladder emptying, with stagnation of urine, secondary infection with urease-splitting organisms, and resultant struvite bladder stones. Pain and haematuria are common as are obstructive symptoms, since stones may impact on the bladder outlet and lead to intermittency and acute obstruction. Bladder stones are often radiolucent (i.e. uric acid stones) and may be found incidentally at cystoscopy or seen on CT or IVP as filling defects. While stones are usually fragmented and removed cystoscopically using a variety of intracorporeal lithotripsy modalities, treatment of infection and underlying obstruction is critical to avoid of recurrence.

The urethral syndrome

While uncommon, most urologists have a small number of female patients in their practice who complain of chronic urethral discomfort and dysuria with no apparent infectious or inflammatory aetiology. Bladder, vaginal, and urethral cultures are all negative and a strong emotional component may exist. Some reviewers consider it a variant of interstitial cystitis.[24] Rarely is there evidence to support an actual obstruction, despite patients' frequent complaints of difficulty voiding.[25] Spasm in the pelvic floor has been suggested but also not proven.[26] Lack of a supportive history or characteristic bladder appearance at hydrodistention makes interstitial cystitis unlikely. Invariably patients have received numerous prescriptions of antibiotics with little or inconsistent results. A period of antibiotic suppression with low-dose sulfa, quinolone, or nitrofurantion preparations should minimize the risk of bacterial infections as an aetiology for future reference. Symptomatic relief may be achieved with NSAIDs, muscle relaxants, or tricyclic antidepressants with variable results. While there is no scientific evidence to support it, dilatation of the urethra in females with urethral syndrome produces months or even years of symptomatic relief in some patients.

Penile pain

Isolated pain in the penis is rare and usually associated with priapism, disease of the glans and prepuce, Peyronie's disease, or genital herpes.[27]

Priapism from self-injection of vasoactive drugs in the penis for impotence is the most common cause of penile pain. If the erection persists beyond 6 hours pain develops, and without prompt detumescence permanent damage to the corporeal erectile tissues may result. Aspiration of the corpora and irrigation with vasoconstrictors reverses priapism in most cases; however, surgical shunting is occasionally required if conservative measures fail.

Peyronie's disease consists of a fibrous plaque between the erectile bodies of the penile shaft and is seen in as many as 1% of adult males.[28] Typical presenting complaints are penile pain and curvature (i.e. most commonly dorsal) and, less commonly, new onset of erectile dysfunction. Aetiology is a fracture of the tunica albuginea or of a communicating vessel between the corpora leading to a localized haematoma; as the injury resolves, it is replaced by fibrous scar tissue, rendering that portion of the corpora inelastic; hence the penis shortens and points to the side of the lesion as the rest of the penis expands with tumescence. Patients are treated conservatively, as pain often diminishes within 6 months and up to 25% will go on to resolution of the plaque and reduction of curvature within 2 years. A multitude of topical, oral, and injectable treatments have been tried for treatment of Peyronie's disease, mostly with anecdotal and disappointing results. Vitamin E is commonly recommended at dose of 800–1200 IU per day in divided doses due to its safety and low cost; however, no good clinical data support its use. Significant deformity and sexual dysfunction beyond 1 year may require a penile straightening procedure, either plaque excision with grafting or plication of the tunica opposite the lesion. Both are successful in straightening, but carry the risk of worsening erectile dysfunction. If significant erectile dysfunction accompanies Peyronie's disease, fracture of the plaque and insertion of a penile prosthesis is a practical alternative. Reports on the use of shock wave lithotripsy in Peyronie's disease are emerging with improvements in pain and curvature as high as 64%.[29]

Occasionally, men will describe pain and bleeding on erection or retraction of the foreskin as a result of a tight ventral frenulum; incision of the frenulum (i.e. frenuloplasty) is curative. Recurrent fungal infections of the glans and prepuce can lead to cracking, bleeding, and scarring of the foreskin (i.e. phimosis). In the early stages this can be managed with topical antifungal preparations and optimal glucose control, if diabetic. Recalcitrant cases require circumcision.

Genital herpes is of concern due to a recent rapid rise in prevalence and ease of transmission. The virus can be passed to the fetus at birth with severe consequences, and is increasingly associated with cervical cancer. Herpes is ten times more common than other sexually transmitted diseases and men present with painful lesions on the penis after a 2–7 day incubation period. Dysuria from associated urethritis is seen in roughly half of men and most women. Urinary retention occurs in approximately 1% of patients, sometimes requiring weeks of catheter drainage or clean intermittent catheterization.[30] Treatment with oral acyclovir or one of its analogues shortens the duration and severity of subsequent outbreaks if treatment is begun at the very first sign of symptoms. Given the permanent residence of the virus in the host, counselling of patients regarding disease transmission is important.

Referred pain to the penis can result from inflammation of the prostate or bladder neck, and occasionally from a ureteric calculus stuck at the ureterovesical junction. A tender prostate, haematuria, or history of stone disease should prompt further evaluation.

Orchalgia and epididymalgia

The incidence and prevalence of orchalgia (i.e. pain in the testicle) and/or epididymalgia (i.e. pain in the epididymis) are unknown, but most affected men are in their mid to late thirties.[31] It can be one of the most difficult and frustrating symptoms to evaluate. Anxiety, frustration, and emotion are likely to be evident. Testicular and/or epididymal pain can have a profound impact on quality of life, relationships, and sexual function. Patients often have encyclopaedic knowledge and copious notes describing their pain from day to day. They may have been evaluated in a superficial manner by prior physicians. The patient must be made to feel that their case will be heard and leave with definite conclusions as to management.

Pain may be chronic or intermittent and may radiate to the perineum, inguinal canals and abdomen, suprapubic area, legs, or back. Pain on ejaculation may be experienced in the testes/epididymis or deep in the perineum or rectum. Patients may become obsessed with their pain and make things worse by frequent self-examination (i.e. self-palpation orchitis).[32] The delicate epididymis will often respond favourably to a physician-ordered reprieve.

A thorough history and physical examination must include a digital rectal exam, as many patients will be found to have a tender prostate indicating one of the prostatic syndromes is present and referring pain to the testis. If not already employed at this point, a full treatment course of antibiotics and anti-inflammatories should be prescribed. A scrotal support may or may not help. Other causes of referred pain to the testes include muscle strain, back pain, or prior surgery such as appendectomy or hernia repair. Sadly, no clear cause of pain is found in at least 25% of people who experience this. If it is severe, epididymectomy or even orchiectomy may be necessary.

Testicular torsion

Testicular torsion refers to twisting of the testicle on its cord, strangulating the blood supply and leading to pain, oedema, and later infarction. Most cases occur around puberty, when the testicles increase in size and may have a more transverse lie making them more prone to rotation. Patients frequently recall prior episodes of pain that resolved as suddenly as they occurred. Pain is sudden in onset, like being kicked or shot in the scrotum. Patients are in severe pain and on exam the affected, swollen testis sits higher in the scrotum due to shortening of the twisted cord.

Testicular torsion is one of the few true urological emergencies, and immediate action is necessary if the testis is to be salvaged. While the typical history and physical exam are enough to warrant immediate surgical exploration, if the diagnosis is in any doubt a Doppler ultrasound or nuclear flow study confirms the diagnosis by revealing reduced blood flow to the testis. Surgical detorsion and bilateral orchidopexy are performed, although though orchiectomy is occasionally required if the testis is not viable. Concerns that an infarcted testis might liberate antigens leading to the later development of antisperm antibodies and reduced fertility have not been substantiated; the testis is simply removed if it appears to be non-viable.[33]

Torsion of testicular appendages

The appendix testis and appendix epididymis are two of the vestigial structures of the testis that may undergo torsion. These small structures cause milder pain that gradually worsens and the patient often doesn't present for several days after onset. The 'blue dot sign' refers to the torted swollen appendage visible through the scrotal skin. Given the later presentation there is often swelling of the hemiscrotum obscuring detail on physical exam and reducing the value of the Doppler scan or nuclear study. The urologist may have no option but surgical exploration, to rule out testicular torsion. If the history is suggestive and the testis is in a normal lie patients require nothing but supportive care. Symptoms resolve completely in several weeks. The torted appendage will infarct, calcify, and float about the scrotum as a 'scrotal mouse'.

Varicocoele

A varicocoele refers to a cluster of dilated branches of the internal spermatic vein atop the testicle and extending up the spermatic cord, mostly affecting the left testicle. While usually asymptomatic, some patients will present with a dull, achy pain or heavy sensation on the affected side. The presumed aetiology is a failure of the venous valves allowing blood pooling in the dependent scrotum; distention is more often seen after standing or strenuous activity. The varicocoele is typically least noticeable after a period of recumbency. The presence of a varicocoele is sometimes associated with infertility. Proposed mechanisms include increased testicular temperature and alterations in hormone metabolism. Varicocoeles are usually repaired in teenagers and young adults to avoid later impaired fertility but varicocoeles are seen in men with perfectly normal fertility. Given the high prevalence of both varicocoele and non-specific orchalgia, one must take a careful history to ensure the reported testicular pain is specifically related to the varicocoele—evidence of worsening pain during strenuous activity correlating with the varix being noticeably enlarged. Surgical ligation or obliteration of the dilated venous branches by a variety of open, laparoscopic, and percutaneous approaches often succeeds in eliminating the pain, though the dilated venous plexus may not completely return to normal size.[35]

Hydrocoele

Hydrocoele refers to a scrotal swelling from an accumulation of fluid within the tunica vaginalis. In the adult, hydrocoeles are usually idiopathic but may result from testicular trauma, infection, or tumour; in severe ascites, communicating hydrocoeles may develop. The normal cycle of production and resorption goes awry, and fluid builds up in the elastic scrotum. Hydrocoeles usually enlarge slowly and become uncomfortable due to their sheer size or from stretching of the scrotal wall. Symptoms such as heaviness and aching are described and acute pain is uncommon.

The hydrocoele transilluminates easily; however, scrotal ultrasound is often necessary to image the impalpable testis and rule out malignancy. If symptomatic, aspiration is to be avoided due to the risk of bleeding and infection with significant morbidity as well as the high recurrence rate. Men with orchalgia and a small hydrocoele are cautioned that their symptoms may not be relieved by surgical correction of the swelling. Surgical correction of a hydrocoele should only be considered if significant discomfort exists, as even minor surgery to the scrotum all too frequently results in several weeks of post-operative bruising and discomfort. A figure-of-eight pressure dressing for 48 hours may dramatically reduce this complication.

Post-vasectomy pain

While only 1 in 100 men will experience significant discomfort post-vasectomy, patients need to be cautioned about this serious complication of an otherwise simple out-patient procedure.[36] After vasectomy, the testes continue to produce sperm and can demonstrate painful distention of the epididymes. Conservative measures of heat, NSAIDs, tight-fitting underwear, and time are adequate for most. Problems arise when pain persists beyond 6 months. Reoperation for chronic pain should only be with a clear indication and an implicit understanding that the pain may persist after surgery. As many as 30–90% of patients have been reported to have persistent pain following epididymectomy.[37, 38] Orchiectomy carries the risk of recurrent pain on the opposite side. The clinical presentation of post-vasectomy pain is far from clear, and many men have minimal findings on examination. Inguinal neuralgia has been proposed as a cause of such chronic pain.[39]

Sperm granuloma

A variant of post-vasectomy pain, a sperm granuloma presents as a palpable swelling at the site of vas ligation; most are asymptomatic. If pain clearly arises from the lesion and swelling persists beyond 6 months, reoperation and wide excision can be expected to provide relief of symptoms.

Chronic epididymitis

Patients described as suffering from chronic epididymitis complain of pain, swelling, and tenderness in the epididymis. Semen cultures are unreliable. The clinician should be on the alert for obstructive symptoms from benign prostatic hyperplasia or stricture which might identify a reversible factor. Epididymitis, is by definition, an ascending infection from the bladder or prostate, and occurence is less likely following vasectomy. True bacterial epididymitis responds to appropriate antibiotic therapy such as a sulfonamide or quinolone for a minimum of 6 weeks. Patients are cautioned that symptoms may require many weeks to resolve. In reality, the clinical picture of most patients fails to meet criteria of a true infectious disease, and the lack of response to antibiotics is no coincidence. A tender prostate would mandate a full therapeutic antibiotic trial to rule out a bacterial prostatitis syndrome. Patients simply describing tenderness in the epididymis with no clear infectious cause and lack of response to an antibiotic trial are better labelled as suffering from epididymalgia.

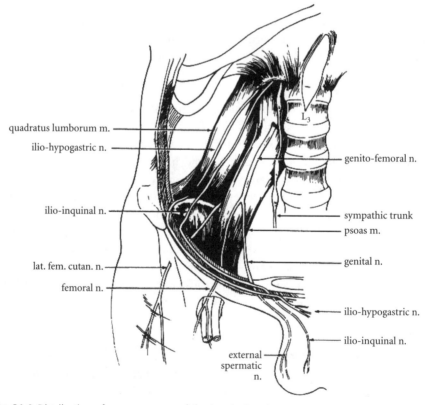

Fig. 21.4 Distribution of sensory nerves of the inguinal region.

Benign non-specific orchalgia

Chronic orchalgia is defined as chronic scrotal pain, unilateral or bilateral, of at least 3 months' duration.[31] This diagnosis of exclusion is made once all other aetiologies have been ruled out, and no other cause of referred pain to the testes can be found. Scrotal ultrasound is of little value if the testes can be easily palpated. Many patients have seen numerous physicians prior to referral. Treatment with input from specialists in chronic pain is invaluable. Diagnostic local anaesthetic nerve blocks and neurectomy, when indicated, can offer these patients real hope of permanent relief from their pain.

Persistent pain and burning sensations caused by irritation of the ilioinguinal and genitofemoral nerves is a common cause of referred pain to the scrotum and testes. Nerve irritation or entrapment can occur following hernia repair, appendectomy, blunt trauma, vasectomy, or seemingly innocuous muscle strain involving the inguinal canal. Such referred pain is seen in roughly 1% of all hernia repairs.[40] An absolute cause of pain may never be found. Figure 21.4 outlines the neuroanatomy of the inguinal canal and genital region and Fig. 21.5 illustrates the dermatomes of the individual nerves

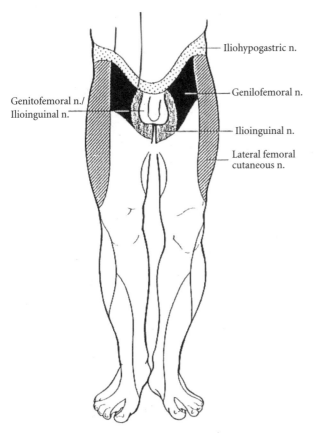

Iliohypogastric n.

Genilofemoral n.

Genitofemoral n./
Ilioinguinal n.

Ilioinguinal n.

Lateral femoral
cutaneous n.

Fig. 21.5 Peripheral nerves of the inguinal region.

supplying the area. Physical exam may reveal a normal testis tender to manipulation or to traction of the spermatic cord. Trigger points are commonly found at some point along the inguinal canal, suggesting neuralgia at that level.

After time and conservative measures have failed, patients undergo a diagnostic local anaesthetic block (e.g. 0.5% bupivicaine without epinephrine) at the site of point tenderness along the canal, or as a spermatic cord block. Anaesthetists may also employ lumbar paravertebral blocks. The patient is seen several weeks later and the response to block noted as well associated numbness. Some patients will experience prolonged relief from such blocks and they can be repeated as necessary; adding a steroid to the local anaesthetic often provides longer-term improvement. Rarely, a neurectomy is indicated and patients must be willing to trade numbness for their pain. Neurectomy is a simple low-risk procedure with a 70% success rate in genitofemoral and 90% success rate in ilioinguinal neuralgia, respectively. Results are admittedly less dramatic in patients with obvious testicular pathology such as sperm granuloma or chronic epididymitis, when surgical excision of the pathology will have higher yield. Developing an algorithm of diagnostic blocks and neurectomy when indicated will offer these patients real hope for relief from their pain. Specialists in pain have much to offer in the management of such patients, and results can be very rewarding.

Conclusions

There are a variety of benign genitourinary conditions which can occur and cause significant pain and impaired function and quality of life; some are self-limited and some are chronic and debilitating; many have significant psychological overtones and impact due to fear and frustration. A clear understanding of the nature of these problems and referral to a urologist or specialist in pain management by the health-care professional can often provide significant improvement.

References

1 Rosenquist R (2003). Evaluation of the pain patient: history, physical examination and diagnostic testing. *American Society of Anesthesiologists Annual Meeting Abstracts*, section 172.

2 Uribarri J, Carrol HJ (1989). The first kidney stone. *Ann. Intern. Med.* 111: 1006–9.

3 Giamberardino MA, de Bigontina P, Martegiani C, Vecchiet L (1994). Effects of shock wave lithotripsy on referred hyperalgesia from renal/ureteral calculosis. *Pain* 56: 77–83.

4 Press SM, Smith AD (1995). Presence of negative hematuria in patients with acute urinary lithiasis presenting to the emergency room with flank pain. *Urology* 45: 753–7.

5 Smith RC, Rosenfield AT, Choe KA, Essenmacher KR, Verga M, Glickman MG *et al.* (1995). Acute flank pain: comparison of non-contract-enhanced CT and intravenous urography. *Radiology* 194: 789–94.

6 Peters HJ, Eckstein W (1975). Possible pharmacological means of treating renal colic. *Urol. Res.* 3: 55–9.

7 Jones DA, Atherton JC, O'Reilly PH, Barnard RJ, George NJ (1989). Assessment of the nephron segments involved in post-obstructive diuresis in man, using lithium clearance. *Br. J. Urol.* 64(6): 559–63.

8 Brown T, Mandell J, Lebowitz RL (1987). Neonatal hydronephrosis in the era of ultrasonography. *Am. J. Roentgenol.* **148**: 959–63.

9 Williams DI, Kenawi MM (1976). The prognosis of pelviureteric obstruction in childhood: a review of 190 cases. *Eur. Urol.* **2**: 57–63.

10 Dunn MD, Portis AJ, Naughton CK, Shalhav A, McDougall EM, Clayman RV (2001). Laparoscopic marsupialization in patients with autosomal dominant polycystic kidney disease. *J. Urol.* **165**: 1888–92.

11 Bokenkamp A, von Kries R, Nowak-Gottl U, Gobel U, Hoyer PF (2000). Neonatal renal vein thrombosis in Germany between 1992 and 1994: epidemiology, treatment and outcome. *Eur. J. Pediatr.* **159**: 44–8.

12 Hamilton G (1996). Fibrinolytic therapy in renovascular disease. In: *Renal Vasular Disease* (ed. A Novick, J Scoble, G Hamilton), pp. 417–30. W. B. Saunders, Philadelphia, PA.

13 Little PJ, Sloper JS, de Wardener HE (1967). A syndrome of loin pain and hematuria associated with disease of peripheral renal arteries. *Q. J. Med.* **36**: 253–9.

14 Lipsky BA (1989). Urinary tract infections in men. *Ann. Intern. Med.* **110**: 138–50.

15 De la Rosette JJMCH, Hubregste MR, Karhaus HFM, Debruyne FMJ (1992). Results of a questionnaire among Dutch urologists and general practitioners concerning diagnosis and treatment of patients with prostatitis syndrome. *Eur. J. Urol.* **22**: 14–19.

16 McGuire EJ, Shi-Chun Z, Horwinski ER, Lytton B (1983). Treatment of motor and sensory detrusor instability by electrical stimulation. *J. Urol.* **129**: 78–9.

17 Stoller ML (????). Afferent nerve stimulation for pelvic floor dysfunction. In: *Campbell's Urology*, 8th edn, Vol. 2 (ed. PC Walsh, AB Retik, ED Vaughan, AJ Wein), pp. 1085–6. W. B. Saunders, Philadelphia, PA.

18 Govier FE, Litwiller S, Nitti V, Kreder KJ Jr, Rosenblatt P (2001). Percutaneous afferent neuromodulation: results of a multicenter study. *J. Urol.* **165**: 1193–8.

19 Oravisto KJ (1975). Epidemiology of interstitial cystitis. *Ann. Chir. Gynaecol. Fenn.* **64**: 75–7.

20 Greenlee RT, Murray T, Bolden S, Wings PA (2000). Cancer statistics 2000. *CA-Cancer J. Clin.* **50**: 7.

21 Mufson MA, Belshe RB, Horrigan TJ, Zollar LM (1973). Causes of acute hemorrhagic cystitis in children. *Am. J. Dis. Child.* **126**: 605–9.

22 Schwartz BF, Stoller ML (2000). The vesical calculus. *Urol. Clin. North Am.* **27**(2): 333–46.

23 Charlton CAC (1986). Historical review: confusions in definition. In: *Sensory Disorders of the Bladder and Urethra* (ed. NJR George, JA Gosling), pp. 81–3. Springer, Berlin.

24 Hanno PM (1995). Interstitial cystitis and the female urethral syndrome. In: *Clinical Urological Practise* (ed. BS Stein), pp. 611–22. W. W. Norton: New York.

25 Mabry EW, Carson CC, Older RA (1981). Evaluation of women with chronic voiding voiding discomfort. *Urology* **18**: 244–6.

26 Raz S, Smith RB (1976). External sphincter spasticity syndrome in female patients. *J. Urol.* **115**: 443–6.

27 Gee WF, Ansell JS, Bonica JJ (1990). Pelvic and pereineal pain of urologic origin. In: *The Management of Pain*, Vol. 2 (ed. JJ Bonica), pp. 1368–94. Lea and Febiger, Philadelphia, PA.

28 Carson CC, Jordan GH, Gelbard MK (1999). Peyronie's disease: new concepts in etiology, diagnosis and management. *Contemp. Urol.* **11**: 44–64.

29 Manikandan R, Islam W, Srinivasan V, Evans CM (2002). Evaluation of extracorporeal shock wave lithotripsy in peyronie's disease. *Urology* **60**(5): 795–800.

30 Corey L, Benedetti J, Critchlow C, Mertz G, Douglas J, Fife K *et al.* (1983). Treatment of primary first episode genital herpes simplex virus infections with acyclovir: results of topical, intravenous and oral therapy. *J. Antimicrob. Chemother.* **12**(Suppl. B): 79–88.

31 Davis BE, Noble MJ, Weigel JW, Foret J, Mebust WK (1990). Analysis and management of chronic testicular pain. *J. Urol.* **143**: 936–9.

32 Schneiderman H, Voytovich A (1988). Self palpation orchitis. *J. Gen. Intern. Med.* **3**: 97.

34 Anderson MJ, Dunn JK, Lipshultz LI, Coburn M (1992). Semen quality and endocrine parameters after acute testicular torsion. *J. Urol.* **147**: 1545–50.

35 Peterson AC, Lance RS, Ruiz HE (1998). Outcomes of varicocoele ligation done for pain. *J. Urol.* **159**: 1565–7.

36 McConaghy P, Paxton LD, Loughlin V (1996). Chronic testicular pain following vasectomy. *Br. J. Urol.* **77**: 328.

37 Selikowitz AM, Schned AR (1985). A late post-vasectomy syndrome. *J. Urol.* **134**: 923–36.

38 Padmore DE, Norman RW, Millard OH (1996). Analysis of indications for and outcomes of epididymectomy. *J. Urol.* **156**: 95–6.

39 Yeates WK (1985). Pain in the scrotum. *Br. J. Hosp. Med.* **33**: 101–4.

40 Starling JR, Harms, BA (1989). Diagnosis and treatment of genitofemoral and ilioingional neuralgia. *World J. Surg.* **13**: 586–91.

Further reading

Books

American Society of Anesthesiologists Annual Meeting Refresher Course Lectures; Pain Management, sections 132–172. (2003). American Society of Anaesthesiologists. Parkridge, Illinois.

Decker BC (1990). *Decision Making in Urology*. CV Mosby, St. Louis.

Genitourinary pain. In: *Textbook of Pain*, pp. 689–709. Churchill Livngstone.

Apkarian AV, Ayrapetian S (1997). *Pain Mechanisms and Management*. F. A. Davis, Philadelphia.

Walsh PC, Retik AB, Vaughan ED, Wein AJ (eds) (2002). *Campbell's Urology*, 8th edn. W. B. Saunders, Philadelphia, PA.

Journal articles

Choi PD, Nath R, MacKinon SE (1996). Iatrogenic injury to the ilioinguinal and iliohypogastric nerves in the groin: a case report, diagnosis, and management. *Ann. Plastic Surg.* **37**(1): 60–5.

Hahn L (1989). Clinical findings and results of operative treatment in ilioingiunal nerve entrapment syndrome. *Br. J. Obstet. Gynaecol.* **96**: 1080–3.

Knockaert DC, D'Heygere FG, Bobbaers HJ (1989). Ilioinguinal nerve entrapment: a little known cause of iliac fossa pain. *Postgrad. Med. J.* **65**: 632–5.

Martyn P (2004). Update on chronic pelvic pain. *Can. J. Diagn.* January 2004: 57–60 (available at www.stacommunications.com/journals/pdfs/2004/diagnosis/DXpdfjan04/womenshealth-pelvicpain..pdf).

Melville K, Schultz EA, Dougherty JM (1990). Ilioinguinal-iliohypogastric nerve entrapment. *Ann. Emergency Med.* **19**(8): 925–9.

Miyazaki F, Shook G (1992). Ilioinguinal nerve entrapment during needle suspension for stress incontinence. *Obstet. Gynecol.* **80**(2): 246–8.

Chapter 22

The patient presenting with malignant genitourinary pain

Florian Heid and Jürgen Jage

Introduction

Supportive care aims to maintain or improve a patient's level of comfort and function. In attempting to achieve these goals, health-care professionals may be confronted with one of the most challenging tasks—mitigation and therapy of malignant pain. In contrast to more or less defined acute pain syndromes (e.g. renal colic, post-operative status), malignant pain syndromes are usually more complex and require tailoring of therapy to the individual patient. To perform this task well, a fundamental understanding of the symptoms is necessary. This chapter will describe the basic pathophysiology of pain, highlight the importance of pain measurement and documentation, and illustrate the decision-making process in choosing the proper therapeutic approach from among a variety of analgesic methods. Finally, the interdisciplinary approach which is essential for a coordinated treatment plan in these patients will be emphasized by outlining a clinical case. The importance of these tasks for urology patients is outlined by the following:

- 70% of prostate cancer patients suffer from pain,[1]

- 60 to 80% of cancer patients experience significantly reduced quality of life due to pain,[2]

- adequate pharmacotherapy can provide satisfying pain control in 85 to 90% of patients.[3]

Pathophysiology of pain

The perception of pain represents a complex interaction of biological, emotional, and behavioural factors. This section will be limited to the underlying biological mechanisms, while recognizing that psychological factors also play an important role in the management of malignant pain.

Nociceptors are stimulated by neoplastic infiltration or compression. Nociceptors are highly specialized terminal endings of sensory nerve fibres and are found in skin tissue, muscles, connective tissue, bones, and joints (i.e. somatic nociceptors), as well as in organs (i.e. visceral nociceptors).[4,5] Primary nociceptive impulses are transmitted via A delta and C fibres from the periphery to the dorsal horn of the spinal cord where the first synapses occur. Persistent inflammation, destruction, or compression can cause nociceptor activation and regional hyperalgesia. The primary nociceptors enter the dorsal horn of the spinal cord via interspinal nerve roots, which are susceptible to blockade with epidural and spinal local anaesthetics at their site of entry (i.e. dorsal root entry zone).

The dorsal horn interneurons are modulated via descending efferent impulses from the cerebral cortex and other higher centres in the brain. It is here that spinal opioids, alpha-adrenergic agents, N-methyl-D-aspartate antagonists (NMDA), and some non-steroidal anti-inflammatory drugs (NSAIDs) have their modulating effects on the transmission of pain. From the dorsal horn, secondary neurons decussate across the midline and ascend via the medial and lateral spinothalamic tracts to the thalamus. From the thalamus, nociceptive information is transmitted to the cerebral cortex. Inhibitory or excitatory impulse processing occurs at each level in this pain pathway.

At the level of the cerebral cortex, pain can be specified with respect to location, intensity, and character (e.g. burning, twinging, twitching, and oppressive). Pain generates spinal reflexes that increase the fasciated muscle tone and, in a similar fashion, the smooth muscle tone. Strong pain increases sympathetic tone resulting in tachycardia and arterial hypertension. Other pain-related vegetative symptoms, such as nausea and vomiting, may be observed. Depression, anxiety, insomnia, and irritability affect mood and behaviour.[6]

These biological mechanisms do not show a clearly defined stimulus–response correlation. Tissue traumatized from neoplastic infiltration, radiation, or surgical intervention liberates peripheral mediators of inflammation such as bradykinins, prostaglandins, and cytokines. These molecules decrease the specific threshold of the nociceptor neuron.[7] Consequently, the flow of afferent impulses to the spinal cord is intensified, thus causing a *primary hyperalgesia*. For example, painful stimuli in the area of the nociceptor will be perceived more intensely than under normal circumstances.[8] Anti-inflammatory agents such as NSAIDs exert their analgesic effects at this peripheral site and in parts of the central nervous system (CNS).

In addition to this 'protective' function, a prolonged state of increased afferent flow causes changes in the CNS. There is evidence that different mechanisms including increased Ca^{2+} release and increased expression of excitatory NMDA receptors, as well as immediate-early gene expression, contribute to these alterations. The result is summarized as the *sensitization of the spinal cord* which causes a lower threshold for switching the peripheral stimulus to the second neuron in the dorsal horn.[7] Electroencephalographic traces reveal amplified impulses, even after extinction of the noxious stimulus. This extension of pain with respect to *time* is referred to as *long-term potentiation*[9] reflecting part of the *pain memory*. Moreover, the receptive area of the spinal neuron becomes enlarged, so that pain is perceived in non-traumatized, lesion-associated regions. This extension of pain in respect to *place* is termed *secondary hyperalgesia* and contributes to the patient's *pain memory*. Thus, long-term potentiation and hyperalgesia reflect the plasticity of the central nervous system. As a result of peripheral and central plasticity, pain becomes more difficult to treat; this represents one of the reasons for the poor treatment success of malignant pain;[10] however, psychological factors also play an important role.[11]

Pain caused by bone metastases is *nociceptive pain*, but can become complicated with *neuropathic pain*, if the tumour invades or compresses a nerve, neural plexus, or the spinal cord. Both, intense *nociceptive* and *neuropathic* afferent stimulation may induce spinal cord sensitization. Combinations of nociceptive and neuropathic pain are common. In a large population of patients with different types of cancer, one-third of patients with tumour-related pain were affected with neuropathic pain components.[12] Although there are no exact data, this probably applies to urological cancer pain as well. Diagnosis of neuropathic pain is important, because it leads to therapeutic consequences regarding the choice of analgesic technique. This needs to be made as an active and accurate diagnosis, not simply as diagnosis of exclusion when interventions seem ineffective.

Neuropathic pain frequently has a constant burning character. Further sensory disturbances might occur and include paraesthesia, tingling, allodynia, hyperalgesia, and intense lancing pain that radiates into the area of the affected peripheral nerve or root. Some patients with neuropathic pain from tumour compression of a nerve or nerve plexus will present with escalating pain requiring increased opioid doses, sometimes several-fold over a few days. The efficacy of opioids is diminished as neuropathic pain progresses and in patients with a high degree of spinal sensitization, hence additional co-analgesics are necessary.[13] At this point, consultation with a specialist in pain management is often helpful. Malignant neuropathic pain syndromes are some of the most challenging cases to confront the pain management team. Therefore, recognition of the syndrome is of principal importance.[14,15]

The impaired activity of patients suffering from severe neuropathic pain represents an enormous strain. Psychiatric alterations frequently occur and specific therapeutic intervention is required often because neuropathic pain is difficult to describe. The WHO recommends a stepwise protocol for the treatment of malignant pain syndromes. This also applies to neoplastic bone pain with neuropathic components in urological patients. Non-opioid co-analgesics are essential. In addition they can improve opioid efficacy in antinociceptive therapy.[16] Bisphosphonates are helpful in stabilizing bone metabolism. Epidural and intrathecal opioids are sometimes useful in the management of malignant pain from metastases.

Nerve destruction by intrathecal or epidural phenol may be useful in selected patients and has the advantage of long-term benefit from a single injection. The risks of spinal neurolytic blocks include loss of motor and sensory function of the extremities, loss of bowel and bladder function, and, in patients with a longer prognosis, severe neural regrowth pain. Clear weighting of the risk/benefit ratio must be done for each individual patient by a physician experienced in these techniques and after discussion with the patient and family. The procedure warrants consideration in some circumstances such as poorly controlled malignant pain in a patient who is confined to bed, has already lost bowel and bladder function, and may not lose any more function by undergoing a peri-spinal neurolytic block.

Goal of pain therapy

The main goal of malignant pain therapy is to provide pain relief for the individual patient with only minimal side-effects. Individual responsiveness to opioids and other agents is a widely variable parameter. In order to improve or at least maintain the patient's quality of life (QOL), balancing of the therapeutic benefit and adverse effects (e.g. dizziness, nausea/vomiting, or cognitive impairment) is important. Well-proven and helpful instruments to measure the effect and make these fundamental goals objective are the Short-Form 36 (SF-36),[17] the Brief Fatigue Inventory (BFI),[18] the Schedule for the Evaluation of Individual QOL-Direct Weighting (SEIQOL-DW),[19] and the Brief Pain Inventory (BPI).[20] In contrast to traditional, mainly functional 'health-related' scales these also focus on the subjective impression (e.g. satisfaction level concerning family, sport, cultural life, or profession). Working with these scales can sometimes be very time-consuming. Thus, simple but effective strategies for improving analgesia for malignant pain syndromes are outlined below (see Fig. 22.1):

1 Interviewing the patient using a numeric assessment Numeric Rating Scale (NRS, 0 = no pain, 10 = unbearable pain).

2 Interviewing the patient using a visual assessment with a Visual Analogue Scale (VAS, 0 = no pain, 10 = unbearable pain).

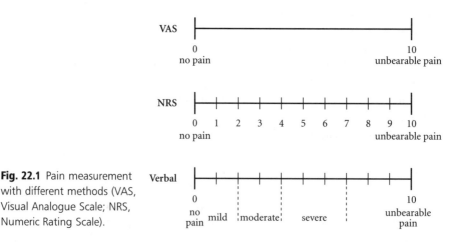

Fig. 22.1 Pain measurement with different methods (VAS, Visual Analogue Scale; NRS, Numeric Rating Scale).

3 Interviewing the patient using verbal assessment correlated to the VAS as follows:

'mild pain' → VAS 1–2

'moderate pain' → VAS 3–4

'severe pain' → VAS 5–7

'unbearable pain' → VAS 8–10.

4 If the patient is not able to answer to any of the above-listed possibilities, the following can be tried: 'Is your pain therapy sufficient?' Yes or No.

5 Given the difficulty of describing pain, it may be worthwhile using the question: 'Are you 100% comfortable around the clock?'

Pain measurement and documentation

Pain is a subjective symptom and every patient has their own individual sense and expression of it. Therefore, the individual patient remains the best resource for pain measurement, self-assessing his or her pain intensity which should be specifically elicited during ward rounds or in the office setting. Placing a numerical score on the intensity allows physicians and nurses to communicate with patients about their pain and to judge the efficacy of analgesic therapies. Keeping a patient pain diary provides even more detailed information, helps detect therapeutic deficits, and simplifies therapeutic adjustments. Using one of these strategies, the nursing staff on the ward should routinely measure and chart the pain intensity once or twice per shift. As long as pain requires treatment, measurment of pain intensity must be continued. Most importantly, the physician must constantly review the data and adjust the analgesic therapy accordingly. Criteria of success include the following:

◆ Sufficient pain therapy:

pain level less than or equal to 3 (at rest),

pain level less than or equal to 5 (dynamic pain, e.g. coughing or ambulation),

patient is satisfied with pain therapy.

◆ Insufficient pain therapy:

pain levels greater than or equal to 4 (at rest),

pain level greater than or equal to 6 (dynamic pain, e.g. coughing or ambulation),

patient perceives pain control to be unsatisfactory.

Documentation of pain scores plays a key role in adequate and timely treatment. Pain scores are documented in a patient's chart (clinical setting) and/or in a patient's pain diary (out-patients). During ward rounds or the out-patient visits pain scores should always be interpreted and, if required, the pain therapy adjusted.

Analgesic methods

It is reasonable to combine substances with different pharmacological mechanisms during treatment of pain, regardless of it being benign or malignant in origin. This concept aims to inhibit nociception at different locations in the pain pathway using structurally different agents (e.g. NSAIDs, opioids, co-analgesics, and local anaesthetics). An added benefit is the ability to keep dosages of the individual medications as low as possible and decrease the incidence of adverse effects. In addition, synergistic or at least additive effects of analgesic combinations can provide more effective analgesia than a single agent alone. Referring to this knowledge, the WHO recommends treating malignant pain by means of a stepwise therapy for nociceptive pain (Fig. 22.2).

Basic analgesic medications

Information regarding common medications used in pain therapy is listed below under the headings indication (I), pharmacological mechanism (P), dosage (D), adverse effects (A), contraindications (C), and recommended (R) or not recommended (N) combinations.

Non-opioids

Acetaminophen Acetaminophen is a suitable basic analgesic with almost no adverse effects but it is less effective than NSAIDs. Therefore, combination with other agents is preferable. It can be used as an alternative if NSAIDs are not indicated. Acetaminophen has opioid-saving potency with added benefit even when patients are on opioids and NSAIDs.

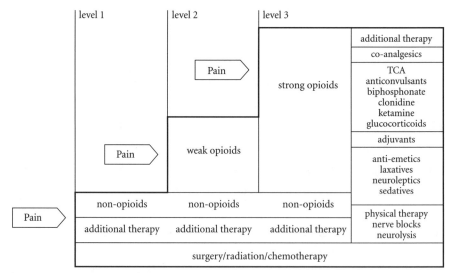

Fig. 22.2 Stepwise concept for cancer pain.

I: Somatic pain.

P: Central antinociceptive by stimulating inhibitory parts of the spinal cord.

D: 1000 mg every 4–6 hours oral/rectal/intravenous; maximum dosage 60–80 mg/kg/ 24 hours (adult: 4–6 g/24 hours).

A: Hepatic or renal impairment if dosage is exceeded.

R: NSAIDs, opioids.

Non-steroidal anti-inflammatory drugs (NSAIDs)

I: Somatic pain.

P: Peripheral effect by inhibition of prostaglandin synthesis and/or release in traumatized tissue (e.g. mixed inhibition of cyclo-oxygenase-1 and -2). Central effect by stimulating inhibitory areas of the spinal cord.

A: Gastrointestinal ulcers, minor and major gastric bleeding, impaired renal function, inhibition of platelet function (e.g. acetylsalicylic acid (ASA) irreversible, other NSAIDs reversible); bronchial obstruction.

C: Gastric or intestinal ulcer, impaired renal function, chronic obstructive pulmonary disease (COPD), potential for bronchoconstriction.

R: Acetaminophen, opioids.

N: Combination of two NSAIDs.

Cyclo-oxygenase-2 (COX-2) inhibitors

I: Somatic pain, in patients where platelet quantity/quality would not allow NSAID use; opioid-saving potency.

P: Peripheral effects by inhibition of prostaglandin synthesis and/or release in traumatized tissue (e.g. effects are limited to COX-2).[21]

D: Celecoxib 400–600 mg/24 hours.

A: Renal impairment.

C: Impaired renal function, increased cardiovascular risk.

R: Opioid.

N: Combination with NSAIDs or combination of two COX-2 inhibitors.

Dipyrone

I: Visceral pain with spasmodic components, colics; alternative if NSAID is contraindicated, opioid-saving potency.[22,23]

P: Central effects by stimulating inhibitory parts of the spinal cord.

D: 1000 mg every 4–6 hours oral/rectal, maximum dosage 60–80 mg/kg/24 hours (adult: 4–6 g/24 hours).

A: Anaphylactic shock after rapid intravenous (IV) injection, agranulocytosis, aplastic anaemia.

C: Severe allergy, leucopenia, and low platelets.

R: Acetaminophen, NSAIDs (either NSAIDs or COX-2 inhibitors), opioids.

Opioids

I: Somatic and visceral pain.

P: Activation of μ and other opioid receptors at different sites of nociceptive transmission; antinociceptive effects by stimulating inhibitory neurons of the spinal cord.

Weak opioids are inferior to strong opioids because they have dosage limits. Above these limits analgesia cannot be increased ('ceiling effect'):

Weak opioids: tramadol

I: Visceral and somatic pain.

P: Weak μ-receptor agonist.

D: 100 mg every 4–6 hours oral/rectal; 100–300 mg every 12 hours oral (i.e. controlled release); IV infusion 20–30 mg/hour; maximum 600 mg/24 hours.

A: Vertigo, nausea, vomiting, sedation, and confusion.

C: Epilepsy, MAO inhibitors, caution in the elderly or patients with reduced constitution, use in combination with other serotonergic medications.

R: Acetaminophen, NSAIDs, and dipyrone.

Weak opiods: codeine, hydrocodone Frequently used in combination with acetaminophen for post-operative analgesia after out-patient surgery and as step 2 of the WHO analgesic ladder. Ten per cent of the Caucasian population do not metabolize codeine to its active metabolites.

Strong opioids Morphine is the reference opioid for acute and chronic cancer pain therapy; however, some European physicians prefer piritramide for acute pain.[23] Hydromorphone is more frequently used in North America. Diamorphine (heroin) is used in the UK to treat post-operative and cancer pain, especially by subcutaneous infusion. Meperidine (i.e. pethidine) has the disadvantage that its major metabolite nor-meperidine (nor-pethidine) accumulates in patients with renal dysfunction and can provoke seizures. In the last decade, the transdermal administration of fentanyl has become popular, mainly in patients with impaired oral uptake, frequent nausea/vomiting, or severe constipation. The individual opioid responsiveness (i.e. relation of analgesic effect versus adverse effects) may vary during long-term therapy. In these cases, switching from one strong opioid to another can significantly improve a patient's analgesia (Tables 22.1, 22.2):[16]

I: Severe visceral and somatic pain.

A: Sedation and CNS depression, ileus, nausea/vomiting, constipation, respiratory depression, urinary retention, and pruritus.

Table 22.1 Classification of strong opioids

Opoid type	Analgesic dosage limit
Pure μ opioid-receptor agonists: morphine, fentanyl, hydromorphone, methadone, oxycodone, piritramide	No
Partial agonist: buprenorphine	Yes
Mixed agonists/antagonists: pentazocin, butorphanol	Yes

Table 22.2 Pharmacological characteristics of equianalgesic strong opioids

Opioid	Dose (mg)[a]		Half-life (h)	Half-life (h)
	Oral	SC/IM		
Morphine	20–30	10	2–3	Immediate-release 2–3 Sustained-release 8–12
Oxycodone	20–30		2–3	Immediate-release 3–4 Sustained-release 8–12
Hydromorphone	7.5(8)	1.5(2)	2–3	Immediate-release 2–3 Sustained-release 8–12
Methadone	20	10	>24	4–12
Fentanyl transdermal	*	**	16–21	48–72

SC, subcutaneous; IM, intramuscular.

[a] When using these values note that because of first-pass hepatic metabolism, the oral dose of each opioid is several times higher than the parenteral dose.

* Relation of morphine p.o. versus fentanyl transdermal is about 100:1 (daily dosage).

** Based on clinical experience, 100 μg/hour fentanyl SC/IM is roughly equianalgesic to morphine 4 mg/hour IV/SC.[14]

C: Caution in the elderly or in patients with reduced physical status; respiratory impairment.

R: Acetaminophen, NSAIDs, and dipyrone.

N: Pure μ agonist with partial agonist (e.g. nalbuphine or butorphanol).

Co-analgesics

Co-analgesics are agents which have proven analgesic efficacy in randomized controlled trials, although their primary indication was not as a pain killer.

Tricyclic antidepressants

Tricyclic antidepressants have anxiolytic, analeptic, or sedative effects. In addition, they have proven analgesic benefits, and are especially useful in the treatment of malignant pain syndromes. They inhibit the reuptake of serotonin and noradrenalin in the synaptic gap, especially of the corticospinal tract inhibitory pathways. The resulting increase of inhibitory transmitters in the antinociceptive tracts induces analgesia. These agents are adjuncts to stepwise therapy, but are never suitable as monotherapy. The most studied agent is amitriptyline and it is the first choice among the variety of agents in this class. When selecting the medication, one must remember that tricyclics differ in regard to their mental side-effects. As a result, analeptic substances should always be administered in the morning and more sedative agents at night.

Amitriptyline (sedative)

I: Neuropathic pain due to nerve infiltration.

P: Central analgesic effect by stimulating antinociceptive tracts.

D: Start with 0–0–10 to 25 mg/24 hrs; increase within 2–3 weeks to full antidepressant dose for optimal analgesic effect.

A: (Over)-sedation, hypotension, cardiac arrhythmias, constipation.

C: Glaucoma, cardiac dysrhythmias of higher degree, cardiac failure, recent myocardial infarction.

R: Opioid, NSAIDs.

Desipramine (analeptic)

I: Neuropathic pain due to nerve infiltration.

P: Central analgesic effect by stimulating antinociceptive tracts.

D: Start with 10–0–0 mg/24 hours; increase within 2–3 weeks to full antidepressant dose for optimal analgesic effect.

A: Hyperactivity, hypotension, cardiac arrhythmias, constipation.

C: Glaucoma, cardiac dysrhythmias of higher degree, cardiac failure, recent myocardial infarction.

R: Opioid, NSAIDs.

Anticonvulsive agents

Patients with neuropathic pain frequently suffer from allodynia (i.e. a normal sensation is perceived as painful) as a sign of secondary mechanical hyperalgesia and from intensive, lancing, pain attacks. From the electrophysiological aspect, these feelings resemble central seizure activity; thus, anticonvulsive agents can play a role in inhibiting them. It is not always possible to mitigate the intensity of pain, but the incidence of pain attacks is frequently decreased making anticonvulsive agents a valuable supplement to the stepwise therapy concept based on opioids.

Carbamazepine and phenytoin have been used for decades. Both activate inhibiting central neurons but carbamazepine also acts peripherally as a sodium-channel blocker to lower spontaneous firing of the affected nerve. Due to a broad spectrum of adverse effects, a new agent has been developed; it is gabapentin (i.e. a synthetic GABA (gamma-aminobutyricacid) analogue). It increases GABA (i.e. the main inhibitory neurotransmitter) production and decreases glutamate production (i.e. the main excitatory neurotransmitter) in the central nervous system and thereby reduces central sensitization. Additionally, gabapentin ligates to Ca^{2+} channels in the dorsal horn which are thought to be associated with effects on hyperalgesia and allodynia.[24] Similar to carbamazepine, ectopic neuronal impulses are suppressed.[25]

Gabapentin

I: Neuropathic pain with lancing pain attacks.

P: Central effect by altering transmitter balance (i.e. GABA↑, Glutamate↓) and ligating to Ca^{2+} channels; peripheral effect by suppressing ectopic activity.

D: First day 100–100–100 mg; second day 200–200–200 mg; third day 300–300–300 mg up to a maximum of 1200–2400 mg/day ; adapt to adverse effects.

A: Sedation, dizziness, rarely nausea, acute confusional states.

C: Acute pancreatitis, dosage reduction in renal impairment.

R: Opioid, NSAIDs.

Carbamazepine

I: Neuropathic pain with lancing pain attacks.

P: Central effect by activating inhibitory neurons; peripheral effect by blocking sodium channels.

D: Start with 100–0–100 mg; increase every week by 100 to 200 mg per day.

A: Sedation, cardiac arrhythmias, hypotension, leucopenia, agranulocytosis.

C: Higher (II, III) atrioventricular block, severe bone marrow impairment, cardiac, hepatic, or renal impairment.

R: Opioid, NSAIDs.

Steroids

Steroids are effective in the treatment of metastatic bone pain and in nociceptive or neuropathic pain by reducing neoplastic compression and lessening perineural oedema. Furthermore, steroids reduce spontaneous impulse rates of affected nerves and may have a central effect leading to improved appetite and mood in cancer patients. In contrast to other co-analgesics, the administration of steroids should be targeted and intermittent; for most patients, therapy lasting a few days to 3 weeks is sufficient.

Dexamethasone

I: Metastatic bone pain, neuropathic or nociceptive pain due to compression.

P: Peripheral: antiphlogistic, anti-oedemic; central: appetizing, mood lifting.

D: Initially 20 to 60(100) mg IV; afterwards 8 to 24 mg oral per day.

A: Adrenal suppression, increased risk for infection and gastric ulcer, osteoporosis, hypertension, glucose intolerance, psychotropic effects.

C: Pre-existing infections, gastric ulcer, diabetes, osteoporoses, thrombosis.

R: Opioid, co-analgesics.

N: NSAIDs.

Bisphosphonates

Neoplasms of the prostate and kidney tend to develop bony metastases. These can cause huge defects in bone tissue, impair mechanical stability, and may lead to spontaneous fractures. They are often responsible for severe pain. By inhibiting the osteoclastic activity, bisphosphonates like pamidronate or ibandronate reduce the liberation of pain mediators. Furthermore, osteoblastic activity is stimulated by bisphosphonates and some osteolytic defects might be repaired.

Pamidronate

I: Metastatic bone pain, severe hypercalcaemia.

P: Inhibition of osteoclasts, stimulation of osteoblasts.

D: 60–90 mg in 500 ml saline, intravenous 100–200 ml/hour every 4 to 6 weeks.

A: Hypocalcaemia.

C: Hypocalcaemia, renal impairment.

R: Opioid, NSAIDs, co-analgesics.

Clonidine and ketamine

These agents are routinely used for anaesthetic purposes but, recently, their analgesic potential has come into focus. Clonidine develops analgesic effects by acting as an agonist at spinal alpha-2 adrenoceptors and by stimulating antinociceptive neurons. Ketamine, a dissaociative anaesthetic, acts as an non-competitive NMDA receptor antagonist. Activated NMDA receptors play a key role in the process of spinal sensitization. Ketamine is especially useful in patients with neuropathic or intense nociceptive pain. Due to a broad spectrum of potential adverse effects both medications should be administered under supervision of a pain specialist in carefully selected patients.

Local anaesthetics

Local anaesthetics are used for diagnostic or therapeutic nerve blocks. Indications include neuropathic pain syndromes which have failed to respond to opioids and co-analgesics. Ropivacaine and bupivacaine are the commonly used substances. All local anaesthetics produce a reversible conduction blockade of impulses along peripheral or central nerve pathways. They prevent impulse transmission by inhibiting passage of sodium ions through sodium channels located in nerve membranes. Due to their high systemic toxicity (e.g. seizures, heart block) accidental intravenous injection of ropivacaine or bupivacaine must be avoided. On the other hand, low-dose infusion of lidocaine shows analgesic effects, especially in neuropathic pain syndromes.[26]

Nerve blocks/regional anaesthesia

This section cannot do justice to the enormous variety of techniques and approaches but will summarize some of the fundamental aspects of nerve blockade and regional anaesthesia. Nerve blocks can sometimes be very effective and keep the patient free of pain for months but they do represent an invasive procedure with possible risks and potentially severe adverse effects. A diagnostic block (i.e. short-acting blockade to determine the effect) always proceeds the therapeutic block (i.e. neurolysis with 90% phenol). Keeping in mind that 85 to 90% of all patients with malignant pain experience sufficient pain relief from adequate systemic pharmacotherapy, nerve blocks should be considered the second choice.

Nerve blocks can be classified as peripheral or central and include blocks targeting the sympathetic system. Peripheral approaches target single nerves or nerve plexi such as the lumbosacral plexus. Central nerve blocks include intrathecal (i.e. spinal) and epidural infusions of local anaesthetics (i.e. diagnostic block) followed by ethanol (i.e. therapeutic block, neurolysis). Since there is potential for respiratory depression and/or haemodynamic instability, these regimens require adequate monitoring during the procedure (Fig. 22.3).

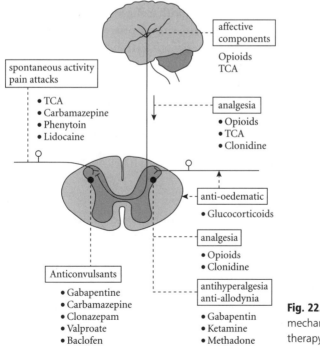

Fig. 22.3 Different mechanisms of analgetic therapy.

Radiotherapy/chemotherapy

Patients with renal neoplasms develop painful spinal metastases in 25 to 50% of cases rising to as many as 80% in those with prostate cancer. Most have disseminated metastases, while only 18% of patients demonstrate a single lesion. As a result, palliation rather than cure is the usual goal. In contrast to curative approaches, potential adverse effects with a longer latency (e.g. fibrosis, ulcers, radiogenic neuropathy) can be accepted in favour of high-dose regimes that lead to faster pain relief. Early adverse effects, such as fatigue or nausea and vomiting, are common, but can be effectively controlled using adjuvant therapy. Chemotherapy in advanced cancer patients follows the same principles concerning dose and adverse effects.

Surgical options

Urogenital tumours frequently cause bony metastasis, especially to the spine, and significant pain and neurological dysfunction often follow. Because radiotherapy sometimes only shows limited effects in controlling the progress of the spinal disease, surgery occasionally becomes an option. Depending on the location and extent of the metastasis, anterior, posterior, or combined approaches are used to perform internal fixation. In selected patients, significant pain relief and preservation of neurological function can be obtained.[27]

Adjuvant therapy, symptom management

One essential aspect in managing the patient with malignant pain is the adequate treatment of adverse symptoms, resulting from cancer progression, radiotherapy and chemotherapy, or other pharmacological agents. Gastrointestinal disturbances, especially nausea and vomiting, frequently occur during chemotherapy, and often impair the patient's quality of life. Opioids negatively affect gastric emptying. Central nervous disturbances such as cognitive impairment, sedation, agitation, and insomnia often require treatment. However, evidence-based symptom management remains difficult because few randomized controlled trials have been published.[15,16]

Patient controlled analgesia (PCA)

Unfortunately, some patients with urological cancer complain of intractable pain unresponsive to well-proved analgesic regimens. In this situation, involvement of the acute pain service and establishment of an intravenous PCA strategy can often help. This technique requires an interdisciplinary team approach and organized supervision to minimize specific adverse effects of administered analgesics.[28,29] The patient controls the degree of pain relief by initiating small intravenous opioid dosages (e.g. morphine 1–2 mg) upon demand by means of a microprocessor-controlled device. Adverse effects such as sedation, nausea/vomiting, ileus, or constipation and urinary retention are possible but not common. The dose-dependant respiratory depression is limited by dose and lock-out schedules. Dosages must be individualized to the age of the patient, previous opioid tolerance, and site and character of the pain syndrome. Requisite for this technique are cooperative alert patients who can learn how to use the PCA device and nursing staff who must monitor respiratory rate and level of consciousness at least every 4 hours.

The worst pain can be treated without undue risks using PCA and the opioid demand of each patient can be quickly and exactly determined by titrating to the individual's response. For hospitals without access to this technology, the principle of titrating opioid doses to VAS pain scores can also be applied by intravenous injection of small doses (e.g. morphine 3 mg) every 5 to 10 minutes without a PCA device.

PCA can also be important in the post-operative management of urology patients with advanced cancer. As a result of their disease progression, drug tolerance, or a combination of both, these patients may already be taking large doses of opioids pre-operatively.[30,31] When they require surgery, post-operative pain control may be a potential problem. For example, consider the prostate cancer patient with spinal metastases who is used to oral opioids but has no bowel movements after anterior internal fixation. He needs opioids, but he cannot swallow, hence, parenteral administration is required. Standard dosage regimens will not accommodate this patient and a background infusion of opioids equivalent to the patient's pre-operative consumption should be instituted to prevent physical withdrawal. In addition, implementation of the PCA technique will help avoid analgesic undersupply because pain levels are now controlled directly by the patient. After restitution of gastrointestinal function, drug administration should be oral. Dose calculation and titration should be done by an experienced pain specialist to prevent adverse events.

Box 22.1 **Clinical case**

This 62-year-old man underwent a radical prostatectomy 2 years earlier for prostate cancer staged as T2, N2, M0. Early rehabilitation was uneventful and the patient lived with his family. However, over the last 2 months he has complained of lower back pain. Initially, it was triggered by ambulation but was managed well by self-medication with NSAIDs; now, the pain has increased and NSAIDs fail to give relief. The acute pain service was consulted and concluded that he had somatic pain localized to the lower spine that was increased by pressure to this area. In addition, there was a constant pain radiating to the right thigh with a lancing quality, aggravated by ambulation. Whereas the pressure-evoked pain was rated 5 on a 0 to 10 NRS, the lancing pain had a much higher intensity of 8 out of 10 and effectively confined the patient to bed. CT of the spine revealed multiple osteoblastic bone metastases in the lumbar region explaining the direct cause for both pain syndromes—the localized *nociceptive pain* due to bone destruction and the lancing

> **Box 22.1** *(continued)*
>
> *neuropathic pain* caused by spinal nerve compression. Initial pain treatment consisted of intravenous PCA with morphine (i.e. bolus 1.5 mg; lock-out rate 10 min) and oral diclofenac. After 24 hours the patient had self-administered 90 mg of intravenous morphine and the localized back pain decreased to a 3 on the NRS; the lancing pain was unaffected. Amitripyline was added in an increasing dosage (i.e. week 1, 25 mg; week 2, 50 mg; week 3, 75 mg). In parallel, bisphosphonate was added to stabilize bone metabolism. After 3 days beneficial effects were noted and the patient's opioid consumption and NRS ratings decreased significantly. Five days after initiation of therapy the patient was switched to sustained release oral morphine (i.e. 300 mg/day). After 1 week with continuous medication (i.e. morphine, amitripyline, and diclofenac), the lancing pain disappeared and the NRS ratings settled down to 1 for pain at rest and 3 for pain with ambulation. After receiving a course of androgen blockade, he was discharged home without any significant impairment.

Conclusion

Mitigation and therapy of malignant pain is critical to maintaining and improving the level of patient function and comfort. It is a fundamental component of supportive care. Adequate analgesic control requires regular pain assessment and documentation plus ongoing therapeutic adjustments depending upon response and tolerance. Optimization of malignant pain therapy requires an energetic and knowledgeable interdisciplinary team to care for these delicate patients.

References

1 **Bonica JJ** (1985). Treatment of cancer pain: current status and future needs. In: *Advances in Pain Research and Therapy*, Vol. 9 (ed. HL Fields, R Dubner, F Cervero), pp. 589–616. Raven Press, New York.

2 **Larue F, Colleau SM, Brasseur L, Cleeland CS** (1995). Multicentre study of cancer pain and its treatment in France. *Br. Med. J.* **310**: 1034–7.

3 **Schug SA, Dunlop R, Zech D** (1992). Pharmacological management of cancer pain. *Drugs* **43**: 44–53.

4 **Koltzenburg M, McMahon SB** (1995). Mechanically insensitive primary afferents innervating the urinary bladder. In: *Visceral Pain. Progress in Pain Research and Management*, Vol. 5 (ed. GF Gebhardt), pp. 163–192. IASP Press, Seattle, WA.

5 **Sengupta JN, Gebhardt GF** (1995). Mechanosensitive afferent fibers in the gastrointestinal and lower urinary tracts. In: *Visceral Pain. Progress in Pain Research and Management*, Vol. 5 (ed. GF Gebhardt), pp. 75–98. IASP Press, Seattle, WA.

6 **Giamberardino MA, Vecciet L** (1999). Recent and forgotten aspects of visceral pain. *Eur. J. Pain* **3**: 77–92.

7 **Woolf CJ, Chong MS** (1993). Pre-emptive analgesia—treating postoperative pain by preventing the establishment of central sensitisation. *Anesth. Analg.* **77**: 362–79.

8 **Woolf CJ, Salter MW** (2000). Neuronal plasticity: increasing the gain of pain. *Science* **288**: 1765–9.

9 Sandkühler J (2000). Learning and memory in pain pathways. *Pain* **88**: 113–18.

10 Wesselmann U, Burnett AL, Heinberg LJ (1997). The urogenital and rectal pain syndromes. *Pain* **73**: 269–94.

11 Eccleston C (2001). Role of psychology in pain management. *Br. J. Anaesth.* **87**: 144–52.

12 Grond S, Zech D, Diefenbach C, Radbruch L, Lehmann KA (1996). Assessment of cancer pain: a prospective evaluation in 2266 cancer patients referred to a pain service. *Pain* **64**: 107–14.

13 Sindrup SH, Jensen TS (1999). Efficacy of pharmacological treatments of neuropathic pain: an update and effect related to mechanism of drug action. *Pain* **83**: 389–400.

14 Portenoy RK, Payne D, Jacobson P (1999). Breakthrough pain: characteristics and impact in patients with cancer pain. *Pain* **81**: 129–34.

15 Ripamonti C, Dickerson ED (2001). Strategies for the treatment of cancer pain in the new millennium. *Drugs* **61**: 955–77.

16 Mercadante S, Portenoy RK (2001). Opioid poorly responsive cancer pain. Part 3. Clinical strategies to improve opioid responsiveness. *J. Pain Sympt. Manage.* **21**: 338–54.

17 Ware JE, Sherbourne CD (1992). A 36-item short form health survey (SF-36): conceptual framework and item selection. *Med. Care* **30**: 473–83.

18 Mendoza TR, Wang XS, Cleeland CS, Morrissey M, Johnson BA, Wendt JK et al. (1999). The rapid assessment of fatigue severity in cancer patients: use of the Brief Fatigue Inventory. *Cancer* **85**(5): 1186–96.

19 Hickey AM, Bury G, O'Boyle CA, Bradley F, O'Kelley FD, Shannon WA (1996). A new short form individual quality of life measure (SEIQoL.DW): application in a cohort of individuals with HIV/AIDS. *Br. Med. J.* **313**: 29–33.

20 Cleeland CS, Ryan KM (1994). Pain assessment: global use of the Brief Pain Inventory. *Ann. Acad. Med.* **23**: 129–38.

21 Jackson LM, Hawkey CJ (2000). COX-2 selective non steroidal anti-inflammatory drugs. Do they really offer any advantages? *Drugs* **59**: 1207–16.

22 Steffen P, Drück A, Krinn E (1996). Investigations on the use of non-opioid analgesics in postoperative pain therapy II. Quantification of the analgesic efficacy of metamizol (dipyrone) in combination with diclofenac using patient-controlled analgesia. *Anästhesiol. Intensivmed. Notfallmed. Schmerzther.* **31**: 216–21.

23 Kuman N, Rowbotham DJ (1999). Piritramide. *Br. J. Anaesth.* **82**: 3–5.

24 Rose MA, Kam PC (2002). Gabapentin: pharmacology and its use in pain management. *Anesthesia* **57**: 451–62.

25 Pan HL, Eisenach JC, Chung JM (1999). Gabapentin suppresses ectopic nerve discharges. *J. Pharmacol. Exp. Ther.* **288**: 1026–30.

26 Woolf CJ, Mannion RJ (1999). Neuropathic pain: aetiology, symptoms, mechanisms and management. *Lancet* **353**: 1959–64.

27 Jackson RJ, Loh SC, Gokaslan ZL (2001). Metastatic renal cell carcinoma of the spine: surgical treatment and results. *J. Neurosurg.* **94**: 340.

28 Kehlet H, Holte K (2001). Effect of postoperative analgesia on surgical outcome. *Br. J. Anaesth.* **87**: 62–72.

29 Miaskowski C, Crews J, Ready B, Paul SM, Ginsberg B (1999). Anesthesia-based pain services improve the quality of postoperative pain management. *Pain* **80**: 23–9.

30 Heid F, Eysel P, Jage J (2002). Postoperative morphine excess or rational therapy? An exceptional case of applying the morphine equivalent. *Anaesthesist* **51**: 263–8.

31 Heid F, Jage J (2002). The treatment of pain in urology. *BJU Int.* **90**(5): 481–8.

Chapter 23

Evaluation and treatment of the infertile male

M. A. Fischer

Introduction

Developments in the area of reproductive medicine have focused on technologies in which the primary objective is pregnancy. However, couples with infertility face significant emotional and psychological hurdles. Both couples with infertility who are successfully treated and couples who do not conceive may need assistance to overcome some of these issues. The extent of treatment therefore must be broadened to include the emotional and psychological needs of patients being evaluated and treated for infertility.

The objective of this chapter is to present a summary of the evaluation and treatment of male factor infertility with additional emphasis on supportive care of the infertile couple during evaluation and treatment of the infertile couple.

Physiology

Production and maturation within the male and transport of spermatozoa to the female genital tract to fertilize the oocyte involves the interaction of several body systems. These environments can be conveniently divided into pre-testicular (generally hormonal), testicular (seminiferous tubule), post-testicular (from seminiferous tubule to female genital tract), and spermatic (interaction of sperm and egg to achieve fertilization) portions for the purpose of understanding both the normal physiology of reproduction and perturbations to normal reproduction.

Male fertility depends to a great extent on the proper functioning of the hypothalamic–pituitary–gonadal (HPG) axis. The simple yet elegant cooperative function of the aspects of this axis provides the necessary stimuli for production of testosterone and spermatozoa while simultaneously self-regulating these vital activities. The hypothalamus provides stimulus for pituitary and gonadal hormonal output by integrating input from various higher brain centres along with influences from circulating blood hormones and extrinsic mediating factors. Gonadotrophin-releasing hormone (GnRH) from the hypothalamus is delivered via the portal venous system to the anterior pituitary gland, where it acts to stimulate release of luteinizing hormone (LH) and follicle-stimulating hormone (FSH). LH stimulates the Leydig cells in the testicular interstitium to produce testosterone. Testosterone is then bound by binding proteins and secreted into the lumen of the seminiferous tubule. FSH is necessary for the proper initiation of sperm production during puberty and is probably also required to ensure ongoing quantitatively normal sperm production in the adult. The testis also produces inhibin which serves to down-regulate the action of the hypothalamus and the pituitary.

The secretion of these stimulating hormones is tightly regulated by the activity of additional hormones in a classic feedback loop. Secretion of GnRH is down-regulated by the actions of LH, FSH, testosterone, and also probably inhibin. The pituitary is also negatively influenced by the action of testosterone and also probably inhibin. Finally the hypothalamus may also be negatively affected by excess production of the pituitary hormone prolactin, which may occur due to various pathological conditions. In this manner, gonadal function is tightly regulated by the actions of the HPG axis and the 'pre-testicular' environment is optimized for normal spermatogenetic function.[1]

The production of sperm incorporates the hormones described above at the site of spermatogenesis in the seminiferous tubules within the testis. Sertoli cells border the membrane of the seminiferous tubule and are of central importance for the production of sperm. These cells produce proteins and hormones which support sperm production, act as a barrier preventing immune cells from reacting to sperm production, and interact directly with developing spermatogonia. The production of spermatozoa occurs in an ordered cycle from the primary spermatogonia stage at the basement membrane to the spermatozoa stage within the lumen of the seminiferous tubule. Formation of spermatozoa involves development of the sperm tail (flagella), compaction and binding of genetic material in the nucleus, and removal of virtually all cytoplasm from the cell. Several cycles of spermatogenesis are under way in each tubule of the testis at a given time. Furthermore, different cycles of spermatogenesis are systematically arranged in steps, called spermatogenic waves. A complete cycle of spermatogenesis, from spermatogonia to mature spermatozoa, requires approximately 75 days. The interaction of the pre-testicular hormonal environment and the testicular compartment in which sperm production occurs provides the required sperm for the post-testicular transport of sperm from the seminiferous tubules to the epididymis for further development and maturation. During passage through the epididymis over a period of up to 2 weeks, spermatozoa undergo several important changes which further develop sperm structure and render sperm capable of penetrating and fertilizing the egg. These changes include alterations in membrane lipid and protein content, surface charge, and enzyme activity. Without these vital changes, sperm remain essentially immotile and incapable of fertilizing an oocyte.

Epididymal fluid containing sperm makes up a small portion of ejaculate volume. The ejaculate contains approximately 0.1 ml of sperm-rich epididymal fluid, 1.5 ml of seminal vesicle fluid, 0.5 ml from the prostate and up to 0.2 ml from the Cowper's and

Littre's glands. Once ejaculated into the female genital tract, the ejaculate forms a clot to prevent rapid leakage from the vagina. Within the ejaculate, sperm undergo a further set of functional and physiological changes called capacitation. Finally, once the sperm contacts the egg, lytic enzymes are released from around the head (acrosome) of the sperm to enable the sperm to merge with the egg and fertilization occurs.

Overview

Successful pregnancy outcomes for infertile couples using expensive and advanced technologies often results in little or no evaluation of the male partner. Unfortunately this approach ignores potentially treatable causes of male infertility (e.g. varicocoele, genital tract obstruction) and also overlooks potentially life-threatening causes of infertility, such as testicular cancer and pituitary tumours. Combined with greater understanding of the genetics of male infertility, these issues mandate an appropriate and systematic approach to the evaluation and treatment of infertile couples.[2]

It is suggested that between 20 and 25% of couples with normal fertility status conceive within month, with almost 90% succeeding within 1 year. Nevertheless, of couples with unknown fertility status, approximately 15% of couples are unable to achieve pregnancy within 1 year. In cases of infertility, approximately 20% are entirely attributable to male factor infertility and in an additional 20–30% due to combined male and female factor infertility, suggesting that male factor infertility is causative in approximately 50% of cases couples unable to achieve pregnancy.[3]

In many cases, the chances of successful conception decrease as couples remain unable to conceive. Unnecessary delay in evaluation and treatment add to the angst and trepidation most couples experience when faced with difficulty conceiving. It is recommended that the evaluation of the couple should begin immediately at presentation and should be rapid, comprehensive, and cost-effective. Evaluation of the infertile male seeks to identify the cause of infertility (if possible), rule out potentially serious medical causes of impaired fertility, and to suggest if assisted reproductive technologies (ART) will be required and/or may be effective for the couple to achieve the goal of pregnancy. Furthermore, detection of conditions for which there is no treatment will spare the couple the unnecessary burden of treatments which will fail. Similarly, genetic conditions associated with male infertility may be identified during evaluation which may preclude paternity. Finally, because of the emotional and psychological impact of male infertility, many men want to uncover the aetiology of their infertility.[4] Given the important issues, it is imperative that the evaluation be conducted in a forthright but sensitive manner. The emotional and psychological aspects of the experience of infertility for couples should be recognized and health professionals treating these couple should recognize these issues. The process of evaluation and treatment can initiate conflict in a previously stable marriage or exacerbate an already strained relationship. Attention tends to be singularly focused on the goal of achieving pregnancy while neglecting other important parts of life. This can result in depression due to loss of self-esteem, self-confidence, and sense of prestige. The diagnosis of male factor infertility is often linked to a profound sense of decreased virility and is often emotionally devastating. Evaluation of male infertility violates the privacy of the most intimate aspects of a relationship and needs to be recognized and dealt with in an appropriate manner.

Evaluation of the infertile male

Recently, best practice polices for the evaluation and treatment of male infertility were published. These recommendations make suggestions about the optimal evaluation of the infertile male and provide a logical framework for understanding the diagnostic evaluation of the infertile male.[5] The availability of both partners throughout the process helps to ensure accuracy of information about the history of infertility and past medical problems and enables the physician to gain valuable insight into the effect of infertility on the couple and their interactions.

The evaluation of an infertile male includes complete reproductive and medical history including all areas related to fertility status. Efforts should be made to ensure that all information, results and treatment plans are understood by both partners. Perhaps more importantly, this engages both partners in the process of the infertility experience and enables the treatment team to gauge the psychological response of the couple to the treatment process. This in turn allows for psychological and counselling interventions before an issues arise.

Reproductive history should include an inquiry of developmental history, childhood illnesses, significant medical illnesses, and surgical procedures. Specific childhood illnesses may have an impact on fertility. A history of cryptorchidism may impair fertility in some men.[6,7] Mumps orchitis in the post-pubertal period or testicular injury due to torsion or trauma may be associated with subfertility.[8] Corrective surgery including hernia repair, orchidopexy, and some bladder surgeries may result in impairment of normal spermatogenesis, obstructive azoospermia, or abnormal ejaculation. A developmental history focusing on sexual development and onset of puberty may elucidate an endocrinopathy associated with male infertility.[9]

Further inquiry should be directed to evaluating frequency and timing of coitus, sexual history including sexually transmitted diseases, and evaluation of sexual and/or ejaculatory dysfunction. The couple should be educated that sexual activity during the middle of the menstrual cycle is essential for pregnancy. Despite some controversy, it is suggested that coitus every 48 hours during the period of ovulation is recommended to ensure viable sperm are present to fertilize the oocyte. Use of sexual lubricants should be detailed. Lubricants which do not impair sperm motility include various natural oils (e.g. peanut, safflower, vegetable) and raw egg whites.[10]

Diagnostic and treatment procedures, in addition to the powerful stressors associated with infertility, may have an adverse impact on the sexual life of the infertile couple. This may be manifested as male sexual disorders including erectile dysfunction, ejaculatory dysfunction, impaired libido, and a decrease in the frequency of intercourse. Particular attention should be paid to the experience of infertility on the couple and how this affects sexual function.[11,12]

Detailed assessment of past medical and surgical history and inquiry into medication and exposure to gonadotoxic agents is essential. Erectile and ejaculatory dysfunction may be impaired with pelvic or retroperitoneal surgery or medical illnesses such as diabetes mellitus, while inguinal or scrotal surgery may be associated with obstruction of sperm transport. Certain therapeutic medications can adversely affect male fertility. These include gonadotoxic agents, which may severely damage spermatogenesis, perturb the hormonal regulation of spermatogenesis via the hypothalamic–pituitary–gonadal axis, and interfer with normal sexual function. If possible, these medications should be stopped or adjusted and fertility reassessed after 3 to 6 months.[13] Environmental exposures may also be significant. Hyperthermia may impair sperm quality. A recent history of fever should prompt reassessment of sperm quality 3 to 6 months after resolution of the fever, while exposure to excessive heat including hot baths and occupational sources of heat should be limited wherever possible. Patients trying to achieve pregnancy should be encouraged to stop smoking, stop using illicit drugs, and limit alcohol intake. Patients who may be in contact with harmful occupational and environmental toxins should limit their exposure.[14]

Physical examination

A focused physical examination is performed to identify abnormalities associated with impaired fertility. Abnormalities of body habitus, a reduced degree of virilization, and the presence of gynaecomastia may indicate an endocrinological cause of impaired fertility. Specific evaluation of the genitalia is of particular importance in the physical examination. Both hypospadius and congenital penile curvature (chordee) may impair both sexual function and ejaculation. Examine scrotal contents in the standing position, in a warm room, to promote relaxation of the cremasteric muscle. Testis volume should be estimated with an orchidometer and should be greater than 20 ml. Reduced testis volume and/or testes which are of a soft consistency strongly suggests a reduced number of or impaired function of spermatogenic components within the testis. Testicular masses suggestive of neoplasia should be ruled out. The epididymis should be examined for the presence of scarring or obstruction. Other intrascrotal abnormalities (e.g. hydrocoele, spermatocoele, epididymal cysts) should be noted but usually do not have a negative impact on fertility. Palpation of both vasa deferens must be performed to rule out obstruction of sperm due to congenital absence of the vas deferens, vasectomy, or iatrogenic causes of obstruction. The spermatic cords should be examined to identify the presence or absence of a varicocoele, which may be graded according to size (Table 23.1). Subclinical varicocoeles identified by ultrasound or venography are controversial and are not considered to be clinically significant.[15] Following the history and physical examination, routine investigations are performed; however, the

Table 23.1 Classification of varicocoele

Grade I: Palpable during Valsalva manoeuvre only
Grade II: Palpable in standing position without Valsalva manoeuvre
Grade III: Visible through scrotal skin

Table 23.2 WHO normal semen parameters

Semen parameters	WHO normal range
Volume	1.5–5 ml
Sperm density	> 20 million/ml
Sperm motility	> 50%
Sperm morphology	> 30% normal forms
Leucocyte density	< 1 million/ml

prudent physician will spend additional time evaluating the psychological effects of infertility on the couple being assessed.

Investigations

Along with history and physical examination, semen analysis forms the basis of the evaluation of the infertile male. Normal values for semen analysis as suggested by the WHO are shown in Table 23.2. Although these values are suggested as reference ranges, recent data suggest that different semen analysis values may be more accurate at distinguishing infertile from fertile males. Nevertheless, most clinical research, infertility clinics, and guidelines for evaluation of the infertile male use WHO values as reference ranges during the evaluation and treatment of infertile couples.[16]

In order to standardize semen analysis testing, physicians should provide detailed instructions for patients to collect their specimens. It is suggested that at least two semen analyses should be performed for each patient so that a baseline of sperm quality may be established. If semen results are very different, then additional specimens may be required to establish the pattern of semen quality. Either masturbation or intercourse with a condom that does not contain components which interfere with sperm may be utilized. The specimen should be collected in a sterile jar after 2 to 3 days of sexual and ejaculatory abstinence. Longer periods of abstinence result in increased sperm concentration but reduced motility and worsening sperm morphology. Sperm motility decreases after ejaculation so if the specimen is produced at home, the specimen should be transported at room temperature and must be analysed within 1 hour of collection.

Although the semen analysis provides very important information about the potential for a given male to produce offspring, it does not test fertility *per se*. This should be emphasized to patients during the evaluation and treatment cycle. Often patients are searching for a specific number or result in the semen analysis in order for them to become pregnant. The reference ranges for semen analysis do not necessarily correlate with the values that are required for fertilization of an oocyte. Similarly, patients often ask what the likelihood of establishing a pregnancy is based on a given semen analysis. It should be emphasized to these patients that men with semen parameters that are not within the reference range may be fertile while men with 'normal' results may be infertile. Recent data suggest that there is extensive overlap between sperm concentration, motility, and morphology between fertile and infertile men. Generally, fertility potential is reduced in patients with a deficit in any of these parameters although normal morphology may have the best discriminatory power for determining fertility potential.[16]

Normal semen volume should be between 2 and 5 ml. Low ejaculate volume or absence of ejaculate on semen analysis despite orgasm may be due to improper collection methods, retrograde ejaculation, hypogonadism, or genital tract obstruction. After ensuring appropriate collection of the semen specimen, a post-ejaculate urine analysis for sperm is indicated for all men with low ejaculate volume who do not have genital tract obstruction or hypogonadism. The urine specimen should be centrifuged and the pellet examined with a microscope. Although there is no consensus about the precise number of sperm required to diagnose retrograde ejaculation, five to ten sperm per high-powered field is suggestive of retrograde ejaculation. If the post-ejaculate urine does not contain sperm, then ejaculatory duct obstruction should be ruled out with transrectal ultrasound of the prostate, seminal vesicles, and ejaculatory duct.

Sperm concentration should be above 20×10^6 per ml. As described above, men with sperm counts below this number can still be fertile, and even very low numbers of sperm can be used for treatment with *in vitro* fertilization. If no sperm are noted after two semen analyses, a third specimen should be centrifuged and the pellet resuspended and carefully examined for the presence of spermatozoa. If no sperm are seen, then the diagnosis of azoospermia can be made. Sperm motility is assessed by determining the percentage of sperm that are motile and at least 50% of the sperm should be motile. In addition, the quality of sperm motility, termed progression, is determined based on a scale of 0 (no motility) to 4 (rapid progression) and at least 25% of sperm should have rapid progression. If no motile sperm are observed, sperm viability may be assessed by staining or the hypo-osmotic swelling test to determine if the sperm are non-viable.[17] Sperm morphology is an important determinant of sperm quality. Morphology parameters take into consideration the shape, length, width, acrosome size and shape, and defects in the shape of different parts of the sperm including head, neck, body, and tail. The most frequently used system is the Kruger system, in which the lower limit of normal morphology is 14% of a specimen.[18]

Attempts to improve on the reproducibility of semen analyses have resulted in the deployment of computer systems to quantify sperm concentration, motility, and morphology. However, these tests have limitations based on technological variabilities.

These techniques are used predominantly in research protocols but are gaining more clinical acceptance.

While some inflammatory cells may be noted in the ejaculate, the presence of increased numbers of white blood cells in the semen is suggestive of infection and/or inflammation in the genital tract. Other potential causes include immune system activation and toxin exposure. Specific stains are required to distinguish inflammatory cells from immature spermatozoa. The presence of more that 1×10^6 white blood cells per high-powered field (leucocytospermia or pyospermia) is deemed significant and should prompt the culturing of the semen and urine to confirm infection.[19]

Immunological causes of infertility include the presence of antisperm antibodies. Given the separation of the seminiferous tubules from the immune system by the blood–testis barrier (Sertoli to Sertoli cell tight junction) exposure of the immune system to sperm may occur after trauma, infection, or most commonly after vasectomy. Semen analysis with isolated reduced or absent sperm motility (aesthenospermia) with other parameters normal should be evaluated for the presence of antisperm antibodies. A history of testis trauma, sperm agglutination, and idiopathic infertility may also be an indication for this antibody testing. Direct testing on the surface of sperm is the recommended method for testing for antisperm antibodies.[20] Sperm viability testing may be indicated to determine whether viable sperm are present in a sample of non-motile sperm. Dyes such as eosin may be used to detect viability. Assays utilizing the hypo-osmotic swelling test are used to identify viable sperm that may be utilized in assisted reproductive technologies (ART).[21]

As the semen analysis does not specifically evaluate sperm function, numerous additional tests of semen parameters and sperm function have been studied. Tests such as the sperm–cervical interaction assay, the hamster egg penetration test, the acrosome reaction of human sperm assay, sperm creatine kinase assay, and reactive oxygen species assay are not routinely performed although the may be indicated in certain circumstances. These tests should be reserved for patients in whom the results would influence treatment and should be performed in specialized andrology laboratories.[22]

Recent data have indicated that sperm chromatin structure can significantly influence the outcome of sperm–egg interaction, during both IVF and natural conception. The sperm chromatin structure assay measures the integrity of the DNA structure within sperm and has been shown to correlate with outcomes of ART. This test provides important information about the potential outcomes of ART and ongoing studies have evaluated the effects of various toxic factors on sperm DNA integrity.[23]

Endocrine testing

Endocrine testing for the male with subfertility is based upon an understanding of the HPG axis and provides important information about sperm production. Endocrine evaluation includes determination of serum FSH, LH and testosterone (T) concentrations, although determining FSH and T levels will detect most endocrinopathies

Table 23.3 Summary of physical exam and hormone testing

Dignosis	Semen analysis	Hormones	Testis size
Oligospermia	Variable	Normal or ↑	Normal or ↓
1° NOA	Azoospermia	↑FSH/LH	↓↓
2° NOA	Azoospermia	↓FSH/LH	↓↓
Obstructive azoospermia	Azoospermia	Normal	Normal

Abbreviations: 1° NOA, primary (testicular) non-obstructive azoospermia; 2° NOA, secondary (hormonal) non-obstructive azoospermia ; FSH, follicle-stimulating hormone; LH, luteinizing hormone.

associated with male infertility. Serum LH and prolactin levels may be added if T and FSH levels are abnormal. The FSH level is indicative of the status of spermatogenesis while T levels are useful for judgeing overall hormonal function. Additional tests including estradiol levels, serum prolactin, and thyroid-stimulating hormone (TSH) should be reserved for men with clinical symptoms and/or signs of poor virilization, gynaecomastia, or manifestations of endocrine deregulation. More recently, an endocrinopathy involving decreased serum testosterone in comparison to estradiol levels in subfertile males has been identified. This may extend the indication for serum estradiol levels.[24] Common patterns for hormone abnormalities have been identified and are summarized in Table 23.3.

The psychological and emotional reactions to infertility begin developing once couples realize that they are having difficulty conceiving. Numerous variables shape the subject-ive sense of well-being of infertile couples. The experience of infertility is affected by gen-der and expectations of the different partners' roles in the relationship. Kowalcek *et al.*[25] demonstrated that infertile and childless women express significantly more psy-chological symptoms and decreased sense of well-being compared with their male partners. The same author also showed that female partners in infertile couples report increased rates of depression and self-distraction. Interestingly, involuntarily childless men were found to utilize fewer coping strategies for their infertility than men with other types of somatic illnesses.[26] Other studies suggest that women in infertile couples experience greater levels of general stress than men in addition to heightened stress related to social issues, sexual function, and the desire for parenthood. The stress of social pressures, in addition to concerns about sexual and relationship dysfunction associated with infertility, are effective predictors of depression and marital dissatisfaction.[27]

Aetiological factors for depression in adults have been adapted for infertile couples by Mahlstedt.[28] These include loss of intimacy in a relationship, a sense of loss of health status, loss of social standing due to a perceived stigma of being infertile, loss of self-esteem and self-confidence, and loss of an expected and important part of many marital relationships. For most couples infertility is a major crisis which can severely disrupt a previously stable relationship. Recognizing these issues and encouraging partners to discuss them is an important part of the treatment process for infertile couples.

The cause of infertility (male, female, or mixed) also affects the psychological impact of infertility. Lee et al.[29] found that female partners experience more stress from infertility tests and treatment than their husbands, regardless of whether a female factor for infertility is present. In addition, female partners in couples with mixed or idiopathic infertility experienced less stress compared with situations with only a female factor for infertility. In contrast, males with mixed or idiopathic infertility experience less stress than cases with only male infertility or female infertility. However, other studies of the psychological effects of infertility on couples have found that male and female partners confronted with a diagnosis of male infertility experience higher global stress in addition to more social and sexual concerns than do couples who are undergoing evaluation and treatment of female infertility.[27] The response to stress incited by a diagnosis of infertility differs depending on gender and infertility diagnosis.

Couples' expectations of societal roles and pressures affect on psychological responses to infertility. For men, the expectations of fulfilling the aspects of the 'male role' and social pressures were identified as the most significant stressors during evaluation and treatment. However, while having a child was of secondary importance for men, child bearing was of prime importance for females and social expectations and pressures were of secondary importance. The impact of fertility on the sexual life of partners was deemed to be of less significance than societal role expectations and pressures both for men and women.[30]

The stages of crisis due to infertility following diagnosis include disbelief, denial, feelings of decreased self-esteem, anger, and helplessness. Counselling can focus on these relevant issues addressing areas of inappropriate self-blame or blame directed towards the partner, stresses and trauma to the relationship, and behavioural issues including obsessive behaviours, depression, and anxiety due to infertility. Patients with changes in mental status or significant psychological and psychiatric symptoms, history of pregnancy losses, problems with substance abuse, sexual dysfunction, and martial disruption should be referred for evaluation by a psychologist or counsellor.

Differential diagnosis of male infertility

Pre-testicular causes of reduced sperm quality are usually hormonal in nature and are due to perturbations in the balance of the endocrine control of sperm production. These conditions may be clinically subtle and infertility may be the first presentation of some of these diseases. These patients may present with abnormal virilization and may be azoospermic with small-volume testes. Diseases at the hypothalamic level include gonadotrophin-releasing hormone deficiency (Kallman's syndrome) which is accompanied by anosmia and other congenital abnormalities. Other rare conditions which are associated to secondary hypogonadism include Prader–Willi syndrome, Bardet–Biedel syndrome, cerebellar ataxia, and isolated LH and/or FSH deficiency. Hypogonadotrophic hypogonadism many also be due to abnormalities at the pituitary level. Pituitary dysfunction may be caused by infiltrative diseases, tumours, vascular infarcts, sickle cell disease, and haemochromatosis. Pituitary dysfunction may also be due to excess circulating prolactin resulting in hypogonadotrophic hypogonadism which may be manifested by abnormal libido, galactorrhoea, and sexual dysfunction. Other pituitary abnormalities may be as a result of thyroid dysfunction or overactive adrenal glands. Excess androgens may result in secondary hypogonadism due to suppression of pituitary function. Excess androgens may be due to adrenal gland abnormalities, in particular congenital adrenal hyperplasia. Unfortunately, excess exogenous anabolic androgens commonly utilized in young male athletes are a common cause of abnormal pituitary function. Excess glucocorticoid production (adrenal hyperplasia) and hyper- or hypothyroidism are unusual causes of male infertility.[9]

Defects at the level of the testis directly affect the function of the seminiferous tubules. Unfortunately many of the genetic causes of this type of infertility are irreversible at the current time. Genetic abnormalities are now commonly understood to be a cause of male infertility. Given that ARTs bypass normal barriers to conception in men with poor quality sperm, it is vital that appropriate genetic counselling and testing be performed prior to proceeding to ART. Severe oligospermia and azoospermia may be linked to genetic abnormalities of autosomes, sex chromosomes, including the Y chromosome, and mutations in the cystic fibrosis transmembrane conductance regulator gene (CFTR). Abnormal karyotypes may in found in up to 15% of men with severe oligospermia or azoospermia including a variety of autosomal abnormalities such as translocations and inversions. Numerical sex chromosome abnormalities, in particular Klinefelter's syndrome (XXY), are the most common sex chromosome abnormalities in men with infertility. Men with severe oligospermia (7%) and azoospermia (15%) may also have deletions in a portion of the long arm (Yq) of the Y chromosome associated with their infertility. The area of the Y chromosome associated with male infertility has been termed the AZF region and the most common deletions involved in the AZFc region are called the DAZ (deleted in azoospermia) (60%) followed by deletions in the AZFb (15%) and AZFa (5%). Phenotype–gentoype studies have shown that conclusions about the likelihood of a patient having a mutation cannot be conclusively made based upon clinical presentation or parameters and thus all men with severe oligospermia or non-obstructive azoospermia should be evaluated with karyotype and Y microdeletion studies.[32]

Men with obstructive azoospermia, in particular men with congenital bilateral absence of the vas deferens (CBAVD), commonly carry mutations in the CFTR gene. This condition is almost universal in men with clinical cystic fibrosis while men with isolated CBAVD are recognized to have a variant of this problem. More than 80% of men with CBAVD will carry a CFTR mutation. In addition, men with unilateral

Table 23.4 Recommendations for genetic testing for infertile males

Severe oligospermia ($<10 \times 10^6$ sperm/ml)	Y microdeletions, karyotype
Non-obstructive azoospermia	Y microdeletions, karyotype
Obstructive azoospermia/congenital absence of vas deferens	*CFTR* mutation

absence of the vas deferens (CUAVD), idiopathic epididymal obstruction (IEO), and Young's syndrome (chronic sinusitis, bronchiectasis, and obstructive azoospermia) are also at increased risk of being carriers of *CFTR* mutations. In contrast, men with non-obstructive azoospermia do not have an increased rate of *CFTR* mutations.[32] Other syndromes resulting in azoospermia include myotonic dystrophy, bilateral anorchia (vanishing testis syndrome), and Sertoli cell only syndrome. Systemic illnesses including renal failure and hepatic cirrhosis can lead to an abnormal hormonal environment and thus have a negative impact on testis function. These genetic tests apply to a large number of infertile men. The development of ART has raised the possibility of transmission of these genetic defects. Recommended genetic testing for infertile males is summarized in Table 23.4.

Spermatogenic function may also be affected by gonadotoxic agents. The effects of radiation and chemotherapeutic agents have dramatic effects on rapidly dividing spermatogenic cells often resulting in irreversible eradication of the germ cell population. If spermatogenesis does recover after chemotherapy, a waiting period of 6 to 12 months prior to resuming attempts at pregnancy is recommended due to concerns about the lingering effects of these agents on sperm chromatin. The testis may also be injured by post-pubertal viral infection (mumps orchitis) and less commonly by bacterial orchitis (epididymo-orchitis). Testicular torsion can injure the testis by initiation of immunological mechanisms and by direct injury to the spermatogenic stem cells. Similar injury may occur after trauma to the testis.

A varicocoele is a series of dilated and tortuous veins of the pampiniform plexus of the testis within the scrotum and is the most commonly diagnosed cause of male infertility. Approximately 15% of healthy fertile men have a varicocoele compared with 40% of infertile men. These enlarged veins result in reflux of blood into the pampiniform plexus and are associated with atrophy of the affected testis. Furthermore, there is good evidence that the presence of a varicocoele is associated with depressed semen parameters.[15]

Post-testicular obstruction results in impaired transport of sperm from the seminiferous tubules to the female genital tract. Obstructions can occur along any point of the male reproductive tract and include congenital absence of the vas deferens (unilateral and bilateral), absence or atrophy of the seminal vesicles, and atrophy of the ejaculatory duct. Each of these congenital conditions is strongly associated with mutations of the cystic fibrosis gene. Idiopathic obstruction of the epididymis is also associated with *CFTR* mutations (see above). Acquired causes of obstruction include vasectomy, iatrogenic vasal injury during groin or scrotal surgery, and bacterial infection, including sexually transmitted diseases.

Sexual and ejaculatory dysfunction may also impair sperm delivery to the female genital tract. Dysfunction at the level of the seminal vesicle may be due to medications or injury to the nerve supply resulting in impaired seminal emission into the urethra. Similar agents may impair the nerve supply to the penis resulting in impaired or abnormal ejaculation and erectile dysfunction. Abnormalities of the urethra, in particular hypospadius, may impair delivery of sperm to the female genital tract.[13]

Dysfunction at the level of the sperm may impair fertility. Immotile cilia syndrome results in defective axonemal formation of the sperm tails and results in immotile but viable sperm. Various sperm maturation defects may occur following obstruction within the epididymis. Seminal infection my result in the formation of reactive oxygen species and/or formation of antisperm antibodies which can impair sperm function.

Treatment for male infertility

Counselling

Some routine advice which may improve fertility potential can be given to all infertile patients. Cigarette smoking, excessive alcohol use, and recreational drugs which negatively affect spermatogenesis should be avoided. Medication usage should be reviewed, and drugs which have a negative impact on spermatogenesis or ejaculatory and sexual function should be adjusted or stopped.

Review of coital timing and frequency can improve fertility. It is important to review timing of coitus to coincide with ovulation. Detection of the LH surge prior to ovulation using a urine dip kit or body temperature monitoring may assist in determining the appropriate timing for intercourse. Usually coitus is recommended every 2 days during the period leading up to and including ovulation. This can significantly reduce the incidence of stress and sexual dysfunction associated with coital timing.

Medical therapy

Effective medical therapy is available for some men with subfertility. Retrograde ejaculation may be treated with sympathomimetic agents including pseudoephedrine, phenylpropanolamine, or imipramine. Patients that fail this treatment can be treated with harvesting of sperm with intrauterine insemination.[33]

Wherever possible, men with an endocrine dysfunction as a cause for infertility should be treated with medical therapy. Patients with elevated prolactin levels should have complete endocrine work-up and may be treated with agents to reduce prolactin levels. These include bromocriptine and newer agents including cabergaline, which have fewer side-effects. Significant hypothyroidism or hyperthyroidism may be treated with either replacement or reduction of hormone levels as appropriate. Hypogonadotrophic hypogonadism (low FSH and/or LH) due to lack of GnRH stimulation (Kallman's syndrome) can be treated with replacement human chorionic gonadotrophin (hCG) and FSH. Men with pituitary dysfunction and low gonadotropins may be treated with hCG and human menopausal gonadotrophin (hMG).[9]

Empirical medical therapy for male infertility provides limited success. If these therapies are to be used, limitations on the duration of therapy should be established so that couples avoid unnecessarily delaying other treatments. Clomiphene citrate is an anti-oestrogen drug which increases gonadotrophin output and may be used for men with oligospermia. Serum testosterone should be monitored to be kept in the normal range and semen analysis should be closely watched as semen quality may decrease on this medication in some cases. The outcomes with this therapy are limited.[33]

Low motility may be due to antisperm antibodies. Treatment may be instituted with oral corticosteroid therapy to suppress antibody production. This treatment may have significant side-effects and patients should be appropriately counselled. Usually *in vitro* fertilization is recommended.[20]

Surgical therapy

Surgical treatments are effective and recognized for male infertility. Men with varicocoeles may be treated with surgical and interventional radiological procedures to abolish reflux of venous blood via spermatic vessels. Different techniques are available including open repair, laparoscopic, and embolization procedures. These approaches are effective for improving sperm counts in men with differing abnormalities of semen quality and improve fertility rates in infertile males.[15]

Microsurgery to restore sperm to the ejaculate following vasectomy or unintentional iatrogenic vasal obstruction and obstruction of the epididymis due to infection or other causes is a very effective method for treatment of obstructive azoospermia. In regards to vasectomy reversal, magnification with an operating microscope results in higher patency rates and better success. Numerous methods and technical modifications for vasovasostomy exist but no one method has been shown to be better than any other. Success rates vary with duration and cause of obstruction. Longer obstructive intervals may result in epididymal obstruction requiring vaso-epididymostomy. This procedure may also be used for epididymal obstruction due to other causes. Reasons for microsurgical failure include failure to recognize and diagnose female causes for infertility, poor surgical technique, and poor sperm maturation due to epididymal defects and antisperm antibody development.[34]

Ejaculatory duct obstruction results in low semen volume, negative semen fructose testing, and, usually, azoospermia. The diagnosis can be confirmed by transrectal ultrasonography. Transurethral resection of the ejaculatory ducts can be an effective treatment for this condition with improvements in semen volume and return of sperm to the ejaculate in the majority of men leading to credible pregnancy outcomes.

In men with irreversible genital tract obstruction (i.e. CBAVD) or failed microsurgery for male infertility, sperm retrieval with assisted reproductive technologies is indicated. Retrieval procedures seek to retrieve the best quality and most mature sperm from different reservoirs within the male genital tract. Sperm may be retrieved from the vas deferens, epididymis, or testis. Sperm from the vas deferens and epididymis are preferred since they have acquired motility but excellent pregnancy rates can also be achieved using sperm from the testis. Overall, fertilization rates exceeding 50% and pregnancy rates up to 50% are possible using harvested sperm for assisted reproductive technologies (ART). Concerns include cost and potential risks to offspring and the female partner.[35] While pregnancy can be established with ART for many cases of infertility, it is recommended that all steps should be taken to optimize sperm quality rather than moving directly to ART without evaluation and treatment of the male partner. If medical or surgical therapy is not possible, does not succeed, or is not desired by the patient, then ART can be successful in achieving pregnancy. Intrauterine insemination (IUI) is the simplest method of ART. This technique consists of placing a concentrated number of highly motile sperm which have been retrieved from the male ejaculate into the female genital tract at the time of ovulation. This technique is indicated for men with low sperm quality, impaired delivery of sperm, and for certain types of female factor infertility. Pregnancy rates in the 15–20% range can be achieved using this technique.[36] More advanced forms of ART bypass almost all barriers to sperm and oocyte interaction to achieve fertilization. These techniques involve ovarian stimulation and oocyte retrieval with fertilization of the egg in a Petri dish followed by transfer of the fertilized embryo to the female partner. Excellent fertilization and pregnancy rates can be achieved for even the most severe forms of male subfertility. This is a potential concern in that natural barriers to conception are being bypassed with these techniques, and this may have genetic implications for future generations. Recent studies have suggested that children born via these techniques may be at higher risk for chromosomal abnormalities than other children.[35] Artificial insemination with donor sperm (AID) may be indicated to achieve pregnancy for couples with irreversible forms of male infertility (i.e. testis failure). This method is highly successful and provides an option for couples beyond adoption.

Advances in reproductive technologies have dramatically improved the prognosis for many infertile couples. However, these technologies place significant psychological demands on an infertile couple. Issues such as religious and cultural beliefs, beliefs about embryo cryopreservation, potential for multiple pregnancy, and failure of the procedures are significant risks to patients. The medical goals of ART often supercede the important psychological issues. These include becoming closer as a couple and the satisfaction that the couple have utilized all means to reproduce. Treatment with ART should include the commitment to deal with the psychological aspects of infertility by all health professionals involved and may include specialized psychological counselling for some couples. The emotional risks of ART should be reviewed and a couple's beliefs about ART and associated procedures should be explored. This approach can mitigate some of the potential emotional and psychological risks that faced by couples. Plans for follow-up including disposition of frozen embryos should be developed for couples who are unable to achieve pregnancy. Patients who do conceive need continuing care as fears of pregnancy loss are very high in these patients. Unfortunately not all couples have positive outcome after IVF and these couples often experience significant grief and depression reactions. Couples that fail IVF require close follow-up, and support for this group of patients should be an integral part of all IVF protocols.[37]

The use of third-party reproduction is an appropriate treatment option for some patients with infertility. This form of treatment raises a number of different challenges. Discussions prior to use of donor gametes should explore a couple's social and religious attitudes, beliefs about the meaning of genetic versus biological parentage, and identification of how treatment of infertility has affected each member of the couple. Prior to the use of donor gametes, a couple should be allowed to reach an acceptance about the failure to conceive. Sufficient time should be allowed to discuss the relevant issues associated with using donor gametes and, in particular, to understand that using donor gametes is very different, from a psychological standpoint, from using a couple's own gametes. Emotions about the loss of the ability to share parentage with the other partner and grieving the loss of the genetic contribution of the infertile partner can be significant. Further issues include decisions about disclosure of the use of donor gametes to family in the present and the child in the future. There is no optimal solution to many of these issues and couples must have time to discuss these issues with the treatment team and a counsellor skilled in this area prior to initiating treatment.[38]

References

1 Veldhuis JD (1997). Male hypothalamic–pituitary–gonadal axis. In: *Infertility in the Male* (ed. LI Lipschultz, SE Howards), pp. 23–58. Mosby, St Louis, MO.

2 Jarow JP (1994). Life-threatening conditions associated with male infertility. *Urol. Clin. North Am.* **21**: 409–15.

3 Spira A (1986). Epidemiology of human reproduction. *Hum. Reprod.* **1**: 111–15.

4 Kim ED, Lipschultz LI (1999). Evaluation and imaging of the infertile male. *Infertil. Reprod. Med. Clin. North Am.* **10**(3): 377–410.

5 Jarow JP, Sharlip ID, Belker AM, Lipshultz LI, Sigman M, Thomas AJ et al. (2002). Best practice policies for male infertility. *J. Urol.* **167**: 2138–44.

6 Rusnack SL, Wu HY, Huff DS, Snyder HM 3rd, Carr MC, Bellah RD et al. (2003). Testis histopathology in boys with cryptorchidism correlates with future fertility potential. *J. Urol.* **169**: 659–62.

7 Cortes D, Thorup J, Lindenberg S, Visfeldt J (2003). Infertility despite surgery for cryptorchidism in childhood can be classified by patients with normal or elevated follicle-stimulating hormone and identified at orchidopexy. *BJU Int.* **91**: 670–4.

8 Lin YM, Hsu CC, Lin JS (1999). Successful testicular sperm extraction and fertilization in an azoospermic man with postpubertal mumps orchitis. *BJU Int.* **83**: 526–7.

9 Jarow JP (2003). Endocrine causes of male infertility. *Urol. Clin. North Am.* **30**: 83–90.

10 Stanford JB, White GL, Hatasaka H (2002). Timing intercourse to achieve pregnancy: current evidence. *Obstet. Gynecol.* **100**: 1333–41.

11 Lenzi A, Lombardo F, Salacone P, Gandini L, Jannini EA (2003). Stress, sexual dysfunctions, and male infertility. *J. Endocrinol. Invest.* **26**(3, Suppl.): 72–6.

12 Jain K, Radhakrishnan G, Agrawal P (2000). Infertility and psychosexual disorders: relationship in infertile couples. *Indian J. Med. Sci.* **54**(1): 1–7.

13 Nudell DM, Monoski MM, Lipshultz LI (2002). Common medications and drugs: how they affect male fertility. *Urol. Clin. North Am.* **29**: 965–73.

14 Hruska KS, Furth PA, Seifer DB, Sharara FI, Flaws JA (2000). Environmental factors in infertility. *Clin. Obstet. Gynecol.* **43**: 821–9.

15 Jarow J (2000). Effects of varicocele on male fertility. *Hum. Reprod. Update* **7**: 59–64.

16 McLachlan RI, Baker HW, Clarke GN, Harrison KL, Matson PL, Holden CA *et al.* (2003). Semen analysis: its place in modern reproductive medical practice. *Pathology* **35**: 25–33.

17 Jeyendran RS, Van der Ven HH, Zaneveld LJ (1992). The hypoosmotic swelling test: an update. *Arch. Androl.* **29**(2): 105–16.

18 Van Waart J, Kruger TF, Lombard CJ, Ombelet W (2001). Predictive value of normal sperm morphology in intrauterine insemination (IUI): a structured literature review. *Hum. Reprod. Update* **7**: 495–500.

19 Bar-Chama N, Goluboff E, Fisch H (1994). Infection and pyospermia in male infertility. Is it really a problem? *Urol. Clin. North Am.* **21**(3): 469–75.

20 Lombardo F, Gandini L, Dondero F, Lenzi A (2001). Antisperm immunity in natural and assisted reproduction. *Hum. Reprod. Update* **7**: 450–6.

21 Jeyendran RS, Van der Ven HH, Zaneveld LJ (1992). The hypoosmotic swelling test: an update. *Arch. Androl.* **29**: 105–16.

22 Montoya JM, Bernal A, Borrero C (2002). Diagnostics in assisted human reproduction. *Reprod. Biomed. Online* **5**: 198–210.

23 Evenson DP, Larson KL, Jost LK (2002). Sperm chromatin structure assay: its clinical use for detecting sperm DNA fragmentation in male infertility and comparisons with other techniques. *J. Androl.* **23**: 25–43.

24 Liu PY, Handelsman DJ (2003). The present and future state of hormonal treatment for male infertility. *Hum. Reprod. Update* **9**(1): 9–23.

25 Kowalcek I, Wihstutz N, Buhrow G, Diedrich K (2001). Subjective well-being in infertile couples. *Psychosom. Obstet. Gynaecol.* **22**: 143–8.

26 Kowalcek I, Wihstutz N, Buhrow G, Diedrich K (2001). Coping with male infertility. Gender differences. *Arch. Gynecol. Obstet.* **265**(3): 131–6.

27 Newton CR, Sherrard W, Glavac I (1999). The Fertility Problem Inventory: measuring perceived infertility-related stress. *Fertil. Steril.* **72**: 54–62.

28 Mahlstedt PP (1997). Psychological issues of infertility and assisted reproductive technology. In: *Infertility in the Male* (ed. LI Lipschultz, SE Howards), pp. 462–75. Mosby, St Louis, MO.

29 Lee TY, Sun GH, Chao SC (2001). The effect of an infertility diagnosis on treatment-related stresses. *Arch. Androl.* **46**(1): 67–71.

30 Hjelmstedt A, Andersson L, Skoog-Svanberg A, Bergh T, Boivin J, Collins A (1999). Gender differences in psychological reactions to infertility among couples seeking IVF- and ICSI-treatment. *Acta Obstet. Gynecol. Scand.* **78**: 42–8.

31 Kainz K (2001). The role of the psychologist in the evaluation and treatment of infertility. *Women's Health Issues* **11**: 481–5.

32 Mak V, Jarvi KA (1996). The genetics of male infertility. *J. Urol.* **156**(4): 1245–56.

33 Siddiq FM, Sigman M (2002). A new look at the medical management of infertility. *Urol. Clin. North Am.* **29**(4): 949–63.

34 Nagler HM, Rotman M (2002). Predictive parameters for microsurgical reconstruction. *Urol. Clin. North Am.* **29**: 913–19.

35 **Braude P, Rowell P** (2003). Assisted conception. II—*in vitro* fertilisation and intracytoplasmic sperm injection. *Br. Med. J.* **327**: 852–5.

36 **Adamson GD, Baker VL** (2003). Subfertility: causes, treatment and outcome. *Best Pract. Res. Clin. Obstet. Gynaecol.* **17**: 169–85.

37 **Peters K** (2003). In pursuit of motherhood: the IVF experience. *Contemp. Nurs.* **14**: 258–70.

38 **Daniels KR** (2002). Toward a family-building approach to donor insemination. *Obstet. Gynaecol. Can.* **24**:17–21.

Chapter 24

The patient presenting with an overactive adrenal gland

Franco Mantero and Nora Albiger

Introduction

The adrenal gland can be the site of hormonally active or inactive lesions, benign or malignant tumours, metastases, and infections. The prognosis in patients having an adrenal abnormality depends not only on the benign or malignant character of the lesion but also on its hormonal activity. For example, patients with primary aldosteronism can suffer from resistant hypertension with its chronic complications, patients with phaeochromocytoma can present in a hypertensive crisis that can be fatal and patients with Cushing's syndrome have high risks of atherosclerosis, thrombosis, and osteoporosis. These situations can often be prevented or reversed by an accurate assessment including careful evaluation of clinical, biochemical, and morphological features. Matching the optimal therapy with the cause can usually often produce a definitive solution.

Primary aldosteronism

Primary aldosteronism (PA) is characterized by hypertension, hypokalaemia, low plasma renin activity, and increased aldosterone secretion. The introduction of the plasma aldosterone concentration/plasma renin activity ratio (PAC/PRA ratio) as a screening test in normokalaemic hypertensive patients has increased the prevalence rates to 5–10% of all hypertensive patients.[1,2]

Classically, PA subtypes are considered as:

- unilateral aldosterone-producing adenoma (APA) accounting for 65–75% of cases and including angiotensin II responsives;
- idiopathic adrenal hyperplasia (IHA)—bilateral (25–30%) or unilateral (1–2%);
- primary adrenal hyperplasia;
- glucocorticoid-remediable aldosteronism (GRA); and
- aldosterone-producing adrenocortical carcinoma.

More widespread screening for PA has increased the proportion of patients having probable IHA compared with APA.[3]

New concepts in aldosterone biology

Aldosterone has a fundamental role in extracellular volume regulation and potassium metabolism through its renal actions. Since mineralocorticoid receptors have been found in non-epithelial tissues, new horizons have opened on aldosterone actions, principally at a cardiovascular level. Hyperaldosteronism induces perivascular fibrosis that is preceded by a pro-inflammatory vascular phenotype that features invading monocytes/macrophages and lymphocytes and adhesion molecule expression. These findings are independent of blood pressure values.[4] An induction of oxidative stress with inflammatory cell activation at vascular sites that precedes the fibrogenic response has been described.[5] Co-treatment with spironolactone and/or an antioxidant prevents the appearance of these cells and associated molecular responses, as well as the subsequent perivascular fibrosis. Aldosterone also induces endothelial vasomotor dysfunction that is normalized by spironolactone alone or in combination with an angiotensin-converting enzyme (ACE) inhibitor.[6]

Diagnosis

Initial and confirmatory diagnosis

Initially, hypokalaemia was considered a hallmark in the diagnosis of PA; however, it is now known that most patients are normokalaemic. A raised PAC/PRA ratio in the upright posture is widely accepted as screening test for PA because of its high sensitivity.[7] It is still debated whether all patients with hypertension should be screened for PA, but there is no debate regarding those patients with hypertension and hypokalaemia (i.e. regardless of presumed cause), patients with resistant hypertension, those with a family history of hypertension, those who have had a stroke at a young age, or patients with adrenal incidentaloma. A large study on adrenal incidentalomas revealed that 1.6% were aldosteronomas.[8]

The cut-off value for the PAC/PRA ratio to consider the possibility of a PA should be calculated on the basis of normal reference ranges for PAC and PRA in each centre. PAC and PRA should be respectively expressed in ng/dl and ng/ml/h. A ratio greater than 20 with a PAC $\geq$ 15 ng/dl has been considered suspicious for a diagnosis of PA.[3] In our experience a PAC/PRA ratio > 40, with minimum PRA levels of 0.2 ng/ml/h, has a sensitivity of 100% and a specificity of 84.4% in screening patients with suspected PA.

Several drugs can interfere with PAC and PRA determinations. Classically, it was recommended that patients undergoing this evaluation should be off of all antihypertensive treatment for at least 2–3 weeks. However, if severe hypertension is present, total washout could be unsafe. In these cases, use of calcium channel blockers and alpha-blockers seems is a valid option. Some authors permit antihypertensive therapy, except anti-aldosterone drugs, while doing the test.[3,9] If hypokalaemia is present, plasma potassium should be normalized and the ratio remeasured 2 weeks later.

Dynamic tests are usually necessary to confirm PA. A sodium-loading test using fludrocortisone or saline infusion is employed. Fludrocortisone is administered at a dose of 0.1 mg four times daily for 4 days during dietary supplementation with 20–30 mmol sodium four times daily, with measurements of aldosterone at the beginning and on days 3 and 4. PA is confirmed if upright PAC is ≥ 5 ng/dl. Oral potassium supplementation may be needed. A saline infusion test is performed with an intravenous infusion of 2 litres of 0.9% (isotonic) saline over 4 hours while the patient is in the supine position. PA is confirmed if PAC levels at the end of the test remain > 10 ng/dl, is highly probable with levels > 7.5 ng/dl, and is excluded when PAC levels are < 5 ng/dl.[10] The captopril test has also been evaluated as a screening or confirmatory test. It is administered orally, 25–50 mg, and the PAC/PRA ratio is measured after 2 hours, or after 1 hour if 50 mg is used, with the patient in the upright position. A ratio > 20 is highly indicative, while a ratio > 30 in a patient with a previously raised PAC/PRA ratio confirms PA.[11,12]

Subtype differentiation

Subtype differentiation is important because of its therapeutic implications. Patients with APA are usually more hypertensive, have higher plasma and urinary levels of aldosterone, and are younger (i.e. < 50 years old) than patients with IHA. However, these data are not absolute in discriminating between the two.

Computed tomography (CT) is the first step in subtype evaluation. An abdominal CT scan with 3 to 5 mm slices through the adrenal regions will demonstrate the majority of adenomas, although very small lesions might be missed. Magnetic resonance imaging (MRI) of the abdomen gives good resolution of the adrenal glands but usually adds little to the information gained by CT. Scintigraphy with iodocholesterol provides morphological and functional data for the adrenals and can be useful in some cases.[13]

Nodules < 1 cm in diameter can be misleading if only a CT is done. Adrenal venous sampling (AVS) remains the gold standard for the differential diagnosis of PA but catheterizing of the right adrenal vein is difficult, and a procedure success rate of 70–80% has been described in experienced hands. It should be performed when other tests are inconclusive (e.g. normal adrenal, thickened limb, micronodularity, and atypical or bilateral masses).[14,15] Considering the age-dependent risk that a solitary unilateral adrenal adenoma may be a non-functioning cortical adenoma, some authors recommend performing AVS in all patients older than 40 years with diagnosis of PA.

Some dynamic tests can help in subtype differentiation, but their sensitivity and specificity are low. After 2 hours supine, PAC values show an increase of ≥ 50% over baseline in patients with IHA or angiotensin II-responsive adenomas, while it does not increase in patients with GRA or APA. A similar response is obtained after the infusion of angiotensin II. A partial response could be seen in patients with IHA after administration of captopril.[11]

Treatment

The optimal management for each patient depends on subtype differentiation. Classically, surgery has been considered the treatment of choice in patients with APA and unilateral adrenal hyperplasia and medical management for the hyperplasia sub-types. In some cases (e.g. where there are contraindications to surgery, patients who refuse surgery, or as pre-operative treatment), medical management of APA can be a reasonable option.[16]

The rationale for aldosterone normalization or mineralocorticoid receptor blockade is to prevent the morbidity and mortality associated not only with hypertension and hypokalaemia but also with the known effects of aldosterone excess on the cardio-vascular system. Clinical evidence has demonstrated the beneficial effects of aldosterone antagonism in patients with heart failure. In the randomized aldactone evaluation study (RALES), aldosterone blockade with spironolactone produced a 30% reduction in mortality in patients with stage IV congestive heart failure.[17] In the international trial, Eplerenone Heart Failure Efficacy and Survival Study (EPHESUS), the use of eplerenone demonstrated a reduction in morbidity and mortality in patients after acute myocardial infarction.[18]

Surgical treatment

Surgical treatment is the treatment of choice in patients with APA. A laparoscopic approach is preferred because it is associated with a shorter hospitalization and less morbidity. Pre-operative blood pressure response to mineralocorticoid receptor antag-onism often predicts the subsequent response to adrenal surgery.[19] A careful analysis of parameters such us family history, age, pre-operative levels of hypertension, type of tumour, and presence of signs of end-organ damage are important to understand the persistence of hypertension that is seen in some patients after successful surgery.[20]

Medical treatment

Several drugs have been used in PA treatment (see Table 24.1).

Aldosterone receptor antagonists These drugs reduce the extracellular volume con-tributing to a lowering of blood pressure, normalize serum potassium levels, and activ-ate the suppressed renin–angiotensin system. Used as pre-operative treatment, the function of the contralateral adrenal is activated in the hope that post-operative hypoaldosteronism may be avoided. Spironolactone is a non-selective mineralocorti-coid receptor antagonist. The starting dose is 25–50 mg twice daily increasing to a maximum of 200–400 mg. Its use may be limited because of dose-dependent side-effects including gynaecomastia, erectile dysfunction, and menstrual irregularities that result from its affinity for androgen and progesterone receptors. In about 30% of patients the drug must be changed because of adverse effects. Another 30–50% of patients need additional antihypertensive drugs to obtain an adequate reduction of blood pressure.[21]

Table 24.1 Medical therapy for primary aldosteronism

Class of drug	Name
Aldosterone receptor antagonists	Spironolactone, potassium canrenoate, canrenone, eplerenone
Sodium epithelial channels blockers	Amiloride, triamterene
Calcium channel blockers	
Angiotensin converting enzyme inhibitors (ACEI)	
Angiotensin II receptor blockers (ARB)	
Aldosterone synthesis inhibitors	Trilostane, metyrapone, heparin, dopamine agonists

Potassium canrenoate is a water-soluble spironolactone derivative, which appears to induce fewer adverse effects than spironolactone in chronic treatment regimens.[22] Our group assessed the biological anti-androgen activity of spironolactone and potassium canrenoate in a mouse kidney cytosol receptor assay and demonstrated that spirono-lactone is four times as potent an anti-androgen as potassium canrenoate.[23] Potassium canrenoate is used in doses of 100 mg daily. In our experience therapy was changed due to adverse effects in only 11% of patients.[21,24]

Eplerenone is a competitive and selective aldosterone receptor antagonist. It has less affinity for androgen and progesterone receptors than spironolactone. It has demonstrated efficacy in the treatment of essential hypertension at doses of 50 to 400 mg per day.[25] The evaluation of eplerenone efficacy in the treatment of PA is in progress.

Sodium channel blockers Although there are no randomized double-blind studies on the use of amiloride in primary aldosteronism, some clinicians use them. A daily dose of 40 mg of amiloride is typical but is less effective as monotherapy when compared with spironolactone.[26] About 75% of patients need other antihypertensive drugs to control blood pressure.

Calcium channel blockers Calcium channel blockers may reduce aldosterone secretion, but this action is neither significant nor sustained despite a significant reduction of blood pressure.[27] Calcium maintains raised systemic vascular resistance and plays a role in aldosterone secretion. A study examining the acute and chronic effects of oral nifedipine and intravenous verapamil in patients with hyperaldosteronism showed a slight decrease of plasma aldosterone values only when nifedipine was chronically administered in IHA subjects, whereas no significant decrease was noticed in APA subjects.[27] There was a greater reduction in aldosterone values in patients with IHA following verapamil but these changes were not significantly different from those seen in control patients.[28] In a separate study, calcium blockers were given to 16 patients as first choice but 15 required the addition of another antihypertensive drug.[21]

Drugs with effect on angiotensin II levels or action ACE inhibitors block angiotensin II generation and reduce blood pressure levels in patients with IHA more than in those with APA, due to greater adrenal sensitivity to angiotensin II in IHA. Similar responses were seen with captopril (75 mg/day)[11] or enalapril (80 mg/day).[29] There is less experience with angiotensin II type I receptor blockers but they may be used in combination with other drugs in primary aldosteronism.[30]

Aldosterone synthesis inhibitors There is no high-level evidence to recommend the use of these medications in primary aldosteronism because their ability to reduce plasma aldosterone is not clearly associated with reduced blood pressure.[31,32]

Phaeochromocytoma

Phaeochromocytomas represent the cause of hypertension in 0.1–0.5% of patients; 4% of patients present with an adrenal incidentaloma.[8] They are neuroendocrine tumours arising from chromaffin cells in the adrenal medulla. Paragangliomas are chromaffin cell tumours derived from the paraganglia and can be of sympathetic or parasympathetic origin. The most common location of paragangliomas include the para-aortic region, urinary bladder, thorax, carotid body, and pelvis.[33]

Sporadic phaeochromocytomas are the most frequent form of disease but up to 30% may be a component of hereditary syndromes. This percentage is higher than the historically reported 10% due to our increasing knowledge from genetic studies. These syndromes include multiple endocrine neoplasia type 2 (MEN2), von Hippel–Lindau (VHL) disease, and neurofibromatosis type 1 (NF-1), and are associated with an autosomal dominant inheritance pattern with variable penetrance. Recently, genes related to subunits of the mitochondrial complex II have been identified as a cause of phaeochromocytoma and/or paraganglioma. These genes are called the SDHX genes (e.g. *SDHD*, *SDHB* and *SDHC*) for the succinate oxido-reductase subunit.[34,35] The short arm of chromosome 1 harbours one or more genes implicated in the development of phaeochromocytoma.[36]

Clinical presentation

As a result of catecholamine excess, there is a stimulation of adrenergic receptors with expression of clinical symptoms and signs of overactivity of the sympathetic system. The most consistent sign is hypertension that may be sporadic or persistent and suggestive symptoms are marked sweating (71%), pallor, anxiety, profound headaches (80%), palpitations (64%), and weight loss[37]. It is also suspected in patients with unexplained shock or marked hypertensive response during parturition, surgery, induction of anaesthesia, or severe trauma. In the presence of familial history of phaeochromocytoma, screening is mandatory.

Diagnosis

The diagnosis of phaeochromocytoma consists of demonstrating an increased catecholamine or metabolite production and locating the tumour.

Biochemical diagnosis

Biochemical assessment requires measurement of catecholamines (i.e. epinephrine and norepinephrine) and their metabolites (i.e. metanephrine and normetanephrine) which are present in plasma or urine in free and conjugated forms. A single measurement of fractionated plasma metanephrines may be superior to combinations of other biochemical tests in detecting or excluding phaeochromocytoma. In a multicentre study, sensitivities of plasma free metanephrines (99%) and urinary fractionated metanephrines (97%) were higher than those for plasma or urinary catecholamines, urinary total metanephrines and urinary vanillylmandelic acid. Specificity was highest for urinary vanillylmandelic acid (95%) and urinary total metanephrines (93%), while it was intermediate for plasma free metanephrines (89%) and urinary and plasma catecholamines (88 and 81% respectively).[38] Because of the high sensitivity, the determination of plasma free metanephrines by high-performance liquid chromatography (HPLC) is recommended as the initial biochemical test of choice. Measurements of 24-hour urinary fractioned metanephrines (i.e. with a sensitivity of 97% and a specificity of 93%) would be the second choice when plasma determinations are not available.[39] False positive results are likely to remain a problem when refer ence intervals are established using the 95% confidence intervals of values from a reference population. To provide an acceptable level of specificity of testing, the diagnostic cut-off for urinary catecholamines or metanephrines in the diagnosis of phaeochromocytoma used at the Mayo Clinic are approximately two-fold higher than those for the normal population range.[40]

HPLC, coupled with electrochemical or fluorometric detection is the most common method for detecting urinary or plasma catecholamines and metanephrines. Spectrophotometric or fluorometric assays of urinary metanephrines are used in many laboratories but are limited by not separating the fractioned forms. New methods like mass spectrophotometry (e.g. gas chromatography–mass spectrometry and liquid chromatography–tandem mass spectrometry) should provide higher specificity than HPLC.[41,42]

In the assessment of the biochemical diagnosis, it is important to be aware of medical conditions or medications that can interfere with catecholamine or metanephrine determinations. Catecholamines may be secreted episodically by a phaeochromocytoma, and so normal values may be found between episodes. Some dietary constituents can stimulate catecholamine or dopamine secretion (e.g. caffeine, cereals, cheeses, bananas); tricyclic antidepressants, antipsychotics, levodopa, ethanol, acetaminophen, and phenoxybenzamine, drugs containing cathecolamines and withdrawal from clonidine may cause false positive results. Labetalol can cause spurious elevations of epinephrine and interfere with spectrophotometric or HPLC assays for catecholamines or metanephrines.[40] It is recommended to stop medications for at least 2 weeks before doing the tests in order to avoid this problem.

In order to distinguish true from false positive forms, the clonidine test may be helpful. Plasma normetanephrine or norepinephrine is measured at baseline and after 3 hours of 0.3 mg oral clonidine administration. Clonidine decreases norepinephrine release from sympathetic nerves and a positive test is considered when the plasma concentration of normetanephrine falls to less than 40% of basal with a final concentration remaining above the upper normal reference limit. Considering these criteria, the sensitivity is 96% and specificity 98%.[43] Glucagon testing should be avoided.

Imaging studies

CT has a good sensitivity (e.g. 93–100%) but limited specificity for the detection of phaeochromocytomas and the sensitivity is less for extra-adrenal forms. Characteristic images consistent with phaeochromocytoma include enhancement with intravenous contrast medium, variable size, and bilaterality. Cystic and haemorrhagic changes also suggest a phaeochromocytoma. MRI can be helpful by showing a high signal intensity on T_2-weighted images. The presence of bilateral, multiple, and multicentric forms suggests an inherited form.[44] ^{123}I-metaiodobenzylguanidine scintigraphy, which exploits the functional characteristic of chromaffin cells in the uptake of precursor amines, has excellent specificity (e.g. 95–100%) and is useful in the diagnosis of extra-adrenal tumours. When all of these imaging studies are negative, positron emission tomography (PET) with 6-(^{18}F)fluorodopamine may be helpful.[45]

Treatment of phaeochromocytoma

Surgery is the treatment of choice. Medical treatment is recommended to improve pre-operative status, to reduce intra-operative complications, when surgery is not possible, or in cases of extended diseases where surgical procedures are only palliative.

Medical treatment

Pre-operative antihypertensive therapy is useful to reduce intra-operative complications as a consequence of catecholamine release from tumour manipulation. The peri-operative course is smoother and there is a reduction in peri-operative mortality when α-adrenergic receptor antagonists are given pre-operatively.[46] A single paper suggests that adequate intra-operative management may eliminate the need for preparing patients for surgery since no patients died or had cardiovascular complications as a consequence of surgery[47] but this is not currently considered an adequate standard of care.

Adequate pre-operative α-adrenergic receptor blockade produces vasodilatation leading to orthostatic hypotension and increased blood volume causing a reduction in haematocrit; 1–2 weeks of treatment may be necessary to reach these objectives.[48] Phenoxybenzamine is a non-selective α-adrenergic receptor antagonist that inhibits of presynaptic α_2-adrenergic receptors and may produce enough reflex tachycardia that β-adrenergic receptor antagonism is necessary. Due to its long half-life (>24 hours) prolonged hypotension can be observed post-operatively and large volumes of intravenous fluids may be required. The initial dose is 10 mg that is increased by 10 mg increments daily until there is orthostatic hypotension and a drop in the haematocrit; typical requirements are 1 mg/kg/day in divided doses.[49]

Selectively competitive α_1-adrenergic receptor antagonists offer potential advantages compared with phenoxybenzamine. For example, prazosin and doxazosin do not produce reflex tachycardia because of their selectivity on α_1-adrenergic receptors. Since their half-lives are shorter than phenoxybenzamine, the likelihood of post-operative hypotension is decreased.[46,48] Doxazosin can be administrated in single daily doses of 1 to 16 mg. Prazosin and terazosin require more frequent dosing because they have a shorter half-lives. The prazosin dose is 1 mg three to four times daily and it may be increased up to 10 mg daily; the maximal terazosin dose is 20 mg at night.[50]

One definition of adequate pre-operative blockade includes the following criteria:[51]

- no blood pressure over 160/90 mmHg 24–48 hours before surgery,
- mild orthostatic hypotension, but not blood pressure below 80/45 mmHg,
- no ST–T changes in the electrocardiogram within the last 1–2 weeks, and
- fewer than two premature ventricular contractions within 5 minutes.

Calcium channel antagonists may be used in patients with paroxysmal hypertension because they do not produce orthostatic hypotension; they probably reduce arterial pressure by inhibiting norepinephrine-mediated transmembrane calcium influx in vascular smooth muscle. The usual effective dose of nifedipine is 30 to 90 mg/day.[48] The use of calcium channel antagonists alone is ineffective for the protection of intra-operative hypertension and tachycardia.[52]

Pre-treatment with β-adrenergic receptor antagonists may be necessary in patients with tachycardia but it should only be initiated in the presence of an adequate α-adrenergic receptor blockade.[46] α-Methyl-p-tyrosine competitively inhibits tyrosine hydroxylase, which is the rate-limiting step in catecholamine biosynthesis. The initial dose is 0.5 mg up to a maximum of 4 mg daily given for about 5 days pre-operatively. There is a high incidence of adverse effects including weakness and fatigue when α-methyl-p-tyrosine is used.[53]

In cases of malignant phaeochromocytoma, when radical surgical resection is impossible, other supportive treatment modalities such as ^{131}I-metaiodobenzylguanidine (^{131}I-MIBG) should be considered. ^{131}I-MIBG generates a symptomatic response rate of 45% and a tumour response of 30%.[54] Applied doses range from 3.7 to 9.8 GBq given intravenously over 2–3 hours with intervals of 3 to 6 months. Cumulative doses range between 3.8 and 85.9 GBq.[55] It is usually well tolerated but can induce toxic effects on bone marrow so that the cumulative dosage should be limited to 40–45 GBq. ^{131}I-MIBG therapy should be used when there is tracer uptake in tumour tissue or the majority of known tumour lesions. Some reports have demonstrated a complete remission of disease with a long period of follow-up.[56]

Somatostatin receptor expression has been found in phaeochromocytoma tissue (sst2 receptors) so that the combination of long-acting octreotide with ^{131}I-MIBG may have a future role.[57] Chemotherapy should be considered in cases of inadequate nuclide uptake or lack of ^{131}I-MIBG response. The most frequent protocol employed is based on the use of cyclophosphamide, vincristine, and dacarbazine. With this regimen a complete remission was reported in two out of 14 patients, a partial remission in six and progression in one.[58] A combination of ^{131}I-MIBG with chemotherapy is also a reasonable approach since cisplatin and doxorubicin have been demonstrated, *in vitro*, to improve ^{131}I-MIBG uptake.[59] Phenoxybenzamine is useful in doses of 30–50 mg daily divided in four to five doses to control hypertension and other symptoms. In cases of excessive production of catecholamines, the use of α-methyl-p-tyrosine may help.[53]

Surgical treatment

Laparoscopic adrenalectomy is the preferred approach because of the short hospital stay needed, but open surgery is still occasionally necessary when the lesion is very large or there are intra-operative difficulties.[60] Patients with hereditary phaeochromocytoma usually present with multifocal and/or bilateral tumours requiring excision of all lesions including the possibility of bilateral adrenalectomy; this would require adrenocorticoid and mineralocorticoid replacement after surgery. Theoretically, this could be prevented by performing autotransplantation of adrenocortical tissue or subtotal adrenalectomy. Experience with autotransplantation has been disappointing;[61] a variable rate of recurrence has been reported following subtotal adrenalectomy.[60,62]

Cushing's syndrome of adrenal origin

ACTH-independent Cushing's syndrome (CS) represents 15–20% of cases with classic CS mainly due to an adrenal adenoma. Adrenal carcinoma, ACTH-independent macronodular adrenal hyperplasia (AIMAH), which depends on the abnormal or ectopic adrenal expression of receptors for various ligands, and primary pigmented nodular adrenocortical disease (PPNAD), which is often associated with Carney complex, are rare forms of CS. Nine per cent of patients with an adrenal incidentaloma may harbour an adenoma with autonomous glucocorticoid production.[8] These patients lack the characteristic signs or symptoms of glucocorticoid excess, so this entity is termed subclinical or pre-clinical CS.

Clinical presentation

Characteristic features of Cushing's syndrome are the moon face, central obesity, hirsutism, supraclavicular fat accumulation, buffalo hump, thinned skin, striae, ecchymosis, oligomenorrhoea, and neuropsychological disturbances (e.g. depression, emotional irritability, sleep disturbances, and cognitive deficits). There is a high prevalence of atherosclerosis due to visceral obesity, systemic arterial hypertension, impairment of glucose tolerance, hyperlipidaemia, and thrombotic diathesis that can persist after long-term cure. Osteopenia and osteoporosis are seen frequently.[63]

Diagnosis of Cushing's syndrome

Biochemical evaluation[64]

Screening tests *Urinary free cortisol (UFC)* Twenty-four-hour UFC gives an integrated index of the free cortisol that circulates in blood. To validate the results, up to three 24-hour urine collections should be performed in conjunction with urinary creatinine. Measurements using HPLC have a high sensitivity and specificity. Milder elevations of urinary cortisol can be found in conditions such as chronic anxiety, depression, and alcoholism, all of which are known as pseudo-Cushing states.

Low-dose dexamethasone suppression test (DST) DST consists of administering 1 mg of dexamethasone orally at 11.00p.m., followed by measurement of fasting plasma cortisol between 8.00 and 9.00a.m. the following morning. The classical criterion for normal suppression is a plasma cortisol level below 5 μg/dl (138 nmol/l). More recently, this cut-off level has been reduced to less than 1.8 μg/dl (50 nmol/l). In some centres, a 2-day 2 mg DST (i.e. 0.5 mg dexamethasone orally every 6 hours) is used as the first screening test. Urine is collected for UFC on two baseline days and on the second day of dexamethasone administration, or alternatively serum cortisol is measured at 9.00a.m. and 48 hours after the first dose. A normal response consists of a decrease of UFC to less than 10 μg (27 nmol) per 24 hours on the second day of dexamethasone administration or of plasma cortisol to less than 1.8 μg/dl (50 nmol/l) on the morning after the last dose of dexamethasone.

Cortisol circadian rhythm Patients with CS often have early morning serum cortisol concentrations within or slightly above the normal range, but lack a normal circadian rhythm. Plasma cortisol levels are above a cut-off value of 1.8 μg/dl (50 nmol/l) when measured at midnight in hospitalized, sleeping CS patients (i.e. requires in-patient admission for a period of at least 48 hours). Salivary cortisol is highly correlated with free plasma cortisol and since it has high sensitivity and specificity it is another simple way to screen for CS and may replace plasma cortisol determination to evaluate circadian rhythm.

Low-dose DST and combined DST-CRH test This has been shown to be highly accurate in distinguishing CS from pseudo-CS (i.e. when there is a blunted response to exogenous CRH after dexamethasone administration due to a chronic CRH stimulation). After administrating 2 mg DST for 2 days, CRH (1 μg/kg) is injected intravenously (IV) at 08.00a.m. (i.e. 2 hours after the last dose of dexamethasone). The plasma cortisol value 15 min after CRH is greater than 1.4 μg/dl (38 nmol/l) in patients with CS, but remains suppressed in normal individuals and in patients with pseudo-CS.

Differential diagnosis

ACTH measurement Fasting morning ACTH concentrations below the level of detection or below 10 pg/ml (2 pmol/l) suggest an ACTH-independent cause of CS. Plasma ACTH values greater than 20 pg/ml (4 pmol/l) suggest an ACTH-dependent cause. For values between 10 and 20 pg/ml (2–4 pmol/l), a CRH stimulation test is indicated, with measurement of plasma ACTH.

High-dose DST Two different oral protocols are used (i.e. 2 mg every 6 hours for eight doses or 8 mg overnight). Plasma cortisol is measured at 8:00a.m. after the last dose of DST or the following morning if the overnight protocol is used. High doses of glucocorticoids partially suppress ACTH secretion from most corticotroph adenomas (80–90%), whereas ectopic tumours and adrenal tumours are resistant to feedback inhibition. A cut-off of plasma cortisol suppression above 50% is present with most pituitary adenomas.

CRH stimulation test Intravenous 1 μg/kg or 100 μg synthetic ovine or human CRH is administrated and plasma ACTH and serum cortisol are measured every 15 min for 2 hours. Most pituitary tumours, and a few ectopic ACTH-secreting tumours, respond to CRH administration with an increase in plasma ACTH and cortisol levels. In adrenal CS, there is usually little or no cortisol or ACTH response to CRH. The criteria used are an increase above baseline in ACTH of 35–50% and cortisol of 14–20%.

Desmopressin test Desmopressin (i.e. 10 μg IV) increases ACTH secretion in 80–90% of patients with CS and only rarely in normal individuals or patients with pseudo-CS. However, 20–50% of ectopic ACTH-secreting tumors respond to desmopressin, thus limiting its usefulness in distinguishing the source of excess ACTH.

Several dynamic tests are used in the diagnosis of AIMAH and help to evaluate the regulation of cortisol production resulting from an abnormal adrenocortical response either to food intake (e.g. in cases of ectopic adrenal expression of the gastric inhibitory polypeptide receptor), vasopressin, beta-adrenergic receptor agonists, hCG/LH, or serotonin 5-HT-4 receptor agonists.

Imaging studies

A pituitary MRI with gadolinium enhancement should be performed in all patients with ACTH-dependent CS. This will reveal a discrete pituitary adenoma in up to 60%. In those in whom biochemical studies are not conclusive for a pituitary origin, bilateral inferior petrosal sinus (IPS) sampling may be helpful. Blood samples for ACTH are obtained at baseline and at 3 and 5 min after 1 μg/kg or 100 μg IV of CRH, simultaneously from both IPSs and a peripheral vein. An IPS to peripheral ACTH ratio (IPS/P) greater than 2.0 in the basal state and/or greater than 3.0 after CRH is consistent with a pituitary origin.

An abdominal CT will help in the diagnosis of adrenal forms. Adrenal adenomas differentiate from carcinomas because the latter are usually >5 cm, invade surrounding structures, and demonstrate necrosis, cystic degeneration, or calcification.[65] PPNAD can reveal a normal adrenal gland or unilateral or bilateral nodularity, bilateral enlargement, a unilateral mass, or asymmetric bilateral nodularity. AIMAH usually presents with bilateral, nodular, enlarged adrenal masses.

Scintigraphy with ^{131}I-norcholesterol will show unilateral tracer uptake due to increased glucocorticoid production by the tumour while the contralateral adrenal gland will be scintigraphically silent due to atrophy. Malignant forms can reveal some bilateral silent uptake. Fluorodeoxyglucose-positron emission tomography (FDG-PET) imaging may be helpful to differentiate adrenal metastases from benign adenomas.[66]

A chest CT or MRI should be done when an ectopic form is suspected. Occasionally, occult ACTH-secreting tumours express somatostatin receptors that can be identified by somatostatin analogue scintigraphy using with ^{111}In-pentetreotide.

Treatment

Surgical treatment

Surgical treatment is the first choice in all forms of Cushing's syndrome when the origin of cortisol excess has been identified. Unilateral adrenalectomy is performed for both adrenal adenoma and carcinoma. Post-operative glucocorticoid replacement is necessary because the secretion of the contralateral gland is suppressed. Bilateral adrenalectomy is an option for ACTH-dependent forms after unsuccessful pituitary surgery or when the patient has persistently elevated glucocorticoids following pituitary radiotherapy. Life-long glucocorticoid and mineralocorticoid replacement is necessary after bilateral adrenalectomy. The principal long-term complication is hyperpigmentation due to the development of an enlarging pituitary tumour (Nelson's syndrome). In cases of PPNAD and AIMAH, bilateral adrenalectomy is curative.[67]

Medical treatment

Medical management is indicated in preparation for surgery, after unsuccessful surgery, while waiting for a radiotherapy response, or in cases of adrenal carcinomas. Ketoconazole, metyrapone, aminoglutetimide and o, p'-DDD (Mitotane) act principally on the adrenal cortex to reduce cortisol secretion. Centrally acting agents such as bromocriptine, cyproheptadine, and sodium valproate can occasionally induce remission but should be reserved for patients with pituitary forms refractory to the more effective medications mentioned. Ketoconazole acts on the cytochrome P-450 enzyme system and, in doses of 200 to 1200 mg/day, normalizes cortisol secretion in patients with CS. Its major adverse effect is hepatotoxicity that usually resolves after withdrawal of the drug. Metyrapone acts on the cytochrome P-450 enzyme responsible for the final step in cortisol synthesis. Its efficacy in controlling cortisol excess in patients with adrenocortical and ectopic tumours is well established.[68] Adrenocortical insufficiency is the major risk if doses are not closely monitored. Women may develop hirsutism or mild acne.

Management of adrenocortical carcinoma

Approximately 60% of all adrenal carcinomas are functioning. They often present with rapid onset of symptoms and signs of hormonal excess. CS is the most frequent form of presentation but these lesions can also secrete excess androgens, oestrogens, and mineralocorticoids. Surgery continues to be the treatment of choice whenever possible, and margin-free resection is a predictor of long-term survival. In cases of a presumable carcinoma, an open surgical approach is preferred since invasion of or adherence to adjacent organs may require a more extensive excision. In metastatic forms, primary and/or localized metastatic tumour removal can help to control hormone excess and improve the response to other therapies. Radiotherapy is the treatment of choice for bone metastases and may have a role as adjuvant post-operative therapy in patients with high risk for local recurrences.[69]

Mitotane is an adrenolytic compound with specific activity on the adrenal cortex. It is usually used after surgery for an adrenal carcinoma alone or in combination therapy but its role as adjuvant therapy after complete surgical removal is still a matter of debate. Doses > 3 g/day are usually administrated, but monitoring of serum drug levels is mandatory since levels > 14 mg/l are necessary to induce tumour regression. Metastatic responses range from 31 to 80%.[70] Highest levels are achieved only after several months of treatment. Side-effects of mitotane which occur frequently and are often dose-limiting include gastrointestinal or central nervous system (e.g. lethargy, somnolence, ataxia, and dizziness) ones. Long-term mitotane induces adrenal insufficiency and may require hydrocortisone replacement. Several other cytotoxic agents have been used in the treatment of patients with advanced adrenal carcinoma. These include *cis*-platinum, etoposide, doxorubicin, vincristine, 5-fluorouracil, and streptozocin. Combined therapy with cytotoxic agents and mitotane has been proposed but response rates using different combinations of cytotoxic agents with or without mitotane are variable (11–46%). A multicentre study using etoposide, doxorubicin, and *cis*-platinum every 4 weeks together with mitotane in doses of 2–3 g/d as tolerated, demonstrated the highest overall response rate (53%).[69]

References

1 Rossi E, Regolisti G, Negro A, Sani C, Davoli S, Perazzoli F (2002). High prevalence of primary aldosteronism using postcaptopril plasma aldosterone to renin ratio as a screening test among Italian hypertensives. *Am. J. Hypertension* **15**: 896–902.

2 Gordon RD, Stowasser M, Tunny TJ, Klemm SA, Rutherford JC (1994). High incidence of primary aldosteronism in 199 patients referred with hypertension. *Clin. Exp. Pharmacol.* **21**: 315–18.

3 Young WF Jr (2003). Minireview: primary aldosteronism-changing concepts in diagnosis and treatment. *J. Clin. Endocrinol. Metab.* **144**: 2208–13.

4 Rocha R, Rudolph AE, Frierdich GE, Nachowiak DA, Kekec BK, Blomme EA *et al.* (2002). Aldosterone induces a vascular inflammatory phenotype in the rat heart. *Am. J. Physiol.* **283**: H1802–H1810.

5 Sun Y, Zhang J, Lu L, Chen SS, Quinn MT, Weber KT (2002). Aldosterone-induced inflammation in the rat heart: role of oxidative stress. *Am. J. Pathol.* **161**: 1773–81.

6 Bauersachs J, Heck M, Fraccarollo D, Hildemann SK, Ertl G, Wehling M *et al.* (2002). Addition of spironolactone to angiotensin-converting enzyme inhibition in heart failure improves endothelial vasomotor dysfunction: role of vascular superoxide anion formation and endothelial nitric oxide synthase expression. *J. Am. Coll. Cardiol.* **39**: 351–8.

7 Ignatowska-Switalska H, Chodakowska J, Januszewicz W, Feltynowski T, Adamczyk M, Lewondowski J (1997). Evaluation of plasma aldosterone to plasma rennin activity ratio in patients with primary aldosteronism. *J. Hum. Hypertens.* **11**: 373–8.

8 Mantero F, Terzolo M, Arnaldi G, Osella G, Masini AM, Ali A *et al.* (2000). A survey on adrenal incidentaloma in Italy. Study Group on Adrenal Tumors of the Italian Society of Endocrinology. *Clin. Endocrinol. Metab.* **85**: 637–44.

9 Mulatero P, Rabbia F, Milan A, Paglieri C, Morellow F, Chiandussi L *et al.* (2002). Drug effects on aldosterone/plasma renin activity ratio in primary aldosteronism. *Hypertension* **40**: 897–902.

10 Holland OB, Brown H, Kuhnert L, Fairchild C, Risk M, Gomez Sanchez CE (1984). Further evaluation of saline infusion for the diagnosis of primary aldosteronism. *Hypertension* **6**: 717–23.

11 Mantero F, Fallo F, Opocher G, Armanin D, Boscaro M, Scaroni C (1981). Effect of angiotensin II and converting-enzyme inhibitor (captopril) on blood pressure, PRA and aldosterone in primary aldosteronism. *Clin. Sci. (Lond.)* **61**: S289–S293.

12 Agharazii M, Douville P, Grose JH, Lebel M (2001). Captopril suppression versus salt loading in confirming primary aldosteronism. *Hypertension* **37**: 1440–3.

13 Pagny JY, Chatellier G, Raynaud A, Plouin PF, Corvol P (1988). Localization of primary hyperaldosteronism. *Ann. Endocrinol. (Paris)* **49**: 340–3.

14 Young WF. Stanson AW, Grant CSM, Thompson GB, van Heerden JA (1996). Primary aldosteronism: adrenal venous sampling. *Surgery* **120**: 913–20.

15 Omura M, Sasano H, Fujiwara T, Yamaguchi K, Nishikawa T (2002). Unique cases of unilateral hyperaldosteronemia due to multiple adrenocortical micronodules, which can only be detected by selective adrenal venous sampling. *Metabolism* **51**: 350–5.

16 Ghose RP, Hall PM, Bravo EL (1999). Medical management of aldosterone-producing adenomas. *Ann. Intern. Med.* **131**: 105–8.

17 Pitt B, Zannad F, Remme WJ, Cody R, Castaigne A, Perez A *et al.* (1999). The effect of spironolactone on morbidity and mortality in patients with severe heart failure. *N. Engl. J. Med.* **341**: 709–17.

18 Pitt B, Remme W, Faiez Z, Neaton J, Martinez F, Roniker B *et al.* (2003). Eplerenone, a selective aldosterone blocker, in patients with left ventricular dysfunction after myocardial infarction. *N. Engl. J. Med.* **348**: 1309–21.

19 Brown JJ, Davies DL, Ferriss JB, Fraser R, Haywood E, Lever AF *et al.* (1972). Comparison of surgery and prolonged spironolactone therapy in patients with hypertension, aldosterone excess, and low plasma renin. *Br. Med. J.* **2**: 729–34.

20 Sawka AN, Young WF, Thompson GB, Grant CS, Farley DR, Leibson C *et al.* (2001). Primary aldosteronism: factors associated with normalization of blood pressure after surgery. *Ann. Intern. Med.* **135**: 258–61.

21 Mantero F, Opocher G, Rocco S, Carpenè G, Armanini D (1995). Long-term treatment of mineralocorticoid excess syndromes. *Steroids* **60**: 81–6.

22 Dupont A (1985). Disappearence of spironolactone-induced gynecomastia during treatment with potassium canrenoate. *Lancet* **2**: 731–4.

23 Armanini D, Karbowiak I, Goi A, Mantero F, Funder JW (1985). *In-vivo* metabolites of spironolactone and potassium canrenoate: determination of potential ant-androgenic activity by a mouse kidney cytosol receptor assay. *Clin. Endocrinol.* **23**: 341–7.

24 Scaroni C, Armanini D, Fallo F, Opocher G, Boscaro M, Mantero F (1981). Treatment of primary aldosteronism with oral potassium canrenoate. *Riv. It. Biol. Med.* 1239–43.

25 Epstein M, Menard J, Alexander JC, Roniker B (2000). Eplerenone, a novel and selective aldosterone receptor antagonist: efficacy in patients with mild to moderate hypertension. *Circulation* **98**: S198–S199.

26 Hoefnagels WH, Drayer JI, Smals AG, Kloppenborg PW (1980). Spironolactone and amiloride in hypertensive patients with and without aldosterone excess. *Clin. Pharmacol. Ther.* **27**: 317–23.

27 Carpenè G, Rocco G, Opocher G, Mantero F (1989). Acute and chronic effect of nifedipine in primary aldosteronism. *Clin. Exp. Hyper. Theory Prac.* **A11**: 1263–72.

28 Opocher G, Rocco S, Murgia A, Mantero F (1987). Effect of verapamil on aldosterone secretion in primary aldosteronism. *J. Endocrinol. Invest.* **10**: 491–4.

29 Griffin GT, Melby JC (1985). The therapeutic effect of a new angiotensin-converting enzyme inhibitor, enalapril maleate in idiopathic hyperaldosteronism. *J. Clin. Hypertens.* 1985;1:265–276.

30 Stokes GS, Monaghan JC, Ryan M, Woodward M (2001). Efficacy of an angiotensin II receptor antagonist in managing hyperaldosteronism. *J. Hypertens.* **19**: 1161–5.

31 Nomura K, Demura H, Horiba N, Shizume K (1986). Long term treatment of idiopathic hyperaldosteronism using trilostane. *Acta Endocrinol.* **113**: 104–10.

32 Ford HC, Bailey RE (1966). The effect of heparin on aldosterone secretion and metabolism in primary aldosteronism. *Steroids* **7**: 30–40.

33 Grossman AB, Kaltsas GA (2002). Adrenal medulla and pathology. In: *Comprehensive Clinical Endocrinology*, 3rd edn (ed. GM Besser, MO Thorner), pp. 223–37. Elsevier Science, Philadelphia, PA.

34 Gimm O, Armanios M, Dziema H, Neumann HP, Eng C (2000). Somatic and occult germline mutations in SDHD, a mitochondrial complex II gene, in nonfamilial pheochromocytoma. *Cancer Res.* **60**: 6822–5.

35 Opocher G, Schiavi F, Conton P, Scaroni C, Mantero F (2003). Clinical and genetic aspects of phaeochromocytoma. *Horm. Res.* **59**: S56–S61.

36 Opocher G, Schiavi F, Vettori A, Pampinella F, Vitiello L, Calderan A *et al.* (2003). Fine analysis of the short arm of chromosome 1 in sporadic and familial pheochromocytoma. *Clin. Endocrinol.* **59**: 707–15.

37 Bravo EL (1994). Evolving concepts in the pathophysiology, diagnosis and treatment of pheochromocytomas. *Endocr. Rev.* **15**: 356–68.

38 Lenders JWM, Pacak K, Walther MM, Linehan WM, Mannelli M, Friberg HR *et al.* (2002). Biochemical diagnosis of pheochromocytoma: which is the best test? *J. Am. Med. Assoc.* **287**: 1427–34.

39 Sawka AM, Jaeschke R, Singh RJ, Young WF Jr (2003). A comparison of biochemical tests for pheochromocytoma: measurement of fractionated plasma metanephrines compared with the combination of 24-hour urinary metanephrines and catecholamines. *J. Clin. Endocrinol. Metab.* **88**: 553–8.

40 Kudva YC, Sawka AM, Young WF Jr (2003). The laboratory diagnosis of adrenal pheochromocytoma: the Mayo Clinic experience. *J. Clin. Endocrinol. Metab.* **88**: 4533–9.

41 Chan EC, Ho PC (2001). High-performance liquid chromatography/atmospheric pressure chemical ionization mass spectrometric method for the analysis of catecholamines and metanephrines in human urine. *Rapid Commun. Mass. Spectrom.* **14**: 1959–64.

42 Taylor RL, Singh RJ (2002). Validation of liquid chromatography-tandem mass spectrometry method for analysis of urinary conjugated metanephrine and normetanephrine for screening of pheochromocytoma. *Clin. Chem.* **48**: 533–9.

43 Eisenhofer G, Goldstein DS, Walther MM (2003). Biochemical diagnosis of pheochromocytoma: how to distinguish true-from false-positive test results. *J. Clin. Endocrinol. Metab.* **88**: 2656–66.

44 Brandi ML, Gagel RF, Angeli A, Bilezikian JP, Beck-Peccoz P, Bordi C *et al.* (2001). CONSENSUS: guidelines for diagnosis and therapy of MEN type 1 and type 2. *J. Clin. Endocrinol. Metab.* **86**: 5658–71.

45 Pacak K, Linehan WM, Eisenhofer G, Walther MM, Goldstein DS (2001). Recent advances in genetics, diagnosis, localization, and treatment of pheochromocytoma. *Ann. Intern. Med.* **134**: 315–29.

46 Kinney MA, Narr BJ, Warner MA (2002). Perioperative management of pheochromocytoma. *J. Cardiothorac. Vasc. Anesth.* **16**: 359–69.

47 Boutros AR, Bravo EL, Zanettin G, Straffon RA (1990). Perioperative management of 63 patients with pheochromocytoma. *Cleve. Clin. J. Med.* **57**: 613–17.

48 Bravo EL (1997). Pheochromocytoma. *Curr. Ther. Endocrinol. Metab.* **6**: 195–7.

49 Kinney MA, Warner ME, vanHeerden JA, Horlocker TT, Young WF Jr, Schroeder DR *et al.* (2000). Perianesthetic risks and outcomes of pheochromocytoma and paraganglioma resection. *Anest. Analg.* **91**: 1118–23.

50 Prys-Roberts C (2000). Pheochromocytoma—recent progress in its management. *Br. J. Anaesth.* **85**: 44–57.

51 Roizen MF, Scheider BD, Hassan SZ (1987). Anesthesia for patients with pheochromocytoma. *Anesthesiol. Clin. North. Am.* **5**: 269–75.

52 Munro J, Hurlbert BJ, Hill GE (1995). Calcium channel blockade and uncontrolled blood pressure during pheochromocytoma surgery. *Can. J. Anesth.* **42**: 228–30.

53 Lehnert H, Hahn K, Dralle H (2002). Benign and malignant pheochromocytoma. *Interninst* **43**: 196–209.

54 Loh KC, Fitzgerald PA, Matthay KK, Yeo PB, Price DC (1997). The treatment of malignant pheochromocytoma with iodine-131 metaiodobenzylguanidine. A comprehensive review of 116 patients. *J. Endocrinol. Invest.* **20**: 648–58.

55 Troncone L, Rufini V (1999). Nuclear medicine therapy of pheochromocytoma and paraganglioma. *Q. J. Nucl. Med.* **43**: 344–55.

56 Lehnert H, Mundschenk J, Hahn K (2004). Malignant pheochromocytoma. *Front. Horm. Res.* **31**: 155–62.

57 Reubi JC, Waser B, Liu Q, Laissue JA, Schonbrum A (2000). Subcellular distribution of somatostatin sst2A receptors in human tumors of the nervous and neuroendocrine systems: membranous versus intracellular location. *J. Clin. Endocrinol. Metab.* **85**: 3882–91.

58 Averbuch SD, Steakley CS, Young RC, Gelman EP, Goldstein DS, Stull R *et al.* (1988). Malignant pheochromocytoma. Effective treatment with a combination of cyclophosphamide, vincristine and dacarbazine. *Ann. Intern. Med.* **109**: 267–73.

59 Sisson JC, Shapiro B, Shulkin BL, Urba S, Zempel S, Spauldin S (1999). Treatment of malignant pheochromocytoma with [131]I- metaiodobenzylguanidine and chemotherapy. *Am. J. Clin. Oncol.* **22**: 364–70.

60 Jaroszewski DE, Tessier DJ, Schlinkert RT, Grant CS, Thompson GB, van Heerden JA *et al.* (2003). Laparoscopic adrenalectomy for pheochromocytoma. *Mayo Clin. Proc.* **78**: 1501–4.

61 Okamoto T, Obara T, Ito Y, Yamashita T, Kanbe M, Iihara M *et al.* (1996). Bilateral adrenalectomy with autotransplantation of adrenocortical tissue or unilateral adrenalectomy: treatment options for pheochromocytomas in multiple endocrine neoplasia type 2A. *Endocr. J.* **43**: 169–75.

62 Lee JE, Curley SA, Gagel RF, Evans DB, Hickey RC (1996). Cortical-sparing adrenalectomy for patients with bilateral pheochromocytoma. *Surgery* **120**: 1064–70.

63 Orth DN, Kovacs WJ, DeBold CR (1998). The adrenal cortex. In: *Williams Textbook of Endocrinology* (ed. JD Wilson, DW Foster, HM Kronenberg, PR Larsen), pp. 517–664. W. B. Saunders, Philadelphia, PA.

64 Arnaldi G, Angeli A, Atkinson AB, Bertagna X, Cavagnini F, Chrousos GP *et al.* (2003). Diagnosis and complications of Cushing's syndrome: a consensus statement. *J. Clin. Endocrinol. Metab.* **88**: 5593–602.

65 Rockall AG, Babar SA, Sohaib SA, Isidori AM, Diaz-Cano S, Monson JP *et al.* (2004). CT and MR imaging of the adrenal glands in ACTH-independent Cushing syndrome. *Radiographics* **24**: 435–52.

66 Rao SK, Caride VJ, Ponn R, Giakovis E, Lee SH (2004). F-18 fluorodeoxyglucose positron emission tomography-positive benign adrenal cortical adenoma: imaging features and pathologic correlation. *Clin. Nucl. Med.* **29**: 300–2.

67 Imai T, Kikumori T, Shibata A, Fujiwara M, Nakao A (2002). Laparoscopic bilateral adrenalectomy for Cushing's syndrome due to ACTH-independent macronodular adrenocortical hyperplasia. *Biomed. Pharmacother.* **56**: S120–S125.

68 Beardwell CG, Adamson AR, Shalet SM (1981). Prolonged remission in florid Cushing's syndrome following metyrapone treatment. *Clin. Endocrinol.* **14**: 485–92.

69 Allolio B, Hahner S, Weismann D, Fassnacht M (2004). Management of adrenocortical carcinoma. *Clin. Endocrinol.* **60**: 273–87.

70 Baudin E, Pellegriti G, Bonnay M, Penfornis A, Laplanche A, Vassal G *et al.* (2001). Impact of monitoring plasma 1,1-dichlorodiphenildichloroethane (o,'p'DDD) levels on the treatment of patients with adrenocortical carcinoma. *Cancer* **92**: 1385–92.

Chapter 25

The patient presenting with frequently recurring urinary tract calculi

Hans-Göran Tiselius

The annual incidence of urinary tract stone disease varies between geographical areas but is estimated to be 1500 per million in Europe and North America. If a stone of diameter >6 mm is used as the limit for considering active stone removal, approximately 30% of these patients will qualify for such procedures. Out of these 450 patients who need treatment, roughly 270 will have one or more stones in the kidney and the other 180 in the ureter. Most patients will have one stone and 30% or fewer will have more than one.

Removal of stones from the kidneys and ureters has become a fairly easy, low-invasive, and straightforward procedure. We have, during the past two decades, witnessed a dramatic technical development in this field. Extracorporeal shock wave lithotripsy (ESWL), ureteroscopy with intracorporeal laser, or electrohydraulic lithotripsy as well as percutaneous surgical techniques have almost completely replaced open surgical approaches for stone problems. Most patients can now be managed on an out-patient basis. The result has been a marked improvement in the treatment of these patients, particularly in those with recurrent stones.

This paradigm shift in stone surgery over the past two decades has negatively influenced, for some, the importance of evaluating risk factors for stone formation and the implementation of a strategic plan for stone prevention. It is critical to appreciate that although most stones can be removed in a safe and easy manner, the risk of recurrent stone formation has not decreased. Moreover, a substantial number of patients have a very bothersome disease including severely painful episodes of renal colic, haematuria, and urinary tract infections despite conservative approaches to spontaneous stone passage.

For patients who form only one stone during their life-time identification of possible risk factors as well as dietary and pharmacological recurrence preventive treatment does not seem to make sense.[1] Unfortunately, it cannot be predicted with certainty who will or will not form only one stone. It is clear that all recurrent stone formers start off as single stone formers and most initial stone formers will develop another one within 5–7 years. We can often identify stone formers with predisposing diseases

Table 25.1 Subgrouping of patients according to the chemical composition of stones formed in the urinary tract

Subgroup	Stone composition
Urate stone formers	Uric acid, ammonium urate
Infection stone formers	Magnesium ammonium phosphate, carbonate apatite, hydroxyapatite
Cystine stone formers	Cystine
Calcium stone formers	
Calcium oxalate	Calcium oxalate monohydrate, calcium oxalate dihydrate
Calcium phosphate	Carbonate apatite, hydroxyapatite, brushite, whitlockite

(e.g. hyperparathyroidism), pharmacological treatments (e.g. indinavir), or anatomical abnormalities (e.g. medullary sponge kidney) that are clearly associated with recurrent stone formation and, in whom, future problems can be anticipated.

An important component of patient evaluation is determination of the type of stone disease under consideration by radiological appearance or, preferably, chemical analysis. The most common types of stone are shown in Table 25.1. Their relative occurrence is subject to pronounced geographical variations but, in Sweden, 55% of stone patients treated with active stone removal had a mixture of calcium oxalate and phosphate. Pure calcium oxalate or calcium phosphate stones were seen in 35 and 5%, respectively. Only about 3% had pure infection stones, 3.5% uric acid, and 0.5% cystine.

Surgical considerations

Symptomatic stones in the kidney should always be actively removed. The same strategy is applicable for asymptomatic stones that show metabolic activity (i.e. growth) or those that are associated with recurrent urinary tract infections. There is also an indication for prophylactic removal of such stones in patients with frequent episodes of stone passage and renal colic. Most asymptomatic fragments ($\leq$4 mm) that remain stable can be left with regular follow-up and intervention if they grow.

Ureteric stones must not be left in the ureter. The rule is to proceed to active stone removal when the stone diameter is 7 mm or greater because it is unlikely to pass spontaneously. Smaller stones can be treated conservatively and followed for 4–6 weeks if there are few symptoms and minimal obstruction. If there has been no progress in stone movement by that time, intervention is required by ESWL or ureteroscopy and basket extraction with or without intracoporeal lithotripsy. The principles regarding stone intervention are summarized in Fig. 25.1.

To whom should active stone prevention be given?

For the individual patient, announcement of a urinary tract stone usually means severe suffering whether it eventually passes spontaneously or requires removal. Therefore

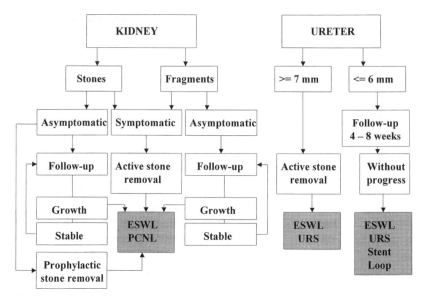

Fig. 25.1 Strategic principles for surgical considerations in patients with urinary tract stones.

the standard questions raised by the stone former are: Why did I get a stone? What can I do to avoid further episodes of this kind?

Since some stones will almost always recur, aggressive prophylaxis is recommended. For example, patients with cystinuria always need fluid/diet/pharmacological advice. The same is true for patients who have formed uric acid or infection stones.[1–4]

For the majority of patients, that is those who form calcium-based stones, it is necessary to apply a more targeted therapeutic approach. A fundamental step in the care of the stone-forming patient is to determine the type of stone that has formed, if it is available. This is done using X-ray crystallography or infrared spectroscopy. If neither of these methods is available, it is worthwhile sending the stone(s) to a laboratory that has the capability since knowledge of the stone composition will enable categorization of patients according to the principles outlined in Table 25.1. It is a clinical reality, however, that stone analysis is not available for many patients (e.g. the stone might still reside in the body or a passed stone has been lost). In these circumstances, an educated guess can often be made based on the following indirect clues:

1 Uric acid stones are not visible on plain X-ray films (i.e. kidney–ureter–bladder, KUB) but are clearly demonstrated on spiral computed tomography (CT). For this reason, it is the author's habit to obtain a plain X-ray film when stones have been shown with CT.

2 The presence of a high serum level of uric acid with a normal creatinine gives support to the likelihood of uric acid stones. The urinary pH in these patients is always low (<5.2).

3 The presence of urease-producing bacteria (e.g. *Proteus*) makes the diagnosis of an infection stone (i.e. struvite) likely. The urinary pH in these patients is always high (>7.5). The demonstration of typical coffin-like crystals of magnesium ammonium phosphate in the urinary sediment is diagnostic.

4 Staghorn (i.e. branched) stones should be considered to be of infectious origin until proven otherwise. These usually have a multilayered appearance on the radiograph. A high content of carbonate apatite makes them very opaque on the plain X-ray film unless magnesium ammonium phosphate is the dominating crystal phase.

5 Cystine stones are less opaque than calcium-based ones but do show up on plain X-rays because of the –SH groups in the cystine molecule. The diagnosis is proved by microscopic demonstration of hexagonal cystine crystals or a positive a sodium nitroprusside reaction.

6 If none of these criteria is met and the stone is visible on a plain X-ray, it is assumed that the composition is calcium oxalate and/or calcium phosphate.

Infection stones

Stones composed of magnesium ammonium phosphate and/or carbonate apatite cannot form unless the urinary tract is, or has been, infected with urease-producing bacteria because pre-requisites for precipitation of this type of solid phase are a supra-physiological alkaline urinary pH and high concentrations of ammonium and carbonate ions. The high pH is the most important determinant and a level exceeding 7.5 is usually necessary in order to get an ion–activity product of magnesium ammonium phosphate above its formation product.[5,6]

The fundamental requirement of preventing recurrence in these patients is eradication of the bacteria. Surgery must remove all infected stone fragments. Meticulous cleaning of the collecting system is essential. Despite this goal, it is not always possible to get a kidney completely free of residual stone fragments harbouring bacteria. Percutaneous irrigation and chemolysis with a 10% concentration of hemiacidrin (Renacidin®) or Suby's solution is often used as adjuvant method to dissolve and eliminate residual magnesium ammonium phosphate, carbonate apatite, and hydroxy-apatite crystals from the renal collecting system.[7,8]

Since the urease-producing bacteria also might reside in the kidney without evidence of residual stone material, it is recommended to give these patients long-term suppressive antibiotics, typically for at least 3–6 months. This may even sterilize small residual stone fragments. Unfortunately, many of the bacterial strains responsible for struvite stones are resistant to all oral antibiotics. A short but intensive course of intravenous antibiotics based on sensitivities is often helpful. It is emphasized that apparently resistant strains of *Proteus* and *Pseudomonas* may respond to oral penicillin, ampicillin, or tetracycline.[6] In fact, most *Proteus* strains can be successfully treated with penicillin or ampicillin and *Pseudomonas* with tetracycline. Tetracycline is also the drug of choice for infections with *Ureaplasma urealyticum* which requires special culturing for diagnosis.[9,10] Even a reduced number of bacteria gives a remarkable reduction in urease production.[6]

Further attempts to counteract struvite stone formation can be made with oral acidification, although the value of this approach has not been proven. The author prefers intermittent acidification by giving ammonium chloride 1 g three times a day, once or twice a week. Acidification of urine can also be achieved with methionine 500 mg three times daily.[3] In highly selected cases with particularly severe disease, administration of a urease inhibitor such as acetohydroxamic acid (Lithostat®) may be used at 500 mg twice daily.[6,11] Promising results have also been recorded with similar agents such as propiono-hydroxamic acid and nonhydroxymate flurofamide (N-(diaminophosphinyl)-4-fluoro-benzamide). Use of urease inhibitors is limited because of side-effects including loss of hair, headaches, and venous thrombosis.

Close follow-up of patients with infection stones should include urine cultures and plain x-rays at 3, 6 and 12 months because of the high risk of recurrence. Subsequently, annual evaluations are wise until the condition appears stable.

Stones containing urate

The two major types of stones with urate as the dominant constituent are uric acid and ammonium urate ones. Of these crystal phases, uric acid is by far the most common. In addition an association between a high urate excretion and calcium oxalate stone formation has been identified.[12]

Uric acid stones

Three urinary risk-factors are responsible for uric acid precipitation and stone formation—low urine volume and pH and high uric acid excretion.[3,5,13] The formation product of uric acid can be exceeded at a normal urate excretion if the pH is low and the urine volume small. The typical patient presents with renal colic but without a visible stone on a plain X-ray film. Excretory pyelography usually reveals a radiolucent filling defect, while the CT examination always demonstrates radio-opaque stone material. A 24-hour urine collection might show a urate excretion of 4.5 mmol, pH of 5.1, and volume of 900 ml. Such a urine composition gives an ion–activity product of uric acid above its formation product and leads to precipitation of uric acid crystals.[5]

The basic principle for prevention is a reduction in the ion–activity product below the formation product. Initially this should be accomplished by drinking more fluids and aiming for 2.5 litres or more of urine output per day. Fluid intake should be at least half water and the patient should strive to keep his/her urine colourless; intake should be even higher on hot days or days on which the patient is physically active. Urinary uric acid can be reduced and pH increased modestly by limiting the intake of purines; help from a knowledgeable nutritionist is indispensable with this counselling.

When fluid and dietary measures are not helpful, or the patient can/will not comply, should pharmacological intervention be entertained. For example, the urinary pH can be increased by administration of alkali such as potassium citrate or sodium potassium citrate 7–10 mmol two to three times daily.[14] High urinary uric acid can be reduced by giving 300 mg of allopurinol daily. If there is normal uric acid excretion, allopurinol is not needed for prophylaxis.

It is of importance to know that uric acid stones are the only ones that can be dissolved by oral chemolysis. The aim is to get the ion–activity product of uric acid as far below its solubility product as possible.[2] This can be accomplished by encouraging a very high fluid intake (e.g. 3–4 litres of water per day, aggressively raising the urinary pH (e.g. acetazolamide 125–250 mg three to four times per day), and reducing urinary uric acid regardless of its level (e.g. allopurinol 300 mg per day). The therapeutic effect is followed with repeated CTs. Once the stones have disappeared, the drugs regimen can be adjusted to the principles for prevention.

Percutaneous chemolysis of uric acid stones can be accomplished by irrigation of alkaline solutions such trihydroxyaminomethan (THAM).[15]

Ammonium urate stones

This stone constituent is seen in patients with pre-requisites for uric acid precipitation and a simultaneous infection with urease-producing bacteria. Preventive steps in these patients should combine a reduction of the ion–activity product of uric acid and eradication or at least suppression of the urease-producing bacteria. Formation of ammonium urate has also been reported in patients with laxative abuse.[16] There is no oral or percutaneous chemolytic method that can be used for dissolution of ammonium urate stones.

Hyperuricosuric calcium oxalate stone disease

This syndrome has to be considered as a possible explanation for recurrent stone formation in some patients.[12] It is more common in some geographical areas than in others.[1,5] The physicochemical mechanism in this disease has not been definitely clarified, but present knowledge supports the idea of a salting out effect. Uric acid crystals may also act as a nidus for calcium oxalate growth and/or reduce the activity of inhibitors of calcium oxalate crystal agglomeration. Fluid and dietary modification of the urinary risk factors of calcium oxalate stone formation (e.g. low volume, fixed/high urinary pH, excessive excretion of calcium, oxalate, and uric acid and/or inadequate excretion of inhibitors) are indicated.[3] Daily allopurinol may be necessary.[17]

Cystine stones

The increased excretion of cystine seen in patients with cystinuria is usually associated with severely recurrent formation of stones. It is essential to exclude the diagnosis of this metabolic abnormality in recurrent stone formers, particularly in children, in whom no stone has been analysed and in whom cystinuria cannot be excluded for other reasons.

Treatment of patients with cystine stones aims to keep the cystine concentration less than 400 mg or 1.7 mmol/l by three prongs of attack—hydration, reduced cystine excretion, and alkalinization.[6,18–20] Since cystine is so insoluble compared with other types of stone forming materials much higher urinary outputs are the goal (i.e. >3 litres per day). Dietary reduction of methionine and sodium can have an important benefit in reducing urinary cystine; help from a knowledgeable nutritionist is indispensable with this counselling. When the ion–activity product is low (i.e. roughly corresponding to a cystine concentration of 1 mmol/l or less), fluid and dietary changes are often all that are needed.

For patients with a cystine concentration between 1 and 2 mmol/l, alkali may need to be added to the hydration and dietary regimen. Potassium citrate 7–10 mmol two to three times daily is recommended with the goal of getting the pH above 7.5. At this level the solubility of cystine increases dramatically, but it is often difficult to maintain satisfactory long-term alkalinization. Alkalinizing agents containing sodium should be avoided because of the increased cystine excretion that is associated with administration of sodium.

At cystine concentrations above 2 mmol/l (>500 mg/l) the condition is considered severe and complex-forming agents should be added to the previous therapeutic measures. Administration of tiopronin (Thiola® α-mercapto-propionylglycine), which forms a soluble cysteine–thiol complex, is most commonly used. Treatment with tiopronin should be started in daily doses of 250–2000 mg and titrated up depending upon response and tolerance. Supplemental vitamin B_6 should be given and close monitoring for potential haematological or renal side-effects instituted.

Some authors have reported good experience with captopril which also forms soluble complexes with cysteine at doses of 75 and 150 mg per day. Bucillamine (Rimatil) is a new dithiol which is able to bind two cysteine molecules. Although this is a theoretically attractive alternative, the clinical experience with bucillamin is limited. D-penicillamine is use infrequently because of frequent side-effects.

In order to maintain compliance and reduce the likelihood of recurrences, frequent out-patient visits are required. Patients require education regarding their stone disease and regular feedback as to their improvements or lack thereof.

Because of the increased solubility in alkaline urine, the stone-free rate following active stone removal can be improved by treating any residual fragments with percutaneous chemolytic irrigation using THAM-solutions.[21] In combination with solutions containing 200 mg/l of acetylcystein, dissolution is further improved.[22]

Identification of risk factors for calcium stone formation

In all patients, and particularly in those with recurrent stone formation, a careful medical history is essential for identification of any disease or any pharmacological treatment known to be associated with stone formation (Tables 25.2 and 25.3). In

Table 25.2 Diseases associated with stone formation

Enteric hyperoxaluria: intestinal resection, Crohn's disease, jejunoileal bypass, malabsorption, ileostomy
Primary hyperoxaluria
Renal tubular acidosis (complete and partial)
Hyperparathyroidism
Hyperthyroidism
Sarcoidosis
Immobilization
Hypertension (?)
Cystinuria

Table 25.3 Pharmacological treatment associated with stone formation

Corticosteroids
Vitamin D
Calcium supplements
Thyroid hormone
Acetazolamide
Indinavir
Cytotoxic agents
Vitamin C (excessive doses)

addition to the valuable information on the situation of the stone, the radiographic examination may also demonstrate any anatomical abnormalities that might be of importance for stone formation (Table 25.4).

Analysis of urine in patients with calcium stone disease

A 24-hour urine collection is necessary to get information on the excretion of those urine variables that are considered important for calcium stone formation.[1–3,20,23] Although urinary macromolecules might be highly important as promoters and/or inhibitors of crystallization[24] there are so far no clinically useful routine methods by means of which such abnormalities can be demonstrated. Neither do we have any simple techniques that give information on the crystal cell interaction.

Analysis of urine is most commonly carried out in samples collected overduring 24 hours (Table 25.5). Two or more collections should be made at least 2–3 months following an episode of renal colic and at least one should be made on a weekday and one at the weekend.[2,20,25] The patient's urine should be free from haematuria and

Table 25.4 Anatomical risk factors for stone formation

Calix diverticulum
Calix cyst
Narrow calix neck
Horseshoe kidney
Pelviureteric junction obstruction
Hydronephrosis
Tubular ectasia (medullary sponge kidney)
Ureterocoele
Vesico-ureteral reflux

Table 25.5 Analytical procedures in calcium stone formers

Type of analysis	Test	Patients analysed
Analysis of blood	S/P calcium, albumin, creatinine, urate	All patients
Fasting morning urine	pH (Brand's test if cystinuria has not been excluded)	Rs, S_{res}, Rm_{res}
Urine collection: 24-hour sample (alternative 1)	24 hours. HCl 30 ml, 6 mol/l: calcium, oxalate, citrate, magnesium, phosphate, urea, sodium, creatinine, volume	Rs, Rm_{res}, S_{res}
	24 hours. NaAz 30 ml, 0.3 mol/l: pH, urate, volume	Rs, Rm_{res}, S_{res}
Urine collection: 16-hour + 8-hour sample (alternative 2)	16 hours (06.00–22.00). HCl 20 ml, 6 mol/l: calcium, oxalate, citrate, magnesium, phosphate, sodium, creatinine, volume	Rs, Rm_{res}, S_{res}
	8 hours (22.00–06.00). NaAz 10 ml, 0.3 mol/l: pH, volume, urate	Rs, Rm_{res}, S_{res}

S/P, serum/plasma; Rs, recurrent stone former with severe disease; S_{res}, first time (single) stone former with residual fragments/stone; Rm_{res}, recurrent stone former with mild disease and residual fragments/stones; NaAz, sodium azide

infection. There should be a low risk of passage of fragments (i.e. collections not made immediately after ESWL). In order to reflect the crystallization and stone-forming propensity in an appropriate way the patients should be told to follow their normal dietary and drinking habits. Often it is useful for patients to record their dietary and fluid intakes while collecting their 24-hour urine; this can be helpful during subsequent dietary counselling.

It is of value to measure the following variables: pH, calcium, oxalate, citrate, magnesium, phosphate, sodium, urate, urea, and creatinine. In order to dissolve any calcium salt and to counteract the oxidation of ascorbate to oxalate, the collection should be made in a bottle with hydrochloric acid as preservative (i.e. 30 ml of 6 mol/l hydrochloric acid per 24-hour collection). This acidification results in uric acid precipitation and, therefore, it must be measured either in a separate 24-hour urine collection or after alkalinization of the acidified sample. A separate urine sample is necessary to measure pH.

The different urinary variables can be used to derive approximate estimates of the ion–activity products (i.e. supersaturation) of calcium oxalate and calcium phosphate and to serve as a guide for specific fluid and dietary advice. Creatinine is used as an indicator of the completeness of the collection.

In whom should urine be analysed?

The vast majority of patients with urinary tract stone disease form stones that are dominated by calcium oxalate, either as calcium oxalate monohydrate or dihydrate. A small fraction of patients form pure calcium phosphate stones of which brushite (i.e. calcium hydrogen phosphate) needs particular attention because of its very high tendency to recur. Although some patients will remain single stone formers, most will go on to form more. The overwhelming majority are keen to learn why they have developed a stone and how they can prevent others. Since the evaluation of dietary intake and urinary excretion is done as an out-patient, is economical and relatively simple, and acts as the background for developing preventive advice, most patients, whether single or recurrent stone formers, undergo these tests. Those with specific risk factors as listed in Table 25.6 require a more detailed evaluation. It is the author's routine to analyse serum concentrations of calcium, creatinine, and uric acid to exclude hyperparathyroidism and confirm satisfactory kidney function.

For patients with frequently recurring stones there is a need for an extended analysis of risk factors in order to be able to design an efficient recurrence prevention programme. It may be difficult to decide who has severe recurrent stone disease (Rs) and who has mild recurrent disease (Rm). This is an important discrimination, because there may be little indication for a preventative programme in the case where there are very long periods of time between stone episodes.

Table 25.6 Specific risk factors to be noted in patients with calcium stone disease

Diseases associated with stone formation (Table 25.2)
Medication associated with stone formation (Table 25.3)
Anatomical abnormalities (Table 25.4)
Early start of stone formation (below the age of 25)
Brushite in the stone
A pronounced family history

As a result, strict rules cannot be formulated for discrimination between recurrent stone formers with severe and mild disease. This step is a function of the clinical course of the disease and the patient's attitude. Another factor that might indicate a need for risk factor analysis is the presence or absence of residual stones or fragments in the urinary tract. Patients with residual stone material are at potential risk of forming new stones or having stone fragments grow, and attention should be directed to those problems.

Preventative treatment in patients with calcium stones

The start of long-term, possibly life-long, pharmacological treatment, with its potential cost and adverse events, requires careful consideration that must be influenced by the severity of the disease and the patient's desire and motivation. It must not be instituted until adequate fluid and dietary advice have been given, tried, and failed.

An attempt to estimate the severity of stone formation in an objective way (i.e. frequency of stone formation, f_{SF}) may be useful but is often difficult to calculate and is imprecise. It is the author's opinion that information on the total number of stones formed (N_{tot}) in relation to the patient's age (stone age index, SAI) can serve as good measure of the stone activity:[23]

$$SAI = (100 \times N_{tot})/age.$$

For a 40-year-old patient who has formed four stones the SAI thus will be 10. As a rough guide, pharmacological treatment should be considered and discussed with the patient who has failed fluid and dietary regimens and who has an SAI above 7.5.

Another group who might be considered for early pharmacological intervention, if they have failed fluid and dietary regimens, are those with residual stone fragments in the kidney after surgical intervention. Such fragments may remain silent without growth or they may grow. It is the author's routine to consider early pharmacological treatment if the presence of residual stone material is associated with an obvious biochemical risk or if stone growth has been shown. Under these circumstances, it might be reasonable to also treat patients with a history of less severe disease (i.e. with an SAI below 7.5).

General recommendations

Increased fluid intake is the foundation of therapy for all patients with stone disease. In the case of calcium stone formers, the goal should be to get the 24-hour urine volume to at least 2 litres. Ideally, the fluid intake should be distributed evenly throughout the day. It is no longer felt that dietary restriction of calcium is beneficial and, in fact, it probably increases the risk of calcium oxalate stone formation. Therefore, calcium-containing products should *not* be reduced. The diet should, moreover, be mixed and balanced and it is better to eat several small meals than one large one. Nuts and chocolate should be avoided as snacks because of their high oxalate content. The intake of fruits, vegetables, and fibre should be encouraged, whereas excesses of sugar, fat, and salt should be avoided. As a rule vegetable fat is superior to animal fat.[1–3] These general recommendations should be given to *all* calcium stone formers. The regimen also should provide a basis for additional treatment in those who qualify for specific dietary advice and pharmacological treatment. Help from a knowledgeable nutritionist is indispensable with this counselling.

Dietary considerations and specific dietary advice

Drinking

Dilution of urine most certainly is the best method of reducing the risk of salt precipitation in urine. Once the ion–activity product has been reduced to a level below the formation product it is less likely that crystallization will occur. Analysis of urine composition and calculation of approximate estimates of the ion–activity products of calcium oxalate and calcium phosphate and comparison of these levels with the formation products is an important part of the risk evaluation. One weakness of this procedure is that the urine analysis only reflects the average composition during the collection period. Arbitrary risk levels of AP(CaOx) index and AP(CaP) index of 1.5 and 50, respectively, might, however, serve as a rough guide[23] and based on this assumption, urine volumes necessary to reach this goal can be calculated. The benefits of an increased intake of fluid have been clearly shown.[24]

Sodium

Although sodium affects the ion–strength and ion–activity products of calcium oxalate and calcium phosphate, the most important effect of a high sodium intake is the associated increased excretion of calcium and sodium. At levels above 200 mmol/24 h, the patient should be advised to reduced his or her salt intake.[3] Reduced sodium load might favourably affect stone formation.

Calcium

For decades patients with calcium stone disease were advised to decrease their intake of calcium-rich products in order to reduce urinary calcium. Unfortunately, it has now been shown that such measures will result in an increased absorption of oxalate, because of reduced calcium oxalate complex formation in the intestine. Moreover, a low calcium intake can lead to a negative calcium balance and bone loss. An inverse relationship between dietary calcium and urolithiasis has been demonstrated in large epidemiological studies.[27,28] It was concluded that the calcium intake in stone formers should be at the level of 20–25 mmol (800–1000 mg) per day and no lower. The approximate calcium content of some dairy products is shown in Table 25.7.

This altered view on calcium in the stone-forming process does not mean that urinary calcium is without importance for calcium stone formation. There are still occasional patients in whom a reduced intake of calcium-rich products is necessary.

Table 25.7 Approximate calcium content in some calcium rich products (from Hesse et al.[3])

Food	Calcium content
Milk and yoghurt	30 mmol/l
Soft cheese (e.g. brie, camembert)	10–15 mmol/100 g
Hard cheese	20–30 mmol/100 g

Whether in other patients an extra load of calcium is beneficial remains a matter of debate. It has, however, been suggested from epidemiological studies that supplements of calcium given together with meals are not associated with an increased risk of stone-formation, whereas for patients who take calcium supplements between meals the situation is different. Calcium citrate is probably best. The combined treatment of supplemental calcium and vitamin D may cause much higher levels of calcium excretion. Among other forms of pharmacological agents that result in increased calcium excretion, corticosteroids should be remembered.

High intake of animal protein

With increased affluence, the intake of a diet rich in animal protein has become common. Such a diet might give rise to the urine abnormalities seen in the patient in the following case history.

Box 25.1 **Case history 1**

A 24-hour urine collection was completed and analysed in a 48-year-old women with a history of five spontaneously passed stones. She had an SAI = 10.4 and a body weight of 90 kg. The following 24-hour excretion levels were recorded: calcium 7.5 mmol, oxalate 0.48 mmol, citrate 1.20 mmol, magnesium 3.50 mmol, urate 5.1 mmol, urea 420 mmol, volume 1800 ml, and pH 5.5.

The pattern of a high excretion of calcium and oxalate, a low citrate and pH as well as an increased excretion of urate is typical for an excessive intake of protein. Although measurements of dietary intake are best, it is possible to get an approximate idea of the daily protein intake using the formula below:[29]

protein (in g) = [urea (mmol/24 h × 0.18)] + 13.

In this patient the protein intake is too high at around 126 g per day. The amount of dietary protein taken daily should not exceed 0.8 g/kg body weight,[3] which in this patient above means 72 g. Advice should be given to reduce the intake of animal protein such as meat, fish, sausage, eggs, and other products in which the protein content is high. Again, a nutritionist is helpful in this regard.

Correction of individual urine abnormalities

Hypercalciuria

Administration of a thiazide (e.g. hydrochlorothiazide, bendroflumethiazide, inda-pamide) is the standard procedure for reducing urinary calcium. In order to minimize side-effects, the dose should be as low as possible (e.g. hydrochlorothiazide 25–50 mg per day). Potassium supplements are often required to prevent the development of hypokalaemic hypocitraturia. The effect of thiazide treatment is well documented and there are several randomized studies that support its use.[30–35]

Another pharmacological agent with calcium-reducing properties is orthophosphate but it is poorly tolerated and low compliance is an issue.

Hyperoxaluria

Urinary oxalate is a powerful determinant of the ion–activity product of calcium oxalate and even small increments in oxalate concentration are important in terms of abnormal crystallization and stone formation. Three different forms of hyperoxaluria are recognized—mild, enteric, and primary hyperoxaluria.

Mild hyperoxaluria

The upper normal limit of 24-hour urinary oxalate is 0.45 mmol for men and 0.40 mmol for women. Mild hyperoxaluria is defined as an excretion slightly above those levels. Although most urinary oxalate is derived from endogenous synthesis, recent results have indicated that increased oxalate absorption might be responsible in some patients. A supernormal intake of food stuffs rich in oxalate and/or a low calcium diet might result in hyperabsorption of oxalate.

Box 25.2 **Case history 2**

A 32-year-old man with several small stones in both kidneys was considered for preventive measures. He was recently treated for a 8 × 10 mm stone in the renal pelvis found to be composed of calcium oxalate monohydrate (70%) and dihydrate (30%). Composition of a 24-hour urine sample was as follows: calcium 3.80 mmol, oxalate 0.52 mmol, citrate 2.90 mmol, magnesium 3.50 mmol, phosphate 25 mmol, urate 2.60 mmol, volume 1300 ml, and pH 5.72.

It was recommended that he increase his fluid intake to achieve a 24-hour urine volume of 2–2.5 litres and decrease his intake of foodstuffs particularly rich in oxalate (see Table 25.8). In addition, he was advised to maintain a daily calcium intake of 20–25 mmol. This last step is essential, not only to form intestinal com-plexes between calcium and oxalate and thereby reduce oxalate absorption, but also to maintain a positive calcium balance. Our nutritionist was instrumental in con-veying this information to him and his spouse (i.e. the person responsible for most of the cooking in this family).

The importance of large doses of vitamin C as a source of oxalate has been a matter of debate because of the conversion of ascorbate to oxalate. The current opinion is that daily doses of up to 4 g do not lead to undesirable effects on urinary oxalate.[20] One must also be careful of patients in whom urinary uric acid is a problem because high doses of vitamin C acidify the urine and make the uric acid less soluble.

Enteric hyperoxaluria

Enteric hyperoxaluria is seen in patients with diseases associated with malabsorption of fatty acids. The formation of calcium soaps (i.e. calcium and fatty acids) in the intestine leaves less calcium available to bind to oxalate and leads to more free oxalate and accordingly increased absorption. It needs to be emphasized that part of this oxalate absorption occurs in the colon.

Box 25.3 Case history 3

This patient is a 47-year-old man with Crohn's disease. An ileocaecal resection was carried out a few years ago, after which he started to produce stones of various sizes. Stone analysis showed 95% calcium oxalate monohydrate and 5% dihydrate. The following recordings were made in a 24-hour urine sample: calcium 2.1 mmol, oxalate 0.95 mmol, citrate 0.80 mmol, magnesium 2.2 mmol, phosphate 20 mmol, urate 3.1 mmol, volume 800 ml, and pH 5.2.

This urine composition is typical for patients with intestinal fat malabsorption. There is a low excretion of calcium, citrate, and magnesium, a high excretion of oxalate, a small urine volume, and a low pH. All of these factors contribute to a markedly increased risk of calcium oxalate crystallization.

Several measures can improve the urinary environment for patients with enteric hyperoxaluria. Foremost, it is essential to restrict the intake of products with a high content of oxalate (Table 25.8). Reduced dietary fat is useful. Calcium supplements, especially calcium citrate, should be given in order to decrease the oxalate absorption

Table 25.8 Foodstuffs with a particularly high content of oxalate (from Hesse et al.[3])

Food	Oxalate content (mmol/100 g)
Cocoa	7
Tea	3–15
Nuts	2–7
Spinach	6
Rhubarb	6
Beetroot	1

by calcium oxalate complex formation within the gut. Another option for complex formation is Oxabsorb®.[36] This is a marine hydrocolloid that binds oxalate. Treatment with this agent has proved to be particularly beneficial by also decreasing diarrhoea.

Although it always is wise to try to increase the fluid intake in these patients, such a goal is not always achievable due to the worsening of diarrhoea with increased fluids. The hypocitraturia, a common feature of enteric hyperoxaluria, should be corrected by administration of potassium citrate if the calcium citrate has not been sufficient; both favourably increase the pH.

In patients with low urinary magnesium, supplements should be given as magnesium hydroxide or oxide.

For the patient presented in Case history 3 the following regimen would be appropriate to start with:

- Restricted dietary oxalate.
- Increased fluid intake to achieve a 24-hour urine volume of at least 2–2.5 litres (if possible).
- Restricted fat intake.
- Supplements of calcium 0.5 g × 3 with meals.
- Oxabsorb 1.5 g × 3.
- Potassium citrate 7 mmol × 2–3 and magnesium hydroxide 250 mg × 2.

Repeated analysis of urine composition should be made to confirm the effects and, when necessary, adjust the doses.

The therapeutic goal is to decrease the activity product of calcium oxalate. It is clinically important to know if patients with intestinal diseases have their colon intact or not. For example, in patients with an ileostomy the oxalate concentration usually is not high and, because of the low urine volume and fixed low urinary pH, these patients typically form frequent uric acid stones.

Primary hyperoxaluria

Fortunately primary hyperoxaluria is a very rare genetic disease in which the urinary excretion of oxalate usually exceeds 1.0 mmol/24h/1.73 m^2 body surface area. There are two types, Type 1 and Type 2.[37,38] In Type 1 patients, there is a deficiency of alanine glyoxylate aminotransferase and in Type 2 of D-glycerate dehydrogenase.

The treatment of patients with primary hyperoxaluria is very difficult and unpredictable; sometimes, the cause of stone formation can only be eliminated by liver transplantation. The aim of the medical treatment is to reduce the concentration of urinary oxalate. Dietary restriction is of little help in this group. Very high fluid intake generating a urine output of more than 5 litres can be of significant benefit but is difficult to achieve. Some patients with Type 1 hyperoxaluria respond to large doses of pyridoxine (i.e. 2.5–15 mg of pyridoxine/kg bodyweight per day).[38] Positive results have been reported with orthophosphate but experience is limited. Magnesium and alkaline citrate might prove useful if the oxalate can be reduced first.

Hypocitraturia

Low urinary citrate is a common and important metabolic abnormality in calcium stone formers. Apart from effects on the ion–activity products of both calcium oxalate and phosphate, citrate inhibits growth and aggregation of such crystals.[39] It is seen in the malabsorptive conditions encountered in patients with gastrointestinal disturbances and as a result of the tubular defect in patients with complete or partial distal tubular acidosis. A diet high in protein or any diet that gives a high acid load leads to hypocitraturia.

In patients treated long-term with carbonic anhydrase inhibitors (e.g. acetazolamide), the ensuing hypocitraturia is associated with a very alkaline urinary pH and, accordingly, these patients form calcium phosphate and not calcium oxalate stones. The biochemical abnormalities seen in patients treated with carbonic anhydrase inhibitors cannot be adequately corrected unless the treatment is stopped.[40]

For other patients with hypocitraturia the treatment of choice is administration of alkaline citrate. Potassium citrate should be chosen instead of sodium citrate or sodium potassium citrate because of the negative effects of sodium on calcium excretion.[41,42] There is no consensus on how much potassium citrate is required, but a daily dose of 14–20 mmol is usually necessary in order to increase the 24-hour urinary citrate to levels above 2–2.5 mmol. The dosage should be determined by the effects on urinary citrate that are recorded during treatment. It is suggested that the therapy starts with 7 mmol of potassium citrate given twice daily and gradually increased to three times daily or even 10 mmol two or three times a day depending upon response and tolerance. In order to reduce gastrointestinal side-effects, it should be taken with meals. There are two randomized studies showing reduced stone recurrence in patients treated with potassium citrate.[42,43] Promising results have also been reported with potassium magnesium citrate, particularly in patients with malabsorptive conditions, but it is not yet generally available.[45]

Hypomagnesuria

Low urinary excretion of magnesium, usually a result of gastrointestinal disease or low dietary intake, is a common finding in stone patients. Although the benefits of magnesium supplementation in reducing stone formation are controversial, it is probably helpful. Because of common tubular handling of calcium and magnesium ions, supplements of magnesium might increase calcium excretion and it is wise to combine magnesium with a thiazide. Magnesium is administered as magnesium oxide 200 mg $\times$ 2 (5.0 mmol/day) or magnesium hydroxide 250 mg $\times$ 2 (4.3 mmol/day).

Hyperphosphaturia

Urinary phosphate is subject to considerable daily and diurnal variation associated with dietary variations. High phosphate excretion is seen in patients with a high consumption of meat and/or cheese. There is no evidence that pharmacological reduction of urinary phosphate is effective in reducing the risk of stone disease.

Conclusion

Patients with frequently recurring urinary stones have benefited over the last few decades from the many technological advances that have been made to facilitate the acute management of a symptomatic stone in a safe and minimally invasive manner. However, this does not exempt the health-care professionals from seeking out potential causes for the stone formation and developing a strategy to help reduce the risk of reoccurrence. Information regarding stone composition and predisposing diseases, work environments, medication, or anatomical abnormalities as well the results of blood tests, fluid, and dietary records and 24-hour urinary risk factor excretions are pivotal. It is important to have strong support from the laboratory and X-ray department plus a knowledgeable and interested nutritionist. If a well-developed increased fluid intake and dietary modification plan does not work or cannot be adhered to, pharmacological treatment should be instituted and targeted toward correcting abnormal urinary variables (Fig. 25.2). The important biochemical risk-factors for stone formation are summarized in Fig. 25.3. Close follow-up with sharing of progress with the patient and spouse can provide the best support and optimize compliance and success.

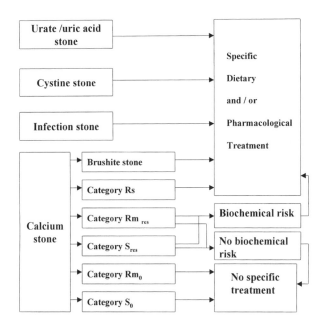

Fig. 25.2 Principles for specific dietary and pharmacological treatment to prevent recurrence in patients with urinary tract stone formation. Rs, severe recurrent stone disease; Rm, mild recurrent stone disease; S, first time (single) stone former; 0, without residual stone material; res, with residual stone material.

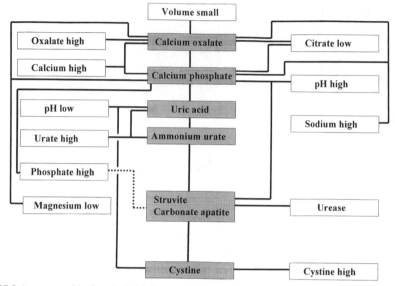

Fig. 25.3 Important biochemical risk factors in urinary tract stone formation.

References

1 Tiselius H-G (2003). Epidemiology and medical management of stone disease. *BJU Int.* **91**: 758–67.

2 Tiselius H-G and Advisory Board of European Urolithiasis Research and EAU Health Care Office Working Party for Urolithiasis (2001). Possibilities for preventing recurrent calcium stone formation: principles for the metabolic evaluation of patients with calcium stone disease. *BJU Int.* **88**: 1–16.

3 Hesse A, Tiselius H-G, Jahnen A (2002). *Urinary Stones-Diagnosis, Treatment and Prevention of Recurrence*, 2nd revised and enlarged edition. Karger, Basel.

4 Pak CYC, Resnick MI (2000). Medical therapy and new approaches to management of urolithiasis. *Urol. Clin. North Am.* **27**: 243–53.

5 Tiselius H-G (1996). Solution chemistry of supersaturation. In: *Kidney Stones: Medical and Surgical Management* (ed. FL Coe, MJ Favus, CYC Pak, JH Parks, GM Preminger), pp. 33–64. Lippincott-Raven, Philadelphia, PA.

6 Wong HY, Reidl CR, Griffith DP (1996). Medical management and prevention of struvite stones. In: *Kidney Stones: Medical and Surgical Management* (ed. FL Coe, MJ Favus, CYC Pak, JH Parks, GM Preminger), pp. 941–50. Lippincott-Raven, Philadelphia, PA.

7 Michaels EK (1996). Surgical management of struvite stones. In: *Kidney Stones: Medical and Surgical Management* (ed. FL Coe, MJ Favus, CYC Pak, JH Parks, GM Preminger), pp. 951–70. Lippincott-Raven, Philadelphia, PA.

8 Tiselius H-G, Hellgren E, Andersson A, Borrud-Ohlsson A, Eriksson I (1999). Minimally invasive treatment of infection staghorn stones with shock wave lithotripsy and chemolysis. *Scand. J. Urol. Nephrol.* **33**: 286–90.

9 Birch DF, Fairley KF, Pavillard RE (1981) Unconventional bacteria in urinary tract disease: *Ureaplasma urealyticum. Kidney Int.* **19**: 58–64.

10 Grenabo L, Brorson JE, Hedelin H, Pettersson S (1984). *Ureaplasma urealyticum*-induced crystallization of magnesium ammonium phosphate and calcium phosphate in synthetic urine. *J. Urol.* **132**: 795–9.

11 Griffith DP, Gleeson MJ, Lee H, Longuet R, Deman E, Earle N (1991). Randomized double-blind trial of lithostat (acetohydroxamic acid) in the palliative treatment of infection-induced urinary calculi. *Eur. Urol.* **20**: 243–7.

12 Coe FL, Lawton RL, Goldstein RB, Tembe V (1975). Sodium urate accelerates precipitation of calcium oxalate in vitro. *Soc. Exp. Biol. Med.* **149**: 926–9.

13 Gutman AB, Yü TS (1968). Uric acid nephrolithiasis. *Am. J. Med.* **45**: 756–79.

14 Pak CYC, Sakhaee K, Fuller C (1986). Successful management of uric acid nephrolithiasis with potassium citrate. *Kidney Int.* **30**: 422–8.

15 Heimbach D, Jacobs D, Müller SC, Hesse A (2000). Influence of alkaline solutions on chemolitholysis and lithotripsy of uric acid stones. An *in vitro* study. *Eur. Urol.* **38**: 621–2.

16 Dick WH, Lingeman JE, Preminger GM, Smith LH, Wilson DM, Shirrell WL (1990). Laxative abuse as a cause for ammonium urate renal calculi. *J. Urol.* **143**: 244–7.

17 Coe FL, Raisen L (1973). Allopurinol treatment of uric-acid disorders in calcium-stone formers. *Lancet* **1**: 129–31.

18 Sakhaee K, Sutton RAL (1996). Medical management of cystinuria. In: *Kidney Stones: Medical and Surgical Management* (ed. **FL Coe, MJ Favus, CYC Pak, JH Parks, GM Preminger**), pp. 1007–17. Lippincott-Raven, Philadelphia, PA.

19 Barbey F, Joly D, Rieu P, Méjean A, Daudon M, Junger P (2000). Medical treatment of cystinuria: critical reappraisal of long-term results. *J. Urol.* **163**: 1419–23.

20 Tiselius H-G, Ackermann D, Alken P, Buck C, Conort P, Gallucci M (2001). Guidelines on urolithiasis (abbreviated version). *Eur. Urol.* **40**: 362–71.

21 Schmeller NT, Kersting H, Schüller J, Chaussy C, Schmiedt E (1984). Combination of chemolysis and shock wave lihtotripsy in the treatment of cystine renal calculi. *J. Urol.* **131**: 434–8.

22 Smith AD, Lange PH, Miller RP, Reinke DB (1979). Dissolution of cystine calculi by irrigation with acetylcysteine through percutaneous nephrostomy. *Urology* **8**: 422–3.

23 Tiselius H-G (2002). Medical evaluation of nephrolithiasis. *Endocrinol. Metab. Clin. North Am.* **31**: 1031–50.

24 Tiselius H-G, Broghi L, Brändle E, Buck C, Coe FL, Hautmann R *et al.* (2003). Biochemistry. In: *Stone Disease. 1st International Consultation on Stone Disease* (ed. **J Segura, P Conort, S Khoury, C Pak, GM Preminger, D Tolley**), pp. 33–121. Health Publications, Paris.

25 Hess B, Hasler-Strub U, Ackermann D, Jaeger PH (1997). Metabolic evaluation of patients with recurrent idiopathic calcium nephrolithiasis. *Nephrol. Dial. Transplant.* **12**: 1362–8.

26 Borghi L, Meschi T, Amato F, Brigati A, Novarini A, Giannini A (1996). Urinary volume, water and recurrences in idiopathic calcium nephrolithiasis: a 5-year randomised prospective study. *J. Urol.* **155**: 839–43.

27 Curhan GC, Curhan SG (1997). Diet and urinary stone disease. *Curr. Opin. Urol.* **7**: 222–5.

28 Curhan GC (1999). Epidemiologic evidence for the role of oxalate in idiopathic nephrolithiasis. *J. Endourol.* **13**: 629–31.

29 Mitch WE, Walser M (1986). Nutritional therapy of the uremic patient: In: *The Kidney*, 3rd edn, Vol. II (ed. **BM Brenner, FC Rector Jr**), pp. 1759–90. Saunders, Philadelphia, PA.

30 Laerum E, Larsson S (1985). Thiazide prophylaxis of urolithiasis. A double blind study in general practice. In: *Urolithiasis and Related Clinical Research* (ed. **PO Schwille, LH Smith, WG Robertson, W Vahlensieck**), pp. 475–8. Plenum Press, New York.

31 Wilson DR, Strauss AL, Manuel MA (1984). Comparison of medical treatments for the prevention of recurrent calcium nephrolithiasis. *Urol. Res.* **12**: 30–40.

32 Ettinger B, Citron JT, Livermore B, Dolman LI (1988). Chlorothiazide reduces calcium oxalate calculus recurrences but magnesium hydroxide does not. *J. Urol.* **139**: 679–84.

33 Ohkawa M, Tokunaga S, Nakashima T, Orito M, Hisazumi H (1992). Thiazide treatment for calcium urolithiasis in patients with idiopathic hypercalciuria. *Br. J. Urol.* **69**: 571–6.

34 Borghi L, Meschi T, Guerra A, Novarini A (1993). Randomized prospective study of a nonthiazide diuretic, indapamide, in preventing calcium stone recurrences. *J. Cardiovasc. Pharmacol.* **22**(Suppl. 6): 78–86.

35 Ahlstrand C, Sandwall K, Tiselius H-G (1996). Prophylactic treatment of calcium stone formers with hydrochlorothiazide and magnesium. In: *Renal Stones—Aspects on Their Formation, Removal and Prevention. Proceedings of the Sixth European Symposium on Urolithiasis* (ed. H-G Tiselius), pp. 195–7. Akademitryck AB, Edsbruk.

36 Lindsjo M, Fellstrom B, Ljunghall S, Wikstrom B, Danielson B-G (1989). Treatment of enteric hyperoxaluria with calcium-containing organic marine hydrocolloid. *Lancet* **2**: 701–4.

37 Watts RWE (1998). The clinical spectrum of primary hyperoxaluria and their treatment. *Nephrology* **11**(Suppl. 1): 4–7.

38 Holmes RP (1998). Pharmacological approaches in the treatment of primary hyperoxaluria. *Nephrology* **11**(Suppl. 1): 32–5.

39 Tiselius H-G, Berg C, Fornander A-M, Nilsson M-A (1993). Effects of citrate on the different phases of calcium oxalate crystallization. *Scanning Microsc.* **7**: 381–91.

40 Ahlstrand C, Tiselius H-G (1987). Urine composition and stone formation during treatment with acetazolamide. *Scand. J. Urol. Nephrol.* **21**: 225–8.

41 Jandle-Bengtén C, Tiselius H-G (2000). Long-term followup of stone formers treated with a low dose of sodium potassium phosphate. *Scand. J. Urol. Nephrol.* **34**: 36–41.

42 Preminger GM, Sakhaee K, Pak CYC (1988). Alkali action on the urinary crystallization of calcium salts: contrasting responses to sodium citrate and potassium citrate. *J. Urol.* **139**: 240–2.

43 Barcelo B, Wuhl O, Servitge E, Rousand A, Pak CYC (1993). Randomized double-blind study of potassium citrate in idiopathic hypocitraturic calcium nephrolithiasis. *J. Urol.* **150**: 1761–4.

44 Tuncel A, Biri H, Küpeli B, Tan Ö, Sen I (2003). Efficiency of long-term potassium citrate treatment in patients with idiopathic calcium oxalate stone disease. In: *Urolithiasis. Proceedings of the 2nd Eurolithiasis Society Meeting* (ed. K Sarica, F Kyagci, A Erbagci, Y Inal), pp. 273. ReTa Offset Publishing, Gaziantep, Turkey.

45 Ettinger B, Pak CYC, Citron JT, Thomas C, Adams-Huet B, Vangessel A (1997). Potassium-magnesium citrate is an effective prophylaxis against recurrent calcium oxalate nephrolithiasis. *J. Urol.* **158**: 2069–73.

Chapter 26

The patient presenting with ureteric obstruction

Villus Marshall

The patient presenting with ureteric obstruction provides a significant and often difficult challenge to clinicians. While in principle it seems a relatively simple problem, the cause of the obstruction, whether bilateral or unilateral, the patient's overall health, and anticipated or current treatment all have an important bearing on what needs to be done both initially and in the long term. For example, a patient presenting in acute renal failure due to bilateral ureteric obstruction with no established cause presents quite a different challenge from an individual presenting in chronic renal failure and the terminal phase of life as a result of a malignancy that is no longer responding to treatment. In essence patients presenting with ureteric obstruction fall into a number of broad groups.

- No established pathology with mildly or unimpaired renal function and ureteric dilatation.
- No established pathology and severely impaired renal function and ureteric dilatation.
- Established pathology with normal or mildly impaired renal function and ureteric dilatation.
- Established pathology with severely impaired renal function and ureteric dilatation.

Initial assessment

The clinical presentation of a patient with ureteric obstruction can be very varied. At one end of the spectrum the patient may present with a history of not passing any urine for a significant period of time. At the other end, where there has been chronic obstruction with slow deterioration of renal function, the patient may present with a history of lethargy, tiredness, and simply feeling unwell. Sometimes the presentation may be quite dramatic with sudden onset of severe loin pain, which may be unilateral or bilateral; at others, the presentation may be due to the disease process which is causing the obstruction such as abdominal pain, abdominal mass, or, in the case of a lymphoma, enlarged lymph glands. Severe back pain may be the presenting symptom with retroperitoneal lesions. Occasionally in patients with large ovarian cysts, which can cause obstruction in the pelvis, there may be a palpable suprapubic mass which could be confused with an enlarged bladder. Thus the clinical presentation of patients with ureteric obstruction is varied and there is the possibility that it could be over-looked. Reliance on a history of flank pain or ache to suggest the presence of ureteric obstruction may be misleading. A high index of suspicion is required.

The initial assessment requires a detailed history of current symptoms, particularly the presence of pain, its nature, and its distribution. Of particular relevance is past his-tory of malignant disease, stones, previous surgery or irradiation, urinary tract infec-tion and haematuria, and current health status. Examination should focus on general status, with an emphasis on abdominal findings and lymphadenopathy. Digital rectal examination is important in both sexes and pelvic examination is required in women. The other key step in the initial assessment is to determine overall renal function by estimation of serum creatinine and urea. These need to be done promptly since the extent of creatinine elevation and electrolyte disturbance, especially hyperkalaemia, will influence the next management steps.

Clinically serum creatinine is the best simple guide to renal function and, although influenced by muscle bulk, it tends to be reasonably constant for a given individual. One must remember that it is not truly representative of the glomerular filtration rate (GFR). The rise that occurs in the serum creatinine with a fall in GFR is hyperbolic rather than linear. This means that a rapid rise occurs in late-stage renal disease whereas at an earlier stage there may be considerable renal function loss with very little change in creatinine. Thus, if there is concern about renal function loss, it is helpful to measure creatinine clearance.

Management

If there is no established pathology but ureteric dilatation and normal or only mildly impaired renal function there is no urgency to decompress the dilated systems. There is usually time to establish a cause for the dilatation and to determine the most appropri-ate form of intervention. If the treatment is successful and the obstruction relieved then the dilatation will resolve. In these individuals overall renal function needs to be constantly monitored during the period of treatment of the underlying pathology. Ultrasound provides a non-invasive means of achieving this requirement.

Patients presenting with severe ureteric obstruction require urgent decompression either through an antegrade percutaneous or retrograde endoscopic approach. The decision as to which is most appropriate is dependent upon a number of factors. The first is the general fitness of the patient and the extent of the electrolyte distur-bance, particularly the serum potassium, creatinine levels, and haematological status of the patient. Other factors that can influence the ultimate approach will be the level and cause of obstruction and the availability of experienced radiologists or urologists to perform the procedure. While it is usually possible to insert ureteric stents endoscopically under local anaesthesia it is sometimes difficult and may only be possible if intravenous sedation or general or regional anaesthesia are available; this may be hazardous in a patient with severe electrolyte disturbance. If, on the basis of the clinical history, the obstruction is likely to be at the level of the trigone as a result of a bladder, prostate, or cervical malignancy, one can anticipate that the ureteric orifices may be difficult or impossible to identify; hence, an antegrade approach would be preferable. On the other hand, if there were disturbances in the coagulation profile leading to an increased risk of bleeding, a retrograde approach would be preferable.

In the situation where both ureters are obstructed, the decision has to be made whether one or both of the obstructed units need to be decompressed. In the patient in whom the diagnosis of the primary cause has not been established, antegrade drainage of the most dilated system with the best renal parenchyma should be the first step. This will allow renal function to be restored and an opportunity to adequately assess the patient's primary disease and to put in place the next steps in management. If the patient is well enough and it is appropriate to insert stents in a retrograde fashion, it is reasonable to stent both renal units since complications such as bleeding are less from the retrograde approach.

In the case of established pathology with normal or mildly impaired renal function, observation may be all that is needed while active treatment is undertaken to control the underlying cause of the obstruction. Again, careful monitoring of overall renal function is needed as well as follow-up with regular ultrasounds to monitor the degree of dilatation. Increasing dilatation may occur without an immediate change in renal function and be an indication for intervention.

Relief of obstruction may also be required if chemotherapy with predictable renal toxicity is required. Serum creatinine is a relatively poor indicator of impaired renal function and pre-drug stent placement will ensure that preservation of renal function is maximized.

In the situation of established pathology with severe impairment decompression is required. If the aetiology is advanced malignancy, discussions should be undertaken with the patient and family as to the potential advantages and disadvantages of not relieving the obstruction at this time. Although antegrade and retrograde stents can improve renal function in an obstructed system, they do not correct the underlying cause of the obstruction. The result may be prolongation of life in an inappropriate circumstance (e.g. patient may not want further operative interventions).

Ureteric stents are not a panacea and there are some limitations associated with their use. In a prospective study patients with stents were followed for a maximum of 3 months. The most common initial problem was fever and bacteriuria after stent insertion (30%); however, in 10% the stent fragmented and in 8% the stent migrated.[1] Proper measurements of ureteric length and choice of stent can reduce the likelihood of the latter.[2] One of the most persistent symptoms was flank pain on voiding (i.e. probably related to urine reflux alongside the stent) and it is important to note that in 62% there was no change in the hydronephrosis, but more importantly in 9% the hydronephrosis worsened after stenting and in 9% dilatation appeared *de novo*.

These authors were unable to find a relationship between the pathology that led to the use of a stent and the development or worsening of the hydronephrosis after stenting.[1]

Stents can cause suprapubic pain, haematuria, and frequency.[3] Anticholinergic/antispasmodic drugs such as oxybutynin can often reduce these symptoms and make the stents more tolerable.

The availability of ureteric stents has been a major advance in urology and their placement often offers a rapid and simple solution to a serious problem related to ureteric obstruction (e.g. sepsis, acute renal failure, etc.). Their benefits greatly outweigh the disadvantages in using them. In general, they should only be left in place for as short a time as necessary. Removal is done endoscopically under local anaesthesia or by the patient by pulling on an attached thread.

Typically, ureteric stents are inserted in a retrograde endoscopic approach; less commonly, antegrade placement is used to convert a percutaneous nephrostomy tube from external to internal ureteric drainage.[4] This is much more comfortable for the patient and eliminates the need for an appliance or leg bag for urine collection.

In one series of 373 patients who underwent 412 percutaneous nephrostomies, the procedure was performed in 7–15 minutes with a fluoroscopy time of 30 s. Failure to puncture the collecting system occurred in one patient and a second puncture was needed in 9.2%. There were five major complications—three due to sepsis and two from haemorrhage requiring transfusion. In 50 cases the nephrostomy catheter became dislodged, in three there was malposition, and in 20 pelvicalyceal haemorrhage. Overall there were 119 minor complications.[5]

There can be a challenge in patients with malignant pelvic disease. A review of 65 patients, of whom 58 had urological cancer, described successful retrograde stenting in only 21% of 24 patients in which it was attempted. Antegrade stenting was performed in 41 of the 65 patients using a two-stage procedure, with a success rate of 98%. This led the authors to recommend that obstruction to the pelvic ureter is best managed by a two-stage antegrade approach when a retrograde attempt is unsuccessful.[6]

In a study comparing nephrostomy tubes with double-J ureteric stents the latter patients had more irritative urinary symptoms and local discomfort. However, using the EuroQOL analysis no significant difference was noted on the health-related QOL or the utility between patient groups which led the authors to conclude there was no patient preference for either modality of treatment.[7] Symptoms can often be reduced by using a stent with a small diameter and short length. If there is a necessity for long-term (e.g. many months) nephrostomy tube drainage, particularly if it is bilateral, the tubes can be tunnelled subcutaneously to a position on the anterior abdominal wall where they will be more comfortable and easily managed.

Other authors have been much more successful in the endoscopic insertion of stents. Using flexible cystoscopy and local anaesthesia/intravenous sedation, 89% of 723 patients were stented and 94% tolerated the procedure well. Twenty-eight per cent of 157 cases with malignant ureteric obstruction failed.[8]

The value of a percutaneous nephrostomy tube is sometimes questioned as part of the supportive palliative care of patients with incurable malignancy and ureteric obstruction. The most common indication is renal failure and only occasionally for flank pain. Complications occur in 13% related to blockage or discomfort. Incurable patients survived a mean of 230 days but, importantly, although 49% of the time was spent as an in-patient it was not significantly different from the 31% of time that patients with curable disease spent in hospital during a similar episode of care.[9] Therefore, decompression and drainage of the urinary system is an important option, even in patients with terminal malignant disease. Careful counselling is required since there is not always a favourable outcome.

Currently, the most commonly used stents are not designed to be permanent, and depending on their nature require changing usually every 3 months or until the obstruction is relieved by other means. Metallic stents have been developed as a means of overcoming persistent obstruction from both malignant and benign causes and a variety are available, including thermoexpandable stents that have shape and memory capacity made from a nickel titanium alloy. One experience in 15 patients included a mean follow-up of 10.6 months and reported complete relief of urinary tract obstruction in all patients. There were no problems with pain, sepsis, or incrustation but the stent migrated in three patients.[10]

The definitive treatment of ureteric obstruction depends on the nature of the disease producing the problem. In the case of a malignant process, relief of obstruction may be achieved either by surgery or chemotherapy. For malignant disease attempts to preserve the ureter intact would be the most common and obviously ideal approach. However, the ideal can only be achieved if it is possible to be confident that the ureter is not infiltrated by the malignancy, and attempts to preserve the ureter would not compromise cure. If a direct surgical approach is to be used to overcome the obstruction and part of the ureter has to be removed, then the approach used will depend upon the level of the ureter that is involved. Upper urinary tract involvement is usually managed by ureteroureterostomy, the interposition of an ileal or colonic segment, or the construction of an ileal loop. A similar approach is suitable for middle-third obstruction of the ureter. In the case of the distal third, if there is only a limited segment involved, a direct anastomosis is occasionally possible but almost always reimplantation with a psoas hitch, into a Boari flap, or directly into the bladder will be the most common means of restoring the continuity of the urinary tract. (With a Boari flap a U-shaped incision is made in the anterior wall of the bladder with the apex of the 'U' towards the bladder neck and this tongue is folded back and turned into a tubular extension which can usually reach to the level of the iliac vessels; the ureter can then be tunnelled into this tubular structure. In patients with large-capacity thin-walled bladders the Boari flap may even extend a few centimetres above the iliac vessels and provide an important means of bridging the gap if a long segment of the distal ureter is not available.)

Summary

In conclusion, the management of ureteric obstruction requires a comprehensive assessment of the overall health of the patient, the cause of the obstruction, and the need to preserve and protect renal function. Stents provide a simple means by which this can be achieved. However, they are in most cases temporary and patients need to be aware of the complications associated with their use and be aware of the implications of the relief of obstruction, particularly where no effective therapies are available to control or eliminate obstruction due to cancer (e.g. in someone who is cachectic with a frozen pelvis and WHO status 4 and who has progression of underlying malignancy despite surgery, chemotherapy, and radiotherapy). Patients and families must always be given the option of no intervention.

References

1 Richter S, Ringel A, Shalev M, Nissenkorn I (2000). The indwelling ureteric stent: a 'friendly' procedure with unfriendly high morbidity. *BJU Int.* **85**: 408–11.

2 Breau RH, Norman RW (2001). Optimal prevention and management of proximal ureteric stent migration and remigration. *J. Urol.* **166**: 890–3.

3 Pollard SG, MacFarlane R (1988). Symptoms arising from double J ureteral stent fragmentation. *J. Urol.* **139**: 37–8.

4 Mazer JM, LeVeen RF, Call JE, Wolf G, Baltaxe HA (1979). Permanent percutaneous antegrade ureteral stent placement without transurethral assistance. *Urology* **14**: 413–19.

5 Agostini S, Dedola GL, Gabbrielli S, Masi A (2003). A new percutaneous nephrostomy technique in the treatment of obstructive uropathy. *Radiol. Med. (Tonino)* **105**(5–6): 454–61.

6 Chitale SV, Scott-Barrett S, Ho ET, Burgess NA (2002). The management of ureteric obstruction secondary to malignant pelvic disease. Clin. Radiol. 57(12): 1118–21.

7 Joshi HB, Adams S, Obadeyi OO, Rao PN (2001). Nephrostomy tube or 'JJ' ureteric stent in ureteric obstruction: assessment of patient perspectives using quality-of-life survey and utility analysis. *Eur. Urol.* **39**(6): 695–701.

8 MacFarlane JP, Cowan C, Holt SJ, Cowan MJ (2001). Outpatient ureteric procedures: a new method for retrograde ureteropyelography and ureteric stent placement. *BJU Int.* **87**: 172–6.

9 Little B, Ho KJ, Gawley S, Young M (2003). Use of nephrostomy tubes in ureteric obstruction from incurable malignancy. *Int. J. Clin. Pract.* **57**(3): 180–1.

10 Kulkarni RP, Bellamy EA (1999). A new thermo-expandable shape-memory nickel-titanium alloy stent for the management of ureteric strictures. *BJU Int.* **87**(7): 755–9.

Chapter 27

Supportive care for the urology patient and family in the future

David C. Currow

Introduction

It is a dangerous thing to try to predict future trends in any context. Clinical practice is evolving in many parts of the world at speeds and in directions not thought possible even 10 years ago. Perhaps it is possible to gain glimpses of the future of patient- and caregiver-focused supportive care by exploring trends across society, clinical services, and the professions in the recent past.

Miles Little, a retired academic surgeon reflects in his book *Humane Medicine* that the practice of clinical medicine has made enormous inroads into the short- and long-term morbidity and mortality of many conditions.[1] Trauma, acute infectious diseases, many malignancies, and chronic complex diseases have their course changed substantially by current clinical interventions. Where current clinical practice continues to fail is where biomedical pathology cannot be demonstrated. Painful conditions that have an adverse impact on level of function and level of comfort where history, physical examination, a myriad of investigations, and potentially empirical treatment fails to resolve or relieve the problem still account for a great deal of clinical practice. It is often practitioners from other paradigms that appear to make the greatest impact in this area. Does the fact that we cannot define a mechanism for their apparent success diminish the improvement experienced by the patient and their family? The treatment of problems where no biomechanical problem can be identified continues to challenge clinicians worldwide. As we saw in Chapter 6, the relationship between empirical medicine and other approaches to chronic problems is less well defined now than it has been for the last half century. It is almost as though there is a coming of age, where the strengths and weaknesses of each approach to a problem can be put into a context where the outcome will be the best possible outcome for that patient. The ability to use the healing power of the mind is underutilized, and better defining those problems that can be supported by improved psychosocial support is an important focus for the future.

There is an expectation that clinical care will not only be provided in a competent way but that it will be provided in a context that recognizes the complexity and individual circumstances of the patient in the context of their life and support network.[2] Although this has been a basic tenet of clinical care since the time of ancient Greece or in the traditions of Chinese medicine, its delivery in the 21st century is more difficult than ever. The increasing complexity of care, the lessening likelihood that any one individual clinician can provide comprehensive care single-handedly, and the continuing struggle to pay for health at a societal or individual level make the process of obtaining integrated care difficult. As fields of clinical endeavour become more specialized, the need for effective teams working cohesively becomes greater.

Patient issues

Introduction

Adequately addressing any threat to a person's identity and sense of self is crucial. The clinical conditions covered in this book are either life-threatening or chronic. Each of the illnesses has a key ability to have an impact on the person, their caregivers, and the role in the social network that they have. Whether it is someone who is confronted by acute gross haematuria for the first time or has come to live with a chronic progressive illness such as Peyronie's disease, as health professionals our technical skills in dealing with the problem will not be sufficient to meet the needs of all aspects of this person. If we are to meet the complex needs of the whole person, addressing the threat to personhood or even existence itself is essential for patients and their families. How we as health professionals support people through these existential crises will be pivotal in how they deal with future function, further deterioration, or loss. Acknowledging the losses will be an important, if at times uncomfortable, first step for health professionals in supporting people.

For the person who needs supportive care, there are a number of key issues that will continue to drive the direction of the development of supportive care into the future. The complex dialogue around whether a person receiving a health service is a consumer, client, or patient will inform more of this process than perhaps we realize. A 'consumer' is likely to make decisions using a different emphasis on information and have both different rights and responsibilities from someone who considers themselves a 'patient'.

Patient information needs and decision-making

Decisions will be informed by personal choices, the availability, costs, and accessibility of various health services, and the presence of co-morbid disease. A person's world view cannot help but influence the decisions that are made as diseases progress.[3] What is the value that they place on their current existence compared with perceived suffering in the future? How has this person dealt with other stressors in life?

Individualizing this process is especially relevant at times of transition—starting treatment and understanding the goal of that treatment as well as stopping, withdrawing, or reducing the level of intervention directly addressing the underlying disease.[4]

A clear patient-focused future trend for good supportive care is going to be the adequate assessment of not only need for knowledge but also the decision-making styles of the patient and his/her support network. The desire to be included in decision-making is well documented.[5,6] Timely, sensitive, and relevant involvement in the process of decision-making about treatment options is no longer the exception. At the same time, there are emerging data that in a post-modern society where consumerism is a way of life, clinical professionals have still not come to terms with the information needs of many people at times of key transition in health decision-making.[7] Supportive care is particularly concerned with transition in the health status of people: from health to treatment; from treatment to periods of 'watchful waiting'; from health to a palliative trajectory; and finally the transition to terminal care.[8,9]

The person who wants to seek all the information available and make a decision themselves can challenge health professionals. There is now a plethora of information available through the internet, almost all of which is unevaluated and whose sources are sketchy at best. Helping someone to sift through this is time-consuming and increasingly outside the skill base of any one individual clinician because of the breadth of the information available.

Conversely, the person who wants a professional to make a specific recommendation for a particular course of action may have a real challenge to find such an individual.[10] The need for informed consent is important but increasingly difficult to deliver. If we seek professional advice, then recommending a preferred course of action may be a reasonable expectation for patients and their caregivers.[7] Such a recommendation can be made without being patronizing. In a society where consumer issues have overriding currency, it is still important to be able to access advice recommending a specific path. In the future defining decision-making styles will become more important for clinicians, especially for people at the time of life-changing transition.

Patient support

As supportive care comes of age, ensuring comprehensive support for people facing major life changes will be expected.[11] For example, patients having procedures like urinary diversions need to have honest discussions about body image and intimacy.[12,13] It is, at times, easy for us as health professionals to assume that people will 'know' about these changes and how to handle them, or assume that another health professional will have had that discussion. How any of us would cope in the short or long term with the need to set an alarm clock every night in order to drain a neobladder is something to ponder. We may argue that it is better than the alternatives, but even the technically best supportive procedures can have a significant burden for patients. Finding ways of continuing to minimize the impact on a person's normal lifestyle is a realistic aim for the future of supportive care.

For people facing transplantation, will it one day be less acceptable to exclude transplantation eligibility on the grounds of poor motivation or the perception of inadequate social support without first demonstrating that there have been real attempts to work with these issues? Treatment of depression, exploration of life goals and life philosophies, together with clinical and technical information in the form most suited to this person must form part of the set of skills need for clinical practice.

Loss is a major issue for patients and their support network in most chronic or life-limiting illnesses, both at diagnosis and in an ongoing way. People may experience significant adjustment disorders throughout the course of such an illness. There is potential for demoralization, which is beyond simply sadness and distinguished from depression.[14] A great range of emotions is encountered which may be out of character for that particular person and may challenge particularly their informal caregivers, as the person is so different from the person they knew. The coping mechanisms to deal with these issues may not yet be in the suite of skills this person has.

Bereavement begins with the threat of loss. Adequate support, often from time of the diagnosis of advanced or progressive illness, is necessary. Bereavement is not limited to people mourning the death of someone—in the supportive care setting it may be about bereavement for the losses encountered with a particular illness or course of treatment. Although many risk factors have been identified for complex or pathological grief after loss (not just death), there is no agreed and validated screening tool, nor subsequently any evidence that a process of screening can actually influence longer-term outcomes by early identification of people who are having problems. Establishing a nexus between risk assessment, interventions as a result of that assessment, and improved long-term outcomes has to be a priority of future research in supportive care.

Social support

Patients talk of 'social death'. Isolation can develop in the setting of either a chronic or a progressive illness. Changes in mobility, motivation, self-image, or even social availability can isolate both the person with the condition and people who have been close to them. Dealing with incontinence, chronic pain, urinary diversion, or impotence all have an enormous impact on how we view ourselves and therefore how we interact with the people around us. Often, more importantly, these changes will influence how other people interact with the person who has this condition. In building a community that is more supportive, there is a need for health professionals to take a leading role in ensuring that a family's range of skills are present, or are developed to support the social needs of someone facing major life changes. This involves time for education of family members and is likely to draw on all the resources of a well-integrated inter-disciplinary care team. The availability of a primary caregiver and support is also a key predictor for community-based care.

Support for sexual needs

Sexual needs, issues of intimacy, and self-image need to be actively addressed by all clinicians concerned with supportive care.[15] These have been identified as topics that health professionals are unlikely to broach with patients or their families.[16] Addressing these issues proactively will help support people as they cope with changes. Many urological interventions will affect people's sense of self or sexual function. Comfortably approaching these questions is a core competency for health professionals working in this area and needs to be better taught as people are training.

Existential support

When faced with unexpected changes in life, or the knowledge that life may end, most people re-explore what life means to them— 'why am I here', 'what does life mean'? Spiritual care concerns these parameters. In a pluralistic society, one's role and one's legacy from life are perhaps less clearly defined in this age than in earlier periods of history. Reconciling key decisions in life with their present reality is a confronting process. Adequate care for the spirit is part of the broader feeling every human has for their fellow beings.[17]

Functional support

Practical needs are of great importance. Clearly defining functional status mirrors the changes in the course of the disease for many disease trajectories.[18] Whether this is measured by Karnofsky or WHO/ECOG performance status scales, without reversible causes as performance decreases so does prognosis.[19,20] People have complex needs, and activities of daily living and finances are specific issues that can be much better supported than they are currently.[5,21] Without specifically seeking information, functional needs will often go unnoticed. Improved screening tools will improve the ability of all health professionals to improve patient care.

Chronicity of disease, survivorship, and death

The chronicity of many urological problems is a challenge to patients, their families, and their health-care professional. Whether present continuously or intermittently, coping with problems such as chronic prostatitis, recurrent calculi, or unresolved urinary tract sepsis is emotionally draining for all concerned.[22,23] Where the course of the illness can, at best, be modified slightly, the remaining symptoms can be overwhelming. Adequately empowering people to deal with the illness by providing relevant coping tools must be a greater part of clinical practice.[24]

The challenge of not only dealing with physical concerns but meeting the psychological, social, sexual, spiritual, and practical needs is an almost overwhelming challenge. Physical issues impinge least on a patient after treatment for cancer while spiritual and psychological issues have continuing impact.[25]

Consequences of the diagnosis of cancer in the context of a chronic or cured disease, as an example, demonstrate the breadth of what supportive care needs to deliver. Survivors of cancer use mental health services more often than people of the same age who have not had cancer, with the rate of use increasing further with the number of co-morbid illnesses.[26] These rates rise further with a younger age at diagnosis of cancer. At a population level, survivors of cancer have poorer global health rating, more limited activities of daily living or other functional limitations, or psychological problems. For younger people after treatment for cancer, working was less likely when compared with similar groups in the population as a whole.[27] Two decades after diagnosis, health problems are still frequently encountered in survivors of cancer including treatment-specific and global issues.[28]

Caregiver issues

Caregivers are the resource around which community-based care is built. The roles that they take on are broad.[29] Training and support for caregivers is not adequate. The breadth of the roles taken on is something for which few feel prepared, including pseudoclinical roles.[30] Although a significant achievement, and for some rewarding, it should not be overlooked that many caregivers resent aspects of the role that they are asked to assume. Caring is a major life stressor which is 'very distressing' when it includes uncontrolled physical symptoms.[31] Caregiver outcomes depend on a number of variables, including the length of time for which care is given and the relationship to the person to whom care is given.[32] Only half the caregivers in one series from the palliative care literature found the role rewarding, with the potential for many unmet needs while trying to maintain the role.[31] For caregivers who have accessed supportive and palliative services at the end of life, there are documented improvement in outcomes for carers long after the person for whom they are caring has died.[33–36]

How caregivers are better equipped for their role in supporting others is probably one of the key challenges of supportive care.[30] Mobilizing communities and informal support networks is likely to make a significant difference.[30]

Working with whole families at the end of life can have a positive impact on caregiver outcomes.[14] Exploring this work across the spectrum of supportive care in properly randomized trials will be important. If such impacts are shown, the longer-term benefits for the *next* time people are confronted with significant life changes could be an important outcome measure. The benefits to family function outside the context of chronic or progressive illness should also be followed.

The economic costs of providing care are substantial, including to carers. In a multisite study in the United States, there was a relationship between complexity of need at the end of life and economic costs. The more complex the care needs the greater the rate of subjective economic burden reflected in higher rates of loans to pay for care, or where more than 10% of household income was spent on health care.[37] Overall cost reductions to funded health services can be seen because of a shift to community care where informal caregiver costs are rarely adequately costed.[38,39] The benefits of the investment in services is understood and appreciated by patients and carers.[40]

Community issues

How supportive care is viewed by the community and health professionals will also have an enormous impact on future trends. Among other implications, this should influence the resources that are committed by the community to supportive care. The impact of supportive care in improving global health outcomes is only just starting to be adequately quantified. At a community level, the demand for such support is becoming an expectation of patients and their families in order to claim that care is 'comprehensive'.[41]

Clinical issues

Introduction

At a clinical level, there are three major factors that have an impact clinical practice in supportive care:

- Treatment of the underlying disease to change the disease trajectory.
- Development of interventions that continue to lower the threshold for intervention (becoming 'supportive') because the burden of the intervention is less invasive, or otherwise more acceptable than previously available options.
- Specific areas of research that are seeking to improve symptom control when the disease course can no longer be modified.

In key areas of urology, significant progress continues to be made in ensuring that procedures that maximize quality of life become more accessible in cost and predictable benefit to the patient.

We also only need look at the history of surgery for the prostate and the enormous changes of the last 50 years. In that time the evolution of the intervention has progressed from either very invasive surgery or no intervention at all to a range of modalities that emphasize the need to obtain good outcomes without unacceptable levels of morbidity associated with the intervention. Minimizing the length of stay in health-care institutions and minimizing the risks of impotence and incontinence have meant a continual drive to modify radical procedures while still delivering the optimal out come of cancer cure. Although in a state of transition, the new modalities that are being explored for the management of benign bladder outlet obstruction include laser surgery (of a variously invasive nature), microwave therapy, increased use of imaging techniques during procedures, and continued improvement in patient selection for any of these procedures. Optimizing level of function after such invasive procedures is a clear aim for the future.

Prostheses for erectile dysfunction or incontinence continue to evolve. The morbidity associated with their placement and use is decreasing. The improving designs also mean that they provide function that more closely resembles normal sphincter and erectile behaviour. From a patient viewpoint, the critical issue is that realistic benefits and adverse effects are well documented and can inform decisions more fully as clinical experience grows with these devices.[42,43] Ultimately, health professionals need to identify the patients who can expect the best outcome from the use of these prostheses.

Likewise, stenting is increasingly used in disciplines right across medicine— cardiology and vascular medicine, pulmonology, gastroenterology, and urology. The growing skill in developing and utiliszing stents that minimize side-effects and long-term morbidity will continue to change the face of supportive care. The increasing sophistication in design and the materials used changes the threshold for what is 'supportive'. The ability to stent the bulbous urethra and also use intra-prostatic stents is going to broaden choices for people who, until recently, often had few options when surgery was no longer possible because of co-morbid disease.

Physical symptom control

Physical symptom control has always been a pivotal starting point for good supportive care. In patient-derived data this is the most important issue when facing a life-limiting illness (and is one of the few biomedical issues that patients highlight).[5,6] Fear of uncontrolled symptoms is still the number one fear of people facing the end of life and of their carers. The developments in this area mimic the developments in other areas of supportive care—those that are driven by less invasive or burdensome procedures replacing existing interventions and those innovations that come from adequately designed research specifically to further the quality of supportive care. For the vast majority of patients, symptoms can be substantially improved. Equally, despite best efforts, there will continue to be a small number of people with significant refractory symptoms.

An improved understanding of the pathophysiology of uncontrolled pain must have an impact on the care that is offered. If current research findings are confirmed, there will be a need for practising clinicians to substantially change the paradigm through which the treatment of pain is approached. The existence and growth of interneurons that bypass the dorsal horn in chronic pain challenges all clinicians to explore how they approach pain relief—delays in initiating adequate analgesia have the potential to cause long-term physical harm.[44] Likewise, accepting patients' accounts of pain is imperative if laboratory evidence for heritable components of neuropathic pain is borne out in human studies.[45] Patients and their families are increasingly expecting that pain will be controlled adequately and early, no matter what the underlying cause.

By way of non-invasive treatments for physical symptoms in supportive care, there are a number of areas where developments continue to take place. Community-friendly ways of delivering medications that otherwise mimic complex drug-delivery systems are starting to be seen. The use of transdermal and transmucosal delivery systems is already commonplace for drug administration. Their increasing use in other delivery systems is likely in the near future. Transdermal delivery systems, in general, need to be used in people whose needs for medication are stable over time. This is because of the significant lead-time in establishing a subcutaneous depot for medication delivery systemically and lag-time if the dose is too high. Computer-controlled inhalers will deliver medications to alveoli.[46] Alveolar administration is important because of the huge absorptive area available, simulating intravenous administration. By controlling drop size and only releasing medication in the phase of inspiration with the required respiratory effort, the drug can be guaranteed systemic delivery almost instantaneously. The use of more sophisticated drug release mechanisms for varying release within a dose interval also widens the versatility of currently available medications and, with decreasing frequency of dose administration, potentially improves patients' compliance.[47] Depot delivery of medications such as octreotide, a somatostatin analogue, point to other mechanisms for people with stable medication needs.

Despite enormous advances in the understanding of the therapeutic use of hormones, current understanding of the full implications of hormone replacement therapy in men is still some way off. Defining the patient who will most benefit from therapy will help foster good outcomes when complex decisions need to be made. As hormone replacement therapy becomes more targeted, it is likely that there can be an ever-increasing approximation of normal physiological function with fewer side-effects.[48]

The emerging field of pharmacogenetics has enormous implications for day-to-day clinical practice. Given current microarray systems, it will be possible to match drug metabolism profiles of individual patients with the medications prescribed. It will be possible to provide this knowledge so that *all* prescribing is informed by a person's own profile of metabolism. Such a process would also inform best prescribing by identifying potential interactions including potentiation and inhibition of drug metabolic pathways. This will further minimize adverse reactions, optimize prescribing to make use of any shared metabolic pathways, and ultimately improve patient outcomes. Nascent work in exploring opioids using this technology also has the potential to explain some of the inter- and intra-person variability in response to frequently used medications and therefore better target interventions.

Biological interventions are rapidly increasing in number for transplants and the treatment of malignancy. Improved target receptor specificity will help to minimize their side-effect profile. The changes in acute transplant rejection treatment have been a major catalyst to more complex multiorgan transplantation. In cancer, identification and blocking of specific pathways that are only manifest by the tumour minimizes the impact on other body systems, making these agents acceptable. Their role in solid tumour and haematological malignancy continues to grow rapidly with small subgroups of patients seeing sustained long-term benefit from currently available interventions.

Professional issues

In order to provide adequate support for people facing chronic complex or life-limiting problems, there is a need for a suitably trained workforce. There are two inherent challenges: preparing new clinicians for practice and influencing the practice of existing clinicians. For all health professionals, practice will be more enjoyable and more sustainable with good communication skills, actively acknowledging the contributions of each health discipline, self-care, and the skills to build, motivate, and sustain a team of health professionals.

For health professionals entering training, it is hoped that more curricula will devote time to these key areas.[49] Curricula that seek to integrate some aspects of learning especially in more junior year, that is across whole schools or faculties, are directly fostering the basic skills required. These are skills that need continued development throughout a professional life particularly as practitioners (generally) become more and more subspecialized.

Most health professionals feel that they have good communication skills. Are these skills innate or are they skills that can be improved? There are data in the cancer literature that clinicians (specifically nurses and doctors) can improve their communication skills in a structured way.[50–52] Randomized trials confirm that there can be a real difference in how people interact, leading to improved satisfaction with care and *shorter* clinical encounters sustained over time. By focusing on the issues that the patient and their family want addressed, the encounter meets more needs for all concerned.

A much bigger challenge is how to best address these issues for people already in (busy) practices. If supportive care is going to continue to grow in the next 20–30 years, people already in practice will need to explore how best to improve key skills. There are good data to suggest that most aspects of clinical practice change little once someone is established in practice. A Cochrane Review does demonstrate that practice can be modified especially with academic detailing—structured evidence-based brief educational encounters presented by specially trained health professionals to colleagues.[53] Much of what we would otherwise consider continuing education or professional development probably has little effect on day-to-day clinical practice. To expect practice to evolve without a significant injection of resource and energy is wishful thinking.

New clinical knowledge

How is it possible for any clinician to keep up to date with the explosion of new knowledge? Although there are attempts through systematic reviews such as the Cochrane Collaboration to sift information for best practice, dispersing this process across all clinical areas will be resource intensive. Clinical pathways based on best evidence will be the practical outcome of well-researched projects. As research continues, all clinicians will need to find more effective ways of sharing the workload of evaluating and assimilating new knowledge.

Interdisciplinary care and teams

Many health professionals would have difficulty in describing the core skills, competencies, and attributes of other health disciplines. This immediately limits their ability to interact as a team because the contribution of each member of the team cannot be used to the full in this setting. Ultimately, the care of people with complex supportive needs is less likely to be met unless there is an effective team.[54] There is an acknowledgement that these needs cannot be met by one person, but adequately engaging appropriate health professionals in a timely way is probably not done ideally.

For true interdisciplinary care, supportive services must move outside the confines of nursing and medical involvement and ensure that the team includes an adequate representation of allied health disciplines.[55,56] More broadly, reflecting the evolution of various professions will continue to be a dynamic process. Nursing and allied health disciplines have both grown and evolved in the last 50 years. This process will continue into the future and influence clinical practice and team dynamics in an ongoing way.

Teams don't just happen—they need specific skills, energy, and nurturing in order to work efficiently. Although many people work in teams, too few health professionals have had the training or invest the effort in ensuring that the colleagues with whom they work have a successful team environment. This is about the ability of members of the team to create an environment where issues can be respectfully and constructively discussed in order to optimize the outcomes for the patient, their family, and the health professionals supporting them. The skills we each bring as a fellow human being, as a health professional, and in our specific discipline can help in providing care for this person. The future may speak of 'pan-disciplinary' skills—an even closer amalgam of the key skills we all need in clinical practice.

Professional support

The practice of good urology confronts clinicians, patients, and their families with the challenges of diagnoses that are not well understood. How we deal with interstitial cystitis, chronic non-infective prostatitis, and other pelvic pain syndromes for which easily defined pathology cannot be demonstrated confronts practitioners on a day-to-day basis. Many of these conditions are diagnoses of exclusion, and although clinical practice is better at excluding other differential diagnoses it is still a negative process.

Part of sustaining practice, and continuing to engage and 'be present' for people with complex problems requiring supportive care, is excellent self-care for all clinicians involved.[57] This includes self awareness:

- when am I communicating well
- when am I so tired or run down that I may be detrimental to this person at this time
- when am I reacting to this person in a way that is not based on their needs (but potentially my own).

Good self-care includes regularly reflecting on practice and potentially debriefing not at times of crisis but on a regular basis to make crises and difficult situations less confronting and less frequent.

Resources and service models

Although there are widely differing models of funding health care around the world, how a community decides to fund supportive care will determine its future more than any other single factor.[41] Supportive care is based almost universally on the referral of a patient to a colleague. There is no automatic provision that someone with complex needs will be seen by a supportive care team. The interface with other services is therefore crucial. Achieving the WHO-style interface between supportive care and its referring services will continue to be a challenge in the future.[58–61]

At every stage of the development of clinical practice there has been a concern about the impact of new technology. On the one hand there is new expense which is real and has a financial impact. On the other hand there is a patient population which benefits from the developments. In between these aspects is the fundamental question about how any progress will affect health spending. For some new technologies and interventions the costs drop as the intervention becomes more widely used. The costs may also drop because the new intervention is replacing something cheaper but less effective. At times, new technologies simply add to the total cost of health or the opportunity cost—that is the ability to spend this resource elsewhere in health. There are clear models where diminishing returns for increasing spending exist. As we look around the world, it is clear that different societies view this dilemma differently. Do we as a community look to ensuring that new technology is available only for those who can afford it, evaluate carefully any new technologies in order to define the net health benefit at a community level, or a combination of both?. Total increases in health spending, in and of themselves, are unlikely to lead to a marked increase in measurable health outcomes for much of the developed world. Balancing this complex equation requires honest consultation with the whole community about priorities and the value system that underpins these priorities. Acknowledging that the health budget is not infinite and that money put into health will affect other parts of society is a challenging notion to us all.

This raises the more complex issue of whether we are truly a global community or a series of smaller segregated communities insulating ourselves from each other. This textbook is not written only for highly industrialized countries. Ensuring that the key interventions for the quality care of *all* people with urological problems is something for which we are *all* ultimately responsible. There are still many parts of the world where the most basic health care is not available and where many urological problems are not recognized or, if recognized, are unable to be treated because of a lack of basic resources. There are also whole communities where significant urological problems exist because of other inadequacies in health-care delivery. One only has to think of the number of people with urological fistulae or incontinence because of inadequate maternal care. How we translate the knowledge in this book to ensure adequate outcomes for all people with these problems is not a dilemma that we can dismiss lightly. It is, however, how future generations will judge the impact of supportive care.

References

1 Little M (1995). *Humane Medicine*. Cambridge University Press, Cambridge.

2 Phipps E, True G, Harris D Chong U, Tester W, Chavin SI *et al*. Approaching the end of life: attitudes, preferences, and behaviours of African-American and white patients and their family carers. *J. Clin. Oncol*. **21**: 549–54.

3 Blanchard CM, Denniston MM, Baker F, Ainsworth SR, Courneya KS, Hann DM *et al*. (2003). Do adults change their lifestyle behaviors after a cancer diagnosis? *Am. J. Health Behav*. **27**: 246–56.

4 Mitchell G, Currow DC (2002). Chemotherapy and radiotherapy: when to call it quits. *Aust. Fam. Physician* **31**: 129–33.

5 Steinhouser KE, Christakis NA, Clipp EC, McNeilly M, McIntyre L, Tulsky JA (2000). Factors considered important at the end of life by patients, family, physician and other care providers. *J. Am. Med. Assoc*. **284**: 2476–82.

6 Steinhauser KE, Clipp EC, McNeilly M, Christakis NA, McIntyre LM, Tulsky JA (2000). In search of a good death: observations of patients, families, and providers. *Ann. Intern. Med*. **132**: 825–32.

7 Butow PN, MacLean M, Dunn SM, Tattersall MNH, Boyer MJ (1997). The dynamics of change; cancer patients' preference for information, involvement and support. *Ann. Oncol*. **8**: 875–83.

8 Arnold EM (1999). The cessation of cancer treatment as a crisis. *Soc. Work Health Care* **29**: 21–38.

9 Gordon GH (2003). Care not cure: dialogues at the transition. *Patient Educ. Couns*. **50**: 95–8.

10 Gattellari M, Butow PN, Tattersall MNH (2001). Sharing decisions in cancer care. *Soc. Sci. Med*. **52**: 1865–78.

11 Harrison J, Maguire P (1994). Predictors of psychiatric morbidity in cancer patients. *Br. J. Psychiat*. **165**: 593–8.

12 Hart S, Skinner EC, Meyerowitz BE, Boyd S, Lieskovsky G, Skinner DG (1999). Quality of life after radical cystectomy for bladder cancer in patients with an ileal conduit, cutaneous or urethral kock pouch. *J. Urol*. **162**(1): 77–81.

13 Webster DC, Brennan T (1995). Use and effectiveness of sexual self-care strategies for interstitial cystitis. *Urol. Nurs*. **15**: 14–22.

14 Kissane D (2003). Family focused grief therapy: the role of the family in the preventative and therapeutic bereavement care. *Bereavement Care* **22**: 6–8.

15 Hordern A, Currow DC (2003). Sexuality at the end-of-life. Implications for practice. *Med. J. Aust*. **179**(6, Suppl.): S8–S11.

16 Maguire P, Faulkner A, Booth K, Elliott C, Hillier V (1996). Helping cancer patients disclose their concerns. *Eur. J. Cancer* **32A**: 78–81.

17 Byrne M (2001). Who cares for the spirit in palliative care. *Prog. Palliative Care* **9**: 129–30.

18 Teno JM, Weitzen S, Fennell ML, Mor V (2001). Dying trajectory in the last year of life: does cancer trajectory fit other diseases? *J. Palliative Med*. **4**: 457–64.

19 Zubrod CG, Schneiderman M, Frei E III, Brindley C, Gold GL, Shnider B *et al*. (1960). Appraisal of methods for the study of chemotherapy of cancer in man: comparative therapeutic trial of nitrogen mustard and triethylene thiophosphoramide. *J. Chron. Dis*. **11**: 7–33.

20 Karnofsky DA, Abelmann WH, Craver LF, Burchenal JH (1948). The use of nitrogen mustard in the palliative treatment of cancer. *Cancer* **1**: 634–56.

21 Taylor K, Currow D (2003). A prospective prevalence study of the unmet activity of daily living needs amongst cancer patients at a comprehensive cancer care centre. *Aust. J. Occup. Ther*. **50**: 79–85.

22 Ku JH, Jeon YS, Kim ME, Lee NK, Park YH (2002). Psychological problems in young men with chronic prostatitis-like symptoms. *Scand. J. Urol. Nephrol*. **36**: 296–301.

23 **Berghuis JP, Heiman JR, Rothman I, Berger RE** (1996). Psychological and physical factors involved in chronic idiopathic prostatitis. *J. Psychosom. Res.* **41**(4): 313–25.

24 **Gupta K, Hooton TM, Roberts PL, Stamm WE** (2001). Patient-initiated treatment of uncomplicated recurrent urinary tract infections in young women. *Ann. Intern. Med.* **135**: 9–16.

25 **Wyatt G, Friedman LL** (1996). Long-term female cancer survivors: quality of life issues and clinical implications. *Cancer Nurs.* **19**: 1–7.

26 **Hewitt M, Rowland JH** (2002). Mental health service use among adult cancer survivors; analyses if the National Health Interview Survey. *J. Clin. Oncol.* **20**: 4581–90.

27 **Hewitt M, Rowland JH, Yancik R** (2003). Cancer survivors in the United States: age, health, and disability. *J. Gerontol. Ser. A—Biol. Sci. Med. Sci.* **58**: 82–91.

28 **Schultz PN, Beck ML, Vassilopoulou-Sellin R** (2003). Health profiles in 5836 long-term cancer survivors. *Int. J. Cancer* **104**: 488–95.

29 **Aranda SK, Hayman-White K** (2001). Home caregivers of the person with advanced cancer. An Australian perspective. *Cancer Nurs.* **24**: 300–7.

30 **Harding R, Higginson IJ** (2003). What is the best way to help caregivers in cancer and palliative care? A systematic literature review of interventions and their effectiveness. *Palliative Med.* **17**: 63–74.

31 **Addington-Hall J, McCarthy M** (1995). Dying from cancer: results of a national population-based investigation. *Palliative Med.* **9**: 295–305.

32 **Schulz R, Beach SR, Lind B, Martire LM, Zdaniuk B, Hirsch C et al.** (2001). Involvement in caregiving and adjustment to death of a spouse: findings from the caregiver effect study. *J. Am. Med. Assoc.* **285**: 3123–9.

33 **McCorkle R, Robinson L, Nuamah I, Lev E, Benoliel JQ** (1998). The effects of home nursing care for patients during terminal illness on the bereaved's psychological distress. *Nurs. Res.* **47**: 2–10.

34 **McCorkle R, Pasacreta JV** (2001). Enhancing caregiver outcomes in palliative care. *Cancer Control* **8**: 36–45.

35 **Ringdal GI, Jordhoy MS, Ringdal K, Kaasa S** (2001). The first year of grief and bereavement in close family members to individuals who have died of cancer. *Palliative Med.* **15**: 91–105.

36 **Christakis NA, Iwashyna TJ** (2003). The health impact of health care on families: a matched cohort study of hospice use by decedents and mortality outcomes in surviving, widowed spouses. *Soc. Sci. Med.* **57**: 465–75.

37 **Emanuel EJ, Fairclough DL, Slutman JBA, Emanuel LL** (2000). Understanding economic and other burdens of terminal illness: the experience of patients and caregivers. *Ann. Intern. Med.* **132**: 451–9.

38 **Goodwin DM, Higginson IJ, Edwards AG, Finlay IG, Cook AM, Hood K et al.** (2002). An evaluation of systematic reviews of palliative care services. *J. Palliative Care* **18**(2): 77–83.

39 **Hearn J, Higginson IJ** (1998). Do specialist palliative care teams improve outcomes for cancer patients? A systematic literature review of the evidence. *Palliative Med.* **12**: 317–32.

40 **Devery K, Lennie I, Cooney N** (1999). Health outcomes for people who use palliative care services. *J. Palliative Care* **15**: 5–12.

41 **Kitzhaber JA** (1993). Rationing in action: prioritising health services in an era of limits: the Oregon experience. *Br. Med. J.* **307**: 373–7.

42 **Chiang HS, Wu CC, Wen TC** (2000). Ten years experience with penile implant prosthesis implantation in Taiwanese patients. *J. Urol.* **163**: 476–80.

43 **Venn SN, Greenwell TJ, Mundy AR** (2000). The long-term outcomes of artificial urinary sphincters. *J. Urol.* **164**: 702–7.

44 Basbaum AI (1999). Spinal mechanisms of acute and persistent pain. *Region. Anesth. Pain Med.* **24**: 59–67.

45 Mogil JS, Wilson SG, Bon K, Lee SE, Chung K, Raber P *et al.* (1999). Heritability of nociception I: responses of 11 inbred mouse strains on 12 measures of nociception. *Pain* **80**: 67–82.

46 Mather LE, Woodhouse A, Ward ME, Farr SJ, Rubsamen RA, Eltherington LG (1998). Pulmonary administration of aerosolised fentanyl: pharmacokinetic analysis of systemic delivery. *Br. J. Clin. Pharmacol.* **46**(1): 37–43.

47 Dezii CM, Kawabata H, Tran M (2002). Effects of once-daily and twice-daily dosing on adherence with prescribed glipizide oral therapy for Type II diabetes. *South. Med. J.* **95**: 68–71.

48 Negro-Vilar A (1999). Selective androgen receptor modulators (SARMSs). A novel approach to androgen therapy for the new millennium. *J. Clin. Endocrinol. Metab.* **84**: 3459–64.

49 Australia and New Zealand Society of Palliative Medicine (1999). *Undergraduate Curriculum.* Australia and New Zealand Society of Palliative Medicine, Sydney (www.anzspm.org.au/education/ugc/index.html).

50 Maguire P (1999). Improving communication with cancer patients. *Eur. J. Cancer* **35**: 2058–65.

51 Fallowfield L, Jenkins V, Farewell V, Solis-Trapala I (2003). Enduring impact of communication skills training: results of a 12-month follow-up. *Br. J. Cancer* **89**: 1445–9.

52 McPherson CJ, Higginson IJ, Hearn J (2001). Effective methods of giving information in cancer: a systematic literature review of randomized controlled trials. *J. Public Health Med.* **23**: 227–34.

53 Thomson O'Brien MA, Oxman AD, David DA, Haynes RB, Freemantle N, Harvey EL (2000). *Educational Outreach Visits: Effects on Professional Practice and Health Care Outcomes.* Cochrane Database of Systematic Reviews, CD0000409.

54 Higginson IJ, Hearn J (1997). A multicentre evaluation of cancer pain control by palliative care teams. *J. Pain Symptom. Manag.* **14**: 29–35.

55 Rashleigh L (1996). Physiotherapy in palliative oncology. *Aust. J. Physiother.* **42**: 307–12.

56 Dawson S, Barker J (1995). Hospice and palliative care: a Delphi survey of occupational therapists' roles and training needs. *Aust. Occup. Ther. J.* **42**: 119–27.

57 Meier DE, Back AL, Morrison RS (2001). The inner life of physicians and the care of the seriously ill. *J. Am. Med. Assoc.* **286**: 3007–14.

58 WHO (2002). *National Cancer Control Programmes: Policies and Managerial Guidelines.* World Health Organization, Geneva (2nd edition available at www.who.int/cancer/media/en/408.pdf).

59 Glare PA, Virik K (2001). Can we do better in end-of-life care? The mixed management model and palliative care. *Med. J. Aust.* **175**: 530–3.

60 Bruera E, Neumann CM (1999). Respective limits of palliative care and oncology in the supportive care of cancer patients. *Support. Care Cancer* **7**: 321–7.

61 Stiefel F, Guex P (1996). Palliative and supportive care: at the frontier of medical omnipotence. *Ann. Oncol.* **7**: 135–8.

Index